MERGING PAST, PRESENT, AND FUTURE IN CROSS-CULTURAL PSYCHOLOGY

MERGING PAST, PRESENT, AND FUTURE IN CROSS-CULTURAL PSYCHOLOGY

Selected Papers from the Fourteenth International Congress of the International Association for Cross-Cultural Psychology

Edited by

Walter J. Lonner
Dale L. Dinnel
Deborah K. Forgays
Susanna A. Hayes

Published for the International Association for Cross-Cultural Psychology

SWETS & ZEITLINGER
PUBLISHERS

LISSE ABINGDON EXTON (PA) TOKYO

Library of Congress Cataloging-in-Publication Data

International Association for Cross-Cultural Psychology. International Congress (14th : 1998 : Western Washington University)
Merging past, present, and future in cross-cultural psychology : selected papers from the Fourteenth International Congress of the International Association for Cross-Cultural Psychology / edited by Walter J. Lonner ... [et al.].
p. cm.
Includes bibliographical references and index.
ISBN 9026515561
1.Ethnopsychology--Congresses. I. Lonner, Walter J. II. Title.

GN502 .I56 1998
155.8'2--dc21

99-049468

Printed in The Netherlands by Krips, Meppel

ISBN 90 265 1556 1

TABLE OF CONTENTS

HISTORICAL AND EPISTEMOLOGICAL CONTRIBUTIONS

COGNITIVE, INTELLECTUAL, AND ASSESSMENT PERSPECTIVES

ACCULTURATION, INDIVIDUALISM-COLLECTIVISM, AND ETHNIC IDENTITY

CLINICAL AND MENTAL HEALTH CONSIDERATIONS

CULTURAL MANIFESTATIONS OF SELF AND SELF-CONCEPT

CONTRIBUTIONS OF SPECIAL RELEVANCE TO CHILDREN AND YOUTH

PERSPECTIVES ON WORK AND ORGANIZATIONAL FACTORS

Merging Past, Present, and Future in Cross-Cultural Psychology: Selected Papers from the 14th International Congress of the International Association for Cross-Cultural Psychology

Introduction and Overview

The 14th International Congress of the International Association for Cross-Cultural Psychology took place on the campus of Western Washington University in Bellingham, Washington from August 3-8, 1998. While official records kept by Conference Services (the WWU office that took care of registration and related matters) indicate that there were 469 paid registrants, more than 525 people actually attended. Attendees who weren't officially registered included many accompanying guests and numerous students from Western Washington University as well as from other universities in the Pacific Northwest of the United States. All told, this was by far the most well-attended IACCP congress in the Association's history. It has been estimated that more than 70 countries were represented, making it the most international of all IACCP conferences. Following the pattern of all previous conferences as well as IACCP membership, there were more people from the United States than any other country. Canada was a distant second, and numerous Western European countries as well as all continents of the world were generously represented.

The Bellingham conference was unusually noteworthy. First, it was the Silver Jubilee meeting of IACCP, the inaugural meeting having taken place at the University of Hong Kong in August of 1972. In much of the Western world, custom dictates that when institutions, marriages, and associations last 10 years it is significant, but lasting for as long as 25 years calls for a celebration. Second, meeting in Bellingham marked the first time that IACCP has met in the United States. It has met previously in 12 other countries (Canada twice). Third, meeting at Western Washington University on this special occasion was most appropriate in view of its connection with IACCP. The **Journal of Cross-Cultural Psychology** was inaugurated at Western in 1970. **JCCP** continues to be copyrighted by the Department of Psychology's Center for Cross-Cultural Research, which was established in 1969. When IACCP was started in 1972, the Center agreed to let it claim **JCCP** as one of its official publications. That important relationship continues to this day, and it was fortunate to be able to observe this connection at the most appropriate place to do so.

Western Washington University was somewhat of an "emergency" or back-up venue for this conference. Traditionally, IACCP has held its biennial meeting in close temporal and geographic proximity to one of two much larger conferences: one sponsored by the International Union of

Psychological Science and the other by the International Association of Applied Psychology, both of which meet every four years but always separated by two years. IACCP was to have met in San Jose, California, one week before the IAAP conference in San Francisco and two weeks before the annual convention of the American Psychological Association in the same city. Unexpected circumstances required a change of venue, and Western volunteered to host the event. The switch resulted in a delay of more than six months in planning time. However, significant conferences require extraordinary attention, and this one was certainly no exception.

Among the first steps taken was to appoint an 11-member Scientific Program Advisory Committee (SPAC). Consistent with IACCP tradition, all members of the main organizing committee were from the host country. Seven of them were from Western Washington University: George Cvetkovich, Dale Dinnel, Deborah Forgays, Sue Hayes, Ron Kleinknecht, Walt Lonner, and Joe Trimble. The other four – all of whom have been active in IACCP – were from universities on the four cardinal points on the compass: Patricia Greenfield from the University of California at Los Angeles (west), Roy Malpass from the University of Texas at El Paso (south), Deborah Best from Wake Forest University in North Carolina (east), and John Adamopoulos from Grand Valley State University in Michigan (north). SPAC members corresponded freely and frequently by e-mail and the WWU members met on a quasi-regular basis to design the conference. We were fortunate to have had the enthusiastic assistance of Kay O'Connor, as well as many voluntary hours of assistance by Katja Boersma, a student from The Netherlands who was attending WWU. We thank Cathie Patrick, especially, and Maria Casarez of the secretarial staff of WWU's Department of Psychology for their help, for their skills in helping to prepare the entire camera-ready document. Cathie's remarkable skills and joyful, high-energy work ethic are remarkable. Thanks also to Michael Kirkelie for his reliable and cheerful help involving computers and logistical support of various kinds. His ready willingness to help with both large and small tasks was a constant source of comfort. An important part of the local team was Ryan O. Murphy, a psychology graduate student. Ryan's knowledge of computers was important throughout the planning phase, especially in preparing the rather elaborate printed program. A number of other WWU students, mainly undergraduate psychology majors, assisted in various ways. Primary among these students was Ryann Haw who was generous in assisting with numerous tables and figures associated with many of the articles that appear in this book.

The conference began with the Founders' Symposium. Consisting of four individuals who have made significant contributions to cross-cultural psychology dating back as far as the mid-1950s, these individuals reflected on the past and explained how they got started in this area. The individuals were Rogelio Diaz-Guerrero (Mexico), Gustav Jahoda (Scotland), Douglass Price-Williams (United States), and Harry Triandis (United States). Durganand Sinha of India was to have been on the program, but sadly he died suddenly and unexpectedly in March of 1998. Ernest Boesch was also to have been on this symposium, but health considerations prevented his travel from Germany. Leonard Doob of Yale University, who was also invited, unfortunately could not attend. This inaugural event was chaired by John Berry, whose introduction to this symposium appears in this volume. Many other individuals could have appeared "on stage" with these people, but both time and resources precluded more extensive involvement. However, a number of them were present throughout the conference, and Berry lists them in his introduction. Truncated versions of the presentations by Diaz-Guerrero, Jahoda, Price-Williams, and Triandis are included.

Another special feature of the conference was a series that featured individuals who represented the extensive breadth of ethnic diversity that has characterized the United States throughout its history. Currently, the four largest non-majority groups in the U.S. are African Americans, people of Hispanic heritage, Asian Americans, and American Indians. Eminent speakers were invited to represent these groups. Respectively, they were James Jones (University of Delaware), Beatrice Medicine (South Dakota), Amado Padilla (Stanford University), and Stanley Sue (University of California at Davis). These individuals were part of the American Jubilee Speakers Series. Joining the group was Carol Tavris (California), a well-known U.S. psychologist and author of several texts that are exceptionally representative of some of the best psychology writing in the United States. All five speakers gave one-hour lectures to large and enthusiastic audiences. With the exception of Carol Tavris, whose talk by prior agreement did not lend itself to a printed version, shortened versions of their talks appear in this book.

Two other impressive symposiums were on the program, and the contents of both are summarized in this volume. One was the Ruth H. Munroe Memorial Symposium. Convened by Deborah L. Best, the participants in this symposium were friends and colleagues of the late Ruth Hagberg Munroe. Like Ruth, all of the individuals on the symposium have made major contributions to an understanding of cultural influences on human development. Representing just two countries, they nevertheless have conducted research in numerous countries. The panel included Daphne M. Keats from Australia, and Carolyn Pope Edwards, Patricia M. Greenfield, Ashley Maynard, Carla Childs, Suzanne Gaskins, and Susan Seymour, as well as Debbie Best, all from the United States. The symposium was a fitting tribute to Ruth who, along with her husband Robert L. (Lee) Munroe, made many innovative conceptual and methodological contributions in the area of human development and culture. Lee was a constant source of support in the planning of this symposium, and served as a silent partner in its development, including Best's overview.

The final symposium was scheduled for the last full day of the conference. The title of the symposium, Millennium Prelude: The Present State and Future of Cross-Cultural Psychology, was convened by Cigdem Kagitcibasi (Turkey) and Ype Poortinga (The Netherlands). Reflecting on the past but devoting most of their time to forecasts on the future, participants included Yoshihisa Kashima (Australia), Ted Singelis (U.S.A.), Heidi Keller (Germany), Patricia M. Greenfield (U.S.A.), Fons van de Vijver (The Netherlands), Kwok Leung (Hong Kong), Sara Harkness (U.S.A.), and Zeyep Aycan (Turkey). This was the most well-attended symposium in the history of IACCP. Incidentally, Kagitcibasi and Poortinga were recognized at the conference by being named Honorary Fellows of the association.

We were also fortunate to have a number of other individuals on the program as invited speakers and discussion leaders in several conversation hours. They included John Berry who gave a talk on research on acculturation, Sid Irvine who discussed the health of nations, and Wayne Holtzman who presented an overview of his recent work on community psychology for family services in schools. Also featured was a lively and informative discussion by James and Jane Ritchie which focussed on 75 years of cross-cultural psychological research in New Zealand (which is included in this volume) as well a discussion by Richard M. Suinn, president-elect of the American Psychological Association, on primary mental health.

A key event of the conference was Marshall H. Segall's presidential address, "On the pernicious concept of 'Race' or Why do we still have racism if there are no such thing as races?" His riveting talk was accompanied by an important, world-class display entitled "All of Us are Related: Each of Us is Unique." We express our appreciation to Marshall for his important address and for arranging the temporary loan of this display. Thanks also to Karen W. Morse, President of Western Washington University, for finding the funds to rent this display. Both Segall's address and the display consisting of 18 large panels dealt with the dubious concept of race. The basic idea of both is that the concept of "race" is often terribly misused, especially in the social and behavioral sciences. Following IACCP tradition, Segall's address entitled "Why is There Still Racism if There is No Such Thing as Race?" appears in its entirety as the first article in this volume.

The bulk of this volume has been committed to a selection of papers that were submitted for possible publication. Approximately 85 papers that appeared on the program were candidates for inclusion. Each was evaluated carefully by the four co-editors of the volume, and limited space permitted the selection and inclusion of 33 of them. These papers were arranged in seven relatively homogenous sections. Following is an overview of the content of these sections.

Section One, *Historical and Epistemological Contributions,* contains three papers that are noteworthy for their perspectives on the field. As indicated earlier, James and Jane Ritchie presented an engaging review of cross-cultural psychology in New Zealand, covering 75 years of rich history. Some of the important earlier contributions to this field were made in that wonderful part of the world, and the Ritchies are uniquely qualified to prepare such a report. In the other two reports contained in this section, Forrest B. Tyler and Josephine Naidoo and her colleagues raise some important issues regarding the cross-cultural perspective as a scientific enterprise. Tyler wonders if it's time to revise the model, while Naidoo and three co-authors from South Africa present some continuing challenges to EuroAmerican psychology. Contributions such as these are welcome, primarily as safeguards against complacency and as reminders that the cross-cultural perspective in psychology, for as long as it lasts, should be considered a work in progress. We must be willing to meet challenges and to facilitate and encourage and revisions that may prove necessary.

In Section Two, *Cognitive, Intellectual, and Assessment Perspectives,* six contributions are included. Samuda and Lewis raise some issues that are important in the area of multicultural assessment. These authors take on one of the most enduring themes in cross-cultural psychology: The appropriateness of administering tests and measures to individuals who may be in environmental and educational circumstances that makes traditional testing questionable and probably inappropriate. Using tasks of varying cognitive complexity and administering them to Iranian and Dutch subjects, Sonke, Poortinga, and de Kuijer investigated the effects of differential stimulus familiarity on simple cognitive tasks. Two papers in this section are directly concerned with intelligence and intellectual development. Srivastava and Misra use the Indian context as a background to show that what they term the "cognitively-loaded psychometric tradition" may well have been outgrown. The authors use notions of social and emotional intelligence, prudence, and other constructs to explore laypersons' conception of intelligence and its use in day-to-day life in India. Using an unusual background and selection of participants along with Wechsler's Intelligence Scales, Dumitrascu analyzed the relationship between parental child-rearing style and intellectual development in the Romanian and Gypsy cultures. The paper by Strohschneider summarizes research that looked into the interaction between culture and problem-solving styles. A simulated problem involving the improvement of living conditions of a small tribe of semi-nomads was presented to university students in Germany and India. Their findings showed that different problem-solving styles are indeed used by these different groups of students. The final paper in this section was concerned with the application of the Cognitive-Affective Processing System (CAPS) theory at the group level. The authors, Mendoza-Denton, Shoda, Ayduk, and Mischel, use a theory that incorporates the idea that a network involving members of a culture or group who share cognitive-affective mediating units within the group members influence decisions, despite the heterogeneity of individual differences that characterize a given group. This has interesting implications for cross-cultural research, for cultures may well apply their own mediating units when reacting to psychological situations.

Section Three, *Acculturation, Individualism-Collectivism, and Ethnic Identity*, includes six papers that are welcome additions to the growing literature in one of the more active and fertile areas of research in the field. Leading off this section Ward presents an overview of models and measures of acculturation. She also describes the development of the Acculturation Index and explains its use in a series of five studies on sojourner adaptation. In another paper dealing with acculturation, Lim, Levenson, and Go used Cambodian refugees to investigate possible relationships between the degree of parental as opposed to adolescent acculturation and adolescent delinquent behavior. Lebedeva used the concept of acculturative stress and how it is experienced by ethnic Russians in the post-Soviet states as they experience possible crises in ethnic identity. Employing correlational analyses, she explains hers findings by using a cluster of features that she has called the "Syndrome of Imposed Ethnicity." Unsurprisingly, many papers and presentations in the Congress were concerned with the ever-popular area of individualism-collectivism. Representing these various contributions in this volume are two papers. The first, by Saha and Ghosh, presented data on the effects of self-orientations, as opposed to group orientations, in a group decision-making task. The study involved participants from India and Bangladesh. In the second paper, Verma and Triandis present data on the measurement of collectivism in India. The last paper in Section Three, by Salazar and Villegas, explored Latin American identity. With university students from Chile and Venezuela serving as participants, they were asked to evaluate such things as their degree of identification with different social categories. Their research suggests that a supra-national Latin American identity may be developing.

Five papers comprise Section Four, *Clinical and Mental Health Considerations*. A familiar area of research, that of stress and coping among immigrants, is represented by a contribution from Niles. With samples of subjects from immigrant groups from Greece and the Philippines in Northern Australia, she examined relationships between acculturative stress and mental health. In the next paper, Hocoy looked at the clinical implications of racial identity as it related to Apartheid in South Africa. The study was based on a 1995 nationwide investigation which included ethnographic analysis and interviews. Hocoy looked at both the positive and negative consequences of apartheid as it related to racial identity as reported by a small saple of subjects. The third paper in this section was also based on research in South Africa. Focussing on health care services provided to historically disadvantaged rural communities in South Africa, Goedeke and Farman surveyed people for the purpose of determining the effects of services brought about by what they refer to as the Primary Health Care Train. They study also sought to assess what effects might be expected in critical areas such as child abuse and sexual abuse if services were to be provided. The fourth paper in this section dealt with depression experienced later in life in ten European countries. The authors, van den Eeden and Braam, used Prince's EURO-D meta-assessment scale. Using a multilevel approach with attempts to correlate depression with other variables, several interesting trends involving age-depression relationships were detected in the analysis of responses from nearly 17,000 respondents. The final paper, authored by Kohli and Dalal, described a study whose main objective it was to examine cultural beliefs that women patients in India used to attribute their cervical cancer. Fate, God, and Karma were seen as the cause of their cancer, but their doctors were seen as the major factor in their recovery.

The area encompassing cultural constructions of self, self-concept, and related topics constitute one of the largest domains of research in attempts to understand connections between culture and the individual. And so it is no surprise that there were many papers on the program that concerned such popular matters. Thus, Section Five, *Cultural Manifestations of Self and Self-Concept*, contains four papers that are highly interrelated. Redford looked at the action tendencies associated with the emotional experience of anger in Hong Kong and the United Kingdom. In a carefully designed study, various cultural differences that were found cast doubt over the theory of display rules, especially as they relate to the emotion of anger as displayed by small samples of individuals in Hong Kong and the UK. The second paper in this section was concerned with culture and gender influences on self-concept and the origins of self-esteem. Using Turkey as the sole source of information and data, Sunar reported on four studies done with Turkish respondents. All studies were concerned with interrelations among self-concept, bases of self-esteem, gender, age, and individualism-collectivism. Sunar emphasizes the importance of contextual variables in understanding these relationships. The third paper reported on relationship harmony that is so important in Chinese interpersonal relationships. Thus Li, Kwan, and Bond report on research to help establish the nomological network surrounding this construct. Such factors as Openness, Emotional Stability,

Helpfulness, Restraint, and Extraversion were found to correlate with relationship harmony. The last article in this section, reported by Germain, examined cultural identity development and ultimately on global self-esteem in indigenous and migrant Australian adolescents. Based on convenience samples of 400 junior and senior high school students, Germain analyzed what her research means with respect to factors such as experiences of racism and cultural exploration.

Section Six, *Contributions of Special Relevance to Children and Youth,* contains five papers that represent what is perhaps the most important area of research for the future: That of trying to understand relationships between culture and child-rearing practices. Leading the section is a cross-cultural longitudinal study that has been ongoing for nine years. The leader of this series of studies is Hans-Joachim Kornadt of Germany. In cooperation with Yoshihara Tachibana of Japan, Kornadt summarized some key findings gleaned from comparative data from participants living in European, East-Asian, and Southeast Asian culture. Highly contextual in nature, the integrated series of studies looks at child-rearing factors that contribute such social motives as aggressiveness and altruism. The second article was written by a team of French researchers, Marie Anaut, Bernard Chouvier, and Jeanne Tyrrell. The focus of their study was the psychosocial and educational consequences of North African and French children who were placed in foster families. A trio of German researchers were authors of the third article in this section. Thus Meischner, Tietze, and Wessels investigated the educational beliefs of mothers and day-care teachers of preschool children in former East and West Germany. Part of the study's aim was to look for what they called "divergent" beliefs in educating young children as a result of political, ideological, and educational separation that covered about a fifty-year period. The fourth article was prepared by Tsai, Yu, and Maynard and looked into mother-child conflict resolution styles amond college students in Taiwan. A 1998 Chinese Model of Conflict Resolution was employed. Compromise, confrontation, face-saving, endurance/forbearance and other styles used to reduce conflict were analyzed by using structural equation modeling. The last paper in this group of papers was written by L. Wong, F. Ishiyama, and P. Wong, a trio of researchers who are affiliated with universities in British Columbia. The topic of their report concerned assessment devices used to explore the world of personal meaning of students who learn English as a second language, or so-called ESL students. Employing these devices with three children of Chinese immigrants, the validity of the devices was demonstrated.

The final five papers are included in Section Seven, *Perspectives on Work and Organizational Factors.* Mainly an applied area, the contributions included here are representative of the research and concerns of those who largely represent industrial and organizational psychology. It is noteworthy that the first author of the first paper in this section is Pieter J. D. Drenth. Drenth can easily be included among the founders of the modern cross-cultural psychology movement, having co-edited a seminal 1972 book in the area with Lee J. Cronbach (**Mental tests and cultural adaptation**). In the current paper, "Culture and Organizational Differences", Drenth and his co-author, D. N. den Hartog, explained the two basic concerns of cross-cultural organizational psychology: Do organizations based in different countries differ with respect to organizational characteristics? And can these differences be explained in terms of culture? A natural paper to follow the Drenth and de Hartog overview is the contributon by Adriaan Viviers who looked into three measures of work orientation in different cultural groups in South Africa. Various questionnaires were administered to a large number of students, both White and Black. The results were examined by using factor analysis and the implications for South Africa were discussed. The third paper in the last section was primarily related to the popular area of multicultural counseling. Wong and Wong point out the need to assess competencies of those who are supposed to be training culturally skilled counselors. The Wongs discuss the development of the 60-item Multicultural Supervision Competencies Questionnaire and present evidence of its reliability. The MSCQ may well prove to be a valuable device for use in the field of cross-cultural counseling. The final paper in this section, and in the proceedings volume, was written by Alexander Thomas of Germany. Using and analyzing more than two hundred interviews with German and Chinese managers resulting in many "critical incidents". The results of his analysis point to continued use of such techniques in intercultural training in areas such as culture assimilator, negotiation strategies, and conflict resolution styles.

We welcome you to read all of the contributions contained in this volume. It has been a pleasure, and a lot of work, to be involved with this Silver Jubilee meeting. However, successful IACCP meetings, like all other conferences, are only as good as the effort expended to make them worthwhile. As we enter the new millennium we are bound to see many changes in the nature and scope of cross-cultural psychology. We hope that future conferences will contribute to increasingly flexible and inclusive ways to view and to use cross-cultural psychology.

Walter J. Lonner
Dale L. Dinnel
Deborah K. Forgays
Susanna A. Hayes

August 17, 1999

Why is There Still Racism If There is No Such Thing as "Race"?

Marshall H. Segall
Syracuse University
The Maxwell School

ABSTRACT

This presidential address is keyed to the exhibition "All of Us Are Related, Each of Us Is Unique." It reveals that there are no biological barriers between the 5.7 billion human beings that today inhabit the earth. We all have the same ancestors and the genetic diversity of contemporary human populations reflects the paths followed by our ancestors in the course of human migrations over the past 100,000 years. I assert that there is simply no such thing as "white people", "black people", "yellow people", or the like, except as social constructs. In a world in which intergroup hostility has long been based on erroneous beliefs in biologically determined characteristics of so-called "races", our habitual way of thinking about how we relate to each other needs seriously to be re-examined.

I acknowledge gratefully the honor you have granted me, allowing me to serve for the past two years as your President. This office carries the privilege of addressing you this evening, on the opening day of the Silver Jubilee Congress of the International Association for Cross-Cultural Psychology. I do not take this privilege lightly; I accept it enthusiastically.

This week the Association honors its past while looking to its future. Since I can look back over forty years as a cross-cultural psychologist, my comments this evening constitute a valedictory. In that spirit, I will look back briefly to a feature of the field that was salient when I first became involved with cross-cultural psychology. I will continue by discussing my current professional concerns, and I'll conclude with a look to the future, which includes a research project on which I will invite your cooperation and participation.

The concept of "race" will be the substantive theme of everything I have to say tonight. To clarify how cross-cultural psychologists in particular, social scientists more generally, and, indeed, all thinking people should treat the concept of "race", will be the goal of my argument.

I begin, as promised, with a glance at the 1950s, when my career began. Many issues and arguments characterized psychology and anthropology in those days. Some of them are now of historical interest only … literally gone from the textbooks and the university curricula. But one that stood out during my years as a student and then a young faculty member persists. It is the question of what determines "racial" differences in behavior, including various indices of competence.

From early on, my teachers and early colleagues, who included the anthropologist Melville Herskovits and the psychologists Donald Campbell and Otto Klineberg, had no trouble convincing me that the conventional answer to that question was patently wrong. There were so many reasons to assert that racial differences in intelligence and in various forms of behavior were *neither* biologically rooted *nor* genetically transmitted. At least, we understood all the reasons why the biology/genetics argument was so weak, including its failure to recognize *interactions* between nature and nurture, the *biases* in the instruments that yielded performance differences between groups, the many social and economic variables *confounded* with "race", and so on. And all of those reasons continue still serve well to counter the continual resurrections of the old biology and genetics arguments from the Jensens, Eysencks, Rushtons and others who, refuse to give up their dogged commitment to biological determinism.

The arguments concerning inadequacies of measuring instruments administered to groups on whom its validity was never established, or the confounds with social and economic variables are fine arguments, as far as they go. But they do not go far enough.

What I wish to underscore this evening is that the question of *what causes "racial" differences* in *anything* we might measure is a meaningless question, because ***there simply are no "races" in the human species***. If this is so, and I will try to convince you that it is indeed so, then there are no racial differences to explain. If we continue to explain differences between *any* human groups while speaking of those groups as "races", then we are pushed into a frame of mind that anticipates a significant role for biological forces to play. This is a mind frame that does not anticipate much in the way of individual differences within the groups being compared, and tends to think of whatever differences emerge as pretty stable over time, if not fixed. All of these expectations, reinforced in my view by the very use of the word "race", contribute not only to serious scientific error but to profoundly dangerous ethnocentric politics both within multi-cultural nations and across ethno-religious groups prone to engage in inter-national conflicts as well. At the very least, when inter-communal conflicts over resources are wrapped in ideas of the primordial, racially distinct, nature of the communities involved, the conflicts are exacerbated and more intractable. Any basis for Us/Them thinking is dangerous; when the concept of "race" is part of it, it is hardened as if set in stone.

I turn now to a quick look at some conventional wisdom about "race" and then, in more detail, the findings from contemporary research in population genetics and paleontology that challenge that conventional wisdom.

The Concept "Race" As Bequeathed to Us

In the second half of the 19th century, through most of the 20th, physical anthropologists (and nearly everybody else) categorized human groups in terms of "race" on the basis of visible physical characteristics, such as skin color, height, hair and facial features. Their taxonomies usually included categories such as, e.g., "Negroid, Mongoloid and Caucasoid", and "black, brown, yellow, red and white". At first glance, classifications like "white, black, brown, red, yellow", seem to reflect a natural phenomenon, linked to geography. None of us today would have any difficulty in distinguishing a native of Senegal from a native of the Netherlands. Nor would we have difficulty distinguishing a Chinese person from an Inuit person, nor guessing where they are from. Since some physical characteristics are correlated, we can usually guess successfully where people (or their ancestors) came from.

However, these visible traits are not highly correlated with each other. The spatial distribution of skin color differs from the spatial distribution of hair form, which in turn is different from facial shapes, or any other visual characteristic.

During colonial times value judgments of superiority and inferiority were attached to these physical characteristics, allowing colonialists and slave owners to justify oppression and exploitation. Despite the end of slavery and colonialism, the concept of "races" is still popular. In many countries in the world, there are even laws couched in terms of "race". While some time ago, South Africa abolished its "apartheid" system, which was, of course, based on "race", in the United States, as we speak, many states still prohibit adoption of children of one so-called "race" by parents of another one! Even the White House "Town Meetings" on "race" relations in the United States fail to include in this all important discourse the fact that there are no "races".

Through history in the West, at least, we have endured "scientific racism." Famous early "scientific racists" were non-anthropologists, like Huston Stewart Chamberlain ("Foundations of the Nineteenth Century"), le Comte A. de Gobineau ("Essay on the inequality of human "races", 1884), and Hans Gunther ("The Racial Elements of European History") in which he said, a "race" is "marked off from every other human group through its own proper combination of bodily and mental characteristics."

Gobineau's essay included such gems as "for a very considerable number of human beings it has been impossible and will be forever to make even the first step toward civilization." and it is impossible "to overcome the natural repugnance which man, like animals, harbors for miscegenation."

Then, with the specter of Nazi racist ideology fouling Europe, the ugliness was expressed so many times, in so many horrible ways, that it is impossible to evoke it in mere words, but the following is quintessentially representative of the rhetoric of the time: e.g. Herman Gauch 1933: "non-Nordics are more closely allied to monkeys and apes than to Nordics.... Non-Nordic man occupies a midway position between Nordic men and animals, next to the apes. ... he is not a man at all...., but only a transition."

Earlier, during the 1920s, some commentators understood that "race" was a construction that served a social and political purpose. Simar, in 1922, said, that the doctrine of "race" "...was originally a doctrine of classes". The doctrine of "race" was used to explain existing class differences. For example, according to Hertz (1925), Count de Boulainvilliers asserted that French people were composed of two "races", with the nobility descended from Germanic conquerors, the rest from conquered Celts and Romans.

Of course, when various European nations colonized Africa and established slavery in the Americas, the two "races", white and black, took on a profound significance. In the context of the Judeo-Christian tradition that prevailed in Europe then as now, colonialism and racism might not have been possible without the underpinnings of a great divide theory of two races, one of masters, the other of slaves.

Contemporary Definitions of "Race"

But all that is history. Or is it? Let's now ask, How is "race" defined today? This month, from Britannica on-line, I learned that a "race" is "a division of mankind possessing traits that are transmissible by descent and sufficient to characterize it as a distinct human type; also .. a family, tribe, people, or nation belonging to the same stock" ...(Britannica Dictionary). Does that strike you as clear, unambiguous, and scientific? Of course not! Cannot individuals from any human group, mating with individuals from any other human group, or from their own, transmit traits that lead some people, somewhere to designate those traits as defining a "distinct" human group...whatever distinct means?

We turn now to "the illusion of "race" and "race" as it is popularly misconceived. We will see that journalists, politicians, and even social scientists, in some countries at least, seem spellbound by the notion of "race". In the United States of America, it is common practice today to perceive and describe people as Black, White or some other "racial"type. Examples:

> "Whatever happened to the white athlete" (cover story with this title in *Sports Illustrated);*
>
> Any day in the *NY Times;*
>
> In academic publications such as the *APA Monitor* which in its January 1998 issue (p. 8) speaks of ""white babies" and "black newborns", "and describes a psychologist who, forty years ago ..."was one of nine black students who integrated" a high school.

The noted African-American scholar, Bruce Hare, tells a story of his two sons, who, years ago, as children, inquired nervously, but with a giggle, why it was that "They call brown people black and pink people white?" This rhetorical question from these child prodigies reminds us that *nobody's* skin color is black or white. So when we say black or white to refer to people, we're obviously not talking about color in the sense of hue, but something else, something metaphorical perhaps. And we must not fail to note that the words *white* and *black* are opposites of each other. The semantic implication of black/white terminology is that the so-called black and white "races" are, at least unconsciously, implied to be in opposition to each other. How more separated and different can any two categories be if they are opposites of each other? And this piece of word magic is apart from the various connotations of these words, black and white, like day and night, visible and invisible, good and evil.

How Many "Races" Do People Think There Are?

Of course, many who believe in the existence of races have in mind more than black and white. We turn now to what various people respond when asked, "How many "races" are there and what are they called?" In the Swiss television film, Six Billion Races, passersby near the Musee de l'Homme in Paris were asked, Combien de "races"? The prototypical response was "Quatre, commes nous etions enseigne a l'ecole; blanc, noir, jaune, et rouge. " (English translation: "Four, as we have been taught in school; white, black, yellow, and red." Incidentally, until recently, the Hall of Man in a museum in New York contained at its entrance four statues designating the black, white, yellow and red "races". A 9-minute film showing interviews videotaped in the student center of Syracuse University in past January, 1998 (shown as part of this address) reveals a shared awareness of human diversity accompanied by profound confusion on the part of American university students as to the basis of that diversity.

Scientific Understanding of Human Diversity

What is the contemporary status of scientific understanding of human diversity? Physical anthropologists have long known and taught the difficulties with the concept of "race", but many social scientists, including many psychologists, don't seem to know about it. Let's review quickly what we know. What does contemporary biology have to say about "race"?

There are no biological barriers between 5.8 billion human beings alive today. External physical features previously used to distinguish "racial groups" are not reliable genetic markers because they represent relatively recent (over the past 20,000 years) adaptations. Skin color and height, for example, are subject to rapid change (in genetic terms) in response to environmental conditions. Skin color is a useful adaptation to the exposure to the sun.

The crucial point about these variations is that they are not categorical but constitute a continuous dimension. They are, to use a technical term to which we will return in a few moments, clinal variations. Variations along the skin color dimension, for example, are due to different, continuous, concentrations of a single pigment called melanin in the skin.

So, is it impossible to classify people by skin color? Of course not; we may classify people however we want... by color of eyes, by height, by income, by religion, by political party affiliation, etc. So, it is also possible to classify human groups according to their average concentration of melanin. But, I ask you to reflect, why would we want to?

Geneticists can now examine many more gene categories than the ones that determine external physical features; the best known of those that determine internal features are blood groups and the Human Leucocyte Antigen (HLA) system. These two also have important implications for our understanding of the diversity of human populations. Consider the following.

While there are only four blood groups in the whole human species, there are many billion possible combinations of genes in the HLA system. If human groupings based on these "hidden" genetic markers were treated as "races", the number of "races" would exceed the number of presently living humans! Genetically, humans are all different (with the exception of identical twins). And, as we are about to see, we are also all related.

Humans everywhere share a lot genetically. There is no gene that is specific to one particular human population, and totally absent in any other. The genetic similarity between populations varies basically with geographic proximity, and reflects the history of population movements in the distant past. While scientists still disagree on the exact way in which this happened, the overwhelming evidence argues for a common origin of all humans. In other words, we are all one single species, called Homo sapiens sapiens, capable of interbreeding, and descendants, over approximately 5000 generations, of the same ancestors.

The gradual variation of a human physical trait across geographical space is a ***cline***. Skin color is clinal, not categorical. For example, the skin color of "Native Americans" or Amerindians is lighter nearer the poles and darker closer to the equator. In Europe, from Scandinavia down through southern Europe and on to North and Central Africa, skin color gets darker gradually, with no sharp breaks.

All genetically determined characteristics, including such visible ones as height, and skin color, are clinal, and, they interact with environmental influences. Invisible ones, like blood types, and HLA, the former with few variations, the latter with many thousands, are also clinal. Moreover, clines do not co-vary. They are not highly correlated with each other. Thus, spatial distribution of hair form differs from that of skin color, both differ from that of blood groups, etc. Because the physical diversity of human populations today is continuous, whatever boundaries have been placed within this continuous diversity are arbitrary. No one knows where one "race" stops and another begins!

Thus, the recent scientific evidence is that "race" is not a useful biological concept at the human level. It is now clear from many recent publications that human genetic diversity defies any simple classification. This is the central point of the exhibition entitled "All of Us are Related, Each of Us is Unique" which I hope you will see in the library sometime this week.[1]

One of the panels deals with the origins of Homo sapiens sapiens, pointing out that 100,000 years ago, out first forebears appeared on earth, most likely in East Africa. Since then, we have fanned out over the inhabitable parts of the Earth.

Present paleontological evidence situates these common ancestors to have lived in the Middle East and Africa between 700,000 and 100,000 years ago. Recent DNA research has shown Neanderthal DNA to be different from Human DNA; it appears that the Neanderthals and we descended from a common ancestor. Moreover, probably all human beings alive today have an African origin. As an article recently in the New York Times had it, "Though modern humans may not look exactly alike, we are indeed all Africans under the skin".

Another panel in the exhibition concerns migration effects on our visible (and invisible) characteristics, making it clear that our contemporary genetic diversity is a product of the migration patterns followed by our ancestors over the past 100,000 years.

Another shows how you are related to everyone in this room, in this city, on this continent, and, indeed, anywhere in the world. We all have the same ancestors (many times over). Consider the following:

Through N generations back, we each have had 2 to the nth ancestors; e.g. back to approx. 1800 AD (about 7 generations) we each have had 2 to the 7th, or 128 ancestors. Let's go back further, to the year we will cite as we ethnocentrically celebrate a so-called millennial change ....the year Christians call year 1 *ano domini*. That's 2,000 years ago. If each of the 5.8 billion of us alive today had *unique* ancestors, since 1 AD that would have been 10 to the 24th power for all of us, requiring 1 million billion billion people. But, there were only 300 million people on Earth in 1 AD; we didn't reach a mere 1 billion until 1800 AD. Therefore, it is a mathematical necessity that we all share, over and over again, the same ancestors. Whoever is seated next to you, from whatever country he or she may have come, is your cousin.

Thus, biologically speaking, "race" is an illusion. Boundaries placed on any dimension of human variation, including "color" are arbitrary; so there really is no such thing as a group of "white people", "black people", "yellow people" or the like, except as social or cultural constructs.

[1] The exhibition is available by rental or purchase from Syracuse University. For ordering details contact mhsegall@maxwell.syr.edu.

"Race" as a Social Construct

The categories in everyday use have been reified and have potent political and economic force. These categories are cultural constructs, varying over time and space.

Consider how we perceive our fellow human beings and how we relate to each other. Do we, most of the time, relate strictly on a person-to-person basis? Do we see everyone we encounter, especially when away from home, strictly as individuals? Or do we view persons as members of groups? When, for whatever reason we perceive "us" (ourselves) as co-members of a group, we see "them" as members of some other groups.

Frequently (nearly always?) we see persons as partly (largely?) defined by group membership (e.g., "blacks", "Asians", "Jews"). This evokes stereotypical characteristics and if a person doesn't fit the stereotype s/he is an exception. "I don't see you as a black person," That's shorthand for "You're not like all those other folks that I see so very negatively." When I was young, I remember being told that I was a "good Jew". I gratefully admit that no one has called me that, to my face, in years. However, would it be paranoid of me to suspect that the thought may have occurred to one colleague or another? My friends who identify themselves, or are identified by others, as African-American invariably tell me that they know that when viewed by others, that their African-American-ness is their most salient characteristic.

A frustrating search for appropriate group labels has gone on for years in my own country. U.S. census categories get changed with every successive census. What will they be this time around? There has been talk that the category "Other" will be dropped, but that people will be instructed that they can, if they wish, claim to belong to more than one "race". Will the categories include Hispanic? Who are Hispanics? Is a recent immigrant to the United States from Spain a Hispanic? In the USA, are Hispanics a "race"? Or do Hispanics cut across "races"? One reads regularly about non-Black Hispanics. And I won't even delve into the morass surrounding the popular term Latino, which one regularly hears in the United States. Wherever Jews live, are they better described as an ethnic group rather than as a "race"? Or as neither? In Australia, who *are* the Black people one hears about? Are they, like so-called Blacks in the USA recent African migrants? I don't think so.

So, it should be obvious that we live with a surfeit of classification labels, a maze of overlapping category systems that include tribes, nationalities, religions, and what have you. What kinds of groups, for example, are the Macedonians in Greece and those in Macedonia?

What does one make of groups defined by the language they speak? Are the Quebecois in Canada a "race"? Or the Basques in France or in Spain? What do we make of the groups defined by religion, or ethnicity, like Catholics and Protestants in Northern Ireland, Arabs and Jews in

Israel/Palestine? Or Croats, Serbs, and Moslems in ex-Yugoslavia. Are these primordial groups? Many groups have origin myths, which assert their primordial status, one that often is linked to a claim for a given piece of real estate.

Whatever these various kinds of groups are, every one of them are often referred to as "races". And everyone of these kinds of groups do in fact satisfy many of the definitions of "race" that one finds in dictionaries and even in some biology textbooks. And, it must be noted, sometimes even in psychology journals, groups categorized by skin color are also referred to as "races", although members of this association are probably less often guilty of this practice than some of our colleagues in other parts of the discipline.

Psychology and "Race"

Although many psychologists continue to treat "race" as a biological fact and continue to debate the nature of racial differences in behavior, a few voices can be heard decrying this repeated airing of what is essentially a meaningless question. I recommend to all of you Jefferson Fish's dramatic challenge to this continuing error in the magazine, *Psychology Today*, in 1995. (This is recounted in detail in the forthcoming 2nd edition of "Human Behavior in Global Perspective" by Segall, Dasen, Berry, and Poortinga.) It features a striking difference across the United States and Brazil in the way terms like Black and White are understood.

In an article in the American Psychologist in July 1998, Comas-Diaz, Lykes, and Alarcon dealt with *racismo*, or Puerto Rican style racism. They say that it "operates differently from its North American cousin in that it is covert, contextual, and subjective. Racial perception is related to individuals' racial self-identification. For instance, a dark-skinned Puerto Rican's race may be perceived differently by two persons according to their racial self-identification. ... the same person's race can be perceived differently according to the race of the observer. ... Regardless of color, the higher the person's social class, the whiter the person is perceived to be, and thus, the less the person is subjected to *racismo*. ... many Puerto Ricans describe themselves as rainbow people ... contrary to the North American dictum that one drop of African blood makes a person Black, one drop of White blood makes a person at least not Black in Puerto Rico."

If "race" does not exist as a biological fact, it is, as we have now seen, a compelling social construct. Since the illusion of "race" is so compelling and so widely held, we have to deal with the fact that many people think it is real and view the world as if it contained "races". When one adds to the belief in "race" the two further ideas that "races" are qualitatively different in terms of talent and capacity and that they should be treated differently, then we have the all-too-familiar form of "racism". Belief in the existence of "race", coupled with widely held beliefs in behavioral differences, is a powerful sociological phenomenon that impacts on intergroup relations. Here

I am arguing that merely treating the social construct of “race” *as if it were* a biological reality is itself “racist” and should be resisted as vigorously as one resists “racial discrimination”.

The American Anthropology Association has gone as record as advocating the elimination of “racial” categories from official forms in the USA. Perhaps this association - the IACCP - will someday find it useful to consider a formal recommendation that the discipline of psychology do the same.

On one of the panels of the exhibition, we see twelve young men, their faces arrayed in a (rough) circle. The differences between any two adjacent faces are scarcely perceptible. Yet, one can probably locate on the circle what appear to be quintessential examples of “black”, “white” and other “races”. But, note that each face flows, continuously, out of the others; so what appear to be “prototypes” are nothing more than variations along a continuum, one without any end points!

These faces take us to my plan for some future endeavors.

A Collaborative Research Project

I want to conduct identical data collection efforts in many different places around the world in order to test the notion that racial categories possess a high degree of consensual "reality" within societies but vary across societies. The research design employs a standard stimulus set and a standard procedure for collecting responses.

The stimuli comprise 13 black and white photographs of young men, derived from a set of morphed photos. (I can provide researcher with a set of photos on firm paper, of appropriate size, so they can be shuffled and presented as if they were a deck of cards.)

One says to the respondent, “You are about to see 13 photographs of some young men. The photographs have been shuffled, so they will be shown to you in no particular order. Each of these persons is unique, but there are relationships of one kind or another among them. I would like you to look through all of these pictures and then sort them into groups, in any way that seems appropriate to you. Do this on the basis of any aspect of these people that seems meaningful to you ”

“Very good! You have sorted these people into x groups. Next, can you name each of the groups? How would you label each group? “*(Respondent states names; collector records them.)*

“Thank you for naming each group. Now, for each group, please choose the one best example of members of that group? Which one is the most typical group member?” *(Respondent designates choice; collector records ID number of best exemplar.)* “Do you personally belong to any of these groups? Which one(s)? “

(If respondent chooses more than one, ask): “If you had to choose one group, which one would it be?” *(Record group, and its name, to which*

respondent claims belonging.) "If you were filling out a form that required you to designate your "race" or ethnicity, what group name would you use?"

"Now we have finished. Thank you very much for participating in this exercise. Your way of sorting these photos was very good, but, as you probably have surmised, there is no necessarily right way to sort them. In this study, we are interested in various ways people categorize individuals, and how much agreement there is among people who do the categorizing. Thank you again for your cooperation."

Time does not permit a presentation of findings already available but let me assure you that they show a dramatic within-group consensus. Seventy-nine of 80 participants sorted the 13 photos into groups. Nearly all of these created 3, 4, or 5 groups. Nearly half constructed three groups, clustered about photos they most often labeled as "Caucasian", "African-American", and "Asian". These emerge as the races students at one university in the USA perceive as a phenomenon of nature. It remains to be seen how other groups of respondents will sort these pictures.

Conclusion

To approach a conclusion, let me remind you of the question we began with in the title. Why do we still have racism if there is no such thing as "race"? In other words, why are intergroup relations so often negative, particularly when they are treated as inter-racial? Ethnocentrism theory provides one answer

Ethnocentrism as discussed by Sumner in 1906 was presented as a universal syndrome of behavior in which positive links with the in-group negative attitudes and behaviors toward out-groups are mutually reinforced. But, as many of us have argued at length elsewhere, however universal it may be, ethnocentrism can vary in kind and degree and is subject to influence from various social policies and political stances. So, there is reason for social scientists to be engaged in efforts to improve intergroup relations. Perhaps one such effort entails challenging the continued unthinking use of the word "race."

Let me try now to conclude by reiterating what we know about the role of the concept of "race" in the story of intergroup relations. Human groups surely exist as more-or-less distinct entities. Some of them even have legal status. For example, insofar as there is such a thing as international laws, most members of the United Nations enjoy the legal status of nation. Some groups, on the other hand, exist, sometimes for short periods, sometimes for centuries, on the basis of their own members' conviction that the group is a meaningful social entity. We have seen that groups may be designated on the basis of the language their members speak, the religion with which their members affiliate, and numerous other bases. Some of these groupings cross national boundaries; some of them also exist as sub-groups within nations. Where does "race" fit into this multivariate matrix of human groupings?

It seems highly likely that the prevailing understanding of "races" around the world is that they are relatively few in number and most often subsume and cross-cut other groupings. Thus, once again using my own nation, the USA, as an example, the "race" called white (or, as many seem to believe is a more polite term, "Caucasian") consists of persons whose recent ancestors migrated from all the different countries of Europe, speaking any of the languages spoken there. A noted African-American scholar once noted how remarkable it was that the English, French, Germans, Turks, Spaniards, Italians et al., once they crossed the Atlantic all became white folks.

Of course, it was also the case that people brought to the United States from Africa were all designated black. Later, as whites and blacks mated with each other, the resultant offspring were all still designated as black, with the various degrees of blackness, such as quadroon and octoroon actually legal categories for many decades in at least some sections of the United States.

This example underscores a second point about "race" and that is that the guidelines for designating groups as "racial" categories can vary markedly from place to place. Thus, as we were reminded, in Brazil and Puerto Rico, as well as in many other places, mating between Europeans and Africans yielded offspring whose racial designations were governed by very different rules.

Another point not to lose sight of is that the racial designation terminology has continually to be readjusted, as various political and economic changes occur. With the white-black categories so salient in the United States, as well as in some other parts of the world, there can emerge such quasi-racial labels as Hispanic or Latino, with attendant ambiguity as to whether some Hispanics are white and some black, or if all of them should be recognized as a third "race".

Membership in a "race" is mostly not a matter of choice, except in relatively few instances for persons who fall near a prevailing boundary of racial categories and who then, to use a term grounded in the language of "race", pass. Passing, of course, is usually unidirectional, from the disadvantaged "race" to the advantaged one.

Despite all of this complexity, most people treat "races" as supercategories of human groups, derived from some primordial division of humankind, fixed and determined in some natural way. "Races are, in this popular view, seen as impervious to environmental influences.

"Race" is thus treated *not* as a cultural construct … which is all it is, but as if it were a biological reality. As such, it is thought to reveal itself in superficial traits, like skin color, and then, more significantly, to carry a deep, biologically-determined structure of behavioral styles, talents, and capacities. It is this sense of "race" that contemporary population genetics has shown to be absolutely invalid.

It is my contention that the continued use of the term "race" hampers the already difficult process of reducing intergroup conflicts. Acknowledging that many such conflicts are not, strictly speaking, inter-racial, but, rather, inter-religious, inter-communal, or otherwise inter-ethnic, I believe that many of them carry at least an overtone of racial thinking. And a sufficient number of intergroup conflicts are overtly described as inter-racial for those conflicts to be lessened if we could spread the realization that the conflicting groups are not, after all, "races".

Culture enters into this story in two distinct ways, so as cross-cultural psychologists, we are in an especially advantageous position to make a contribution to intergroup relations. First, we can help spread the word that "race" is a cultural construct, varying over space and time, differing even from one country to another, and within a single country from decade to decade. Secondly, we can demonstrate in our research and writing that various groups that are anywhere perceived as "races" are better described as ethnic groups, simultaneously shaped by and reshaping their own particular cultures, and influencing other groups with whom they come in contact. These are two related, but separate points, about "race" and culture.

Most of you, of course, know **all** of this. However, if you leave here this evening with these points in mind, intending to instruct others who do not already know it, I'll leave now, finally pleased to have said something, after several decades as a cross-cultural psychologist, that truly needed to be said. Enjoy this Congress. Enjoy the exhibition. Thank you, and good evening.

References

American Anthropology Association (1998). AAA statement on "race." *Anthropology Newsletter, 39,* 3.

Comas-Diaz, L., Lykes, M. B., & Alarcon, R. D. (1998). Ethnic conflict and the psychology of liberation in Guatemala, Peru, and Puerto Rico. *American Psychologist, 53,*778-792.

Fish, J. (1997). How psychologists think about "race." *General Anthropology, 4,* 1-4.

Langaney, A., Hubert van Blijenburgh, N. & Sanchez-Mazas, A. (1992). *Tous parents, tous differents*. Paris: Chabaud.

Segall, M. H., Dasen, P. R., Berry, J. W., & Poortinga, Y. H. (1999). *Human behavior in global perspective: An introduction to cross-cultural psychology.* (Second edition). Boston, MA: Allyn & Bacon.

Founders Symposium

An Introduction by John Berry, Convener and Chair

The relationships between culture and human behavior have been of interest to scholars for centuries. About 80 years ago anthropology, psychology and psychiatry jointly began to advance the field conceptually and empirically. More recently (from the 1960s) there has been an upsurge in interest, rooted in earlier work, and advanced by a group of scholars who may be identified as Founders. From many perspectives and cultural backgrounds, and engaged in diverse research domains, they established a field (or more accurately, a set of related fields) within which culture-behavior relationships can bestudied and interpreted. The Founders' symposium brought together many of these Founders on the occasion of the Silver Jubilee of IACCP. The goal of the symposium was to share personal reflections on the origin, changes and current status of the field. Believing that a balanced sense of our recent past is the only sound basis for understanding our present and anticipatingour future, it was hoped that a living history would unfold during this Symposium.

In developing this Symposium, Walt Lonner and I established some criteria to guide our planning: individuals should have been in the field early (1960s), have been a continuing contributor, and now be into their "retirement" years (but, of course, no one ever really retires from this field!). A long list was created, and from these we selected a few to be invited to make presentations, based on the diversity of their experience, and on the probability of their attendance at the Congress. We originally approached Ernest Boesch (Germany) Rogelio Diaz-Guerrero (Mexico), Leonard Doob (USA), Gustav Jahoda (Scotland), Douglass Price-Williams (USA), Durganand Sinha (India), and Harry Triandis (USA). Unfortunately, Professor Sinha passed away, and Professors Boesch and Doob were unable to attend.

To our great pleasure, many others on our initial founders list were able to come to the Congress. These included Jan Deregowski, Pieter Drenth, Wayne Holtzman, Sid Irvine, Daphne and John Keats, Norman Feather, Hans-Joachim Kornadt, Alastair Mundy-Castle, James and Jane Ritchie, Ron Samuda, Marshall Segall, Ron Taft, John Williams, Robert Serpell, Geert Hofstede, Josephine Naidoo, and Jose Miguel Salazar. Apologies to others whose names could well have appeared along with the others.

The four papers that follow are all personal, candid and critical reflections on our field. We are all better at what we do because of the insights and contributions of these, and the other Founders. Let us hope that our field flourishes as much during the next twenty-five years.

Precursors of Cross-Cultural Psychology and the Context of Culture

Rogelio Diaz-Guerrero
Universidad Nacional Autonoma de Mexico
Facultad de Psicologia

I begin my remarks by making a few biographical comments on some major parts of my career orientation. My mentors at the State University of Iowa, between 1943 and 1947 (Lindquist, Bergman, Knott, Wendell Johnson, Robert Sears, Kenneth Spence and Kurt Lewin), provided me with solid theoretical, methodological and content knowledge about the science of psychology. But culture was not in the psychological vocabulary at that time, much less the term cross-cultural psychology. In Mexico, a mestizo culture, you could hardly avoid the term. For example, an early Mexican scholar, Ezequiel Chavez (1901), wrote an essay on our national character. Upon my return from Iowa in 1948, as Head of the Department of Psychology of Mexico City College, I organized a course with the title "The Psychology of the Mexican People". The bibliography included materials from Mexican philosophers and poets as well as European and American anthropologists and sociologists.

Samuel Ramos (1938), a philosopher, felt that to understand the Mexican culture one had first to understand the Mexican mind. The Mexican mind could be best understood through Adlerian psychology: Mexicans had an inferiority complex that showed best in their Machismo, and the culture showed it particularly in its tendency to imitate other cultures. Octavio Paz (1959), our Nobel laureate poet, wrote that Mexicans were solitary, airtight, simulators, servile and "sons of the nothing". When distinguished Mexican psychoanalysts, both Freudian and Frommian, expressed their views, interesting conceptualizations developed but the view of the Mexican character was still utterly negative.

As a member of a very traditional lower middle class family immersed in Mexican proverbs, and influenced by the Kluckhohns, I decided to try to understand the psychology of the Mexican on the basis of their most important and/or generalized beliefs. For substantial theoretical reasons, these were eventually labelled "Historic-sociocultural premises". The first study with ten of these beliefs was carried out in 1949. Questions such as, "Is the mother for you the dearest person in existence", "Do you believe the place for women is the home", "Do you believe that men should wear the pants in the family", were answered affirmatively by around 90% of individuals over 18 years of age in a weighted random sample in Mexico City in 1949 (Diaz-Guerrero, 1952).

In January, 1951 Werner Wolff came to Mexico City for the World Congress of Mental Health, where he contacted Guillermo Dávila, Manuel Facón , Oswaldo Robles and myself. Werner felt it was important to communicate in psychology across the Americas. An Argentinean, Eduardo Krapf, was drawn, and the InterAmerican Society of Psychology (SIP), was founded.

At the second congress of the SIP, in Mexico in 1953, Theodora Abel noted in a paper dealing with culture change that "we can achieve greater flexibility for our concepts and develop new models through comparative studies of cultures in transformation" (Abel & Metraux, 1954, p. 100). During a conversation with her, this must have been the first time I felt it might some day be possible to isolate what was truly Mexican through some sort of multicultural studies. Soon the SIP was to permit the alliance of a Mexican group headed by Guillermo Dávila and a group led by Wayne Holtzman. Wayne and I became friends and collaborating scientists. Beginning in the middle fifties, we initiated and continued cross-cultural research between Mexico and the U.S. The most notable result of these efforts was a six-year cross-cultural longitudinal and overlapping study of school children in Mexico and the U.S., with systematic use of intracultural variation and a longitudinal design. In that project we followed children with a battery of tests from the first to the sixth, from the sixth to the twelfth, and from the twelfth grade to university entrance. This work led to the simultaneous publication of a now classic book, in English in the U.S. and in Spanish in Mexico, (Holtzman, Diaz-Guerrero, Swartz, et al, 1975).

The InterAmerican Society of Psychology deserves further credit among the antecedents of IACCP, because its Xth Congress in April 1966 in Lima, Peru, had so many symposia and papers on cross-cultural psychology that its proceedings (Hereford and Natalicio, 1967) had the title " Aportaciones de la Psicologia a la Investigacion Transcultural", that is, the contributions of *psychology* to cross-cultural research. There was an invited address on "Cross-cultural Research", by Fred Strodtbeck, who asserted that: "The most easily conceptualized form of transcultural study equates cultural experience with the laboratory treatment administered to an individual subject" (Hereford and Natalicio, 1967, p. 67).

Triandis (1997) and I (1997) appear to strongly agree that the Ibadan Conference was an unintended cornerstone leading to the birth of our Association. The main purpose of the Ibadan Conference, as indicated in its prospectus, was "to encourage and promote research on the psychological aspects of social change and development (with special emphasis on developing countries)". It was definitely not to test cross-culturally the universal validity of psychological principles and data! Actually, the intention of the Ibadan Conference was well recognized in the central theme of the 1967 XIth InterAmerican Congress of Psychology: "La Contribución de las Ciencias Psicológicas y del Comportamiento al Desarrollo Social y Económico de los Pueblos" (Natalicio, Hereford & Natalicio, 1969), that is, "the Contribution of Psychology and the Behavioral Sciences to the Social and Economic Development of Nations". Its Proceedings were published by the National University of Mexico in two volumes, and had on its title page an original and symbolic drawing by the noted Mexican artist Jose Luis Cuevas.

But the two most pragmatic recommendations of the Ibadan conference, a directory and a newsletter, fell on fertile ground: John Berry was then editing a directory of Cross-Cultural Psychologists and the assembly recommended sending the names of the Ibadan members to him; and Harry Triandis volunteered to start a newsletter and with the title **Cross-Cultural Social Psychology Newsletter**. As most members know, this eventually lead to the quarterly **Cross-Cultural Psychology Bulletin**. Thus the Ibadan Conference was, in retrospect, central in the birth of our Association. Two years after the Ibadan conference, Walter Lonner joined the faculty of Western Washington University (then Western Washington State College) and became centrally involved in starting the Center for Cross-Cultural Research and also became founding editor of the **Journal of Cross-Cultural Psychology,** which was inaugurated in 1970. These various efforts were consolidated by John Dawson, leading to the founding of IACCP in 1972. At that time JCCP became associated with IACCP as one of its official publications.

Now to an anecdote and a happening. Triandis (1997) refers to Fredj Stambouli, the Tunisian member at Ibadan whose eloquence convinced him and the entire assembly of the evils of intellectual colonialism. Stambouli possessed a volcanic voice. Sometimes he used it to break into a discussion, often at the end of a discussion and nearly always to express disagreement. In one of my interventions I put my foot in my mouth; I tried to summarize the statements of the speakers, but then I exclaimed, to the loud amusement of the assembly, "Stromboli erupted again!" (Fortunately Stambouli and I had developed a friendly relationship.) But there was also fun in Ibadan; I asked a Danish participant to go to a dance where we entered a competition. I had never danced the local rhythm High Life, but with the guidance of my graceful lady companion we won the competition, receiving as a prize an ice box, which remained in Ibadan!

I have been persistently fascinated by Ruth Benedict's statement that a culture is a gestalt and not a series of isolated characteristics. For many years I hoped to approximate this gestalt through the factor analysis of the Historic Sociocultural Premises or HSCPs (Diaz-Guerrero, 1972, 1986a). A number of studies found these Factors of HSCPs significantly and meaningfully correlated (Diaz-Guerrero, 1977, 1979, 1982) to many cognitive, personality and social variables. These findings led to a school of psychology termed *ethnopsychology* (Diaz-guerrero, 1986b, 1993, 1995, Diaz-Guerrero & Pacheco, 1994) among Mexican social and cross-cultural psychologists.

As an example of the predictive value of the HSCPs, let us take the most generalized belief in Mexican students: "the mother is the dearest person in existence". This belief was held by over 90% of respondents in several studies in Mexico. The extreme contrary of this belief (the insult to the mother) was studied using a pancultural semantic differential (SD) among 200 high school students equally divided by sex and socioeconomic level. Respondents also responded to 20 other SD formats featuring clinical concepts such as suicide, drunkenness, crime, divorce, sickness, craze, fear, aggression, etc. as well as to Spielberger's State-Trait Anxiety Scale. The results showed that the greater the insult to the mother the more highly rated are crime (.57), suicide (.55), drunkenness (.50), aggression (.43), craze (.41), the less positively I evaluate myself (.26), and the higher the anxiety state (.21). That is, to behave brutally against the most cherished belief of the culture appeared to be related to most psychopathology (Diaz-Guerrero, Lichtszajn and Reyes-Lagunes, 1979).

But studies of Mexican ethnopsychology has gone beyond these cultural beliefs: a number of colleagues have shown idiosyncratically descriptive social dimensions and personality traits (i.e., La Rosa & Diaz-Loving, 1986). A recent and possibly critical discovery indicates that all interpretations in intra- and cross-cultural studies of values are at least incomplete (Diaz-Guerrero, Moreno and Diaz-Loving, 1995). It appeared that value scores were dependent on the satisfaction of the needs connected to the values. After recognizing the dynamic complexity involved in the process of need satisfaction and its impact on the connected value, a quasi experimental cross-cultural design is being carried out in Canada by John Adair, in the US by Harmon Hosch and Roque Mendez and in Mexico by Rolando Diaz-Loving and this author. Results, in the three cultures, indicate that value scores are importantly dependent on interesting aspects of the dynamics of need satisfaction. Coincidentally, the local ethnopsychology has been upgraded, from cultural beliefs, social dimensions and personality traits, to apparently idiosyncratic levels of satisfaction of needs, the difficulty encountered in their satisfaction, the pleasure derived in their satisfaction and the importance ascribed to the associated values.

References

Abel, T. M. & Metraux, M. (1954) Pruebas Proyectivas en una comunidad rural: Montserrat. Memorias del II Congreso Interamericano de Psicología. *Criminalia, 12, (2),* 100-108.

Chavez, E.A. (1901). Ensayo sobre los rasgos distintivos de la sensibilidad como factor del carácter mexicano. *Revista Positiva*, Mexico.

Díaz-Guerrero, R. (1952). Teoria y resultados preliminares de un ensayo de determinación del grado de salud mental, personal y social, del mexicano de la ciudad. *Psiquis, 2*, (1-2), 3-56.

Díaz-Guerrero, R. (1972). Una escala factorial de premisas histórico-socio-culturales de la familia mexicana. *Revista Interamericana de Psicología, 6*, 235-244.

Díaz-Guerrero, R. (1977). A Mexican psychology. *American Psychologist, 32*, 934-944.

Díaz-Guerrero, R. (1979). Origines de la personalité humaine et des systemes sociaux. *Revue de Psychologie Appliquée, 29*, 139-152.

Díaz-Guerrero, R. (1982). The psychology of historic-sociocultural premise, I. *Spanish Language Psychology, 2*, 383-410.

Díaz-Guerrero, R. (1986a). Historio-sococultura y personalidad. Definición y características de los factores de la familia mexicana. *Revista de Psicología Social y Personalidad, 2*, (1), 13-42.

Díaz-Guerrero, R. (1986b). Una etnopsicología mexicana. *Revista de Psicología Social y Personalidad, 2*, (2), 1-22.

Diaz-Guerrero, R. (1993). Mexican ethnopsychology. In U. Kim & J. W. Berry (Eds). *Indigenous psychologies* (pp. 44-55). Newbury Park: Sage.

Díaz-Guerrero, R.(1995). Una aproximación científica a la etnopsicologia. *Revista Latinoamericana de Psicología, 27*, (3), 359-389.

Díaz-Guerrero, R. (1997) Harbingers for our Association. *Cross-Cultural Psychology Bulletin, 31*, (2), 6-8.

Díaz-Guerrero, R., Lichtszajn, J. And Reyes-Lagunes, I. (1979). Alienacion de la madre, psicopatologia y la practica clinica en Mexico. *Hispanic Journal of Behavioral Sciences. 1*, (2), 117-133.

Díaz-Guerrero, R., Moreno-Cedillos, A. y Diaz-Loving, R. (1995). Un eslabon perdido en la investigacion sobre valores y su persistencia. *Revista de Psicologia Social y Personalidad, 11*, (1), 1-10.

Díaz-Guerrero, R. & Pacheco, A. (Eds.1994) *Etnopsicologia, Scientia Nova*, San Juan, PR: Servicios Profesionales y Cientificos.

Hereford, C.F., and Natalicio, L. (Eds,1967*). Aportaciones de la psicologia a la investigacion transcultural,* Mexico, D.F.: Trillas.

Holtzman, W.H., Díaz-Guerrero, R. y Swartz, J.D. En colaboracion con Lara -Tapia, L., Laosa, L. M. Morales, M.L., Reyes-Lagunes, I., y Witzke, D.B. (1975), *Personality development in two cultures,* Austin and London: University of Texas Press.

La Rosa, J. & Díaz-Loving, R. (1986). Evaluación del Autoconcepto: una escala multidimensional. *Revista Latinoamericana de Psicología. 23*, (1), 15-33.

Natalicio, F. S., Hererford, C. F. and Natalicio, D. S. (Eds., 1969). La Contribución de las Ciencias Psicológicas y del Comportamiento al Desarrollo Social y Económico de los Pueblos. *Memorias del XI Congreso Interamericano de Psicología* (two volumes). México: D. F.: Universidad Nacional Autónoma de México.

Paz, O. (1959). *El Laberinto de la soledad.* Mexico, D.F.: Fondo de Cultura Economica.

Ramos, S. (1938). *El perfil del hombre y la cultura en Mexico*. Mexico: Editorial Pedro Robredo.

Triandis, H.C. (1997), Bulletin's 30th Anniversary! *Cross-Cultural Psychology Bulletin, 31,* (1), 4-6.

Reflections of a "Pre-Nominal" Cross-Cultural Psychologist

Gustav Jahoda
University of Strathclyde, Glasgow
Department of Psychology

The beginning of my story dates back almost half a century, and can be viewed in the light of chaos theory - you know, the beating of a butterfly wing in Brazil results in a storm across the Atlantic. In my case it was the invasion of the body of a colleague by a virus that resulted in me, rather than him, being asked to look after a visitor from New Zealand. I was much impressed when he told me that to become a good social scientist one ought to learn at first-hand about other cultures. So two years later I got a job in West Africa and started doing cross-cultural psychology. But like Mr. Jourdain, who only later discovered that he was speaking prose, I did not know then that I was doing cross-cultural psychology, since the term had, as far as I know, not yet been invented.

At the time I was very much the odd man out, regarded as something of an eccentric by my colleagues back home. In the intervening years more and more people have become interested, and the area has become relatively respectable. I use the word "relatively", since mainstream psychology is far from having welcomed us warmly. The impact varies greatly according to domains, though not in a logically coherent way. For instance, one would have thought that culture is particularly important for both developmental and social psychology. In the former this has to a considerable extent been taken on board, but social psychologists, notably experimental ones, continue with what in my view are often trivial pursuits. I have tried to show in the past that a substantial proportion of their findings are unlikely to be more than locally valid, but my challenge was almost totally ignored.

The reasons for the resistance have probably more to do with institutional vested interest, conservatism, and practical problems, than with theoretical considerations. Perhaps rather more disturbing to me is an attack from another quarter, namely Michael Cole, many of whose views I share, and whom one might have expected to be an ally. Let me explain. In an excellent book expounding his vision of cultural psychology, Cole (1996) has a chapter headed "cross-cultural investigations". In it he surveys a sample of three areas, namely perception, intelligence, and memory. It is a concise and acute summary, difficult to quarrel with it as regards factual content. However, when it comes to evaluations, the accent is throughout on shortcomings and limitations.

Beginning with the classic work of Rivers, he writes that "these results are what one would expect" (p. 66). Surely this is true only in hindsight! As far as modern studies of illusions are concerned, it has been shown that several complex factors are involved; and if the fact that, as he puts it, "many key issues about causality remain problematic" (p. 52) is taken as rendering the whole project questionable, then the same could be said about many fields of research, and not only in psychology.

The second theme dealt with by Cole, namely intelligence, is certainly problematic; but no more so in cross-cultural than in mainstream psychology. Moreover, it is rather a peripheral issue for cross-cultural psychology. The third and last theme is that of memory, to which Cole himself together with his colleagues made important contributions. It must be admitted that generally cross-cultural research on memory has not been very impressive, and I shall come back to that. At any rate Cole suggests, in accordance with cultural activity theory, that cultural differences in remembering arise from variations in "organization of activity in everyday life". The case for this is convincing, but it is worth noting that the broad drift of the argument is rather similar to that of Rivers in relation to perception: while visual acuity is more or less the same in all cultures, exceptional ability to make use of minimal visual cues is highly context-dependent.

In sum, the contrast between cross-cultural and Cole's cultural psychology is perhaps rather less sharp than he contends in seeking to demonstrate the superiority of the latter. He concludes with some harsh words about what he calls the "standard cross-cultural approach":

> Assuming that my assessment of these three examples more or less characterizes accomplishments in other psychological domains, the marginality of cross-cultural research to mainstream psychology is not difficult to understand. Its substantive offerings appear modest, and the evidence on which they are based is suspect. (p.68)

In sum, Cole's assessment tends to exaggerate the weaknesses and play down the achievements; hence it is rather unfair. On the other hand, there are in my opinion no grounds for complacency. Hence I shall use this opportunity, perhaps inappropriately on such an occasion, to voice some of my misgivings. However, I am not alone: my views are in line with some of those expressed by A. C. Paranjpe (1997). My discussion will initially be focused on the declared objectives of cross-cultural psychology, and I shall suggest that these are, at least in part, misguided. Its threefold goals, as set out in the important volume by Berry, Poortinga, Segall and Dasen (1992), may be summarized as follows: 1) Transport and test: investigating the applicability of western hypotheses and theories in other cultures; 2) Exploring cultural variations in psychological functioning; 3) Arriving at universal laws. As regards the first goal, transport and test, it can hardly be said that a great deal of progress has been made. This is not just the fault of cross-cultural psychology , and can also be attributed to the nature of most psychological theories; they are often formulated in a manner that renders rigorous testing difficult. Moreover, for the mainstream to abandon or even modify theories, the weight of evidence has to be very substantial, and this is usually not feasible given the usually slender resources. Nonetheless, if this were a major goal, results obtained in that direction ought to be more visible after a quarter-century. There should be a chapter or at least just a paper, entitled "Western theories cross-culturally tested and found wanting"; but I have never come across anything like that. Before discussing the second goal, let me first jump to the third, distal one, of a universal psychology based on cross-cultural research. Some of my friends and colleagues believe that this will soon be within our reach, but I do not share that faith, for the following reasons. First of all, I have not met any clear and convincing explication of the way in which a universal psychology might be generated. One proposal has been to, as it were "strip away" culture, which would leave universal human nature. The trouble is that by doing so one also strips away an essential feature of humanity. For as Geertz (1973) graphically put it, humans without culture would be mere unworkable monstrosities. The problem arises from the fact that human behaviour is a complex function of both biology and culture, and the boundaries between the two are uncertain, varying according to domain and context. Cultures themselves differ not merely geographically, but change over historical periods, while the time-scale of biological change is vastly greater. Given this variability, it would seem that a universal psychology would have to rest largely on biology, as is implicit in much of mainstream theorizing. In other words, in so far as one is concerned with certain *partial* aspects of human functioning such as, for instance, information processing or remembering, universal features will be identifiable. But the goals of arriving at a universal psychology via cross-cultural psychology, is, in my opinion, little more than a chimera.

There is, however, an alternative approach adopted by one of the *cultural psychologies*. I use the plural, since its several versions take very different positions regarding universality. What cultural psychologies have in common is the conviction that methodological behaviourism is unsuitable for the study of culture and mind. Shweder's version eschews such an aim altogether, concentrating on the need to understand *particular* cultures in depth. By contrast, Cole and his associates have sought to cut the Gordic knot by returning to the notion of *culture-in-general* as conceptualized by Tylor at the end of the 19th century. This permits the formulation of a universal cultural theory, at least for the important developmental domain. Since all humans have culture, one does not necessarily have to go to exotic places for one's empirical work. The theoretical emphasis is on common processes rather than cultural variations. The cost of this approach, as far as theory is concerned, is that one is forced to remain at a high level of abstraction.

Let me return now to the second goal, namely investigating cultural variations in psychological functioning. Since this is effectively the major area of cross-cultural research, the relevant passage in the Berry et al. (1992)

text will be considered in more detail. The stated objective is an exploratory one, designed to discover variations not present in one's own culture. Two means of achieving this are suggested. One is to keep a sharp lookout for "novel aspects of behaviour". The other could be a by-product of the first aim: if on testing a Western theory in another cultural setting one fails to obtain the expected results, one should seek to uncover the factors responsible for that failure. Thereby novel and interesting cultural variants might be found. The concrete example offered to illustrate both the first and second sub-goal concerns learning and memory. As regards the first, they consider the question whether primacy and recency effects are universal; if such effects are not found, one should investigate further how lists are memorized. It might be, for instance, that "individuals may evidence different mnemonic devices during a memory study". It is noteworthy that there is hardly any further mention of memory in the volume, and the term does not appear in the index.

It is probably no accident that this kind of illustration was selected, since follow-up studies are more readily feasible when dealing with cognitive processes than with such spheres as, say, attitudes, values, personality, or identity. As regards the latter, post-hoc speculative interpretations are most commonly found. There is thus a gap between declared aims and aspirations, and what is actually done. Moreover, it seems to me that the gap has widened over time. This view is based on my impressions, admittedly superficial, of the kinds of changes that have taken place over the decades. They are based mainly on trends discernible in the *Journal of Cross-Cultural Psychology*. This is no doubt a somewhat biased source, since many investigations are published elsewhere. Nonetheless, since it is a kind of flagship, its contents are surely not insignificant.

One thing that becomes apparent is that cross-cultural psychology has become a healthier activity over the years, and this is not just because more and better antibiotics have become available. Let me explain: those of us who laboured as pioneers often worked in remote villages and were thus exposed, in my own case, to such afflictions as malaria or dysentery. We were in direct contact with people, and thus in a position to observe "novel aspects of behaviour". Here is an example: I encountered a superbly skilled illiterate basket weaver, and commissioned him to copy a special kind of basket from a photograph. To my astonishment, the finished product turned out to be totally different from the picture, which he believed to have followed faithfully. This led on to a series of studies of 2D visual space perception.

It would seem that this kind of approach has become increasingly rare. In a large majority of studies there is no direct personal contact between researcher and the people studied. Hence there is little if any opportunity to observe variations in behaviour. Moreover, we commonly criticize the mainstream for basing their theories on such an unrepresentative sample of humanity as is constituted by American college students. But studies reported in the Journal also predominantly rely on college or to a lesser extent high school students, ignoring the fact that a substantial part of the world population still has little or no formal schooling.

The modal style of recent work reported appears to be one of getting together with colleagues in other countries, usually equated with cultures. Some kinds of questionnaires or scales are administered, recording differences and similarities. This is of course something of a caricature, but only in the sense of an exaggeration of characteristic features.

Let me hasten to add that it is of course perfectly legitimate to employ such an approach as part of a coherent research programme; but more usually that is not the case. Or again, one popular exercise consists of attempts to find out whether a particular measure works across cultures, but going no further. One is reminded of Kuhn's (1962) remark that: "In the absence of a paradigm ... all of the facts that could possibly pertain to the development of a given science are likely to seem equally relevant. As a result, early fact-gathering is a far more nearly random activity than the one that subsequent scientific development makes familiar". (p. 15)

There appears to have been a return to what, if I remember rightly, John Berry once called the "anecdotal" approach, which is purely descriptive of "interesting" differences. There is unlimited scope for such exercises, especially if one ignores the warning issued by Campbell and Naroll about the problems of interpreting comparisons between two natural groups. The chances are that any such comparisons will throw up differences, for a wide variety of reasons. More important and instructive would be the discovery of invariances as attempted by Ype Poortinga. In sum, the question arises whether the previously mentioned efforts are really worth while, if their product is not cumulative and fails to contribute to the building up a coherent body of knowledge. Perhaps in our post-colonial and rapidly changing world this would be too much to expect. Nevertheless, we should not shy away from asking ourselves critical questions about fundamental issues.

Although I have taken advantage of this forum to voice some of my misgivings, I would not wish to leave you with the impression that my general attitude is negative. After all, I have spent a good part of my life in cross-cultural psychology, and would like to see it continue to flourish. Nor would I want to gainsay the solid achievements reflected in the three volumes of the new edition of the *Handbook* (Berry, et al, 1997). But we should not rest on our laurels.

References

Berry, J.W., Poortinga, Y.H. Segall, M.H., & Dasen, P.R. (1992). *Cross-cultural psychology: Research and applications.* Cambridge: Cambridge University Press.

Berry, J.W. (et al) (Eds). *Handbook of cross-cultural psychology (3 Vols.).* Boston: Allyn & Bacon.

Cole, M. (1996). *Cultural psychology: A once and future discipline.* Cambridge, Mass: Harvard University Press.

Geertz, C. (1973). *The interpretation of cultures.* New York: Basic Books.

Kuhn, T.S. (1962). *The Structure of scientific revolutions.* Chicago: University of Chicago Press.

Paranjpe, A. (1997). Piles of data that contribute little to the mutual understanding of cultures. *Cross-Cultural Psychology Bulletin,* 31, 11-17.

Cross-, Intra-, Inter-, and Just Plain Cultural

Douglass R. Price-Williams
Departments of Psychiatry and Anthropology
University of California, Los Angeles

About 1980 I made a drastic career change in that I began to think less in terms of a cross-cultural psychology and more in terms of a cultural psychology. This was a few years after I had been given a joint appointment with an Anthropology department and had been engaged in the study of psychological anthropology, becoming a co-editor of the first journal devoted to psychological anthropology. This tends to explain why I began to think of the idea of a cultural psychology. In a paper first presented at a cross-cultural conference in Honolulu in 1978, and published a year after (Price-Williams 1979) I re-introduced the concept of Cultural Psychology as a idea to be considered in its relationship to cross-cultural psychology. I later expanded the theme (Price-Williams 1980). In that paper I claimed that the idea of a ***cross***-cultural psychology logically necessitated the anterior idea of a *cultural* psychology, but that the systematics of their relationship, and indeed to other methodological variants such as psychological anthropology, needed to be worked out. I returned once more to this subject in the contribution to Lindzey's third edition of the Handbook of Social Psychology, where I actually called the chapter as "Cultural Psychology"(Price-Williams 1985), reinforcing the key idea that psychology operated within a cultural medium.

I thought at the time that my idea was fairly innocent, seemingly logical, yet recognizing that there would be a serious division of labor entailed, and giving a little consideration as to how this could be done. But it was at this time that I became more engrossed with psychological anthropology, and missed, with some exceptions, several important developments concerning the idea of a cultural Psychology.

From subsequent reading I have been made aware of key publications which are new to me. In particular there is the important volume of the journal *Culture and Psychology* (Vol. 3, No. 3), in which the fundamental ideas of Ernest Boesch are presented. Further, I found that I had regretfully earlier missed the important contribution by Lutz Eckensberger (1979) in which he advanced the perspective of a cultural psychology about the same time as my Honolulu paper.

In what follows, however, I am going to concentrate on two books that have appeared in the 1990s, both with the leading title of Cultural Psychology, on which to affix my observations on the development of this subject. The first is a book edited by Stigler, Shweder and Herdt (1990), *Cultural Psychology*, in which there is a seminal chapter by Shweder entitled "Cultural Psychology: What is it?", which re-opens the question, and advances a viewpoint which I did not have at the time of exploring this concept. To my surprise, Shweder draws a sharp distinction between cultural psychology, and both cross-cultural psychology and psychological anthropology (also ethnopsychology). As I had regarded cultural psychology as a superordinate title, with cross-cultural psychology and psychological anthropology therefore as subordinate titles, I was taken aback. It was true that in the Social Psychology Handbook chapter I had suggested that in pursuing this domain we should relinquish partly the starting theories and definitions of subjects that mark these fields of study and plunge more daringly into new concepts. Nevertheless I did not envisage a schism between what I was calling Cultural Psychology and these other fields. Yet this is apparently precisely what Shweder seems to be doing.

The second is an important book by Michael Cole distinctly called "Cultural Psychology". Whereas Shweder is coming from the discipline of Anthropology and the philosophy of intentionalism, Cole originates from experimental psychology and adopts, one would say, a more positivist philosophy. Nevertheless their engagement in the same topic allows me to further expand on my previous ideas of a cultural psychology. It is easiest to make my commentary on these two books by invoking key points on which to present their ideas along with my observations.

1. *The Question of Scope.* Cole (1996: 103) made the comment that Shweder "place[s] a greater emphasis on the centrality of interpretation and methods of analysis derived from the humanities than do Price-Williams or the German action theorists". Indeed, one of the surprises that I had on reading the Shweder chapter was the long laundry list that he gives as constituting a Cultural Psychology (Shweder 30-31).

Cole, on the other hand (although only somewhat; it's as if we need three hands for Cultural Psychology), is a little less pantheistic. His broadening focuses on development and history and on everyday activities that do not fit easily into a nice tight nomothetic scheme. Let me quote him directly: "Consistent with the ideas of nineteenth- and early twentieth-century cultural psychologists, as well as the Russian cultural-historical school, I adopt a developmental approach to the study of human nature. Consistent with the broad, contextual underpinnings of cultural psychology, I seek to derive its principles from activities at the level of everyday practices as a grounding for its theoretical claims" (p.349).

In both cases then, we have a radical enlargement of the discipline as we knew it at the beginning of the Jubilee time frame. There is of course no theocratic mandate as to what discipline should be considered under this rubric. Still, we are forced to notice that a discipline, by definition, has its own programmatic mode, its own methods of analysis and its own scope of generalization. Coming from our own discipline, what other discipline shou we take note of, if any? This decision may not, or only partly, influence what we do, but it has to factor in to our final interpretation of the wider field.

2. *The Matter of Definition.* I had hoped to avoid this issue, as I have always found the problem of defining culture a tiresome affair. I am constrained here, alas, to at least tell how Shweder and Cole define culture, as perhaps the previous question of scope depends on the definition.

It is noteworthy that Shweder, in keeping with his philosophy of intentionalism, does not define culture as something apart from the person. Over and over again he stresses this point. Cole (p.301) also stresses the interconnection when he states: "culture comes into being wherever people engage in joint activity over a period of time". Thus, although there are microcultures as well as macrocultures, there is still culture, if one defines it in terms of people implicitly or explicitly engaging in agreements regarding habits of conduct, shared values and the like.

3. *The Historical Factor.* We meet here a theme which Lévi-Strauss has met in the study of myth: namely the diachronic versus synchronic dichotomy. Both Cole's position and the writers in the Stigler et al. book are by admittance clearly on the diachronic and developmental side. The question arises as to the relationship between cross-cultural psychology, which does not necessarily concern itself with history, and cultural psychology, which inevitably involves history. The situation is the same for anthropology, on which Lévi-Strauss (1966, p. 256) has commented, "The anthropologist respects history, but he does not accord it a special value. He conceives it as a study complementary to his own; one of them unfurls the range of human societies in time, the other in space". Perhaps this comment will suffice for our discipline also. We should, however, keep in mind especially in these days of rapid social change, of the time factor when a study is done. We need perhaps to treat the time factor as a sampling variable.

4. *Context.* Context, as Cole (p.338) reminds us, "is a devilishly polysemic concept". Cole's way of handling context, what he calls the "culture as garden" metaphor of context, appears to be a satisfactory way of dealing with it. Earlier I had opted for "necessary" context when dealing with psychological variables within a culture, but I think Cole's essentially Chinese boxes notion, of variables stacked within other variables, is a better way of handling it. It is as he thinks of it, a multi-level methodology, and although there will always be argument regarding the contents of each level, nevertheless I think this is the only way to go.

5. *Comparison.* The consideration of context with the acceptance of the idea that psychological variables are embedded in a cultural medium, undoubtedly complicates our simple- minded idea of comparing psychological factors. Cole (pp.305-309) shows how this can be done, but admittedly it is cumbersome. As Eleanor Ochs, in another chapter of the

Stigler, Shweder and Herdt book (1990, 291), regarding the specific problem of relating language to sociocultural context, states: "We have as well to account for how the sociolinguistic organization of..specific communicative events in turn interfaces with more general systems of social order and cultural knowledge. The jump from situation to the more generalized culture is often complicated". Ochs cites for example the case of traditional Samoan communities, whose "members view activities and tasks as social and not individual accomplishments". Here we have an instance in which cultural values pervade the level of situation at its most elementary level. A reasonable emphasis can be given to what Popper used to call the "logic of the situation". Roger Barker's ecological psychology seemed to indicate that when one goes to a hairdresser or when one goes to a butcher, the situation calls for a certain standard behavior. In any one culture, yes; but situations differ with cultures.

So far, we have discussed the "cross", "intra" and plain "cultural" aspects of the talk. We need now to discuss the "inter". By this I do not mean, for example, how one ethnic group might think of another ethnic group, which could be and has been taken into consideration. I am thinking more of the reflexive aspect of the comparative problem, wherein the nature of the experimenter or researcher needs to be taken placed into the equation, most notably with the possible impact of his or her own culture or gender, and perhaps one's religious affiliation also. It is not so much a simple-minded bias that I have in mind, as the effect of the researcher on subjects. Also, the choice of what should be studied in a target culture may well reflect the nature of the researcher. I have mentioned elsewhere that when women began to be interested in shamanism, the number of women shamans throughout shamanic cultures suddenly began to increase. The question does arise as to the importance for cross-cultural psychology of what, in general psychology, has become understood as the experimenter effect. I do not think we know, there not being sufficient data, whether the results of psychological studies are seriously influenced by the matching of investigator with investigated, or even by type of study. For this problem I suggest that we adopt the spirit of the old Campbell and Fiske (1959) principle for behavioral assessment, namely the multimethod-multitrait approach. We might apply it to cross-cultural psychology as the multimethod-multi researcher principle. This does not necessarily mean that for each individual study we are constrained to employ several researchers from different cultures or genders, and utilize more than one method. It only means that we should not be satisfied with the teasing out of one variable until it has been investigated from different angles and by researchers of different backgrounds, including, though not limited it to, the crucial investigator factor of matching the culture with an investigator from it.

Two questions remain. The first, lamentably and inexorably, concerns the word "culture". The word as used stretches from the diffuse and generalized values of a society to the narrower definitions of the activities of a small group. Perhaps we are better off consistently delineating the term, when we use it, in terms of its appropriate and concrete synonym: that is, either a specific value or a specific custom or a specific way of looking at things or a specific rule or a specific standard or whatever. In all instances however, Shweder's insistence on intentionality is well taken. "Culture" in not something "out there", apart from people. We must be careful not to reify the concept, as the tendency is with common parlance of "history". There is no "history" in the abstract, only what historians write.

The second question is the relationship of cross-cultural or comparative psychology to cultural psychology. Cross-cultural psychology might be conceived of as sampling a variable from two or more societies or groups. If that is the case then the more we know about the society or group under consideration the better off we are, including knowing *what* to study. We not only need more samples, but we need to know, in any one society or group, how one particular variable is connected to other variables. For this we turn to studies under the rubric of cultural psychology. In my own opinion such studies may not necessarily be "psychological" in the scientific sense. Literary studies, for example, can well throw light on any particular culture. For our own studies, of course, we need to translate these literary studies into our own terminology and make then amenable for psychological analysis. Nevertheless, in the first degree of approximation, I do not see why they cannot be plumbed.

References

Cole, M. (1996) *Cultural psychology: A once and future discipline*. Cambridge: Harvard..

Eckensberger, L.H. (1979) A metamethodological evaluation of psychological theories from a cross-cultural perspective. In L.H.Eckensberger, W.J. Lonner and Ype H. Poortinga (Eds,), *Cross-cultural contributions to psychology*, (pp. 255-275) Amsterdam: Swets and Zeitlinger.

Lévi-Strauss, C. (1966). *The savage mind.* Chicago: University of Chicago Press.

Ochs, Eleanor (1990) Indexicality and socialization. In J.W. Stigler, R.A. Shweder, and G. Herdt (Eds), *Cultural psychology: Essays on comparative human development*, (pp. 287-308). Cambridge, Mass: Cambridge University Press.

Price-Williams, D. (1979) Modes of thought in cross-cultural psychology: an historical overview. In A. Marsella, Tharp, R., and Ciborowski, T. (Eds.) *Perspectives on cross-cultural psychology*, (pp. 3-16). New York, Academic Press.

Price-Williams, D. (1980) Toward the idea of a cultural psychology: A Superordinate Theme for Study. *Journal of Cross-Cultural Psychology, 11* (1), 75-88.

Price-Williams, D. (1985) Cultural psychology. In G. Lindzey and E. Aronson (Eds), *The Handbook of Social Psychology*, (pp. 993-1042). New York: Random House.

Stigler, J.W., Shweder, R.A. and Herdt, G. (1990) (Eds.). *Cultural psychology: Essays on comparative human development*. Cambridge: Cambridge University Press.

Shweder, R.A. (1990). Cultural psychology - What is it? In Stigler, J.W., Shweder, R.A. and Herdt, G. (Eds.) *Cultural Psychology: Essays on Comparative Human Development*, (pp. 1-43). Cambridge: Cambridge University Press.

Odysseus Wandered for 10, I Wondered for 50 Years

Harry C. Triandis
University of Illinois in Champaign-Urbana
Department of Psychology

The title of this paper is highly individualistic: It uses "I" and it is very competitive! Yet I was raised in Greece when it was a collectivist culture, as is clear from Triandis (1972). I started as an allocentric and ended up as idiocentric person. In January 1948, at age 21, I came to Canada, to study at McGill University, because the Technical University (Polytechnion) where I was studying in Athens was not in good shape just after the war (e.g., poor labs). I found the contrast between Athens and Montreal as great in temperature (leaving in 50 degree weather and finding -10 F) as well as in social relationships. Montreal had an individualist culture, with people having many, but relatively superficial relationships, and that contrasted with Athens collectivism where one had few but deep relationships. In Montreal my friends talked to their parents once a month, while if I could have afforded it I would have talked to my parents every day. In Montreal social relations were fluid and quick-changing, in Athens they were stable and more or less unchanged. Traces of allocentrism remain, so that when I go back to Athens, each year, I spend time with my old friends, even 50 years after leaving. The contrast between Canada and Greece started me thinking about cultural comparisons.

But I had little trouble adjusting to Canada, because I was already more of an idiocentric than most Greeks. That was because I was not especially ethnocentric, having been exposed to German governesses and a French high school, and having discovered for myself at age 16 that all religions are systems of self-deception. Religion is an important aspect of Greek culture.

After studying engineering, and working as an engineer in Canada for three years, I discovered psychology and was so fascinated that I abandoned engineering for graduate work at Cornell University in social psychology. When I went back to Greece after my first year in graduate school I collected cross-cultural data (Triandis & Osgood, 1958; Triandis and Lambert, 1958). But mainstream psychology was not interested in culture. Culture was quaint, curious, stimulating, but most psychologists claimed that "what we found are the eternal, invariant laws of behavior."But there were exceptions. Brewster Smith, then editor of the most important social psychology journal, favored cross-cultural work, and he published my two cross-cultural papers.

In the early years of my career as a psychologist I worked mostly on attitudes and on industrial psychology. These were "mainstream fields." I received tenure three years after starting in Illinois, and then I started thinking that I could do cross-cultural studies, even if these were not "respected" as much as my other activities. For good measure I wrote a book on attitudes (Triandis, 1971), but my real love was cross-cultural work.

I was encouraged in the cross-cultural direction when Len Berkowitz asked me to do a chapter on culture and cognition, which appeared as the first chapter of his series of *Advances in Experimental Social Psychology* (Triandis, 1964). Before writing that chapter and came across Pike's work on *emics* and *etics*, and structured the chapter around such concepts.

In the early 1960s the U. S. Navy approached Fred Fiedler with a request that he develop a team to study how "every sailor can become an ambassador," a goal that Admiral Elmo R. Zumwalt had set as Chief of Naval Operations. Fiedler asked me to be part of the team, which also included Osgood and Stolurow. We divided the job as follows: I would identify what elements of culture are relevant. Osgood would use those elements to improve the communication of Navy personnel with their hosts; Fiedler would use those elements to improve the leadership behavior of Navy personnel; Stolurow would use these elements to teach people who are going to another culture to perceive social behavior according to their own culture as well as the host culture. It was in that context that we came up with the idea of developing culture assimilators (Fiedler, Mitchell and Triandis, 1971).

In order to find out what elements of culture were needed for the project I worked on the "analysis of subjective culture." I went around the world on my sabbatical, spending significant time in Hawaii, Japan, Hong Kong, Malaysia, Thailand, India, Iran, Israel, Greece, Germany, France, and Belgium, talking with potential collaborators of the project. The data finally came from Japan, India, Greece and the USA (Triandis, 1972).

The analysis of subjective culture included aspects of what is now called cultural psychology, such as the analysis of the meaning of emic concepts, changes in the meanings of concepts, and examining one culture in detail, and cross-cultural psychology, such as equivalence of measurement of etic constructs, examination of universals of meaning, and examining many cultures in one study.

An important event in my intellectual development was a conference that took place in Ibadan, Nigeria, over the New Year holidays of 1966-67. It was in that conference that I became convinced that one must avoid intellectual colonialism, which includes the study of a culture without indigenous collaborators, and without giving credit and co-authorship to local social scientists. This resulted in the inclusion of a section on the ethics of cross-cultural research in *The Analysis of Subjective Culture*, and collaboration with a group of psychologists in the development of a code of ethics for cross-cultural research (Tapp, Kelman, Triandis, Wrightsman, and Coelho, 1974). When I was President of IACCP in 1976, I tried to "sell" that code to the membership, but many members felt that the code was too restrictive and demanding, and therefore limited the options of members. Consequently, it was never adopted.

In Ibadan we also discussed the need for a newsletter that would keep people with intercultural interests aware of the activities of others doing cross-cultural work. I agreed to edit that small publication, which we named the *Cross-Cultural Social Psychology Newsletter.* It started as a simple mimeographed publication and was distributed free to those who were interested (the Navy agreed to pay for the postage). It has since become the quarterly *Cross-Cultural Psychology Bulletin* of IACCP. Another important conference was held in Hong Kong, in 1972, when IACCP was formed.

In the 1970s I became President of Divisions 8 (Personality and Social Psychology) and 9 (Society for the Psychological Study of Social Issues) of the American Psychological Association, and tried to introduce some emphases on cross-cultural research. Then in the 1980s I became President of the Interamerican Society of Psychology and also got very much involved in the International Association of Applied Psychology, serving at its President in 1990-94. Most of these jobs were related to providing a context within which psychologists can meet, and develop collaborative relationships which improve the chances of doing cross-cultural work.

In the late 1970s I reviewed the manuscript of Geert Hofstede's 1980 book, *Culture's consequences.* I was enthusiastic, and recommended its publication. I also started working on individualism and collectivism, which corresponded with the contrast between Americans and traditional Greeks that I had reported in the *Analysis of subjective culture.*

In the 1980s I worked with and for Hispanics in an effort to understand aspects of their culture. The concept of collectivism fit very well our findings (Marin & Triandis, 1985). We identified the *simpatia* script (Triandis, Marin, Lisansky & Betancourt, 1984), which is certainly an element of collectivism.

Thus my main focus became the study of this cultural syndrome (Triandis,1989,1990,1993,1996). In the beginning I was not sure I was right in stimulating Harry Hui to work for his dissertation on the development and validation of a method for the measurement of the construct. What if no one was interested in it? I would have pushed him into a dead-end. Fortunately, it was not a dead-end. In fact, by 1993 I was able to spend my sabbatical at the East-West Center summarizing what was known about that construct, and there was already quite a lot that was known (Triandis, 1995). It has since become even more central, so that in August 1998, Hazel Markus and Michael Morris organized a conference of 50 researchers at Stanford University who talked mostly about aspects of this construct.

I think the future of cross-cultural psychology is going to be bright. I think that culture and social behavior are so strongly interrelated (Triandis, 1994) that no social psychology can be meaningful if it is not cross-cultural.

I want to mention the construct of "cultural syndromes," and their importance. They consist of shared attitudes, beliefs, norms, and values found among those who speak a particular language dialect, in a specific geographic region, during a particular historic period. The shared elements of subjective culture are organized around a theme, such as complexity, or the importance of the collective. Cultural syndromes provide a focus, so that we can get out of the fuzzy construct of "culture" and into a construct that we can probe systematically.

Following are examples of such syndromes:

Cultural complexity, e.g., hunters and gatherers versus information societies. The size of settlements is one of the best ways to index cultural complexity (Chick, 1997).

Tightness. Tight cultures have many rules, norms, and ideas about what is correct behavior in different kinds of situations; loose cultures have fewer rules and norms. In the former cultures also, people become quite upset when others do not follow the norms of the society, and may even kill those who do not behave as is expected, while in the latter cultures people are tolerant of most deviations from normative behaviors. In Japan, which is a tight culture, people are sometimes criticized for minor deviations from norms, such as having too much of a sun tan, or having curly hair (Kidder, 1992). Most Japanese live in fear that they will not act properly (Iwao, 1993).

Individualism and collectivism. Triandis (1994) has suggested that individualism emerges in societies that are both complex and loose; collectivism in societies that are both simple and tight. For example, theocracies or monasteries are both tight and relatively poor; Hollywood stars live in a culture that is both complex and loose. This speculation has not been tested rigorously, but the data seem to hang together reasonably well so that it may be the case that, for instance, Japan that is now quite complex is less collectivist that the Japan of the 19th century.

Vertical and horizontal cultures. Vertical cultures accept hierarchy as a given. People are different from each other. Hierarchy is a natural state. Those at the top "naturally" have more power and privileges than those of the bottom of the hierarchy. Horizontal cultures accept equality as a given. People are basically similar, and if one is to divide any resource it should be done equally.

Active-passive cultures. In active cultures individuals try to change the environment to fit them; in passive cultures people change themselves to fit into the environment. Active cultures are more competitive, action-oriented, and emphasize self-fulfillment; those characterized as more passive are more cooperative, emphasize the experience of living, and are especially concerned with getting along with others.

Universalism-particularism. In universalist cultures people try to treat others on the basis of universal criteria (e.g., all competent persons regardless of who they are in sex, age, race, etc. are acceptable employees); in particularist cultures people treat others on the basis of who the other person is (e.g., I know Joe Blow and he is a good person, so he will be a good employee).

Diffuse-specific. Diffuse cultures respond to the environment in a holistic manner (e.g., I do not like your report means I do not like you). Specific cultures discriminate different aspects of the stimulus complex. (e.g., I do not like your report says nothing about how much I like you).

Ascription-achievement: People can judge others on the basis of ascribed attributes, such as sex, race, family membership, etc. These are attributes people are born with. By contrast, people might judge others in terms of achieved attributes, such as skill, publications, awards.

Instrumental-expressive. People may sample more heavily attributes that are instrumental (e.g., get the job done) or expressive (e.g., enjoy the social relationship).

Emotional expression or suppression. People may express their emotions freely, no matter what the consequences, or they may control the expression of emotion.

One can identify many more syndromes, such as those reflected in the Kluckhohn and Strodtbeck (1961) value orientations, the culture of honor (Nisbett & Cohen, 1996), and others. It should be noted that cultural syndromes are probably correlated. That would be an important research topic for the next generation of cross-cultural psychologists.

References

To preserve space most references were dropped. However, interested readers will find most of them in:
Triandis, H. C. (1994). *Culture and social behavior*. New York: McGraw-Hill.

References not found in Triandis (1994) appear below.
Triandis, H.C. (1995). *Individualism & collectivism.* Boulder, CO: Westview Press.
Triandis, H. C. (1996). The psychological measurement cultural syndromes. *American Psychologist, 51*, 407-415..
Triandis, H. C. & Lambert W. W. (1958) A restatement and test of Schlosberg's theory of emotion with two kinds of subjects from Greece. *Journal of Abnormal and Social Psychology, 56,* 321-328.
Triandis, H. C. & Osgood, C. E. (1958) A comparative factorial analysis of semantic structures of monolingual Greece and American students. *Journal of Abnormal and Social Psychology, 57,* 187-196.

The American Jubilee Speakers Series

Because the United States is such a large nation that can boast a wide range of cultures and ethnic groups, we considered it appropriate to feature a sampling of its diversity at this first-ever IACCP conference in the U.S. The four major "subcultures" that together constitute a sizeable percentage of the entire U.S. population are African Americans, American Indians, Hispanic Americans, and Asian Americans.

There is surely tremendous diversity within diversity. Thus, just as African Americans can be characterized by distinct regional differences, the same can be said of the huge variation there is among American Indians. In other words, there is no such thing as *the* African American or *the* American Indian. The same can be said of both Hispanic Americans and Asian Americans, both of whom have rich legacies and considerable variability based upon country of origin, age, gender, and other factors.

Despite this fact of exceptional within-group variation, we chose to recognize these broad groupings by inviting excellent spokespersons for each. Thus we selected James M. Jones to represent African Americans, Beatrice Medicine to speak for American Indians, Amado M. Padilla to give his commentaries on Hispanic Americans, and Stanley Sue to speak on behalf of Asian Americans. Each of these individuals was given an hour to deliver their prepared speeches spread over a three-day period, and they were encouraged to meet with others after each speech for more informal discussions. We did not have room in this volume for their complete speeches. However, each speaker kindly complied with our request to prepare an overview or summary of their respective talks.

As mentioned in the introduction to this volume, Carol Tavris was the fifth speaker in the American Jubilee Speakers Series. It was, however, agreed that her talk would be general and wide-ranging and not appropriate for summation in this volume. As first of the five speakers, Tavris performed admirably, as usual, as a "kickoff" speaker for the series.

The four presentations that we are pleased to include in this volume should be read as overviews of certain characteristics or traditions of the four major non-white groups in the United States kaleidoscope of ethnicities and cultures. While each should be read on the basis of their own substantial merits, one could be reasonably certain that any other representative of these groups would likely write something substantially different. Such is the nature of human diversity.

Walter J. Lonner

Toward a Cultural Psychology of African Americans

James M. Jones
University of Delaware
Department of Psychology

ABSTRACT

The cultural psychology of African Americans involves the evolution of African patterns of thought, feeling and behavior and their utilization as adaptive mechanisms in a context of racism and oppression. Assumptions about cultural psychology as the intersection of psyche and culture, and African American psychology as the multidimensional response to dehumanization and psychic conflict are discussed. Time, Rhythm, Improvisation, Orature, and Spirituality (TRIOS) are proposed as psycho-cultural mechanisms of adaptation, innovation, and psychological control for African Americans. TRIOS is described as a way to understand the psyche-cultural interactions for African Americans, and to provide a framework for their cultural psychology.

In the first edition of *Prejudice and Racism* (Jones, 1972), in a multi-level analysis I described the persistent effects of dehumanizing and oppressive relationships between Whites and Blacks. Racism defined beliefs about the naturalness of white domination and black subordination. *Individual racism* captured micro-level psychological processes by which individuals internalized and acted upon their beliefs about race. *Institutional racism* was found in the instruments of society that dictated divergent social and economic outcomes on the basis of race. *Cultural racism* represented the cumulative set of beliefs, symbols, meanings and values that defined the meaning of race in our cultural worldview, informed institutional structure and practices and set the context for individual beliefs and actions.

Cultural racism produced the most pernicious racially biasing effects because it was through cultural mechanisms that the meaning of race was defined and implemented. However, "race" was viewed as a biology-based entity created by some naturally ordained force in the Universe. As a result, the culturally-determined meanings of race defined a social hierarchy of human groups based on observable physical features and presumptive psychological attributes. These core assumptions about "race" established a normative set of beliefs and expectations about the superiority of whites and the inferiority of blacks that have been handed down over centuries.

Anti-racism activities have been carried out *within* the racism paradigm. Challenging racist assumptions leads anti-racist activities to eliminate *both* the "superiority" assumption for whites and the "inferiority" assumption for blacks. As a result, the arguments against both assumptions are based on the premise that differences between blacks and whites are trivial. These differences, however, have been measured by human characteristics that are validated on the beliefs that emanate from a western, Anglo-American cultural worldview. Within this perspective, Blacks are validated only to the extent that they are believed to be similar to whites.

My aim in this paper is to consider the implications of this cultural racism analysis for African Americans. Specifically, I consider the possibility that adaptations to racism both create and reflect racial differences in psychological processes. Psychological differences among racial groups derive from different cultural origins, and evolve along different pathways as a result of different experiences with race. Blacks were dehumanized within American culture, and their adaptation to and liberation from that experience required the utilization and evolution of psychological mechanisms founded in their African cultural origins.

This chapter is not a comparative analysis of Blacks and Whites in America, nor is it an attempt to use an analysis of African Americans to make claims for universality of behavioral principles, or human attributes. Rather, what follows is a discussion of the psychological consequences of a situated human experience of a visible group of people that are socially, psychologically, politically and culturally significant in the United States. In the following pages, I will first summarize the basic working principles of cultural psychology, and then the working assumptions of African American psychology. I will then describe the core features that a cultural psychology of African Americans entails.

Assumptions about Culture and Cultural Psychology.

Kroeber and Kluckhohn (1952) define culture as"...patterned ways of thinking, feeling and reacting, acquired and transmitted mainly by symbols ... [and may] on the one hand, be considered as products of action, on the other, conditioning elements of future actions." (p. 181).

The basic elements of this definition suggest several critical features of culture: 1) the importance of symbols; 2) the distinction between, but dual validity of implicit meaning and explicit behavior; 3) the historical influence on contemporary events and their meaning; and 4) the dual nature of culture as a template for and a consequence of behavior.

Triandis (1994) emphasizes the subjective psychological nature of culture-- "A cultural group's characteristic way of viewing the man-made part of the environment." For Triandis, subjective culture is characterized by two important features that are derived from human interaction: 1) an individual's view (expectation; interpretation) is influenced by one's own experiences *as well as* the interactions *others* in the group may have; and 2) an individual may hold *symbolic representations* of the group's values and experiences, which affect behavior at a given moment in time. That is, the interpretative framework of meaning depends not only on the experiences one has directly with others, but what one believes about the experiences others in his or her group have had at various other times. These symbolic and identity-based beliefs play a critical role in what a person thinks, feels, sees or experiences.

Shweder & Sullivan (1992) define cultural psychology as the "..comparative study of the way culture and psyche make each other up." (pp. 497,498). Since culture and psyche are interchangeable, changes in one imply changes in the other. Culture evolves over time as it influences the outcomes of adaptation-coping sequences and is transformed by them. If Blacks and Whites evolved in different cultural circumstances prior to their contact with each other, and continued to have divergent experiences during their interactions over several centuries, it is certain that they would evolve divergent cultural psychologies as a consequence of these circumstances.
Fiske, Kitayama, Markus and Nisbett (1998) offer three specific objectives of cultural psychology: 1) to characterize varied cultural meanings and practices and the psychological structures and processes to which they are linked; 2) to discover the systematic principles underlying the diversity of culturally patterned socialities and psyches; 3) To describe the processes by which psyches and cultures construct each other.

In consideration of these cultural approaches, I take cultural psychology to be those *"symbolic representations that condition and follow from behavior, giving rise to characteristic ways of perceiving, understanding, anticipating, valuing and behaving for members of a socially defined group."* Culture evolves over time, defining the challenges its members must address and providing the interpretative schema and behavioral orientation to do so. Moreover, culture affects the thinking patterns, preferences and performances that, if not taken in cultural context, will be poorly understood.

Assumptions About African American Psychology

My first assumption is that African Americans comprise a multidimensional cultural group; characterized by diversity of experiences around a common core of cultural belief and origin. A more or less common template of cultural heritage, interacting with a diversity of experiences by virtue of one's place in or outside the system of slavery, and over the years, the cumulative consequences of a variety of factors including skin color, regional socialization, educational opportunities and gender. To talk about African Americans in the singular is in some ways to essentialize them in much the same flawed way the concept of race has done.

My second assumption is that the driving force behind the cultural psychology of African Americans is the fact of their systematic dehumanization over centuries, and their continued presence in the society that has dehumanized them. Adaptations to oppression call upon psychological tendencies and capacity to guide their deployment. Since African Americans continue to live within the society that has victimized and dehumanized them, the adaptations are ongoing, and their consequences are cumulative.

My third assumption is that psychological identity mediates the cultural adaptations to the dehumanizing forces and prescribes the means by which humanity is reclaimed or asserted. Psychological identity is not simply a psychological variable or a sense of worth or esteem, but a dynamic organization of the self in relationship to ones cultural group. Psychological identity has the capacity to influence perceptions and judgments, endorse values and rationalize beliefs. In this sense, the psychological processes of African Americans are derived from their socio-cultural context.

My fourth assumption is that the domains within which critical elements of the cultural psychology of African Americans evolve can be represented by TRIOS (Time Rhythm, Improvisation, Oral Expression and Spirituality). These domains comprise the adaptations and expressions of behavior that are fundamental to experience, and give rise to basic cultural psychology as defined by experience-near concepts. Shweder and Sullivan (1992) describe 'experience-near' as those psychological processes that occur so automatically or routinely that the boundary between psyche and culture is obliterated. The following section will briefly elaborate on each of these four assumptions.

Toward a Cultural Psychology of African Americans

A cultural psychology must account in some way for the interplay between psychological processes and cultural dynamics. For African Americans, this means that the cultural symbols, tendencies, values, beliefs, patterned ways of thinking and feeling interact with the psychological adaptations to the experiences of oppression and "otherness" in a racialized world. An individual's experience will to some extent reflect the distinctive pattern of his or her representation and internalization of these complex forces. The following account will describe how this dynamic interplay may aggregate toward a systematic pattern of culture-psyche interaction for African Americans.

African Americans comprise a multidimensional cultural group. African American cultural psychology is necessarily multidimensional in at least three ways: First is the joint function of Africa-originating cultural effects and the adaptive, reactionary mechanisms demanded by slavery and the experience in the Diaspora. Second, the social structure of slavery created multiple levels of African American society first distinguishing slave from free, then among slaves, the field and house slaves. Third, the regional context presented additional dimensions for divergence including North and South distinctions as well as variations caused by western expansion.

African Americans, then, can be characterized by diversity of experiences around a common core of cultural belief and origin. There is evidence that the Africans who came to America had a more coherent cultural system than many believe (Morgan, 1998). For example, Pidgin, a functionally restricted language employed by speakers of different languages usually for trading, emerged among indigenous coastal peoples of Africa. Once established, Pidgin evolved into Creole, which was a unifying language of West coast Africa in Senegambia even before slaves left Africa. According to Morgan (1998) "Africans retained elements of their grammars, phonology, and even parts of their lexicon in the unique languages that they created and bequeathed to their descendants.... Because, therefore, it is inappropriate to speak of the total dismantling of the slaves' indigenous languages, it is equally inappropriate to expect the total destruction of their cultural heritage. In part, at least, the powerless can appropriate a dominant language on their own terms" (p. 580). Sidney Mintz argues the point with respect to the culture-psyche connection in these terms: "The glory of Afro-Americana depended—had to depend—on creativity and innovation more than on the indelibility of particular culture contents" (cited in Morgan, 1998, p. 657).

A cultural psychology must be able to integrate the African cultural origins with the adaptations in the American context. With an emphasis on syncretic processes (merging of two different cultural traditions), and creativity and innovation, African American culture is necessarily context-rich and diverse. Moreover, it is fluid and changeable by virtue of the ongoing mechanisms of adaptation and evolution.

Cultural psychology of African Americans is critically affected by their systematic dehumanization over centuries. One constant in the ever-changing context for African Americans has been the systematic dehumanization and stigmatization they have experienced for centuries. The motivational goal of African American behavior and perception could be described as re-humanization and self-esteem protection and maintenance. The psychological literature is filled with illustrations of the psychology of dehumanization, and contains models of psychic conflict..

Mark of oppression (Kardiner & Ovesy, 1951). The "mark of oppression" analysis argues for the inevitability of degraded sense of self. "The Negro, in contrast to the white, is a more unhappy person; he has a harder environment to live in, the internal stress is greater By "unhappy" we mean he enjoys less, he suffers more. There is not one personality trait of the Negro the source of which cannot be traced to his difficult living conditions. *There are no exceptions to this rule.* The final result is wretched internal life." (p. 81) However, there is no contemporary empirical evidence that supports this damaged self-esteem hypothesis.

Double Consciousness (DuBois, 1903). The societal systems of racial dehumanization and promises of individual liberty and opportunity created a deep-seated psychic conflict which DuBois (1903) described thus: "It is a peculiar sensation, this double consciousness, this sense of always looking at one's self through the eyes of others, of measuring one's soul by the tape of a world that looks on I amused contempt and pity. One ever feels his twoness, --an American, a Negro; two warring ideals in one dark body, whose dogged strength alone keeps it from being torn asunder." As psyche and culture are intertwined, the duality of this psychic conflict drives the mechanisms of adaptation and coping.

Bifurcation of Self (Jackson-Kalb). When Jesse Jackson ran for the democratic nomination for president in 1984, he had an exchange with Marvin Kalb, then host of NBC's *Meet the Press*, that symbolizes what I call the bifurcation of self. Like double-consciousness, racial and American identity are pitted against each other in what appears to be a win-lose scenario.

Kalb: The question …[is]…are you a black man who happens to be an American running for the presidency, or are you an American who happens to be a black man running for the presidency?

Jackson: Well, I'm both an American and a black at one and the same time. I'm both of these…

(Excerpted from Meet the Press, February 13, 1984.

The legacy of oppression, and the ongoing efforts to find a psychological space in which to feel comfortably human, is an ongoing psychological struggle to be explained by cultural psychology. Culture is multifaceted -- black/white; European/African; good/bad -- and in our cultural psychology analysis, psyche must necessarily be also. The duality pits instrumental goals of well-being against expressive goals of life satisfaction.

Psychological identity mediates the cultural adaptations to dehumanization. Social identity theory (Tajfel, 1978) stipulates the close link between one's psychological well being and his or her identification with a group. If psyche and culture make each other up, how then does the culture of racism, stigma, freedom and opportunity conjoin in psyche? Research suggests it is a tricky union.

Fordham and Ogbu (1985) suggested that it is possible that racism and oppression may be joined with freedom and opportunity such that opposing one (say racism) may cause one to oppose the other (say achievement). Thus doing well in school may in some situation be interpreted as "acting white." Arroyo and Zigler (1995) demonstrated that indeed, retreating from one's racial identification was associated with improved performance in school. However, they also showed that it was associated with lowered mental health status (e.g., depression).

Steele (Steele & Aronson, 1995; Steele, 1997) has shown that mental representation of the culture of negative racial stereotypes regarding academic performance could lead otherwise prepared and capable Black students to perform poorly. Other research shows that racial identity has been shown to mediate self-esteem, interaction patterns in interracial contexts and utilization of mental health facilities. Measures of racial identity (cf., Taylor & Rogers, 1993; Cross, 1991; Helms, 1990; Baldwin and Bell, 1986) capture the tension caused by processes used to protect and maintain esteem when they conflict with racism and prevailing principles of freedom and equality.

TRIOS represents the critical elements of the cultural psychology of African Americans. TRIOS provides the means by which African Americans employed African cultural origins in their adaptations to the context of slavery and dehumanization. TRIOS provides the degree of flexibility, creativity and innovation that helps one adapt to changing and unpredictable circumstances, and gain control over the conditions and qualities of one's life (cf., Jones, 1999). I argue here that TRIOS provides the mechanisms of coping and adaptation, and have, over time, become the cornerstones of African American Cultural Psychology. I will briefly describe each of the TRIOS dimensions below.

Time. Time is the substrate of life and consciousness (Ornstein, 1977). More importantly, perceptions of time take on values, which dictate behavior and the valuations of human affairs. The valuing of time has been referred to as "temponomics" (McGrath &Kelly, 1988). In temponomic societies, time may be saved, wasted or invested much as any valued resource. When time is not of value in its own right, none of these attributes pertain. Thus time is not simply a reference for the unfolding of behavior, but constitutes a fundamental value that organizes and dictates societal structures, perceptions and beliefs.

There is an expression in Trinidad, West Indies that "any time is Trinidad time" (Jones, 1986). What this means is that time has no independent status or value and therefore does not dictate behavior and choice. Rather, time is a derivative concept, responsive largely to the feelings, desires and behaviors of individuals. Time is controlling in a temponomic society, but not in a non-temponomic one

The psychological story concerns preparation for the future (what we may call future orientation) by conserving capital and not squandering it (what McDougall called Providence). Orienting to the future requires psychological restraint, denial of preferences, and emotional suppression. One of the most conspicuous losses of freedom impelled by slavery was the loss of temporal freedom, and the disconnection of soul and behavior. The psychological liberation from slavery is the liberation from control in all of its aspects. TRIOS offers specific mechanisms of regaining personal control in a society were external control is difficult to come by. Controlling time is, in its essence, psychological liberation.

Rhythm, Rhythm defines a recurring pattern of behavior within specified time frames. Time is necessarily implicated in rhythms. Behaviors occur within temporal units. The regularity of the behaviors and the values of the temporal units (an *adagio* has broad and an *allegro* narrow time values) create the rhythmic experience. One may gain control over rhythms by changing the temporal units and adjusting the behavior accordingly.

Racism often introduces asynchronies or disharmonious connections between internal and external states. Gaining behavioral control over the environment may require adapting rhythmic control either through accommodation (adjusting the internal aspects) or assimilation (adjusting the external aspects). At its core, rhythm is an ecological variable conceived in a transactional framework with psychological properties and consequences. Following on the Gibsonian model of perception (Gibson, 1979; McArthur & Baron, 1983), environmental affordances merge with psychological attunements to create the rhythmic behavioral act. These acts are significantly affected by the cultural context in which they occur, and the personality characteristics of the acting parties.

Improvisation. Improvisation is "…a combination of *expressiveness* and *invention*, or *creativity*, which occurs *under time pressure* (Jones, 1997, p. 488). Again, we find freedom at the core. Improvisation is inherently free by virtue of its spontaneity. But it is not random and it is not haphazard. Improvisation is inherently "problem-focused." That is, we are inventing or creating toward a purpose. Improvisation takes an underlying foundation, say grammar or musical structure, then, under the constraints of time (a rhythmic order) configures a text or specific scale to make some coherent statement that expresses a point. Because the improvisation is done "on-line" it is unique and bears the signature of the author. This improvisation is necessarily a fusion of the author and performer in the same person. Characteristic patterns of time-based problem solving are expressive and can rise to the level of a "self-signature" we may call style.

Oral Expression. *Orature* (vocality, drumming, storytelling, praise singing and naming) is what Asante (1987) calls the sum total of the oral tradition. Orature captures human creation and life itself. The crucial aspect of Orature is its immediacy. Orature means that all meaningful behavior, values and beliefs are defined by context. It becomes important, then, to share in experience in order to understand it. Experience cannot be abstracted, out of context, in a meaningful way. Morality, even value, is bound up in context.

Another consequence of the context-rich nature of Orature is that it allows for creative freedom in the expression and decoding of the meaning of things. Cole, Gay, Glick and Sharp (1971) found that the Kpelle of Liberia were reliably poorer than Americans at memorizing lists of words. This was true even when the researchers tried to encourage categorization as a mnemonic device. However, when the 20-items to be recalled were embedded in a folk story, the Kpelle subjects not only remembered them all, but in the order in which they appeared in the story. Context gave the words meaning that they did not have independently.

In African American culture, language is also used as an avenue of control through privileged meanings and neologisms. "Bad" becomes "good, "cool" defines an essence of spirit and self, a preference a taste, 'dope' becomes 'bad' which we know is good. "Stupid" is not dumb but smart. The use of language in slavery times required neologisms and privileged uses to hide collective action from slave owners and overseers. Over centuries it has become one of the most stable means of asserting self-control in a potentially hostile or at best indifferent context. Rap is a contemporary extension of this evolutionary process. Rap is more than a style of singing and rhyming. It is an expression of reality and assertion for self that is not filtered through powerbrokers of the mainstream (George, 1998). It creates its own authenticity for those who are "down with it." These mechanisms of self-control and personal freedom have the capacity to bond individuals together in concerted reality, and also distance oneself and one's group from others who are potentially harmful.

Spirituality. Finally, spirituality can be defined as the belief in nonmaterial causation in human affairs (Jones, 1986). That is, what happens to us is determined in some measure by forces or energies that are beyond our control. Those forces are not haphazard but are part of a system of meaning and energy that determines human events. According to Jahn (1961) the basic force is *Ntu*, and influences human beings (*muntu*), all things (k*intu*), all places and all time (h*antu*), and modalities of existence (k*untu*). A person who is spiritual shares cause-effect agency with *ntu*, and does not claim it all for him or herself.

In U.S. society, control is a defining property of wellbeing. In McDougall's (1921) description of the races of Europe, "will" and "introversion" were positive properties, and "extraversion" and "gregariousness" were negative. Self-Actualization implies that the pinnacle of selfhood can be achieved through personal agency. Those who fail to accomplish this actualized state may be thought of as "pawns" rather than "origins" (DuCharms, 1966), or external as opposed to internal in their locus of control (Rotter 1966), or field dependent rather than field independent (Witkin et al, 1962). Moreover, research shows that having control can confer better physical health among nursing home patients (Langer & Rodin, 1976), or that the illusion of control can cause people to overvalue things over which such control is exerted like playing bingo cards (Langer 1983).

Spirituality liberates one from the expectation of personal responsibility in a world that denies the full range of options and opportunities. Thus one can also claim spirituality among the mechanisms that liberate one from the dominance of cultural expectations and constraints. Whether this shared responsibility is seen as a kind of self-handicapping, or a legitimate cultural belief, it is one of the important elements of the psychological evolution of persons of African descent.

Conclusion

TRIOS describes psychological processes and tendencies that provide an "experience-near" template of cultural difference. The mechanisms of TRIOS provide psychological control and affirm the self as well as the collective in a societal context that devalues them both. The challenge of racism for its targets is the creation and preservation of a positive self and an instrumental identity. The historical evolution of African American culture has resulted in large part from the coping-adaptation sequences that derive both from African origins (evolutionary) and challenges of racism in the American context (reactionary). As a result, the psychology of African Americans is heavily context dependent. The psychological manifestations of TRIOS also serve to strengthen the bond within the group and protecting group members from assaults. The cultural psychology of African Americans promises to be an interesting and important study that will expand our understanding of the range of human psychological capacity.

References

Arroyo, C.& Zigler, E. (1995) Racial identity, academic achievement, and the psychological well-being of economically disadvantaged adolescents. *Journal of Personality and Social Psychology*. *69*, 903-914.

Asante, M. K. (1987) *The Africentric idea.* Philadelphia: Temple University Press.

Baldwin J.A. & Bell, Y.R. (1985) The African Self-Consciousness Scale: An Africentric personality questionnaire. *The Western Journal of Black Studies*, *9*, 61-68.

Brill, N. Q. (1999) *Being Black in America. A Multiperspective Review of the Problem.* Springfield, IL: Charles C. Thomas.

Cole, M., Gay, J., Glick, J. & Sharp, D. (1971) *The cultural context of learning and thinking.* New York: Basic Books.

Cross, W.E. (1991) *Shades of black: Diversity in African-American identity.* Philadelphia: Temple University Press.

DuBois, W.E.B. (1903) *The souls of black folk.* Chicago: A.C. McClurg and Company.

Fiske, A. Kitayama, S., Markus, H. and Nisbett, R. (1998) The cultural matrix of social psychology. In D. Gilbert, S. Fiske, & G. Lindzey (Eds.) Handbook of social psychology, 4th Ed., Pp. 915-998. Boston: McGraw-Hill.

Fordham, S. and Ogbu, J. (1985) Black students' school success: Coping with the burden of "acting white'" *Urban Review*, *18*, 176-206.

George, N. (1998) *Hip hop America.* New York: Viking Press.

Gibson, J.J. (1979) *The ecological approach to visual perception.* Boston: Houghton Mifflin.

Helms, J. (1990) *Black and White racial identity: Theory, research, and practice.* New York: Greenwood Press.

Jahn, J. (1961) *Muntu: An outline of the new African culture.* New York: Grove Press.

Jones, J..M. (1972) *Prejudice and racism.* Reading, MA: Addison Wesley.

Jones, J..M. (1997) *Prejudice and racism, second edition.* New York: McGraw-Hill.

Jones, J..M. (1999) Cultural Racism: The Intersection of Race and Culture in Intergroup Conflict. In D. Prentice and D. Miller (Eds.) *Cultural Divides: The Social Psychology of Cultural Identity*. New York: Russell Sage Foundation.

Jones, J..M. (1988) Cultural differences in temporal perspectives: Instrumental and expressive behaviors in time. In J. McGrath (Ed) *The Social Psychology of Time: New Perspectives Pp. 21-38.*. Thousand Oaks, CA: Sage Publications.

Kroeber, A.L. & Kluckhohn, C.(1952) *Culture: A critical review of concepts and definitions*. New York- Random House

Kardiner, A. & Ovesy, L. (1951) *The mark of oppression*. New York: Norton.

Langer, E. & Rodin, J. (1976) The effects of choice and enhanced personal responsibility for the aged: A field experiment in an institutional setting. *Journal of Personality and Social Psychology, 34*, 191-198.

Langer, E. (1983) *The psychology of control*. Beverly Hills, CA: Sage Publications

McArthur, L..Z. & Baron, R. (1983) Toward an ecological theory of social perception. *Psychological Review, 90*, 215-238.

McDougall, W. (1921) *Is America safe for democracy?* New York: Scribner & Sons.McGrath, J. & Kelly, J. (1986) *Time and human interaction: Toward a social psychology of time.* New York: Guilford Press.

Morgan, P.D. (1998) *Slave Counterpoint: Black culture in the eighteenth-century Chesapeake & Low Country*. Chapel Hill, NC: University of North Carolina Press.

Ornstein, R. E. (1977) The*psychology of consciousness*. New York: Harcourt, Brace Jovanovich

Rotter, J. (1966) Generalized expectancies for internal and external control of reinforcement. *Psychological Monographs, 80(Whole No. 609)*

Shweder, R. & Sullivan, M. A. (1992) Cultural psychology: Who needs it? *Annual Review of Psychology, 44*, 497-523.

Steele, C.M. (1997) A threat in the air: How stereotypes shape intellectual identity and performance. *American Psychologist, 52*, 613-629.

Steele, C.M. & Aronson, J. (1995) Stereotype threat and the intellectual performance of African Americans. *Journal of Personality and Social Psychology. 69*, 797-811.

Tajfel, H. (1978) *Differentiation between social groups: Studies in the social psychology of intergroup relations.* London: Academic Press.

Taylor, J. & Rogers, J. (1993) relationship between cultural identity and exchange dispositions. *British Journal of Social Psychology, 19*, 248-265.

Triandis, H.C. (1994) *Culture and behavior.* New York: McGraw-Hill.

Witkin, H. A, Dyk, R B., Paterson, H F., Goodenough, D R. and Karp, S A. (1962) *Psychological differentiation*. New York: John Wiley Publishers.

Directions in Gender Research in American Indian Societies: Two Spirits and Other Categories

Beatrice Medicine
Wakpala, South Dakota

ABSTRACT

Indigenous social role categories that represent third and fourth gender characteristics, such as the Lakota (Sioux) *winkte* and the Din9 (Navajo) *n<dleeh* and other Native terms, mark the status of these individuals. However, they are often blanketed by the term, *berdache*, in social science literature. Contextualization in an ethnographic frame is essential to greater comprehension of these roles. A critical review of contemporary research and the writings of the Native occupants of these categories has resulted in an all encompassing term: "Two Spirits." Coterminously, Native terms for lesbians are also emerging. However, all Native gay males and lesbians have not accepted the term. This article discusses the concerns of indigenous researchers and others or non-indigenous researchers in this discourse.

The *berdache* role was institutionalized among the Lakota, who reside now primarily in the state of South Dakota. It was often stated in early ethnographic writings and stressed in culturally relative terms that many Plains tribes socially constructed sexual "abnormality" (a Western view at that time) in acceptable ways. This term did not reveal the cultural variance that gave the *berdache* role its many forms and functions. This is what many gay and, increasingly, lesbian indigenous persons in North American Native societies find offensive. *Berdache* is a label which obscures tribal variation of Native linguistic terms. The anthropological literature is overburdened with categories for *berdache*. It includes homosexuals, transvestites, hermaphrodites, and transgendered individuals. By examining this term in each unique cultural context one can see how the various gender roles were played out and privileged. Embedded in such frames of ideology and social structure and analyzed linguistically, concepts of gender variation have given new dimensions to this often misconstrued social role. Symbolic structures and marked behaviors resulted in various appraisals of personhood.

Gender studies in anthropology have proliferated since the 1970s. This may be attributed to the impact of feminist theory and, perhaps, post-modern influences. The role of reflexivity in anthropological writings may also have pointed to the role of individual professional's experiences in cross-cultural settings. From the viewpoint of ethnic minority anthropologists, this examination of "imperialistic navels" by anthropologists may herald greater awareness of sub-altern concerns and contributions in the discipline of anthropology.

Life stories and personal narratives of many Natives are proliferating. The University of Nebraska Press, for example, has chosen to collect life stories of many Native peoples. I have referred to these as "I was there-isms!" They are, however, "voices" from the sub-alterns- and in some cases subjugated subjects as in feminine stories. Many of these "stories" are collected and edited by non-Natives, so the question remains, "Whose voice?" Many do provide rich texts to view individual lives in cultural settings. In my view, such collections must go beyond the journalistic. They must be situated within the local social and cultural matrices. Essentially, a framework of realistic and appropriate ethnography should frame the individual. We should be able to view these representations and contextualize them within power relations, racism, economic and social deprivation in our teaching, research, and counseling strategies. Moreover, this collection of life histories can be a powerful means of understanding life cycles in contrasting Native groups.

I shall attempt to examine the term, *berdache*, which has been introduced in every beginning course in anthropology and explained as a *male homosexual.* This, in most classes, has elicited titters and embarrassed glances.

Walter Williams (1986, 1991) traces the origin of the word to Arabic (bardash) meaning "kept boy" or "male prostitute." The term was introduced in the New World and found in the Jesuit relations with Natives who observed men dressed as women among the Iroquois.

As for the Siouan term *winkte*, Williams relied upon his Lakota "informants" at the Pine Ridge Reservation in South Dakota. He defines *winkte* as "woman to become." He places them in supportive families, as having fondness for children (caretakers) and describes them as "sacred people," "half man and half woman," "half and half people." He also elicited the terms "hermaphrodite," and he/she. Many Lakota people feel that Williams has glamorized the *winkte* as being sacred.

In his book, Williams' states that "Many Native Americans also understood that gender roles have to do with more than just biological sex. The standard Western view that one's sex is always a certainty and that one conforms to one's morphological sex is a view that dies hard. Most American Indian world views generally are much more accepting of the ambiguities of life. Acceptance of gender variation in the *berdache* tradition is typical of many Native cultures' approach to life in general" (p. 4). Essentially, this view remained in operation for some time but was gradually eroded in the Europeanization and Christianization processes. After about 1950, homophobia on reservations and in Indian communities caused many gay Indian males to move to San Francisco or other urban centers where gay sub-culture provided some form of safety net.

For purposes of this presentation I rely upon the term *gender* to refer to a social category which is culturally construed, based upon Native ideologies, and accepted behavior for individuals who evidence certain social and sexual characteristics. Persons who occupy this category are located within a range of gender possibilities, which are defined by their cultural prescriptions. Sexuality refers to a range of sexual actions (after Thomas and Jacobs, 1999).

Since I investigated the Lakota term *winkte*, I will elucidate how research might be construed by a Native researcher. I do not often personalize my work as an anthropologist, but in this age of reflexivity, perhaps you will bear with me.

From 1969 to 1972, I taught at San Francisco State University. As an ethnic minority faculty member and in those days of expected community involvement, I participated in many events, including the take-over of Alcatraz Island. However, the most ordinary community events were "Pow-wows" or social events in which Native peoples dressed in Native attire and danced to Native music. At these events, I noticed obviously gay and transgender Indian males who participated. In many instances they were shunned or ridiculed by other Indian participants.

In my childhood, we were aware of this social category, which was referred to as *winkte*. Linguistic analysis of this Lakota word is:

win – "woman"
kte – "to be like"
kte - "to kill" (a deeper structural form)

The common vernacular usage was *winkte* "wants to be like a woman."

We, as children, were instructed, "There are these individuals - in all cases males (*wicasa*). They are different. They are *winkte*. Don't make fun of them. They are also Lakota," said our parents and grandparents.

Later, in San Francisco, a well-known Native woman of another Plains tribe said to me, as I was speaking to a gay male, "Isn't it terrible that so many of our good-looking Indian men are gay?" I replied, "You don't know much about your culture do you?" For many Plains Indian societies, a feminine or transgender role was "institutionalized." Contrary to the common designation of *berdache* to mean male homosexual, there were traditionally several strands to the *winkte* class in traditional Lakota society.

These encounters resulted in a paper "Changing Sex Roles in an Urban Context" which I read at an Anthropology regional conference in 1987) This paper found its way into the Indian and non-Indian gay community. When I later gave the additional linguistic analysis, "to kill women," many non-Indian gay men were offended. But Native gay men somehow viewed me as a mentor, as an accepting person, and therefore were not as critical. As in other parts of North America, gay people came to San Francisco to follow a gay life style and escape a growing homophobia due to Christian influences and the forced legal assimilation to Euro-American life ways due to education away from traditional life.

I rely on the following Native Lakota views on these reasons for the *winkte* role.

1. The perduring notion still extant is that some Lakota males were not destined to be warriors. For example, Lang (1998) makes an erroneous assumption about the ethnographic record when she asserts that men who did not go to war were *winkte.* Not all Lakota men were expected to go to war; "men who didn't want to go war" were not classified as *winkte*, because not all were of this third gender. We have terms that means strong-hearted - *chante-tinza* -- that is also used to refer to warriors. Some men did not choose to be warriors because they did not have the orientation to **killing**. These men were not looked down upon as less manly. Many of these were **not** *winkte.*
2. Many preferred to excel in women's crafts -- tanning skins, embellishing them with quills from the porcupine, making rawhide containers, and sewing tipi covers.
3. Some preferred to take care of children -- naming them in ceremonies where it was believed that a name bestowed by a *winkte* brought good luck and fortune to the child.
4. Some went on the war path with warriors -- to cook, mend moccasins, and perform clairvoyant rituals (by killing a badger and reading its stomach lining). It is uncertain if any sexual encounters occurred, because warriors often fasted, prayed and refrained from sex during this event -- as in preparing for the Sun Dance -- our sacred ritual.
5. Others were obviously sexual partners for men. Lakota believed "they look for each other."

My research into views on birthing, sexuality, and expected behavior of the Lakota reveals some possible pertinent corollary aspects. The word for children in Lakota is *wakan yeša (wakan = sacred* and *yeša - like = "to be").* Thus, children were viewed as "sacred beings" - traditionally, never hit but cherished and nurtured by the *tiospaye* (extended family). Children were seen as autonomous individuals It was thought that bearing many children detracted from the social development of each child. Children made their own life chances and actualized social roles. Thus, some chose to be *winkte.*

In traditional Lakota society, excessive sexuality was not condoned. Women practiced a long lactation period lasting up to 4 to 5 years; this custom persisted into the early reservation period. Of course, as the Lakota practiced sororal polygyny (sisters marrying one man), this social script might also have been a factor. It was a common belief that the Lakota woman's life was difficult in a nomadic society and a yearly pregnancy was debilitating. When men pledged to dance in the sacred Sun Dance, they were **expected** to refrain from sex for a year before this yearly event. Early reservation records revealed one child per family in traditional families. A three-child family was considered "large." Feminine sexuality has not been carefully examined in so-called "Warrior societies."

My perusal of field notes revealed an interesting note. *Akaska* is the name of a town in South Dakota. A narrative from Mrs. Lucy Eagleman reveals: A returning war party encountered a *winkte* in this area, and shouted the Lakota term *akaska* ["to stick to; to accost, to enter (sexually)]." There is no information as to the consequences, but when I asked, "What happened?" I was told, "The *winkte* ran away." So as in most traditional societies, the rate of homosexual activity remains shrouded. Were the returning warriors in a secular state? And therefore able to engage in sex? Or was this a threat?

I present another narrative of gay Lakota men in the 1930s. This was the period of administered human relations on all Indian reservations, where colonialism and Christianization practices prevailed. A superintendent of the Standing Rock Reservation in South Dakota commanded the Bureau of Indian Affairs Police to arrest a *winkte*, Patrick Hail, cut his long hair and put him in jail. This person was an excellent seamstress and craftsperson. He sewed his mother's (and other women's) dresses and was lauded by other women for this ability. He is pictured in an ethnography. As a child, I viewed him dressed in a woman's blouse and slacks, with curled hair, and wearing lipstick. A grandmother said (translated from Lakota) "Don't ridicule him. He's also Lakota."

My linguistic research has **not** uncovered a Lakota term for lesbians. I am not denying that this role was absent from traditional Lakota society. There are few instances in which Lakota women did not marry. Some older widowed women lived together after their husbands died. This was a common practice in the early reservation period and therefore not to be interpreted as lesbianism. Women who chose not to marry usually were embedded in a *tiospaye* (extended family) in which male relatives were able to care for them. Thus there seem to be evidences of feminine individual autonomy.

The world of engenderment is extremely varied among American Indian and Alaska Native societies. There have been few analyses of indigenous words which are contextually placed in the lexicon of the attribution of gender by speakers of Native languages. Rather, there is increasingly a designation of terms for those individuals who fit a third and sometimes a fourth gender category, be they males or females in their outward appearances. These terms are often utilized by outsiders who attribute meaning and gender categories for the occupants of these gender roles. Even though the gender researchers often state that they have checked these words with their "informants," there is seldom a referral to reconfirm the linguistic connotation of these appellations. It is thus encouraging to note that emic analyses are beginning to occur in the field of naming, designating, and attributing the range of gender occupancies in some aboriginal groups (Thomas, 1993). This direction is significant for it is an attempt to deal with the permutations of gender specific categories within a total cultural framework. These attempts should also focus upon the terms; that is, the ways in which they are shared in the cultural group and the ways in which they are seen to differ in the ordinary usage in this cultural group. This latter caveat is necessary in order to give meaning to the cultural construction of gender.

In a recent paper (Medicine, 1997), I noted that the Lakota term for a gay male, *winkte*, was assuming Pan-Indian proportion in its usage and level of understanding in contemporary "Indian country." The latter term is also an accepted description which glosses the more than five hundred tribes on reservations and federally-recognized enclaves of indigenous peoples. The 55% of Native peoples living in off-reservation towns and in cities are often referred to simply as "Urban Indians." Yet, the term *winkte* has meaning in the indigenous gay world.

In an effort to clarify Lakota terminology which gives meaning to words which signify aspects of gender, these words will be examined, and contextualized. *Wičaša* (man*); winyan (woman); koshkalaka (young man-youth); wikoshkalaka (*young woman*); winkte* (gay male); *bloka* (ultimate manliness*); bloka egla wa ke* (thinks being capable of doing manly things); *wean ketch* (ultimate womanhood); *winkte-winyan* (gay female - first heard in 1993). My aim in doing this is to document the various cultural constructs which are used in discourse among contemporary Lakota people. These words also give an adjectival aspect to gender terminology, and speak to the construction of terms to meet emerging gender categories (e.g. Paula Gunn Allen's term who stated in 1986 that "koshkalaka means dyke"). This attempt is also a response to some of the Native participants at the Wenner Gren conference on gender held in Chicago, May, 1994. This was a continuation of the first conference held during the American Anthropological Association's annual meeting held in Washington, D.C. in November, 1993. At the meeting in Chicago, the gay American Indian and Alaska Native males agreed to use the term "Two Spirit" to replace the controversial "berdache" term. The stated objective was to purge the older term from anthropological literature as it was seen as demeaning and not reflective of Native categories. Unfortunately, the term "berdache" has also been incorporated in the psychology and women studies domains, so the task for the affected group to purge the term looms large and may be formidable.

The Lakota term *heyoka* should not be confused as a gloss for *winkte*. The former may be viewed as a "contrary," or one who reverses his behavior and acts in ceremonial activities. But because Williams only witnessed one *winkte* chopping the sacred tree and offering a prayer does not account for his calling *winkte* sacred. A contemporary variation in Sun Dance ritual is idiosyncratic as to who is asked to paint the tree. This also is significant in the role *winkte* play in ordinary Lakota life. They are not considered sacred. At present, *winkte* individuals are generally accepted among the Lakota. There may be instances of ribaldness or teasing. Homophobia is generally not a part of ordinary Lakota life.

However, a new phenomenon is occurring. There has been an influx of males afflicted with AIDS, who return to their communities from urban centers. This is possibly to receive medical help from Indian Health Services. Because of confidentially issues, it is impossible to obtain verifiable data on the numbers. However, family members care for these persons. Only in one instance was a male afflicted with AIDS returned to a metropolitan hospice. A young gay male from the Rosebud reservation, an "opera singer" whose stage name was White Eagle, made a video of his life but concentrated on his singing career and not on AIDS, which resulted in his early demise.

In some Native communities in North America, homophobia has become brutally evident. Sue-Ellen Jacobs documents the horrendous treatment of a feminine male in a Pueblo community. In addition, many indigenous gay people challenged the belief that AIDS is only a homosexual affliction. It appears to be heterosexual in some communities. However, on hears in Lakota communities, "All Indians have AIDS!" -American Indian Drinking Syndrome!" Again, this is a counter to views of the "drunken Indian" syndrome.

In 1993, Sue-Ellen Jacobs and others organized a unique symposium. Entitled "Revisiting the North American Berdache: Empirically and Theoretically," the symposium was an interaction between indigenous gay people and those persons (native and non-native anthropologists) who had written about the issue. This event was undoubtedly a first encounter of its kind among a marginalized group (in U.S. society) and anthropologists. Tribes were Paiute, Shoshone, Yupik, Taos, Pueblo, two Dakota males, one Lakota female, one Navajo male, two Navajo women and "straight me"! This began almost five years of interactive collaboration which resulted in the book, "*Two Spirit People: Native American Gender Identity, Sexuality and Spirituality*" (Jacobs, Wesley, and Lang, 1997).

The major outcome of this unique endeavor was that the term "*berdache*" had evolved from the imperialistic and colonial discourse and was onerous to Native participant's gender and sexual behaviors.

This problem of "naming" was an important part of annual "Native American Gay and Lesbian Gatherings." In meeting annually in various parts of North America, the term "Two Spirit" became accepted by participants. Future meetings were to be called "The International Two Spirit Gathering". The first international meeting was held in Minneapolis in 1989. At the Winnipeg, Manitoba in 1990, the term "Two Spirit" emerged. It supposedly is from the Anishinabe (Ojibway) *neizh manitoog* (*neizh*= two; *manitoog*= spirit). This term needs verification by an Anishinabe or Ojibway -speaking person.

I was told by a Lakota female that the term was Metis. As the Metis ("Half-breed, mixed blood, people in Canada) spoke several Native languages, the Anishinabe referent seems logical. This may give a strong attribution to the spiritual aspects of the social roles of lesbian and gay indigenous individuals as they perceive themselves.

The Native term *neizh manitoog* is not Lakota. Walter Williams has only one "informant" who stated, "A *winkte* is two spirits, man and woman combined into one spirit." (1986b; p. 184). Statements such as these only seem to focus on the individual which is so integral to Lakota personhood and the self-imagery of Lakota gays.

In an unpublished paper, Thomas and Jacobs write: "The term is not intended to mark a new category of gender. Instead indigenously defined pan-Native North American term that bridges Native American Indian diversity and sexualities and those of Western cultures" (1999, p.2). Many apparently feel that issues of self-identity are covered by the term. Two Spirit roles and identities are also referred to by some Native American people as gay, lesbian, transvestite, transsexual, transgender, drag queens and butches," as well as *winkte* and *nádleeh* and other appropriate tribal terms" (p.2-3). This term "two spirit" is a self-imposed category. However, a transsexual of Dakota heritage said she objected to the term as her feminine "spirit was the over-riding one." Thus, as many ask, why not continue using "berdache?" I feel it is a factor in this era of indigenous self-determination. However, some Lakota gays do not accept the term saying, "I feel like a woman!"

Emerging Lesbian Terms

I now pick up the theme of lesbianism in Lakota society. In her M.A. thesis, Evelyn Blackwood uses the term "cross-gender for the female role." I was unable to elicit a Native term for the English designation.

Beverly Little Thunder writes in (Jacobs, Thomas and Lang), "I am a Lakota womyn." In this interesting personal narrative, she speaks of life in urban California, with an alcoholic mother, foster home placements, detentions, and involvement in the American Indian Movement. She returned to South Dakota and became involved in Sun Dance ceremonies seeking "Spirit." Upon rejection by the Sun Dance people (AIM) for her lesbianism, and as part of this homophobia, she was told to "do ceremony for her own kind." She began a Sun Dance for "Wimmin" in the California hills. Her involvement in the second conference on the "Berdache Revisited" in 1994 seemed to be an emotional fulfillment for her.

In a recent publication, she indicates that in Lakota tradition, "there's a story about when someone who was born having the spirit of both male and female being able to understand the male and female components. So they are born "Two Spirit." From that it has become a contemporary term that many lesbian and gay men in the Native Community have adopted as a marker for who they are. However, the term Two Spirit does not translate into any Native tongue." She goes on to say that "In our tribe, lesbians were called *koskalawin.* Historically, they were the women who were trained to take care of the other women who had female problems. They usually opted not to marry. They were the women who adopted orphaned children. They became the aunties and grandmothers to all the children of the tribe. They held prominent positions in ceremony."

Beverly Little Thunder, an Urban Lakota turned "Pipe Carrier" and leader in the Wimmen's Sun Dance, has reinvented Paula Gunn Allen's *koskalaka* Lakota for "young man" to *koskalaka win* - young man woman. Therefore, can we see a complete self-serving use of Native Lakota words? This, despite my correction of Gunn Allen's use of *koskalaa* to mean "dyke" (letter, 1994) to which Gunn Allen replied, "I got the wrong information."

Perhaps, the reconstruction of Native terms may be a part of self-naming of indigenous people who occupy these roles. In any case, the dynamic flux of self-ascription may be ongoing. Meanwhile, back on the reservation, besides the English term he/she, the term *winkte win* has emerged to translate as "male gay woman." However, the term for gay male – *winkte* - continues in the social discourse of contemporary Lakota people.

I wish, however, to outline what the collaboration of Native peoples, occupants of various gender roles and professionals of anthropology, achieved in the 1993 conference. The first benefit was that a sub-altern, disenfranchised group of Native peoples of various genders and nations presented a variable rationale for their own self-naming. The second benefit was that anthropologists listened, but also contributed. Native peoples were not like "my informants" dragged into a professional meeting as had happened so many times before. In general, however, I feel that this honest interchange allowed all of the participants an opportunity to reassess how research can be done to give voice to target populations.

It is important to understand the ethnohistorical record to contextualize contemporary Native life. An understanding of the way gays and lesbians, and others, live and write about their lives adds new dimensions to the discipline of anthropology and to women and gender studies. Some of the participants were interested in categories of gender, others on personhood and the life cycle, and others spoke of spirituality and homophobia. But the discussions were frank, open, and set new standards for participatory research. Many were concerned about the contextualization of the term used for marked individuals in their distinct cultures in contemporary life.

All of us, I believe, viewed this experience as a means of assessing ourselves in our own societies and in the discipline in which we work. I wish to conclude with the directive in research that we examine histories of women that not only openly examines the shifting nature of gender itself, but examines the culture, class, racial and sexual components in differences through temporality. We might attempt to construct histories of ideas regarding women by both genders in Native societies. I take one example, which is the emergence of lesbianism among Aboriginal women. For example, it was not uncommon for Lakota women to choose not to marry.

As an economic necessity, older Lakota women lived together after being widowed or divorced or abandoned (by white partners) in the early reservation period. Thus, one must assess the emergence of contemporary Lakota lesbianism. It is, I feel, by reassessing our theories and research methods of gender roles in any society that the enrichment of anthropology and feminist studies may continue.

References

Allen, P. G. (1986). *The Sacred Hoop: Recovering the feminine in American Indian Traditions.* Boston: Beacon Press.

Jacobs, Ellen, S. Wesley, T. Lang, S. (1997). *Two Spirit People: Native American gender, sexuality and spirituality.* Urbana: University of Illinois Press.

Lang, S. (1998). *Men as women, women as men.* Translated from the German by John L. Vantine. Austin: University of Texas Press.

Medicine, B. (1980). "Indian Women: Tribal Identity as Status Quo". In R. Hubbard & M. Lowe (Eds) , *Women and nature* (pp. 63-75). NY: Pergamon Press.

Medicine, B. (1997). "Changing Native American sex roles in an urban context." In S. E. Jacobs, W. Thomas & S. Lang (Eds.) *Two-Spirit people.* Native American gender identity, sexuality, and spirituality, pp. 145-255. Champaign-Urbana, IL: University of Illinois Press.

Roscoe, W. (1991) *The Zuni Man-Woman.* Albuquerque: University of New Mexico Press.

Seydan, B. Herrera, D. (1998) *Women in love: Portraits of Lesbian mothers and their families.* Boston: Little Brown and Company

Thomas, Wesley (1993) Unpublished manuscript.

Thomas, Wesley, Jacobs, Ellen. (1999). *American Indian Culture and Research Journal*, Vol.23, No.2.

Williams, W. (1986). "Persistence and Change in the Berdache Tradition Among Contemporary Lakota Indians." In E. Blackwood (Ed.) *The many faces of homosexuality* (pp.181-200). New York: Harrington Park Press.

Williams, W. (1996b,1991) *The spirit and the flesh: Sexual diversity in American Indian culture.* Boston: Beacon Press.

Hispanic Psychology: A 25-Year Retrospective Look

Amado M. Padilla
Stanford University
School of Education

ABSTRACT

Hispanic psychology has its roots in ethnic psychology and in cross-cultural psychology. The basic premise is that it is a valuable enterprise both theoretically and empirically to study the behavior of Hispanics. Over the past 25 years, research in Hispanic psychology has given way to a new scholarship or paradigm that calls for the recognition of intragroup variation which values within-group comparisons rather than relying exclusively on between-group effects. Acculturation and biculturalism have taken on special significance in Hispanic psychology. Further, Hispanic psychology must also consider the effects of racism and oppression on people and how these affect ethnic identity, attitudes toward the dominant group, and intergroup relations.

In 1973 Rene Ruiz and I published a monograph entitled "Latino Mental Health: A Review of Literature" (Padilla & Ruiz, 1973). This work represented the first systematic effort to organize the psychological and mental health literature on Spanish-origin people in the United States. In a March 1971 census report the total Spanish origin population was estimated to be just under 9 million. Also at this time, "Hispanic" as an ethnic label had not yet been coined. The word was first introduced by the U.S. Bureau of the Census in 1980 as a replacement term for people of Spanish origin. Further, it was not until the latter part of the1970s that it became clear how rapidly this ethnic group was growing. Today, Hispanics number approximately 30 million and will become the largest ethnic group in the United States shortly after the turn of the century.

At the time of writing "Latino Mental Health" only about 500 articles, chapters and books of a psychological nature on Latinos could be located (Padilla & Aranda, 1974). Of this literature about 25% was only tangentially related to psychology or mental health. Over the ensuing years, research on Latinos has increased substantially. A recent search of PsychInfo using the term "Hispanic" resulted in more than 3,500 citations.

What is Hispanic Psychology?

A definition of Hispanic psychology is important because it sets the stage for theoretical paradigms, research methodologies and instruments used, and the interpretations we give to our findings. Specifically, Hispanic psychology is a branch of ethnic psychology where the population of interest is of Latin American origin, and where the target population resides within the U.S. or

Puerto Rico. Therefore, the study of Hispanics takes place in a context of majority-minority group relations.

It is also important to be clear about the term Hispanic and how it is used. A person who is of Latin American origin (e.g., Mexico, Cuba, Peru, Argentina, Guatemala) is designated for census purposes as Hispanic. Such a person may be an immigrant to the United States or may even be part of the 8th or 9th generation of U.S.-born citizens whose roots extend back to when the American west was part of Spain and later Mexico. However, the ethnic label that an individual uses to self-identify is very important. Many individuals prefer to identify as Latino rather than as Hispanic. Thus, in the remainder of this paper, I will use the two labels interchangeably because this practice is frequently found in the psychological literature.

More important than specific national origin or preferred ethnic label are the shared cultural values and traditions of the population and how these shared values and traditions influence behavior (Padilla, 1995). These shared values and traditions include: Spanish language usage; strong sense of familism; Catholicism; traditional male-female roles; celebrations of Latin national holidays; visual, performing and musical forms; etc. Since the majority of Hispanics are U.S. born citizens, most speak English fluently and are influenced by American values, traditions, and lifestyles. This is also true of immigrants who have resided in the U.S. for more than a few years.

Hispanic psychology also has roots in cross-cultural psychology, but is distinct in that it concentrates less on *inter*cultural group differences (e.g., cognitive differences between Japanese and American students) and more on *intra*cultural group differences. In other words, cross-cultural psychology is usually concerned with the systematic study of experience and behavior as it occurs across cultures in different nation states (e.g., Japan and the United States). Exceptions to this pattern often occur, of course, because the logic of the cross-cultural method can be used both within and across cultures

In contrast, Hispanic psychology seeks to understand the influence of culture, language, and minority-majority group status on people of Latin American origin who reside in the U. S. The *intra*cultural comparison enters because Latinos maintain aspects of their culture of origin while also acquiring American culture. Hispanic psychology then seeks to learn how differences in acculturation level also influence a wide variety of behaviors such as substance abuse, sexual attitudes and behavior, or coping responses to stressful environments.

The Effects of Oppression and Racism

An additional feature of Hispanic psychology is that often the focus is on understanding how oppression and racism influence the behavior of Latinos. As members of an ethnic minority group, many Hispanics have experienced prejudice and/or discrimination. When members of an ethnic group feel that they are the targets of discrimination, there is a natural tendency to form close social networks and to look toward their own group for support. This also affects the perceptions that members of an ethnic group have toward members of the majority group and their willingness to integrate socially, especially if it means giving up their culture and identity.

How oppression and racism influence the perceptions, feelings, and behavioral expressions of Latinos is not easily dismissed in Hispanic psychology, whereas these conditions are less relevant in cross-cultural studies. The reason that themes of oppression and racism are important in Hispanic research is that these topics emerge frequently in the accounts of Hispanics as they relate their experiences with majority institutions and individuals. Also research bears out the fact that racism creates social barriers that pose serious obstacles for Hispanics and these experiences shape their construction of a social identity (Niemann, Romero, Arredondo, & Rodriguez, 1999).

An example of how oppression and racism adversely affects Hispanic youth can be gleaned from data on school completion rates. Demographic information taken from numerous sources including the U.S. Bureau of the Census shows that Hispanics have the largest school dropout rate compared to all other ethnic group. Many majority group researchers attribute the poor showing in school achievement to: (a) their belief that education is not a core Hispanic cultural value, (b) to their belief that parents don't value education because of their culture, (c) and to students who do not invest themselves in schooling because they are not rewarded by the culture for school success.

An alternative explanation and one based on a Hispanic perspective is that underachievement of Latino students has noting to do with the culture, the family, or students. Rather, the root causes of the underachievement of Hispanics lie with the school culture and educational practices that predispose students to failure. This is very different from the "cultural deficit or disadvantage" hypothesis. For example, Valencia (1991) calls for an examination of the discriminatory and institutionalized racist practices of schools that channel Latino students into low educational tracks from which few can exit and which establish the pattern of school failure.

Eurocentric vs. Cultural-Specific Paradigms

Another unique feature of Hispanic psychology is the recognition that universalistic principles of behavior do not always apply when societal structures of dominance and oppression exist that influence a person's experiences and interactions with majority group members and institutions. The nomothetic or universal approach has come under sharp criticism from feminist and minority researchers because of its Eurocentric perspective. The most salient feature of the Eurocentric paradigm is its focus on a monocultural, male-oriented, and comparative approach to research. This approach lends itself to a very narrow database that results in biased conclusions of substantive psychological importance that are problematic for even majority group members who differ from the normative population. Sears (1986) in a provocative article declared that research based on college students tested in academic laboratories on academic-like tasks has resulted in social theories that are incompatible with the ordinary experiences of most non-college age majority-group adults.

The problem is worse for Hispanics who frequently differ markedly from the majority group who, because of privilege and status, are defined as the normative group. Hispanic researchers have recently begun to reject aspects of this Eurocentric approach and have become more active in developing instruments that tap the unique experiences of Latinos. For example, the author with colleagues developed a measure to assess psychological stress in Hispanics that specifically included items not found in other measures of stress. This instrument, the Hispanic Stress Inventory, includes items having to do with the stress of not speaking English well, changes in family values and relationships due to acculturation, and perceptions of discrimination (Cervantes, Padilla, & Salgado de Snyder, 1993). A very useful and thorough discussion on the development and adaptation of psychological instruments for use with Hispanics can be found in a book by Marin and Marin (1991).

In sum, the Eurocentric approach is appropriate so long as the population being studied possesses similar characteristics to the normative group on which instruments and theories were developed. The problem arises when "biased" instruments that favor White middle-class males are used in a comparative research design to examine differences between racial or ethnic groups. As we all know the comparative research design requires a statistical test between at least two groups that have been equated on all variables known to have an influence on the behavior in question. However, if both the construct being assessed and the method or instrument used to assess the construct originate in the same cultural context, then the comparative approach seriously increases the potential for bias.

The "New Scholarship" in Hispanic Psychology

In recent years, we have witnessed a paradigm shift in Hispanic scholarship, which is evident in much of the current psychological research conducted with Hispanics. This "new scholarship" is marked by conceptual models that incorporate Latino cultural and linguistic information, the development of new assessment measures and methods of data collection that are culturally sensitive to the target population. The outcome is better quality information and culturally appropriate interpretations of findings based on the sociocultural and ecological context in which Hispanics live (e.g., Garcia and Zea, 1997).

In a particularly insightful paper, Rogler (1989) asserts that research is made culturally sensitive only after meshing the process of inquiry with the cultural characteristics of the group being studied. This occurs when research from planning of the study, to the instrumentation of measures including translation if necessary, to the collection of data, and to the analysis and interpretation of the data is informed by the culture of the group being studied. Thus, Rogler (1989) calls for a paradigm shift, in which the study of Hispanics is valued for the knowledge that it creates and the incessant need to compare Hispanics to another social group is not always of value or of interest (Marin & Marin, 1991). This approach is a reaction against the general acceptance of comparing Hispanics to members of other ethic groups to determine whether group differences emerge on some dependent variable (e.g., intelligence, cooperative behavior, etc).

The "new scholarship" in Hispanic Psychology has to do with the importance given to the within group variation that had frequently gone unnoticed in conventional research. Hispanic psychologists have pushed for the realization that an understanding of the heterogeneity is important in unraveling the processes of how an ethnic group in America adapts and ultimately becomes incorporated into the fabric of the mainstream society (Marin & Marin, 1991). This approach emerged in the 1970s and has become more prominent in the writing of Latino researchers in this decade.

The cross-cultural approach has produced a great deal of important knowledge about members of many different cultural groups, including Hispanics. However, from a Hispanic perspective there are limitations in this approach when studying Latinos. For example, Hispanic culture promotes a strong sense of familism which means a preference for intrafamilial relationships and a cultural script known as *simpatia* which calls for positive interpersonal relationships. The researcher who does not possess an insider perspective on Latino culture could misconstrue familism and *simpatia* as evidence that Latinos are overly dependent and socially compliant. If I can draw an analogy from the Chomskian view of language, we might think about the workings of culture from a deep structure and a surface structure perspective. In other words, culture is not always what it seems on the surface. The "outsider" is likely to make assumptions about the culture and its influence on members of the social group that the insider knows are inaccurate. On the other hand, the insider has deep cultural knowledge and is able to use this knowledge to draw a more accurate understanding of the interplay of culture and behavior.

Another limitation comes about in assuming that all members of a cultural group share equally in the values, beliefs, customs, and knowledge of the culture that they affiliate with. This assumption does not apply to Hispanics. There is no single monolithic Hispanic culture in the U.S. today. Hispanic culture can be thought of as existing on a continuum ranging from very traditional to a cultural orientation that meshes nearly completely with U.S. culture. Thus, the full spectrum of cultural heterogeneity is critical in understanding Hispanics.

In short, Hispanic psychology is rooted in the cross-cultural approach with its numerous strengths and limitations. In the new scholarship of Hispanic psychology, researchers have evolved theoretical and methodological interests that specifically move away from comparisons of Hispanics with non-Hispanics and that concentrate on understanding the heterogeneity that underlies the different subgroups of Hispanics.

The Role of Acculturation and Biculturalism in Hispanic Research. Acculturation has emerged as the key variable in understanding Latino social behavior. Questions pertaining to how Latinos acquire and adapt to the majority group culture have been a central concern for the past 25 years in Hispanic psychology and figure prominently in many research studies. Numerous papers have been published which present measurement instruments for determining the acculturation level of a respondent (e.g., Cuellar, Arnold, and Maldonado, 1995; Padilla, 1980; Marin and Gamba, 1996). In addition, the process of immigration and acculturation has been conceptualized as stressful because of the intrapsychic conflict created by the necessity of incorporating new cultural knowledge and ways of comportment into a person's existing orientation (Cervantes et.al., 1991). In the traditional view of acculturation, incorporation of a new culture on the part of immigrants was seen through the lenses of a replacement model where the new culture came to dominate and replace the home culture. This view has given way to the conception of biculturalism (Berry, Kin, Power, Young, and Bujaki, 1989). According to this view, members of an ethnic group can maintain two cultural orientations (i.e., that of the dominant group and that of the ethnic group) and use either depending on what the social context calls for. Thus, the bicultural individual is behaviorally competent in the two cultures.

Research also indicates that biculturalism has distinct psychological advantages for ethnic minority populations (LaFromboise, Coleman, and Gerton, 1993; Padilla, 1995). For example, individuals who are bicultural experience less psychological dysfunction, are less likely to abuse drugs and alcohol, and generally do better in school than less acculturated individuals or more acculturated Hispanics who lack the knowledge (e.g., Spanish fluency) and behavioral skills of the culture of origin.

We still have much to learn about intergroup contact and the processes associated with acculturation and how to measure this construct. We need to recognize the significance of biculturalism and its protective role (LaFromboise et. A., 1993) in a society that demands adaptation and adjustment to mainstream behaviors, but which permits discriminatory practices against Hispanics forcing many to seek the comfort and safety of their home culture (Padilla, 1995). This conflicting message does more to motivate bicultural development than any other experiences.

Current Issues in Hispanic Psychology

In order to assess current research being carried out with Hispanics, I ran a search of PsychoInfo using the descriptor term Hispanic. The search resulted in approximately 3,500 hits and nearly two-thirds of the titles (approximately 2,200) appeared between1990 and 1998. Thus, research with Hispanics has shown a remarkable increase in the 1990s. Perusal of the titles indicated a wide range of topics and publication outlets.

Interesting patterns emerged from this bibliographic look at the current psychological literature. I first wanted to know what percent of the 2,200 articles appeared in American Psychological Association publications. My tally showed that only about 3% of the articles appeared in APA journals. The most frequently observed journals were the *Journal of Consulting and Clinical Psychology, American Journal of Community Psychology,* and *Developmental Psychology.* I also looked to see what percent of the materials had been published in the *Hispanic Journal of Behavioral Sciences (HJBS).* The *HJBS* is an interdisciplinary journal and publishes materials in anthropology, economics, education, linguistics, political science, psychology, psychiatry, public health and sociology. Thus, it was not a surprise to see that only 5% of the published papers appeared in the *HJBS.*

A content analysis of the materials publications between 1990 and 1998 showed that 75% of the published articles were in one of five major categories. Nineteen percent of the articles were related to education, academic achievement, testing, special interventions, or special education. Eighteen percent of the articles were in the area of social psychology, intergroup relations, prejudice, or social deviance. Another 15% dealt with clinical or counseling interventions, psychological assessment, support group and/or indigenous helping system. Eleven percent focused on substance abuse interventions primarily with adolescents, while 10% addressed issues of physical health status, utilization of health services, positive health practices, intervention and indigenous helping system. The remaining articles covered such topics as family dynamics, child rearing, aging and care of the elderly including Alzheimer's disease, gender studies, and mental health services and utilization practices.

Importantly, many of the papers reported the use of an instrument to assess the acculturation level of the respondents or implications drawn about the negative consequences of oppression on Hispanic informants. The content analysis also showed that important shifts have taken place over the past 25 years. First, there was the small number of papers on mental health treatment and utilization of services in the 1990s. This topic was the major theme in Hispanic research during the 1970s. Another surprise was the growing interest in the Hispanic elderly and Alzheimers Disease. Not surprising was the large number of papers with adolescents around topics of school achievement, substance abuse or prevention and social grouping (e.g., gangs). Notable in this research was the continued focus on problematic behaviors, rather than on success or hope. In sum, the study of Hispanic psychology has grown over the past 25 years and the field is marked by research questions that indicate the importance of studying an ethnic group that is growing in importance in the United States.

References

Berry, J. W., Kim, U., Power, S., Young, M., & Bujaki, M. (1989). Acculturation attitudes in plural societies. *Applied psychology, 38,* 185-206.

Cervantes, R. C., Padilla, A. M., & Salgado de Snyder, N. (1991). The Hispanic Stress Inventory: A culturally relevant approach toward psychosocial assessment. *Psychological Assessment, 3,* 438-447.

Cuellar, I., Arnold, B., & Maldonado, R. (1995). Acculturation rating scale for Mexican Americans – II: A revision of the ARSMA scale. *Hispanic Journal of Behavioral Sciences, 17*, 275-304.

Garcia, J. G., & Zea, M. C. (Eds.) (1997). *Psychological interventions and research with Latino populations.* Boston: Allyn and Bacon.

LaFromboise, T., Coleman, H. L. K., and Gerton, J. (1993). Psychological impact of biculturalism: Evidence and theory. *Psychological Bulletin, 114*, 395–412.

Marin, G., & Gamba, R. J. (1996). A new measurement of acculturation for Hispanics: The bidirectional acculturation scale for Hispanics (BAS). *Hispanic Journal of Behavioral Sciences, 18*, 297–316.

Marin, G., & Marin, B. V. (1991). *Research with Hispanic populations.* Newbury Park, CA: Sage Publications.

Niemann, Y. F., Romero, A. J., Arredondo, J., & Rodriguez, V. (1999). What does it mean to be "Mexican"? Social construction of an ethnic identity. *Hispanic Journal of Behavioral Sciences, 21*, 47-60.

Padilla, A. M. (1980). *Acculturation: Theory, models and some new findings.* Boulder, CO: Westview Press.

Padilla, A. M. (1995). *Hispanic psychology: Critical issues in theory and research.* Thousand Oaks, CA: Sage Publications.

Padilla, A. M., & Ruiz, R. A. (1973). *Latino mental health: A review of literature.* Washington, D. C.: U.S. Government Printing Office.

Padilla, A. M., & Aranda, P. (1974). *Latino mental health: Bibliography and abstracts.* Washington, D. C.: U. S. Government Printing Office.

Rogler, L. H. (1987). The meaning of culturally sensitive research in mental health. *American Journal of Psychiatry, 114,* 296–303.

Sears, D. O. (1986). College sophomores in the laboratory: Influence of a narrow database on social psychology's view of human nature. *Journal of Personality and Social Psychology, 51,* 515–530.

Valencia, R. R. (1991). *Chicano school failures and success: Research and policy agendas for the 1990s.* Basingstoke, England: Falmer Press.

Asian American Mental Health: What We Know and What We Don't Know

Stanley Sue
University of California, Davis
Department of Psychology

ABSTRACT

This chapter reviews and critically examines issues regarding the mental health of Asians in the United States. As a distinct ethnic group in the United States, Asian Americans have experienced value conflicts between their own ethnic culture and that of mainstream Americans, as well as instances of racial prejudice and discrimination. Given these experiences, it is important to examine the mental health status of Asian Americans. Several consistent research findings have emerged. First, few Asian Americans utilize the mental health system. Second, those who do use services are highly disturbed in terms of psychiatric disorders. Third, cultural factors appear to influence this pattern of low utilization but greater severity of disturbance. Fourth, epidemiological surveys show that the rates of mental disorders among Asian Americans are not extraordinarily low. Fifth, the relatively small population of Asian Americans, their heterogeneity, and the constantly changing demographic characteristics of the population have made it difficult to ascertain rates of mental disorders. More research is needed in order to gain insights into the within-group differences among Asian Americans, the role of acculturation in psychopathology and help-seeking behaviors, and cultural expressions of psychopathology.

The Population of Asian Americans

Asians in the United States represent many subpopulations including Cambodians, Chinese, Japanese, Filipinos, Koreans, Laotians, Asian Indians, Vietnamese, etc. (Asian and Pacific Islanders are often considered among the many subpopulations). Asians comprise only 4% of the United States population but 60% of the world's population. Despite the fact that the groups are heterogeneous, researchers have often studied the subpopulations as an aggregate group because Asians often show similar cultural values that are in contrast to Westerners (e.g., Asian Americans are more likely to exhibit interdependence and family orientation than do White Americans).

In evaluating the mental health of Asian Americans, some inconsistencies are apparent. As an aggregate, Asian Americans appear to be relatively successful in terms of low rates of divorce, crime, and juvenile delinquency and high rates of educational attainments, family income, and socio-economic mobility. On the other hand, they have experienced racial prejudice and discrimination, stereotypic portrayals in the media, and English language and cultural adjustment difficulties. Given the inconsistent data on well being, how adjusted are Asian Americans?

Mental Health Services Studies

Early research on Asian Americans examined their use of treatment services. Research uniformly demonstrated that Asian Americans failed to use mental health facilities in the same proportion as their population (Sue, Sue, Sue, & Takeuchi, 1995). The "underutilization" was apparent regardless of the Asian American subgroup, age, gender, or geographic location. Is it possible that this population is relatively better adjusted than other populations, so that greater utilization of services is unnecessary? In general, every population underutilizes in the sense that not all individuals with psychological disturbance seek help from the mental health system. The important question is whether or not Asian Americans with psychiatric disorders have a greater propensity than other populations to avoid using available services. Considerable indirect evidence suggests that Asian Americans are less likely than the general population to use community resources. Research findings have revealed that few Asian Americans seek mental health treatment and those who do use them exhibit a greater level of disturbance within the client population. A parsimonious explanation is that only the most disturbed Asian Americans tend to seek such resources. Asian Americans who show a moderate degree of disturbance are thus more likely than are comparable White Americans to avoid using services.

A number of factors affect utilization and effectiveness of mental health options. Some of the factors involve accessibility (e.g., including ease of using what's available, financial costs involved, and their location and availability, cultural and linguistic appropriateness of what is offered, knowledge of what's available, willingness to use them, and existence of alternative and competing or alternative treatment possibilities. Obviously, the nature and severity of one's problems also influences utilization.

Culturally-based factors such as shame and stigma, conceptions of mental health, and alternative options are important factors that affect utilization and appropriateness of mainstream services (i.e., those that are available to the general population of Americans).

For many Asian Americans, cultural attitudes and beliefs must be considered in the analysis of service utilization. Particularly important is the concept of "shame" or "face." "Haji" among the Japanese, "Hiya" among the Pilipinos, "Mentz" among the Chinese, and "Chaemyun" among the Koreans are terms that reveal concerns over the process of shame or the loss of face (Sue, 1994). Many Asian Americans tend to avoid the juvenile justice or legal system, mental health agencies, health services, and welfare agencies, because the utilization of services for certain problems is a tacit admission of the existence of these problems and may result in public knowledge of these familial difficulties. In particular, Asian Americans have been found to differ from White Americans in help-seeking behaviors for emotional difficulties. They are less likely to request outside help for these difficulties, turning first to their families for help and then to outside agencies or mainstream services as a last resort. Although most Americans are likely to turn to their families as the first resource, and to feel shame or stigma over certain problems, the avoidance of mainstream services is more pronounced among Asian Americans. That is, there is a differential effect caused by the strong concern over loss of face among Americans.

Because of shame and stigma, several consequences can be hypothesized. First, those behaviors that create shame and stigma are the ones that are most likely to be denied. Services for those behaviors tend to be underutilized. Second, Asian Americans may have needs for certain resources that are not reflected in utilization patterns. Third, if services are avoided and used as a last resort, then problems may be exacerbated, since there is a delay in finding assistance. It should be noted that the shame associated with having health and mental health problems may be more acutely experienced by Asian Americans who tend to reside in immigrant communities. In such communities, there are great expectations for doing well in America for the sake of the family members both in the United States and back in the country of origin. The personal networks in these communities are often extensive in which information about others is easily shared and disseminated. Within this context, the development of a mental health problem that may compromise a person's productivity or status can generate significant loss of face. Moreover, the need to seek outside help for such problems only exacerbates the shame.

Furthermore, cultural influences help to shape the symptoms exhibited when one is emotionally disturbed. Cultural factors also affect interpretations of the causes of disorders and interventions deemed appropriate to overcome health and mental health problems (Leong, 1986). In traditional Chinese culture, many diseases or physical afflictions are attributed to an imbalance of cosmic forces--yin and yang. The task is to restore imbalance through proper diet, exercise, and psychosocial relationships with others. Essentially, this is a holistic approach to health. Kinzie (1985) notes many Southeast Asians have a folk tradition in which illness is believed to be caused by physiological factors or supernatural forces (e.g., the consequence of offending a deity or spirit). Thus, they may have an unwillingness or inability to differentiate between psychological, physiological, and supernatural causes of illness.

Because of these cultural factors that influence symptom expressions and conceptions of illness, it is apparent that Asian Americans are likely to differ from mainstream Americans in the types of interventions used to prevent or treat emotional disturbances and illnesses. The interventions may involve restoration of balance and holistic approaches: Use of herbal medicine, consultations with folk healers or fortune tellers, acupuncture, certain forms of exercise, etc., that are consistent with their cultural beliefs. The extent of utilization of these alternatives among different Americans is unknown, although it is probably higher among recent immigrants or those who are relatively unacculturated to American society.

Asian and White Americans do have different conceptions of mental health and disturbance. Asian Americans tend to perceive more organic or somatic involvement in emotional disturbance. They also believe that the exercise of will power, the avoidance of morbid thoughts, and a focus on pleasant cognitions are means to enhance psychological well-being (Sue, 1994). Since professional mental health treatment often utilizes insight-oriented approaches that require self-disclosure of "morbid" (that is, disturbing and embarrassing) thoughts, Asian Americans may avoid Western forms of mental health treatment and seek medical treatment for emotional problems.

The research on utilization of mental health services and factors that inhibit utilization has been valuable in providing insights into mental health issues. However, to fully address the prevalence of mental disorders, epidemiological research is needed.

Epidemiological Studies

In studying the rates of mental health disturbances for Asian Americans, it is instructive to examine the rates of Asian who reside overseas (e.g., in Hong Kong, Japan, or Indonesia). As noted in Sue's review (1994), the evidence from epidemiological studies of overseas Asians does not support the notion that Asians are better adjusted than are Westerners. Several implications can therefore be drawn from this evidence. First, there is no reason to believe that being Asian is associated with significantly low rates of mental disorders and that Asians coming to the United States are less prone to developing these disorders. Second, Asian Americans are likely to be different from their overseas counterparts. Those who emigrate to the United States are not representative of those who remain (some come from educated, upper classes while others have led impoverished lives in their homelands and flee to the United States for better opportunities). Immigrants and refugees encounter unique experiences in this country such as exposure to different cultural values, English proficiency problems, minority status including racial/ethnic stereotypes, prejudice, discrimination, and a reduction in available social supports. In turn, these experiences can alter the stress-coping formulas for immigrants to the United States.

Indeed, one might speculate that Asian Americans might be under considerable stress because of these experiences. What do the empirical findings reveal? Large-scale and rigorous epidemiological studies have not been conducted on Asian Americans. Under such circumstances, one must form conclusions based on the preponderance of evidence. Until recently, the findings seemed to converge. They revealed that the prevalence of disorders among Asian Americans was as high as or even higher than those of other Americans--findings that were inconsistent with the general stereotypes concerning Asian well-adjustment. The studies of Asian Americans cover broad periods of time, starting from the 1970s to the present.

Many of the available surveys appear to indicate that significant numbers of Asian Americans are experiencing mental and emotional problems. Several studies have examined the rates of depression among Asian Americans using the Center for Epidemiology Studies of Depression (CES-D). Interviewing Asian Americans located through directories, organizations, and snowballing techniques in Seattle, Kuo (1984) found that Chinese, Japanese, Filipino, and Korean Americans on average reported slightly more depressive symptoms than did Caucasian respondents in other studies. Using the CES-D, similar findings of prevalence rates were reported by Hurh and Kim (1990). Korean immigrants residing in Chicago had higher scores for depression than did the Chinese, Japanese and Filipinos in Kuo's study. High rates of depression were also revealed in a telephone survey of Chinese Americans located in the telephone directory in San Francisco. Using the CES-D, Ying (1988) found the Chinese Americans to be significantly more depressed than the Chinese Americans in Kuo's study.

Certain groups such as Southeast Asian refugees and immigrants have extremely high levels of depression and other disorders (Westermeyer, 1988). Studies have also consistently shown that Southeast Asian refugees constitute a high risk group for mental disorders including depression and Post-Traumatic Stress Disorder (Kinzie et al., 1990). The elevated prevalence rates of psychopathology in the Southeast Asian refugee community are attributable to repeated exposure to catastrophic environmental stressors such as torture, combat, witnessing the death of family and relatives, and forcible detainment in harsh refugee camp conditions.

As noted by Leong (1986), studies of college students also suggest that Asian Americans experience major adjustment problems. For example, Okazaki (1997) compared the responses of Asian and White American college students on various measures of depression and anxiety. Results revealed that the Asian American students reported higher levels of depression and social anxiety.

All of these various studies (on students, refugees and immigrants, etc.) go beyond suggesting that, contrary to some stereotypes, Asian Americans are not an extraordinarily well-adjusted minority group. They support a more drastic conclusion--namely, that Asian Americans have lower mental health than do Whites. Before considering this statement, it should be noted that some more recent studies suggest that Asian Americans may indeed be better adjusted.

The Chinese American Psychiatric Epidemiological Study (CAPES) was undoubtedly the most rigorous and large-scale investigation of any Asian group in the United States (see Takeuchi et al., 1998). The project was a five-year community epidemiological study investigating the mental health problems and needs for mental health services among Chinese Americans.

The study had two specific aims: (a) to estimate the prevalence rates of selected mental disorders among Chinese Americans, and (2) to identify the factors associated with mental health problems among Chinese Americans. This study obtained 1,700 completed household interviews with Chinese-Americans residing in Los Angeles County. Followup interviews with the same respondents were conducted one-and-one-half years later which allowed the unprecedented opportunity to note changes in mental health and the factors associated with changes. The target population for the study includes Chinese immigrants and native-born residents of the United States.

The results were contrary to the findings of the studies reviewed earlier. Chinese Americans in the CAPES project did not have higher rates of mental disorders than Whites. While it can be argued that the rates of mood disorders among Chinese Americans were within the bounds of other Americans, the rates for anxiety were somewhat low. Why have the findings been so discrepant? Perhaps the conflicting findings with respect to the mental health of Asian Americans are attributable to the nature of the population.

Research Problems

What is the nature of the Asian American population? It is small, diverse, and ever-changing. Asian Americans represent only about 4% of the U.S. population. Consequently, researchers have had a difficult time finding adequate sample sizes and representative samples of Asian Americans. In many studies, samples of convenience were frequently used, often from quite different sources. Estimates of the prevalence of psychopathology may conflict because they are based on different kinds of samples.

The Asian American population is also extremely diverse and heterogeneous. More than 50 distinct ethnic groups (including Pacific Islander Americans), that may primarily speak one of more than 30 different languages, are included in the Asian American category. Even if we focus on one particular group, the heterogeneity is problematic and not encountered to the same extent by Asians in their homeland. For example, the Chinese American population is far more diverse than the Chinese population in overseas parts of the world. Chinese in the U.S. are composed of both native and foreign born, individuals who come from mainland China, Taiwan, Hong Kong, Singapore, Vietnam, and elsewhere.. Chinese Americans speak many dialects and languages, are exposed to American values, and are members of a minority group. All of these produce a very heterogeneous population. The same is true of nearly all Asian American groups--greater heterogeneity exists for their group in the U.S. than in their homeland. This is an important point to understand. It means that measures (such as the MMPI-2) which have been validated with Chinese in China may not have good validity for Chinese in the U.S. The problem confronting Asian American researchers is that the heterogeneity exists within a relatively small population. Outcomes from research investigations are then highly dependent on the particular samples drawn, and findings may fluctuate widely.

Finally, the Asian American population is undergoing rapid change relative to other populations. The Asian American population has doubled in size each decade for about the last three decades. The composition has changed, too. Whereas Japanese Americans were the largest group of Asian Americans a couple of decades ago, they are now outnumbered by Chinese and Filipino Americans. Today the Asian American population is predominantly overseas born, in contrast to the situation three decades ago. These demographic changes are likely to produce different prevalence rates. Because of the traumas faced by Southeast Asian refugees and their relatively recent entry into the U.S., prevalence rates for mental disorders among Asian Americans have dramatically changed.

In sum, there are some very good reasons why researchers have a difficult time ascertaining the prevalence of mental disorders among Asian Americans and why findings may be inconsistent. The relatively small size, heterogeneity, and changing demographic characteristics of the population pose more basic difficulties in research than do problems of measurement.

The specific prevalence rates of mental disorders among Asian Americans have been difficult to determine. Sufficient evidence does exist to show that Asian Americans are not significantly less prone to mental disorders than other ethnic groups. The relatively small population, heterogeneity, and changing demographic characteristics have hindered a more precise determination of prevalence rates within the Asian American population. Research concerning mental health issues should continue to be based on both the aggregate group (all Asian Americans) and particular Asian ethnicities (e.g., Chinese Americans).

References

Hurh, W. M., & Kim, K. C. (1990). Correlates of Korean immigrants' mental health. *Journal of Nervous and Mental Disease*, *178*, 703-711.

Kinzie, J.D. (1985). Overview of clinical issues in the treatment of Southeast Asian refugees. In T.C. Owan (Ed.), *Southeast Asian mental health: Treatment, prevention, services, training, and research* (pp. 113-136). Washington, DC: U.S. Government Printing Office.

Kinzie, J., Boehnlein, J.K., Leung, P.K., Moore, L.J., Riley, C., & Smith, D. (1990). The prevalence of posttraumatic stress disorder and its clinical significance among Southeast Asian refugees. *American Journal of Psychiatry*, *147*,913-917.

Kuo, W. H. (1984). Prevalence of depression among Asian-Americans. *Journal of Nervous and Mental Disease*, *172*, 449-457.

Leong, F. T. (1986). Counseling and psychotherapy with Asian-Americans: Review of the literature. *Journal of Counseling Psychology*, *33*, 196-206.

Okazaki, S. (1997). Sources of ethnic differences between Asian American and White American college students on measures of depression and social anxiety. *Journal of Abnormal Psychology, 106*, 52-60.

Sue, S. (1994). Mental health. In N. Zane, D.T. Takeuchi, & K. Young (Eds.), *Confronting critical health issues of Asian and Pacific Islander Americans* (pp. 266-288). Newbury Park, CA: Sage.

Sue, S., Sue, D.W., Sue, L., & Takeuchi, D.T. (1995). Psychopathology among Asian Americans. *Cultural Diversity and Mental Health, 1*, 39-54.

Takeuchi, D.T., Chung, R.C., Lin, K.M., Shen, H., Kurasaki, K., Chun, C., & Sue, S. (1998). Lifetime and twelve-month prevalence rates of major depressive episodes and dysthymia among Chinese Americans in Los Angeles. *American Journal of Psychiatry, 155*, 1407-1414.

Westermeyer, J. (1988). DSM-III psychiatric disorders among Hmong refugees in the United States: A point prevalence study. *American Journal of Psychiatry, 145*, 197-202.

Ying, Y. (1988). Depressive symptomatology among Chinese-Americans as measured by the CES-D. *Journal of Clinical Psychology, 44*, 739-746.

The Ruth H. Munroe Memorial Symposium: A Synopsis

Deborah L. Best, Convener
Wake Forest University
Department of Psychology

Participants

Carolyn Pope Edwards (USA) – Chldren's play and the emergence of a gendered division of labor: A reanalysis of the social behavior data collected by Beatrice and John Whiting, Ruth and Robert Munroe, and other collaborators

Daphne Keats (Australia) - Cross-cultural studies in child development in Asian contexts

Patricia M. Greenfield, Ashley Maynard, & Carla Childs (USA) - History, culture, learning and development

Suzanne Gaskins (USA) - The cultural construction of Yucatec Mayan children's activities

Susan Seymour (USA) - Household size and infant indulgence in an Indian town

Deborah L. Best (USA) - Gender concepts: Convergence in cross-cultural research and methodologies

ABSTRACT

The invited symposium honored the long and distinguished career of the late developmental psychologist, Ruth Hagberg Munroe, Research Professor of Psychology at Pitzer College, former Secretary-General and Honorary Fellow of IACCP. Trained by Beatrice and John Whiting, Ruth and her husband and colleague, Robert L. Munroe, carried out major fieldwork projects in American Samoa, Belize, Kenya, and Nepal. Ruth published steadily and widely, focusing primarily on the causes, correlates, and consequences of children's behaviors and designing systematic observational methods to improve our understanding of children. The symposium featured invited presentations by researchers who were her friends and colleagues and who shared her interests in developmental questions in cross-cultural context. The initial presentations in the symposium examined children's behaviors cross-culturally, the first reanalyzing data from the Six Cultures communities regarding gender differences in games and play, and the second looking at a number of different behaviors of Asian children. The next three presentations focused upon a single culture, the first two looking at Mayan culture, one examining weaving as an activity influenced by socialization and development, the other examining factors that influence the organization of children's daily activities. The final presentation compared the methodologies and findings of several large-scale cross-cultural studies of gender with those of the Munroes' observational projects.

Synopsis of the Presentations

The symposium began with a presentation by *Carolyn Pope Edwards* who provided a qualitative and quantitative reanalysis of spot observation data on child's play from the classic "Six Cultures" and "Children of Different Worlds" studies, directed by John and Beatrice Whiting. Among the Whitings' collaborators were Ruth and Robert Munroe, who directed the collection and analysis of spot-observation data. These data, collected primarily in the 1950s and 1960s, offer a portrait of the world of childhood at a time when all of the communities were relatively more isolated than today and when children had less access to the media and to manufactured child-oriented products as well as the trash and refuse of global industry so useful for constructing homemade toys. School, for most of the samples of children, played a less prominent role in children's lives and hopes for the future, and was not an area of daily pressure.

Frequency data on creative, fantasy, role, and competitive play indicated that complex symbolic play was much less evident in cultural communities where children's work involvement was important to the economy; children were provided few toys, bought or homemade, and adults did not join them in play or games. In general, these children, particularly girls, whose work involvement was earlier and more extensive than boys, showed more involvement in sociable work ("playful work") where they practiced adult skills, strategic planning, and cooperative problem-solving, rather than creative or constructive play. However, Edwards pointed out that settlement pattern, the work expectations of children, and access to material goods for making toys, such as cast-off wire and tires, also influenced children's opportunities for play. The running records provide many interesting examples of all types of play from the communities.

Also taking a cross-cultural comparative orientation, *Daphne Keats* reviewed developmental research conducted over a number of years with colleagues in Malaysia, Thailand, Indonesia, and China. These studies have demonstrated cultural influences on formal operational thinking, they have highlighted the importance of values in various cultural groups, and they have shown the similarity between children's and adults' views of intelligent behavior. In each of the countries where Keats and her colleagues have conducted research, there are far-reaching changes that now challenge traditional cultural values in family relations and child-rearing practices.

Moreover, these Asian countries are multicultural with literally hundreds of ethnic groups and indigenous peoples who have many languages and very different cultural backgrounds. Asian children growing up in the twenty-first century will experience both the advantages of such rich multicultural environments as well as the concomitant tensions and stresses that often develop between diverse ethnic groups. Extant western theories of development and child rearing do not address the traditional cultural contexts in these countries nor the vast changes brought about through urbanization and the globalization of industries. Keats cautioned that an important challenge for developmental psychology is to create theoretical and research orientations that are appropriate for such changing non-western contexts.

In the first of the studies focusing upon a single culture, *Patricia Greenfield* described her research that has followed a group of Zinacantec Mayan families for 24 years, spanning two generations. Greenfield and her colleagues investigated weaving as the focal activity through which to examine the relationship of ecological change to socialization and development. Using videos, ethnography, artifacts, and experimental data, the researchers tracked intergenerational change and continuity at the cultural level and the processes of learning, innovation, and cognitive development on the individual level. Predictions were confirmed that as the system in Zinacantan moved from subsistence to an entrepreneurial cash economy, the scaffolded instructional process of weaving education would change to learning by trial and error, and weavers would innovate new patterns. The study points up the importance of adding a sociohistorical or institutional perspective to the traditional emphasis on the individual in developmental research.

In the second of the single culture studies, *Suzanne Gaskins* examined Yucatec Mayan children's daily activities. Her investigation incorporated the Vygotskian insight that children's activities are organized through interpersonal construction of contexts and behavioral options that are consistent over time. Gaskins explored the range and distribution of Yucatec Mayan children□s daily activities from infancy through adolescence, emphasizing how cultural beliefs and practices contribute to the construction of the children's activities. She found that in order to understand the quantitative estimates of maintenance activities, social orientation, play and work, they needed to be interpreted by three "cultural principles of engagement," including adult work, cultural beliefs about children, and the independence of children's motivation. By understanding the cultural meaning brought to the activities by both the children and their caregivers, the differences between Mayan and Western children□s behavior could be understood as part of two different cultural systems rather than as isolated instances of precocity or deprivation.

In the last of the three cultural studies presented, *Susan Seymour* tested John Whiting's "household size/infant indulgence" hypothesis which the Munroes examined in their cross-cultural socialization research. The hypothesis assumes that if there are many hands to care for an infant, high indulgence will be more likely to occur. However, as the Munroes found, increased household size may result in a decline in exclusive maternal caretaking and an increase in multiple caretaking of infants. Previous research support for the hypothesis has been mixed, suggesting that the relationship between ecological factors, such as household size and density, and the care of infants is not a simple one.

Seymour investigated the household size/infant indulgence hypothesis using naturalistic observations of infant caretaking from the initial two years (1965-67) of her longitudinal study of 24 families in Bhubaneswar, India, a town with striking diversity in household size and structure. Families in the Old Town part of Bhubaneswar were compared with those in the New Capital part of Bhubaneswar. Old Town is organized by ties of caste and kinship along traditional patrifocal extended family lines. New Capital is a more recently built nuclear family neighborhood with modern amenities and is organized according to the household head's position in the government service hierarchy. The samples from the two areas were stratified by socioeconomic status. Even though multiple measures of household size and of indulgence were used, Seymour found only modest support for the household size/infant indulgence hypothesis. However, she did find that the amount of maternal caretaking did decline in households where multiple caretakers were available. Seymour concluded that household size cannot be treated independently of other socio-cultural factors, such as social stratification and gender. She speculated that multiple caretaking produces a diffusion of affect and a sense of interdependence in infants and young children that underlies joint family life in India. Seymour's findings have important implications for how researchers conceptualize indulgence as well as "multiple caretaking" and its relationship to the emotional bonds that children develop.

In the final paper in the symposium, *Deborah Best* examined the convergence in cross-cultural findings from the Munroes' studies of gender-related aspects of development with findings from studies she has conducted with her colleagues. These two research programs contrast different methods and multiple behavioral assessments of gender concepts obtained from children and adults. To examine children's gender-relevant behaviors and those of their parents in less developed societies, the Munroes generally have used interviews, narrative forms of field observation, and spot observations, a modification of time sampling developed by Ruth Munroe. In contrast, Best and her colleagues have used primarily self-report measures to study gender concepts, such as stereotypes, with large samples of school-age children and young adults in more developed countries.

Interestingly, the findings from these two methodologically diverse research traditions demonstrate a high degree of correspondence in the gender-related behaviors, attitudes, and beliefs of children and young adults in these different populations that have been studied. For example, the Munroes report that observational data indicate that boys are more aggressive than girls across a wide variety of cultures. Likewise, Best and her colleagues have shown in more developed societies with their picture-story technique that aggression is one of the earliest learned and best known of the male stereotype traits. Turning to girls, the Munroes' observational data show that girls are more frequently involved in infant and child care, and perhaps as a result, they are more nurturant (e.g., offer help and support). Similar to the male findings, Best's research shows that nurturance is a major component of the female stereotype (e.g., affectionate, appreciative, softhearted), and in most cultures, children know this concept well by eight years of age. There were also similarities in the findings of the adult studies. When asked about ideal traits for adults, mothers in American Samoa, Belize, Kenya, and Nepal told the Munroes that women should be shy, obedient, and gentle, while men were described as strong, courageous, and independent. These characteristics correspond closely with those reported by college students in the studies conducted by Best and her colleagues. In her concluding remarks, Best proposed that biological influences establish predispositions and limitations on the development of gender roles and behaviors, but socialization experiences and cultural expectations alter the development of gender differences and concepts.

Epilogue

The symposium highlighted the importance of studying both more proximal influences on development, such as mothers teaching daughters to weave, as well as more distal influences, such as economic changes occurring in Asian nations. It is clear from this collection of papers that current theory and research in developmental psychology must address both western and non-western contexts and cultural values in order to understand and explain the complexities of development how behaviors originate, are maintained, and change.

As is evident from the presentations in this symposium, single culture studies provide a window for examining proximal causes of behavior within one context. It is easy to see the influence of adult priorities on children's daily activities when closely examined within the Mayan context. On the other hand, cross-cultural comparisons broaden the framework and demonstrate the generality of findings across a range of cultural contexts. For example, Edwards' work demonstrates the clear influence of the gendered division of labor on children's play behaviors across a varied set of cultures. When convergence is found between studies that differ in methods as well as samples, such as those considered in the comparison of the Munroes' research and that of Best and her colleagues, cross-cultural "universals" appear robust and stable. It is evident that both single culture and cross-cultural studies of development that use observational, experimental, and self-report methods are all essential to achieve a rich, more complete picture of development and the factors that influence its course.

Ruth Munroe was fascinated by "big picture" questions, such as those discussed in this symposium, as well as by the details that make research challenging. She delighted in attending and participating in sessions at IACCP and other meetings that focused upon these sorts of cross-cultural developmental issues. As a lasting tribute to Ruth Munroe's contributions to the field, the participants in this symposium, representing her many friends and colleagues around the world, hope these presentations will inspire other researchers to explore the role of culture and context in their investigations of developmental questions.

The Millennium Prelude Symposium: A Synopsis

Cigdem Kagitcibasi, Convener
Koc University, Istanbul
Department of Psychology

Ype H. Poortinga, Convener
Tilburg University
Department of Psychology

Participants

Yoshihisa Kashima (Australia) - Conceptions of Culture and the Person for Psychology
Theodore M. Singelis (USA) - Cross-Cultural Analysis of Social Behavior
Uichol Kim (South Korea) - Understanding Culture
Heidi Keller (Germany) and Patricia M. Greenfield (USA) - The History and Future of Development in Cross-Cultural Psychology
Fons J. R. van de Vijver (Netherlands) and Kwok Leung (Hong Kong, PRC) - Methodological Issues in Psychological Research on Culture
Sara Harkness (USA) - Applied Cross-Cultural Psychology: Perspectives on Interventions in Health and Education
Zeynep Aycan (Turkey) - Can Industrial and Organizational Psychology Offer Solutions to Developing Country Problems?

ABSTRACT

The concluding symposium at the IACCP Jubilee Congress, referred to as "the millennium symposium", was aimed at a critical evaluation of the current state of affairs in cross-cultural psychology and an assessment of how and where it can make a contribution in the next 25 years. In this chapter the convenors give a brief account of the preparations and a synopsis of the presentations as they were given during the congress. As stated in the program, some of the basic issues addressed in the symposium included which theoretical and metatheoretical perspectives shape current cross-cultural psychology; which ones of these promise to sustain into the first quarter of the next century; whether these perspectives promise to open up cross-cultural psychology towards broader directions of growth and progress -- or conversely to narrow the outlook of researchers; what are the research and methodology implications of the current debates in the field; what research directions can be envisaged for the coming decades; what may be the future balance of pure and applied research emphasis; how is cross-cultural research expected to relate to the other social and behavioral sciences; how will it relate to applications; and how will it inform humane policies and contribute to human well-being, particularly in the face of increasing globalization.

The concluding symposium at the IACCP Bellingham Congress was titled: "Millennium Prelude: The Present State and Future of Cross-Cultural Psychology". The origin was an invitation extended by the Scientific Program Advisory Committee to the co-convenors. The invitation asked us to convene a symposium that would reflect on the field of cross-cultural psychology as it currently exists as well as on future developments. We were to seek broad representation, both topically and culturally. As convenors we faced what in French eloquently is called "un embarras de choix", the embarrassment of not knowing what choices to make in the face of many attractive alternatives, in respect of both topical coverage and speakers.

In a letter we asked each intended participant for a review of the prospects of a particular field, with on the one hand giving a critical evaluation of the current state of affairs, and on the other hand providing an assessment of how and where cross-cultural psychology can make a contribution in the next 25 years. Given the constraints of time, not more than five topics could be defined, but we allowed, and in some cases even encouraged, double authorship or the division of a topic into two parts. In the selection of speakers two criteria were prominent: a previous record of cross-cultural research and the expectation of continued contributions to the field during the coming years. In short, we looked for speakers who can make their own words come true.

In as much as psychology is a field of research we chose to have presentations on both theory and methodology. For the contribution on theory the main subject seemed to be conceptualizations of culture that had relevance or are expected to have future relevance in cross-cultural psychology. For methodology we sought a presentation that would review difficulties of reaching valid cross-cultural findings without getting caught up in the -- in our opinion not very fruitful -- controversy on quantitative versus qualitative approaches.

Attention had to be paid explicitly to application as the ultimate justification of scientific research. Here we deliberately focused on the Majority World. Two contributions dealt with application, one with health and education and the other with organizational psychology. The first choice to us appeared to be self-evident, in view of the emphasis in the cross-cultural literature. The choice for a contribution on organizational psychology is perhaps less obvious; it reflected our conviction that the main dimension of cultural differences in the world today is associated with the so-called North-South contrast.

The limited number of topics implied restrictions on the selection of thematic issues. Of the two slots still available we designated one to social psychology and one to ontogenetic development. Although cross-cultural research can be said to span the whole of psychology, studies on social behavior form the largest part of our literature. It seemed evident to us that indigenous research had to be represented, as well as the more traditional approaches in which cross-cultural differences in social behavior are mainly examined in function of ecocultural and sociocultural antecedents. The inclusion of ontogenetic development was based on our expectation that culture as the context of behavior, and development as the emergence of differentiation in behavior, will become integrated in future cross-cultural psychology, more than has been the case so far. Also, developmental science provides analytic grounds for studying how and why certain behavioral patterns emerge in certain sociocultural contexts and how changes in these patterns come about.

Synopsis of the Presentations

The symposium started off with a presentation by *Yoshihisa Kashima* on "Conceptions of culture and the person for psychology". In a brief historical overview an outline was given of the contrast between the empiricist and interpretivist conception of the human mind. The former approach sees the mind as part of nature, the latter as separate from nature. Kashima argued that there is an emerging consensus on four points: (i) mind consists of physical matter (ii) culture is part of the evolutionary history of the human species, (iii) ontogenetic development is a process of enculturation, and (iv) context and the human mind constitute each other. This consensus transcends the old controversy and leads to a new conception of the person.

Kashima mentioned three issues that demand attention. First, there are different views on culture. Some authors, like Triandis, take culture as a meaning system, with enduring patterns, whereas others, like Cole, maintain a practice-oriented viewpoint in which culture is seen as a signification process. The second issue is the evolutionary explanation of culture; according to which domain specific modules have arisen that are the outcome of adaptation processes. The third issue is how to explain cultural stability and cultural change. On this point there are various approaches, specifying ecological adaptation (e.g., Berry), cultural evolution (e.g., Campbell), Lamarckian transmission of acquired traits (e.g., Kagitcibasi), or non-linear dynamics (e.g., Sperber). Kashima questioned the heavy reliance on processes of adaptation, submitting that culture may have non-adaptive, or at least adaptation-neutral, consequences.

The first of the two contributions on social cross-cultural psychology had the title "Cross-cultural analysis of social behavior" and was presented by *Ted Singelis.* He argued that in a number of respects the future has already begun. There is an increasing proportion of social psychological publications being concerned with culture. There is also an increasing conceptual input from outside the USA with notions like interdependent self-construal and harmony. Research has become more complex, with increasing concern for the elaboration of contextual variables. Finally, researchers tend to look more at mediating variables, unpackaging differences, rather than to group membership as a source of differences.

Singelis also spoke about future trends that still have to begin, but that he hopes to see developing. There is a need for "middle level theorizing", linking psychological variables with culture level variables as they are studied in cultural anthropology and sociology. Surprisingly few studies look at the actual dyadic interaction of individuals belonging to different cultures. Also, more attention should be paid to application. Singelis made some very concrete predictions. He suggested that topics like individualism-collectivism, acculturation and emotions will remain hot, and that topics like self-presentation, situation-linked and role-linked norms, and masculinity-femininity will become hot.

In the second presentation on social behavior *Uichol Kim* described the pervasiveness of culture, i.e., the context in which we function. Culture is the eyes through which we see reality, easy to see for the outsider but difficult for the insider. Within a culture members share intentions, values and goals. A distinction was drawn between three approaches to culture. First, there are the *universalists* who believe that there is no thing as culture. They will argue for universal values like human rights, but these are abstract principles which universalists cannot define for a particular national context without falling into an ethnocentric stance. Then there is the *comparative approach* based on culture as independent variable and individual behavior as dependent. This dichotomy is unnecessary and fraught with tautology. The third approach, to which Kim subscribes, is the *indigenous approach* in which culture is not something outside, but the way in which we think, feel and behave. It is not a variable, but a superordinate construct that provides meaning, efficacy and coherence to its members.

Indigenous psychology was defined as "the scientific study of human behavior (or mind) that is native, that is not transported form other regions, and that is designed for its people" (Kim & Berry, 1993, p. 2). Various key aspects of the indigenous psychologies approach were listed, like the rooting of understanding in a particular context, taking serious cultural boundaries more than national boundaries, the use of multiple methods appropriate for the phenomena studied, and the empirical discovery, rather the a priori assumption of psychological universals. Finally, Kim cautioned against the uncritical use of religious and philosophical indigenous writings to describe and explain how people thin and feel without empirical verification.

The contribution by *Heidi Keller* and *Patricia Greenfield* started off with a clear mission statement: "Our theme is that better integration of a developmental approach into cross-cultural psychology can enhance the future of our field, both empirically and theoretically". In the view of Keller and Greenfield culture is strongly present in developmental research, but development is not substantially present in the cross-cultural psychology literature. One reason for this is the dynamic orientation of development, a trend that is at variance with the more static orientation of most culture-comparative studies. Other reasons are the dominant position of the questionnaire as a research method and the use of (late adolescent) university students as subjects.

There is a biological grounding of maturation and developmental stages, affecting the acquisition and expression of cultural behavior. A developmental perspective can help to unravel the mechanisms of interplay between biology and cultural influences. This was illustrated with the following example. Babies are born with capacities for contacts with caretakers that have been demonstrated in a wide range of societies, but actual caretaking arrangements vary widely. Keller and Greenfield distinguished two major developmental trajectories. One is the European style of interaction with much face-to-face exchange and independent sleeping arrangements; this leads to the development of an independent self and an individualistic way of life. The other style relies on multiple caretaking and extensive body contacts with the baby; this promotes the conception of an interdependent self as found in collectivistic societies. Thus, basic cultural learning that forms the foundation for a later independent or interdependent style starts very early in life.

In their presentation *Fons van de Vijver* and *Kwok Leung* distinguished two kinds of *parti pris* (preconceived views) that act as impediments to the rate of progress in cross-cultural psychology. There are parti pris that have arisen within cross-cultural psychology, such as the uncritical acceptance of observed differences in social behavior, the uncritical rejection of ("real") differences in cognition, insufficient attention for inequivalence of data and a tendency to overgeneralize findings. There are also parti pris inherited from mainstream psychology, including a focus on significance testing, rather than on estimates of effect size, and poor measurement of the environment. Van de Vijver and Leung presented a table with four types of culture comparative research taken from their recent book (Van de Vijver & Leung, 1997) and outlined the major strengths and weaknesses of each.

For the future they predicted that there will be two groups of researchers: "natives" and "sojourners". Sojourners are researchers from other areas who do an occasional cross-cultural study. Because of the popularity of "culture" their influence will grow and it is important that they are informed about appropriate standards for research. Natives are those who identify with cross-cultural psychology and they will continue to unravel culture-behavior relationships. The natives would do well to utilize recent psychometric advances, like item response theory, structural equation modeling, and multi-level analysis. Another much needed development is a more quantitative approach to inequivalence to overcome the traditional dichotomy between biased and unbiased data.

Views on how cross-cultural research has informed interventions in health and education were offered by *Sara Harkness.* Outstanding examples concern maternal and child health and nutrition, literacy and home-school relations. Over the years two shifts have had a major impact. First, there has been shift away from so-called deficit models. This has been inspired by cultural traditions that foster superior school achievement (e.g., in Asia). The second shift is the growing attention for immigrant populations and minorities within industrialized countries that has blurred the distinction between cross-cultural and intracultural studies. In addition, there is a growing diversity in the cultural and academic background of the researchers, which has an impact not only on theory but also on the issues studied.

Future research based interventions in health and education should seek a balance between the trends towards a global psychology and towards extreme relativism. Cases in point are attention deficit disorders; they have culturally variable elements leading to unique configurations in the form of culture-specific syndromes.

In the talk about industrial and organizational psychology *Zeynep Aycan* expressed her surprise that this popular field of applied psychology is so poorly represented in cross-cultural journals like the *Journal of Cross-Cultural Psychology.* She saw as a major reason the misguided idea that organizational psychology is for businesses and industries that cater to the rich, while the first duty of cross-cultural psychologists is towards the real problems of real people.

However, development as meant in the term "developing countries" refers primarily to the economic sphere. Research in organization and work psychology concerns issues like job design, leadership, and motivation, contributing to improvement in work conditions, satisfaction, health and productivity. It is a complicating factor that applications of North American findings have proved to be problematic elsewhere in the world. Indigenous approaches should be developed to ensure culture fit in areas such as unemployment, work force development, leadership development, child labor, transfer of technology and integration of foreign investment.

The symposium was concluded by one of the co-convenors (CK) with some brief comments addressing challenges that face cross-cultural psychology with respect to position, substantive issues and application.

Cross-cultural psychology needs to sustain its identity as a general methodological and conceptual orientation in psychology. There has to be close interaction with mainstream psychology, otherwise cross-cultural psychology may come to be ignored. On the other hand, it should not be engulfed by the mainstream, as seems to be threatening now in ethnic minority research. Also, cross-cultural psychology needs to keep its international character. We should not return to the earlier pattern of Westerners imposing theory and collecting data in the Majority World.

As far as substance is concerned, cross-cultural psychology needs to be better informed by and come to terms with evolutionary and biological psychology. It should be recognized that cross-cultural psychology is not necessarily searching for cultural differences; both differences and similarities are important. By showing invariance of behavior and variations across a wide range of cultures we can make an important contribution to psychological science. At the same time, there is a need to go beyond the individual-level analyses to develop broader integrated perspectives. For this it is necessary to seek collaboration with other disciplines, such as sociology, economics, health, and education.

A good balance must be found and sustained between research and application. Psychology must be relevant to development efforts, particularly in the Majority World. We should get involved in policy relevant work and strengthen the voice of advocacy of cross-cultural psychology.

Epilogue

As conveners we have appreciated to work on this symposium and we would like to thank the Scientific Program Advisory Committee for the invitation to organize it. We also like to thank the participants for their cooperation and for the efforts they made in the preparation of their presentations. Comments after the symposium from members of the audience have given us the impression that the contributions generally were well received. A special issue of the *Journal of Cross-Cultural Psychology* is being planned with a set of articles based on the presentations of the Millennium Symposium.

Many important fields of cross-cultural research have been shining in absence; we can mention research on migrant and ethnic minorities, on cognition, on emotion, on personality and on the transfer of tests, as glaring examples. An overview of cross-cultural psychology requires simply more time than is available in a single symposium. Still, it appears to us that the contributions have conveyed an impression of cross-cultural psychology as a viable field of research that has potential for further expansion and advancement in the period until IACCP's next jubilee.

Speculation is in many ways at variance with science, though vision is closely associated with it. The task of the participants was not an easy one. It may still turn out to be an ungrateful one as well, if their expectations about the future should prove to contain unwarranted speculations and they will be made to "eat their words" at the Golden Jubilee congress of IACCP. We feel confident that they nevertheless are looking forward to that occasion.

References

Kim, U., & Berry, J. W. (1993). Introduction. In U. Kim & J. W. Berry (Eds.), *Indigenous psychologies: Research and experience in cultural context* (pp. 1-29). Newbury Park, CA: Sage.

Van de Vijver, F. J. R., & Leung, K. (1997). *Methods and data analysis for cross-cultural research.* Beverly Hills, CA: Sage.

Historical and Epistemological Contributions

Seventy-Five Years of Cross-Cultural Psychology in New Zealand

Jane and James Ritchie
University of Waikato
Department of Psychology
Hamilton, New Zealand

ABSTRACT

The Maori, the indigenous people of New Zealand, had a well-developed psychology to explain and govern human behaviour as they perceived it. On contact with Western thought a cross-cultural awareness developed. Early records from missionaries, travellers and gentlemen scholars reveal a curiosity about the metaphysics of both cultures. In the 1920s the inter-cultural dialogue entered the universities and laid the foundation for cross-cultural psychology in New Zealand. Scholars such as Ernest Beaglehole and Margaret Mead in the 1920s used the Maori example in laying the theoretical foundations for this area of study. For seventy-five years New Zealand has had its own distinct tradition which grew from both culture and personality within anthropology and from the psychological study of culture and the individual. Currently, a new theme has emerged as Maori psychologists balance the dialogue as they develop an explicit Maori ethnopsychology. This paper will review this history and indicate its likely future development.

The most profound and yet difficult task that confronts cross-cultural psychologists is to wrench our field of study from its ethnocentric roots in Western science and metaphysics. The indigenous people of New Zealand, the Maori, have developed their own explanations of human behaviour, systems of regulating and controlling it and definitions of the human condition. One effect of the dominance of Western philosophies of science has been to suppress that development and to cast the indigenous model into a role of separation and consign it to history. Post-modernist thinking is a reminder of the multiplicity of methods of inquiry and conceptions of humanity within any culture and between cultures. In this paper we will review the history of cross-cultural psychology in New Zealand. Seventy five years ago New Zealand psychologists recognised that cross-cultural psychology cut to the very core of the discipline and also was a necessity in the local context. Even before this, observations by non-psychologists, but of a psychological nature, were laying the foundations for understanding the Maori viewpoint.

Early Reports

The first generation of scholarship in New Zealand was dominated by the Royal Society Gentlemen Scholars of the nineteenth century who, coming to our shores, wrote of the exotic life and beliefs of the natives. Their accounts are, of course, coloured by their various interests and styles.

Some sought to portray what was strange and exotic, reflecting the interests of their countrymen in barbarous practice and sensational custom (Belich, 1996). Others brought to New Zealand that European tradition of interest in 'the ancients' and in their writings transformed the authenticity of Maori myth and religion, custom and belief, into an antipodean version of the Graeco-Roman tradition. The best records came from the scientists and journal keepers who were part of the early entourage of the voyagers of exploration, such as Cook, Banks and Darwin (Beaglehole J.C. 1962,1967,1974).

After them came the administrators and missionaries (Salmond, 1995, 1997). They were a mixed bag. For the most part, they sought to deny and discount native practices. Records from outstanding observers such as Colenso, Sir George Grey and Kendall offer accounts that reflect Western notions of civilization, progress, social evolutionism and colonial attitudes of superiority. (Belich, 1996).

Maori Psychology Emerges

Maori were themselves acute observers of these new arrivals and, with literacy added to their oral tradition, began to leave records which a new generation of Maori scholars are researching and recovering. Contemporary Maori scholars are, for example, currently building an electronic data base to access the extraordinary range of newspapers published under Maori auspices from the middle eighteen hundreds, right through to the present day. Much of this is written in Maori and it constitutes an important resource, not only for historians, but for those who are interested in the whole range of topics that constitute Maori psychology. There is no greater corpus written in a Polynesian language. One may read there of matters which reveal traditional metaphysics, cosmology, value priorities, motivation, strategies of negotiation and conflict resolution, cultural stance in relation to current issues of the day, matters of status and gender, aspirations - a whole inventory of psychological concerns.

With the formation late in the nineteenth century of the Polynesian Society Maori themselves contributed to the western world of scholarship by writing about their own world view. The Journal of the Polynesian Society, though targeted at the varied scholarly audience of its membership, was, in fact, the earliest anthropological journal to be published anywhere and clearly represents an intention to present to the world a home grown discipline respecting no boundaries but defining its own. An indigenous anthropology was about to be born. The major figures were Sir Peter Buck, who became the director of the Bishop Museum in Honolulu, and Sir Apirana Ngata who, as well as being an important political figure, strongly advocated as far back as 1912 the entry of anthropology to the curricula of New Zealand universities. When this did happen, however, in the early nineteen fifties, it was through the neo-colonial importation of a distinctly British version of that subject, which owed more to Malinowski than to Maori. The opportunity to have a New Zealand based anthropology illuminating both cultures passed us by.

The University: The Foundations

In similar fashion, as psychology began its difficult birth pangs in New Zealand, growing first within the formal teaching of philosophy as mental and moral science, there were advocates for it to take on the task of reflecting the bicultural experience. The pioneers, Sir Thomas Hunter and Ivan Sutherland, were little known beyond their home shores. Hunter was a liberal humanist and rationalist who, influenced by the "scientific psychology" of Wundt, determined to bring the new psychology to the Southern hemisphere. After his visit to Titchener's laboratory at Cornell he quickly established a psychological laboratory at Victoria University College in Wellington. At first it was the experimental psychology which took root. But that was not all. Hunter had read the *Volkpsychologie* of Wundt also. In the 1920's Hunter began to lay the foundation for both social psychology and cross-cultural psychology in New Zealand.

Hunter trained Sutherland who became a strong advocate for the recognition of Maori psychology and saw the contribution New Zealand psychologists might make to correct the ethnocentrism of Western psychology (1940). But Sutherland's energies were caught up in the cultural renaissance which Ngata and a powerful group of Maori political activists had initiated at the turn of the century. Till then the public and political view had been that Maori population and culture were in decline and would ultimately disappear. By the nineteen twenties both the population and the culture of Maori were developing a new vitality. Sutherland took a strong stance, challenging the New Zealand intellectual world to understand and accept a broadened view. With his death in 1949 those efforts to examine Maori cognition lapsed, though a new generation of Maori interested in these matters is emerging (Ritchie, in press).

Two of the students trained by Hunter and Sutherland, Reo Fortune and Ernest Beaglehole, went on to make a truly international contribution and helped to lay the foundations of cross-cultural psychological study. After completing a masters degree in mental and moral philosophy, Fortune left

New Zealand for Cambridge, England in 1926. Under Hunter his graduate thesis had been on dream symbolism, a topic which led him away from psychology toward cultural anthropology.

Fortune never considered himself to be a psychologist. Yet, *The Sorcerers of Dobu* was, in fact, deeply psychological. This was quickly picked up by Ruth Benedict in *Patterns of Culture* as an almost quintessential demonstration of how deeply a psychological trait, suspicion, penetrated every aspect of the life of the people of that island.

Culture and Personality

Ernest Beaglehole, the other renowned student of Thomas Hunter, was part of the founding brotherhood and sisterhood in the study of culture and personality. His whole intellectual focus was to integrate psychology and anthropology in a new field of inquiry, ethnopsychology, and especially to relate it to Maori and Pacific affairs. His university education under Professor Thomas Hunter culminated in a research thesis on propaganda already revealed his distinctive blend of social psychology applied to a vital issue of the day which threatened human liberty and rights.

As was the pattern of the time, he left to join other young New Zealand intellectuals for the exciting world of London where he studied at the London School of Economics under Ginsberg. There, under the socialist ethos which transcended narrow disciplines, he pursued his Ph.D research on acquisitiveness, the psychological basis of property, a matter of deep concern to the Fabians. *Property* (1932) became a classic. Through its tabulation of data from thirty cultures, it predated the Human Relations Area Files at Yale, cross-cultural psychology's first data base. This work came to the attention of George Peter Murdoch visiting from Yale, where Dr. Peter Buck, a Maori, held the Stirling Professorship in anthropology . Beaglehole chose to go to Yale for his post-doctoral study as a Commonwealth Fellow. There he was excited by the new ideas of the founder of psychological anthropology, Edward Sapir. Beaglehole was simultaneously disenchanted with the descriptive anthropology of Franz Boas and, across the Atlantic with Malinowski. He was enthused with the work of Ruth Benedict. Her analysis of Pueblo culture in her article 'Psychological Types in the Cultures of the South West' (1930) initiated a furore of intellectual discussion. *Patterns of Culture* (1934) was already in manuscript when Beaglehole came to Yale.

Sapir drew around him an exciting group of young and old, stimulated by the possibility that psychoanalysis and psychological linguistics could provide anthropology with the theoretical framework it lacked and so desperately needed. Besides Benedict the group included Margaret Mead, Ralph Linton, later Abraham Kardiner, John Whiting, George Peter Murdoch and others. Beaglehole maintained contact with these people throughout his life, but especially with Margaret Mead.

Focus on the Pacific

Mead did her doctoral work on canoe types in Polynesia though her masters degree was in psychology. She then went on to the series of studies in Pacific island cultures and became the doyenne of culture and personality. It was she who promoted the notion that by studying childhood one might best perceive the patterning of culture. (Mead 1978). In 1928, Mead married Reo Fortune and together they went to Manus. The resulting publications showed their separate interests, Mead (1930) in the relationship between childhood and cultural character, Fortune (1935) in ritual and religion.

The South Pacific had become an area of intense interest for anthropologists old and new. At the theoretical level, the work of Malinowski and Radcliffe-Brown had opened questions of the universality of Freudian theory. The question of human universals was of intense interest to the young Ernest Beaglehole, now responding to the challenges which Sapir and his group had thrown to both disciplines, the psychological and the anthropological.

The next phase in this story develops from his association with the great New Zealand anthropologist, Te Rangihiroa, Peter Buck, who held the Sterling Professorship in Anthropology at Yale in association with the Bishop Museum in Honolulu. A close friendship developed and Buck invited Beaglehole and Malsin to join his research team in Hawaii. First he had to fulfil his obligations as a Commonwealth Fellow. He became a consultant to the Bureau of Indian Affairs and with Pearl Malsin, who he later married, researched aspects of the daily life of the Hopi of the second Mesa (1935). Their publications established their reputation as anthropologists. Their articles described economic and ritual life, ownership and inheritance, topics which grew out of the earlier interest in property, but also of childhood and parenting (1935, 1936,1937).

In 1934 Buck arranged for them to go to the remote northern Cook Islands atoll, Pukapuka, as part of his comprehensive Pacific Island ethnographic survey. This visionary enterprise in what was termed 'salvage anthropology' sought to provide a baseline ethnography for every Pacific culture, a project fatally disrupted by World War 11. The Beagleholes completed their research in 1935 and returned to Honolulu to write up their notes, still the most comprehensive of any Bishop Museum expedition, and published as *Ethnography of Pukapuka* (1938). But the transition to psychological anthropology is also evident in their writings about the symbolism in myths, chants and love poetry, courtship, marriage and child rearing. They also continued their series of studies of contemporary

Polynesian life with the fieldwork which resulted in the publication of *Some Modern Hawaiians* in 1939.

In 1937 Beaglehole returned to Hunter's department of Mental and Moral Philosophy as a Senior Lecturer, a position he held until 1948 when Hunter became principal of the college and Ernest was appointed the first Professor of Psychology in New Zealand. Throughout this time he published both from fieldwork and wrote important articles on the concept of character structure in the rapidly developing area of culture and personality (1940a, 1940b, 1941, 1944).

Ernest and Pearl continued their ethnographic work in Tonga (1941) and then in Otaki they applied the concept of character structure to contemporary Maori life. By now, psychological theory and explanation was becoming dominant in their work. It provided a more complex and sophisticated framework than the simplistic theory of needs that dominated orthodox anthropological ethnographies.

From this work they wrote *Some Modern Maoris* (1946), which, with a powerful foreword by Te Rangi Hiroa, exploded into controversy because of its frank revelations about Maori life and its Freudian interpretations. It also drew Ernest into a consultative role on contemporary Maori affairs.

The anthropological record was completed with the publication in 1957 of *Social Change in the South Pacific,* a study of Rarotonga and Aitutaki and the supervision of research on social change in Murupara, the Rakau studies. In these studies his attention was focussing on the worldwide phenomenon of the disappearance of traditional indigenous lifestyles, and the challenge of modernity.

Through all of this work he was known internationally as a psychological anthropologist, deeply committed to the application of knowledge to the improvement of the human condition. But in New Zealand, as well as in the way he viewed himself, he was a psychologist, an observer and appreciator of the quirks and idiosyncrasies as well as the depths of human nature.

As the first professor of psychology in New Zealand, Beaglehole not only established a thriving department, which quickly achieved international standing but also developed strong applied links into mental health, education and industry. He was also one of that influential group at Victoria University College of the University of New Zealand who deliberately set out to shape government policy through the application of social science theory and information.

After 1948 the Department he founded grew and flourished and his students spread out into industry, adult education, education and research, child and family guidance, social work, clinical psychology; six of his students became professors of psychology in New Zealand universities. The

Victoria department became known internationally for its blend of academic and applied social psychology as well as for its ethnopsychology, now more commonly known as cross-cultural psychology.

Throughout Beaglehole's professional life, Pearl continued to be his sharpest editor, a challenging critic and commentator, and his sparkling and outgoing collaborator. Her linguistic ability enabled their fieldwork to penetrate areas of understanding inaccessible to him. For example, the lists of words for parts of the anatomy in Pukapukan are in her handwriting; she, not he, recorded the chants, myths and love poetry, so explicit the Museum did not dare publish them. Her vivacity and charm complemented his rather shy, dry, introverted style.

Beaglehole's Legacy

Despite Beaglehole's early death, within New Zealand his legacy persists in his writings which established the cross cultural tradition there and in the students he trained. Five are important and stand directly in this tradition. Graeme Vaughan developed the research methodology of applying the techniques of experimental social psychology to issues of identity, prejudice and race relations, but his work belongs more in the mainstream of social psychology. Michael Hills has largely used the techniques of attitude measurement to address issues of biculturalism and race relations. David Thomas did the typical 'kiwi' thing by sailing around the Pacific collecting cross-cultural information on parenting. He then developed a strong interest in applied social psychology in cross cultural settings and in community psychology, of which he was the founder in New Zealand.

Our own work began with a re-examination of the child rearing hypotheses of the Beagleholes and exploration of the concept of character structure applied to contemporary Maori. The work in Murupara was characteristic of its time in its use of projective techniques which were liberally applied in a hypothesis testing framework. We have traversed and reassessed this territory in some detail elsewhere (Ritchie and Ritchie, 1979,1984, 1989,1997). What has survived that re-evaluation is the descriptive fieldwork, stripped of the Freudian interpretations and reassessed in a straightforward developmental framework. In a sense, we could now see Maori parenting and family style in the wider context of the corpus of work on Polynesian childhood (Ritchie and Ritchie, 1979) Once we had dropped the baggage of projective methods, the field records could be addressed within a dual framework of Maori contexts and the forces and influences of social change.

This equipped us to enter the action research mode which was developed within the Centre for Maori Studies and Research from 1972 onwards. Others were making the same shift, in particular, Allan Howard and Ron Gallimore had begun their highly creative partnership in Nanakuli, on Oahu, Hawaii. Their work took ours and transformed it into an action programme of early childhood, family education, and community building. (Gallimore, Boggs and Jordan, 1974; Howard, 1974). That work was the foundation for the Kamehameha Early Education Project.

In the Maori Centre we began an early childhood education intervention programme based substantially on language development and cognitive and behavioural skill training. (Ritchie, 1977, 1978) This programme demonstrated that active and intensive direct instruction could achieve learning and language objectives and skill acquisition that would facilitate easy transition to the learning environment of the primary school. In addition, it showed that, by focus on the child, there were measurable and positive outcomes for the family as a whole. The experimental programme ran for three years but at the end of that time funding ceased.

In the mid to late seventies, prevailing public policy concerning Maori development was summed up in the government programmes called 'Tu Tangata'. This title covered a variety of programmes such as the stimulation of small business ventures based on Maori communities, job training and job seeking programmes based on a buddy system, the stimulation of positive identity and self esteem through group cultural activities and other ways of overcoming, in the language of the day, disadvantage. The idea of Maori language based early childhood education came to fruition with the establishment of the Kohanga Reo movement in 1982. There are now 650 such language nests which are the most vital and successful element in the revival of Maori language.

Social Action in the Field

There are many ways in which cross-cultural psychology has developed as an applied aid to social well-being in Aotearoa/New Zealand. There have been two avenues of operation. One addresses issues concerning cross-cultural understanding and biculturalism and the other objectives which Maori themselves define and articulate and to which our discipline can be of service.

Essential to the first of these is the progressive need to inform New Zealanders of the legacy of the past and its continuing effects in institutions that need bicultural definition and the reduction of discriminatory policies, actions and forces (Ritchie, 1994, 1997). This is the bicultural agenda.

The second challenge itself has two parts. Maori now make their own claim upon our profession to develop culturally safe and appropriate procedures all the way from the practice of clinical psychology to the fundamentals of research methodology and ethical conduct. It is now widely recognised that psychology grew from the stem of Western learning and therefore has the legacy of its monocultural past to deal with. The professional branches of psychology now have a new agenda. This can be a joint enterprise but the other part of this challenge is simply to stand aside while Maori themselves repossess and develop their own cultural psychology.

Let us be very clear about this. As psychologists we cannot simply walk away from this and say if Maori psychologists want to do this, then they should get on with it and it is no business of ours. If we do that, then the bicultural agenda itself is severely compromised. The appropriate stance is to contribute to that development as requested, when required, as a contribution of service to rebalancing the bicultural partnership which is currently so heavily weighted in endorsement of Western models and means. Before psychology as a whole can contribute to the post-colonial world, it needs to confront its own colonial history, with positive attitudes replacing positivism.

In professional terms the New Zealand Psychological Society has begun to develop its affirmative stance by incorporating cultural recognition into its charter statement and code of ethical practice. To monitor and attend to implementation it has established a national standing committee on biculturalism. The professional journal of the Society, the Bulletin, regularly includes a section on bicultural issues and several university departments now have added programmes in Maori psychology. Maori psychology research units now operate at the University of Waikato and Massey University.

The development of Maori psychology, in the domains of both academic scholarship and in applied practice, is proceeding rapidly. It is for Maori to speak definitively concerning this. But as they do so, we hear fundamental questions of epistemology, ontology, varieties of logic, cognitive styles and models being addressed by Maori in ways that derive basically from Maori world view and their considerations of the nature of knowledge. Beyond this, there are now many Maori graduates employed in the administration of the justice system, penal institutions, community sentencing, alternative treatment and rehabilitation centres, psychiatric institutions, private practice, social welfare operations, both government and private, in the various health and education services and in government departments.

When the International Association for Cross-Cultural Psychology began twenty five years ago ethnopsychology was still a branch or subset of psychology. That is no longer a tenable position and the Association itself has become a forum to which scholars of many ethnicities may bring their own psychologies, the fulfilment of the recognition that multiple realities coexist, have equal importance and validity and yet, in total, contribute to a common humanity.

References

Barnouw, V. (1973). *Culture and personality.* Illinois: The Dorsey Press.

Beaglehole, E. (1927). *Social aspects of propaganda.* Unpublished Master's Thesis, Wellington, New Zealand: Victoria University College.

Beaglehole, E. (1932). *Property: A study in social psychology.* London: Allen and Unwin.

Beaglehole, E. (1940a). Cultural complexity and psychological problems. *Psychiatry, 3,* 329-339.

Beaglehole, E. (1940b). Notes on the theory of interpersonal relations. *Psychiatry,*

Beaglehole, E. (1941). Social psychology and interpersonal theory. *Psychiatry, 4,* 61-77.

Beaglehole, E. (1944). Character structure, its role in the analysis of interpersonal relations. *Psychiatry, 7,* 145-162.

Beaglehole, E. (1957). *Social change in the South Pacific.* London: Allen and Unwin.

Beaglehole, E. & Malsin, P. (1935). *Hopi of the Second Mesa.* Wisconsin: American Anthropological Association.

Beaglehole, E. & Malsin, P. (1936). Ownership and Inheritance in a North America Indian Tribe. *Iowa Law Review, 20,* 304-316.

Beaglehole, E. & Malsin, P. (1937). *Notes on Hopi economic life.* New Haven: Yale University Publications in Anthropology.

Beaglehole, E. & Malsin, P. (1938). *Ethnology of Pukapuka.* Honolulu: Bishop Museum.

Beaglehole, E. & Malsin, P. (1939). *Some Modern Hawaiians.* Honolulu: University of Hawaii.

Beaglehole, E. & Malsin, P. (1941). *Pangai: Village in Tonga.* Wellington: Polynesian Society Memoir No. 18.

Beaglehole, E. & Malsin, P. (1946). *Some Modern Maoris.* Wellington: NZCER.

Beaglehole, J.C. (1962) (ed). *The Endeavour Journal of Joseph Banks* Sydney: Angus and Robertson.

Beaglehole, J.C. (1967) (Ed). *The Journals of Captain James Cook.* Cambridge: Hakluyt Society.

Beaglehole, J.C. (1974). *The Life of Captain James Cook.* London: Black.

Belich, J. (1996). *Making peoples.* Auckland: Penguin.

Benedict, R. (1930). Psychological types in the cultures of the Southwest. Proceedings of the 23rd International Congress of Americanists. September, 1928, New York.

Benedict, R. (1934). *Patterns of culture* New York: New American Library.

Fortune, R.F. (1932). *Sorcerers of Dobu.* London: Routledge.

Fortune, R.F. (1935). *Manus religion.* Philadelphia: American Philosophical Society.

Gallimore, R., Boggs, J.W., and Jordan, C. (1974). *Culture , behavior and education* . Beverly Hills: Sage.

Howard, A. (1974). *Ain't No Big Thing.* Honolulu: The University Press of Hawaii.

Howard, J. (1984). *Margaret Mead : A life* New York: Simon and Schuster.

Mead, M. (1930). *Growing up in New Guinea* New York: William Morrow.
Mead, M. (1972). *Blackberry winter* New York: Simon and Schuster.
J.E.R. (1965-1966). Obituary Notice Ernest Beaglehole 1906-1965. *Proceedings of the Royal Society of New Zealand , 94.*
Ritchie, J.E. (1966). Obituary Ernest Beaglehole 1906-1965 *Journal of the Polynesian Society, 75*, 109-119.
Ritchie, J. (1994). *Becoming bicultural.* Wellington: Huia Press.
Ritchie, J. (1997). What ever happened to Cross-Cultural Psychology? *The Bulletin, 92,* New Zealand Psychological Society, 17-21.
Ritchie, J. (1998). Ivan Sutherland. *The Dictionary of New Zealand Biography* Volume 4, S 57, 506.
Ritchie, J. (1977). *Tamariki Maori.* University of Waikato: Centre for Maori Studies and Research.
Ritchie, J. (1978). *Chance to be equal.* Picton: Cape Catley.
Ritchie, J. & J., (1978). *Growing up in New Zealand.* Sydney: Allen & Unwin.
Ritchie, J. & J. (1979). *Growing up in Polynesia.* Sydney: Allen & Unwin.
Ritchie, J. & J. (1985). *E Tipu E Rea: Polynesian socialization and psychological development.* University of Waikato: Centre for Maori Studies and Research.
Ritchie, J. & J. (1989). Socialization and character development in Alan Howard and Robert Borofsky (eds) *Recent developments in Polynesian anthropology.* Honolulu: University of Hawaii Press.
Ritchie, J. & J. (1997). *The Next generation: Child rearing in New Zealand.* Auckland: Penguin.
Salmond, A. (1991). *Two worlds: First meetings between Maori and Europeans 1641-1772.* Auckland: Viking.
Salmond, A. (1997). *Between worlds.* Auckland: Viking.
Sutherland, I. (1940). *The Maori people today.* Wellington: NZCER.

Cross-Cultural Psychology: Is it Time to Revise the Model?

Forrest B. Tyler
University of Maryland
Department of Psychology

ABSTRACT

Kuhn focused on the role of exemplars in critiquing science. He argued that they are the core of any theory, teaching the scientist how to recognize and assign meaning to science's subject matter. Science's content does not exist without exemplars to identify and abstract it. Further, a science's laws cannot be tested until there is content against which to test them. The theme of this paper is that cross-cultural psychology's exemplars promote Western biases. For cross-cultural psychology to be culturally and comparatively based, it must incorporate a wider range of exemplars. To support my critique I cite evidence in the current data and paradigmatic forms of cross-cultural psychology supporting the conclusion that it is embedded in a physical science positivist model and actively perpetuates ethnocentric cultural imperialism. In conclusion, changes in direction that will enable the field to counter these biases and move toward a more transculturally balanced approach are highlighted.

The highlighting of the twenty-fifth anniversary of the International Association of Cross-Cultural Psychology (IACCP) and the number of people from all parts of the world who celebrated it confirmed that this anniversary was an important sign of the continuity of the association's shared purposes. However, a twenty-fifth anniversary does not have the same significance to all cultures, so the decision to celebrate this anniversary is an exemplar of an imposed etic promoting a Western bias. That is the point of this paper. It is time to check on IACCP's biases and revise its model of cross-cultural psychology.

Kuhn (1970) focused on the role of examples, or exemplars, as the core of any theory. A science's laws cannot be tested until there is content against which to test them. Exemplars teach scientists how to recognize that content and what meaning to assign it. Mannheim (1936) argued that what competing scientists are trying to do is make a compelling argument that their own paradigm is the *general paradigm.* They can then make the rules for evaluating competing theories while remaining free from critique. If Westen psychologists can define cross-cultural psychology's general paradigm as well as its anniversaries, they can impose their biases on the study of psychology in the world's cultures.

In *The Racism of Psychology* (1994), Moffitt and Owusu-Bempah pointed out that psychology's founders were white European and American racists. Their general paradigm institutionalized their biases. Consequently, active racists are no longer needed to perpetuate them. Such Western biases, including its physical sciences model, have also been perpetuated in cross-cultural psychology's general paradigm. People are defined as objects of study, as devoid of emergent creative capacities and choice, not as creators of meaning. Culture is defined as an external force impinging on people. Cross-cultural psychologists must change their paradigm and incorporate a wider range of exemplars. In the next section, I cite several representative issues in regard to such changes of the field's structure will enable this field to move toward a more defensible pancultural stance.

First, I want to make it clear that I believe in an "objective reality" apart from any limits on our capacities to define it. I agree with Wetherell and Potter, two discursive theorists, who pointed out that "you still die if your plane crashes into a [New Zealand] hill whether you think that the hill is the product of a volcanic eruption or the solidified form of a mythical whale" (p. 65, as cited in Sampson, 1993). However, our "constructed reality", what we did to cause those deaths and how we understand them are products of our cultural discourses, and they are equally important.

Limitations of Current Cross-Cultural Paradigms

The six controversial issues in this section illustrate how our discourses and arguments about cross-cultural psychology's paradigm highlight its current limitations.

Active agent vs. Object - Paranjpe vs. Poortinga: In the 1997 *Cross-Cultural Psychology Bulletin*, Paranjpe reviewed the *Proceedings* of the 1994 IACCP Conference and Poortinga (1997) reacted to the review. Although the review and the reaction covered a number of points, my focus is primarily on one aspect of their differences. Paranjpe commented on cross-cultural psychology's Western imperialistic nature and commitment to objective and quantitative methodology. Specifically, there is a power differential between the subjects who are studied and the psychologists who study them. That power is "epistemic, in the sense that the psychologists are presumed to be the knowers and the so-called 'subjects' are no more than objects of knowledge and not knowers in their own right" (p. 14). Culture is studied as a set of variables influencing the phenomena under observation rather than as different ways to understand, interpret, and evaluate human issues. Poortinga (1997) agreed that misapplication of methodology and the Western imperialistic bias of cross-cultural psychology are distressing. But, he defended objective and quantitative methodologies and argued for incorporating indigenous approaches within a universalist framework.

These two view of people highlight cross-cultural psychology's paradigmatic divide. To Poortinga they are subjects, informants, "donors of data", not participants as there is no equality in the process between them and the researchers. His " professional responsibility makes [him] the person who is accountable for the legitimacy and ethical standards of the project " (p. 12). Poortinga argued in favor of Western positivism; Paranjpe in favor of a general paradigm in which the researcher and the researched are both knowers and known (or at least knowable). Poortinga's general paradigm may be valid and adequate for studying inorganic subjects; along with Paranjpe, I question whether that paradigm is sufficient for studying living humans.

Different epistemologies: Murayama (1997), a Japanese organizational psychologist, challenged both the universalist-positivist model and the more recent postmodernist constructionist approaches to understanding behavior. His point is that any social group is heterogeneous, it is composed of individuals who differ in their epistemological approaches to reality. However, each culture is assumed to have its character because advocates of one of the several possible epistemological types becomes dominant. The others are suppressed and use various strategies to cope with and survive under the dominant mainstream. Consequently, both of these paradigms are based on an assumption of a homogeneity that does not exist. The diversity among people and the differing organizing frameworks of cultures get lost in our studies of them.

Biases in the General Paradigm of Cross-Cultural Psychology's Origins: Gustav Jahoda (1997), one of cross-cultural psychology's founders, identified two important themes in the "Zeitgeist" of that time: (1) With the growing revulsion to racism, culture became a relevant vehicle for organizing the study of differences, and (2) with decolonization and growing interests in social change, the idea emerged that people and/or societies should become more civilized. He added that the word "civilizing" is no longer politically correct, but it was a precursor to the current term, "modernization". Substituting "culture" for "race" and "modernizing" for "civilizing" has not changed the general paradigm of psychology. It is still characterized by the cultural biases of developed societies.

Definitions and Exemplars: Cooper and Denner's (1998) critique of Triandis' focus on individualism and collectivism is of particular importance because his approach has captured much attention among cross-cultural psychologists. Triandis' approach highlights differences between cultures and tends to portray them as holding mutually exclusive, stable, and uniform views. That approach excludes other possible differences between cultures and raises questions about which stable differences to highlight. Hofstede (Hofstede & Vunderink, 1994) identified masculinity/femininity as a distinction that accounted for almost as much difference between cultures as individualism-collectivism. He suggested that individualism-collectivism has received greater emphasis is because it fits readily into the ongoing institutional cross-cultural dialogue between Western societies and those of Asia. In contrast, classifying cultures by the masculinity/femininity distinction yielded a quite different grouping. Masculinity oriented cultures include Japan, the Anglo group, central European, and some Latin countries. Feminist oriented cultures include North European, some Latin American, some Southern European, some Asian, and East African countries.

CDG-NCDG Interactions and NCDG Contributions: Murayama made the point that non-dominant groups get suppressed and find ways to cope within the constraints imposed on them. To some extent, psychologists with non-Western orientations are faced with that situation in this association. Berry (Berry, et al., 1992) proposed that we find etics by starting with emics from dominant culture. Doing so excludes starting with emics originating in non-dominant cultures. Further, psychologists from dominant cultures cannot address contextual aspects of non-dominant cultures of which they are not even aware. Those aspects can only be addressed by psychologists or other members of the non-dominant culture, and, as I just noted, their perspectives are excluded.

Rotter's concept of locus of control (1967) has spawned thousands of studies, and its definition and properties have been explored in many cultural contexts. In the U.S., primary control is *mastery* of the external environment; in Japan, it is *adaptation* to the external environment; in traditional Hinduism and Buddhism, it is *denial* of desire. My colleagues and I compared patterns of locus of control in culture-defining and non-culture defining groups of adolescents in the U.S., India, the Caribbean, and Colombia (Tyler, Brome, & Williams, 1991; Tyler & Sinha, 1988; Zea, Tyler, & Franco, 1991). In general, an internal locus of control served students better; however, being moderately external worked better for our African American students. We also found that males and females were making different choices. U.S. and Indian males saw themselves as active agents, creating and taking advantage of their opportunities. U.S. and Indian females saw themselves as passive agents, controlling their fates by reacting to the choices society provided them. U.S. females thought life would provide each a fair set of choices; Indian women did not. In brief, people's concepts of control are part of their cultural embeddedness, cultural status, and that culture's definition of control; a conclusion that can be arrived at only by incorporating non-dominant culture and group perspectives.

Cross-cultural similarities and differences in development: The Munroe's published the first cross-culturally based text in human development in 1975. In its 1995 reissue, they emphasized that large, overarching theories discount the distinction between what is universal and what is not. However, studies of the lower stages of development, for example Erikson's *basic trust*, have identified characteristics that may approach universality. They recommended that the search for such universals should continue at these primary levels. They also speculated that "perhaps, the next ambitious theoretical system will provide greater understanding of adult humans' ingeniously diverse modes of thought and behavior." (p. 152)

Snarey's (1985) review of Kohlberg's theory of moral development also found cross-cultural similarities at the early developmental stages, and all cultures included the kinds of reasoning that Kohlberg had identified. At more advanced stages, several cultures included other principles, for example, collective principled reasoning. Such differences lead to the conclusion that we can pursue people's "ingeniously diverse modes of thought and behavior" only by starting with holistic exemplars from a number of cultures and attending to their significance for everyone, including the people providing them.

Revising the Model

I believe there are three changes that will enable cross-cultural psychology to transcend some of its current biases and move toward a more defensible multicultural stance. They are summarized as follows:

Add New Exemplars. We cannot get there with our present exemplars. Our current dominant paradigm has provided enormously important information, but using an experimenter defined and controlled approach limits the input of research participants. Human events are not random, independent occurrences, nor devoid of ingenious thought. Different societies organize themselves in different ways and, as Murayama noted, they may emphasize the integration of heterogeneities rather than the maximization of homogeneities. We need to identify and include exemplars which allow us to study these possibilities.

Revise our View of Human Interactions. Our data support that people are not just passive objects of study. On that basis, I advanced the concept of ethnic validity; that is, the idea that people actively organize their understanding of what is valid for their lives in relation to their psychological environments, and they interact by actively managing processes of convergence, divergence, and conflict (Tyler, Brome, & Williams, 1991). By approaching our interactions from that perspective, we can offset some of the paradigmatic biases we inevitably bring with us.

A personal, professional experience provides an example. I became interested in cross-cultural psychology because I wanted to know why a generation of young people in the U. S. found Indian gurus so fascinating, and whether the psychosocial processes of racial integration in the U.S. and caste integration in India were similar. I took what I thought to be the sensible approach of going to India to learn about the cultural context that created and sustained them. Other issues that interested me while there were the psychosocial correlates of religious belief systems, the nature of helping and help-seeking behaviors in children, and the evolving life roles of college women. None of these topics permit of in depth study without the active participation of the respondents. We got complex responses that revealed patterns of convergence, divergence, and conflict in meanings within each of these cultures as well as between them. We found that people's experiences are ecologically and culturally embedded, oriented to their survival and well-being.

Our findings do not mean there are no cross-cultural generalities. It suggests that generalities are embedded in culturally organized holistic configurations, and cannot be identified without stepping outside of particular cultural contexts. At my own university, a Black South African senior fellow in journalism recently wrote an editorial in the university newspaper. She had focused her life on addressing white racist oppression of people of color. In our very multicultural university, she found that oppression comes in many colors and contexts, and is perpetuated by many different kinds of people toward many other different kinds of people. Oppression is the central human issue, not the color of the oppressors or the oppressed. Only by escaping her own culture did she, or does any of us, learn how much of our view of reality is indigenous and culture bound. Incorporating the possibility that all people are knowers will enable us to include more kinds of exemplars and more successfully overcome our current biases.

Research is an Intervention. We are among society's designated agents to advance and utilize psychology in humanity's interest, and bear a responsibility to understand the nature of our impact. Part of that impact is that participating in research changes people. They learn about themselves and their world from their participation. If we treat them like guinea pigs, they learn what that means. If we treat them like "knowers", they learn what that means. It affirms to them that they are important contributors to human knowledge. The data we gather changes us as well. The information it contributes about the nature of peoples' lives as known and as knowers can contribute to our own lives and to improving the quality of people's lives, to such issues as social justice, and to survival of life on the planet However, it can also serve destructive purposes unless applied with a prosocial orientation and relevant knowledge and skills.

Summary

In summary, I have identified three significant research foci in cross-cultural studies; namely, the forces that influence us as "known"; the process of becoming "knowers"; and our functioning as knowers, as creators in our own lives. The first two foci have been dominant in cross-cultural psychology. By limiting our approach to these two, we have severely restricted the scope of inquiry in cross-cultural psychology and, as Poortinga and Van de Vijver (1987) argued, found culture predicts very little of the variance.

By contrast, attending to people's contributions as knowers who are creative agents in their lives and their worlds has had seminal consequences. It was input from a variety of people in a range of cultures that led us to know that internal locus of control can mean "to adapt to or ignore reality" as well as "to manipulate it". It was attention by psychologists from a feminist oriented culture that provided evidence of cultural biases in ignoring masculinist-feminist differences between cultures. Those of us from masculinist cultures had never even noticed. Our growing awareness of elements of cultural imperialism in cross-cultural psychology has stemmed primarily from those we call indigenous psychologists and others who have become responsive to their views.

To accord legitimate status to the third focus of "knower" issues requires that we recognize, as Paranjpe proposed, that our subjects are "knowers in their own right". To do that we must accord equal status to the perspectives of people from different cultures and different statuses in them, and not obscure their differences by averaging them out. We must also accord equal status to appropriate methods for studying the issues they consider important, seeking out the best from a range of cultural perspectives, and providing space at meetings and in our journals for the best work from those perspectives as judged by their criteria as well. Thereby we can revise our cross-cultural model and broaden our contributions to human knowledge and well-being.

References

Berry, J.W., Poortinga, Y.H., Segall, M.H., & Dasen, P.R. (1992). *Cross-cultural psychology: Research and applications*. Cambridge: Cambridge Unilversity Press.

Cooper, C.R., & Denner, J. (1998). Theories linking culture and psychology: Universal and community-specific processes. In J.T. Spence, J.M. Darley, & D.J. Foss, D.J. (Eds.). *Annual Review of Psychology, 49*, (pp. 559-584). Palo Alto, CA: Annual Reviews.

Hofstede, G.& Vunderink, M. (1994). A case study in masculinity/femininity differences: American students in the Netherlands vs. Local students. In A. Bouvy, F. J.R. van de Vijver, P. Boski, & P. Schmitz (Eds.). *Journeys into Cross-Cultural Psychology: Selected papers from the Eleventh International Conference of the Internat ional Association for Cross-Cultural Psychology*. (pp. 329-347). Lisse, Belgium: Swets & Zeitlinger.

Jahoda, G. (1997). On the Origins of IACCP. *Cross-Cultural Psychology Bulletin, 31*(3), 4-7.

Kuhn, T. (1970). *The structure of scientific revolutions.* Chicago: University of Chicago Press.

Mannheim, K. (1936). *Ideology and Utopia.* New York: Harcourt, Brace, & World, Inc.

Moffitt, D. & Owusu-Bempah, J. (1994). *The Racism of Psychology*. London: Harvester Wheatsheaf.

Munroe, R.L. & Munroe, R.H. (1994). *Cross-Cultural Human Development*. Prospect Heights, IL.: Waveland Press, Inc.

Murayama, M.. (1997). Beyond post-modernism: Trends since 100 years. *Cybernetica, XL*(3), 169-178.

Paranjpe, A. (1997). Piles of data that contribute little to the *Mutual* understanding of cultures. *Cross-Cultural Psychology Bulletin, 31*(2), 11-17.

Poortinga, Y.H. (1997). Paranjpe's Review of the Pamplona Proceedings: Some Comments. *Cross-Cultural Psychology Bulletin, 31*(4), 8-11.

Poortinga, Y.H. & Van de Vijver, F.J.R. (1987). Explaining cross-cultural differences: Bias analysis and beyond. *Journal of Cross-Cultural Psychology, 18,* 259-282.

Rotter, J.B. (1967). Generalized expectancies for internal versus external control of reinforcement. *Psychological Monographs, 80(609)*, 1-23.

Snarey, J.R. (1985). Cross-cultural universality of social-moral development: A critical review of Kohlbergian research. *Psychological Bulletin, 97*, 202-232.

Tyler, F.B., Brome, D.R., and Williams, J.A. (1991). *Ethnic Validity, Ecology, & Psychotherapy*. New York: Plenum.

Tyler, F.B., & Sinha, Y. (1988). Psychosocial competence and belief systems among Hindus. *Genetic, Social and General Psychology Monographs, 114*(1), 33-49.

Sampson, W. (1993). Identity politics: Challenges to Psychology's understanding. *American Psychologist, 48,* 1219-1230.

Zea, M.C., Tyler, F.B., & Franco, M.C. (1991). Psychosocial competence in Colombian university students. *Revista InterAmericana de Psicologia/InterAmerican Journal of Psychology, 25,* 135-145.

Challenging EuroAmerican-Centered Psychology: The Voices of African Psychologists

Josephine C. Naidoo
Wilfrid Laurier University
Department of Psychology

Akinsola Olowu
Obafemi Awolowo University
Department of Psychology

Andrew Gilbert
Rhodes University
Department of Psychology

Charity Akotia
University of Ghana
Department of Psychology

ABSTRACT

Developments in cross-cultural and indigenous psychology in Sub-Saharan Africa have important implications for the discipline. Findings in Euro-American cultures cannot be assumed to be universal. Scales and testing measures developed in the West may not be the most useful for studying non-Western cultures. This study examines the status of cross-cultural psychology from the viewpoint of the indigenous cultures, traditions, and needs of peoples in Sub-Saharan Africa. African cross-cultural researchers, psychology departments and journals with a cross-cultural focus, emerging movements towards indigenous psychology and their schools of origin, and controversies in the "First World versus Third World" psychological debate are identified. Contributions of African cross-cultural psychology to the global study of the discipline await exploration in the context of Berry & Kim's 1993 framework for pursuing a universal psychology.

Challenging Euro-American Centered Psychology: The Voices of African Psychologists

Recent developments in cross-cultural and indigenous psychology in Sub-Saharan Africa have important implications for the discipline: theoretical, methodological, and applied. As pioneers in the "indigenization" movement in psychology have pointed out, Western psychology has limited applicability to Third World issues because of its individualistic orientation, emphasis on narrow aspects of larger social problems, and lack of conceptual tools for exploring these problems (Sinha, 1990). Findings from Euro-American cultures cannot be assumed universal. Scales and testing measures developed in the West have limited usefulness for the study of Non-Western cultures. When alien schemata are applied to Africa, important phenomena may not be noticed since such models may be insensitive to their recognition (Nsamenang, 1997). Nsamenang calls for African psychologists to endeavor to reverse the dependence on foreign models. Key contemporary cross-cultural psychologists agree that general psychology is both culture blind and culture bound (Berry & Kim, 1993). They argue that the development of indigenous psychologies is an essential remedy for this state of affairs in the discipline. Others focus on the concept of "appropriateness" in the transfer of social science knowledge from developed to developing nations (Moghaddam & Taylor, 1986). Psychological knowledge and models imported by the developing world from the West must be achieved within a framework of creating scientific independence and self-reliance by professionals and their institutions. There is a need to restore the true identity of people who have lost it due to imperialistic subjugation and intellectual domination (Sinha, 1994). This study examines the status of cross-cultural psychology from the viewpoint of the indigenous cultures, traditions, and needs of peoples in Sub-Saharan Africa.

Status of Psychology in Sub-Saharan Africa

Interest in the study of psychology in Africa, south of the Sahara, extends from Mauritania across to the Sudan and down to South Africa, a vast area enormously diverse in its ecology, ethnicity, linguistics, politics, and history. However, "a certain common quality" deriving from similarities in historical experiences, cultural traits and adaptation to environmental forces, characterizes the many peoples of **Afrique Noire** (Nsamenang, 1995a).

The 1998 volume of "The World of Learning" indicates over 100 universities have been established across the sub-continent, led by Nigeria and South Africa, (29 and 21 respectively). Since 1962, many universities have established psychology departments. Nigeria with 12 and South Africa with 19 have done best at promoting the discipline. These two countries also have the most visible international representation of Africans in cross-cultural psychology: 13 South African and 9 Nigerians are active members of the International Association for Cross-Cultural Psychology (IACCP; membership list, 1998).

Nsamenang attributes the fledgling status of psychology in Afrique Noire to lack of recognition of psychology, inadequate finances, political instability, political interference, unstable research leadership, a paucity of psychologists, poor infrastructure, and low incentives for scholarship. Added to these problems of emerging nationhood, is the over dependence on Western models of psychology and Euro-American values and epistemologies more generally. Eurocentrism, lack of indigenous concepts and measures to capture local knowledge, and low cultural relevance of the discipline exacerbate the present day situation (Nsamenang, 1995a; 1993). Alfred Awaritife (1997) identified the numerous tasks that fall to overburdened editors of scientific journals in Sub-Saharan Africa. Problems to be contended with include frequent electric power cuts, poor postal and telephone services, and acute shortages of water.

However, despite the multiplicity of Africa's needs, by 1995 Nigeria could boast of the publishing and management of 9 psychology journals. These include publication of cross-cultural and indigenous psychological studies of high caliber. Elias Mpofu of the University of Zimbabwe points out (1998) that the efforts of African psychologists could be augmented appreciably by tangible support from Western-based cross-cultural organizations. He appeals for professional interaction, the encouragement of African participation in international activities of the discipline, and for some necessary financial support.

Controversies in the Cross-Cultural Debate

Psychologist Andrew Gilbert of Rhodes University in South Africa pondered over the issue of what constitutes cross-cultural psychology. He grappled with the issues of culture and cross-cultural research in the African context. He asks the question: Is cross-cultural psychology determined by its goals, methods, professional affiliations, or its orientation? (Personal communication, August 22, 1997.)

The goal of cross-cultural psychology is invariably stated in the literature as follows: "to generate a more universal psychology that will be valid for a broader range of cultures" (Berry, Poortinga, Segall, and Dasen, 1992, p.3), and, "to pursue more effectively the universal validity of psychological theories in all branches of psychology and related disciplines" (IACCP Brochure, 1997). Gilbert asks whether these are descriptions of what cross-cultural psychologists actually do or whether these are prescriptions for what psychologists should be doing. Given the growing push towards indigenous psychology in Asia and Africa, one may ask whether the pursuit of universals is basically generated by First World psychologists. Berry (1993) offers a potential, if long drawn out route, to resolving the indigenous (emic) /universal (etic) controversy. Out of numerous indigenous studies arises the possibility of deriving a universal psychology. In Berry's terms, psychology conducted **in** a particular country is frequently an imposed etic, while psychology done **by** a country is usually emic in character. He envisions that from the integration of these two sources of data will emerge a derived etic and eventually produce a pan-human, universal psychology. African psychologists concur with this goal. Says Michael Durojaiye (1993, p.219), "Human nature, human culture, and the uniqueness of each human being lead to the conclusion that each person is in some ways like all other persons, like some other persons, and like no other person."

Sometimes cross-cultural psychology delineates its discipline by its methodology. Certainly cross-cultural psychologists have been in the vanguard of attention to concerns such as cultural biases of standard research methods, the problems of accuracy of translation equivalents, the sensitivity of field work, and the interpretation of data by scholars with understanding of a given culture. In Gilbert's assessment, a large amount of research in Southern Africa does not take into account the rigorous methodological guidelines provided by cross-cultural psychology. However, this review of psychological studies emanating from Sub-Saharan Africa revealed praiseworthy care, innovation, and execution of studies drawing on samples from African ethnic populations. Their findings enhance our understanding, both emic and etic, of the psychology of peoples whom researchers world-wide ordinarily cannot access. Thus, for example, psychologist E. Egwu of the University of Jos in Nigeria (1996) demonstrated the importance of identifying and utilizing indigenous cultural metaphors in work organizations to elicit optimal performance from workers.

Metaphors that are meaningful in one culture or society may be meaningless in others. By testing well known subgroups in Nigeria, (the Yoruba, Igbo, and Hausa), as well as lesser known groups (the Tiv, Tarok, Bajju), Egwu demonstrates commonalities in cultural metaphors of work, time and money for all Nigerians. These shared metaphors for the Nigerian sub-samples contrast sharply with Euro-American metaphors for similar concepts. Nigerians do not conceptualize work as an activity that takes place in "modern organizations" under managers, foremen and supervisors, i.e., in Egwu's terms, a "machine" metaphor of work. Rather, work is conceptualized in an environment of freedom, independence and maturity. Indeed, work is directly related to time, money, life itself. Egwu describes the Nigerian worker as disoriented in the modern organization.

Citing other ethnic researchers of cultural metaphors, such as Yoshihisa Kashima, who identifies the family metaphor as the focus of organizational life in Japan (Kashima, 1994), Egwu calls for integrating Nigerian cultural metaphors into modern organizations in his country. His research suggests that Nigerian cultural ontological metaphors of work, time, and money may aid his people in the development of a viable, healthy, indigenous organizational form in Nigeria, possibly generating new solutions to current problems of work organization and associated behavior.

If, however, cross-cultural psychology is determined by affiliation via membership in organizations such as IACCP or publication in international journals (Gilbert, 1997), then the psychologists of Afrique Noire origins need resources, funding, and interest from Euro-American and Asian colleagues. Membership from the sub-continent in IACCP is comprised of a mere 32 psychologists, almost half of whom hail from the ranks of White South African psychologists. However, there is a growing presence of Black African researchers in international and African national social/cross-cultural psychology journals. The writings of A. Bame Nsamenang, Michael Durojaiye, R. Cecil Bodibe, Pumla Gobodo, and Akinsola Olowu, deserve mention. The focus of this paper is on these and other Black African voices.

Despite the long-term criticisms of Western-based cross-cultural research by Third World psychologists, such as Durganand Sinha (Sinha, 1993), little has changed in the psychological world has changed. As Gilbert (1997) points out, there lingers a tacit acceptance of Western mainstream psychology in African universities generally. Academic trends move from North to South. Psychology theory and methodology is derived from Europe and America. Psychology departments and current curricula are modeled after those in existence in Britain, Europe and America. Textbooks are largely imported from the United States; most psychologists are trained overseas and their North-South networks are retained. Psychological studies and knowledge emerging from Africa and Asia have "second class" status. Ethnocentrism, Western individualistic values, and general failure to draw on indigenous perspectives continue to permeate mainstream psychology.

African psychologists are not necessarily uncritical of the contextual appropriateness of the discipline (Gilbert, 1997). However, these critiques are primarily aimed at refinements and minor revisions of psychology theory and practice for the African context. The positive outcome of this approach is that students and practitioners can benefit from the sensitivity to culture, methodological rigor, and networking among cross-cultural psychologists that the discipline brings with it.

At the brink of the 21st century, the challenge for African psychologists is two-fold. On the one hand, with globalization of Africa, African peoples will become more like those in the "West" and the assumed universals of Euro-America will become more widely applicable (Gilbert, 1997). On the other hand, the countries of Africa, Asia, and the Middle East resist the pervasive impact of such globalization, homogenization, and Americanization. Indigenous cultures, values, traditions, and customs are profoundly interwoven with ethno-cultural identity. Perhaps African/Asian cross-cultural psychologists will bring new momentum to grappling with the universal nature of psychology within indigenous local contexts.

African Viewpoints

Theory, Methods, Applications

In contrast to the tacit acceptance of Western psychology, the global/local tension in psychology may be resolved by moving towards a relativism (Gilbert, 1997). In Africa, there have been two approaches to this issue, either by (1) rejecting the assumed universal base of psychology or (2) questioning it and arguing for a psychology based on the local context.

The first approach is illustrated by freedom fighters such as Franz Fanon (Naidoo, 1997) and Steve Biko (1978) both of whom adopt strong ideological positions to demonstrate how personal identity is determined by the structure of social relations operating within local contexts. Fanon's analysis of the psychology of the oppressed evolved from his structural analysis of racism in Algeria. Biko sought to explain Black identity in relation to the structural components of "Apartheid" society. In this approach, there is little place for contemporary cross-cultural psychology seeking universals in human behavior.

The second relativist approach is found in the "indigenous psychologies" which seek to identify the unique (emic) characteristics of the psychological life of "cultural" groups from a more empirical perspective. This approach is usually not based on ideology but rather studies the "emic" nature of the selected cultural group. In recent years, many new insights about the African world view have emerged from these studies.

Cecil Bodibe (1993) discussed the cultural hierarchy that colors the contemporary global scene in which African countries have been relegated to "Third World" and by extension Black people and Black culture to an inferior status, viewed in terms of a deficit model. Probing the underlying dynamics to African behavior, (South African context in particular), he asserts that "Africans have a cosmology, ontology, eschatology, epistemology and axiology that is quintessentially their own", (p. 54). These "ologies" form a metaculture from which the manifest behavior of Africans evolves. He sees African behavior as wholistic, a product of the reciprocal interaction between the metaculture and the socio-political/economic milieux in which Africans find themselves. Research conducted on African samples illustrate Bodibe's contentions, as the following studies indicate.

Akinsola Olowu's (1997) studies of the Black self-concept among the Ashantis of Ghana, and the self-concept of Nigerian adolescents reveal the centrality of self as deriving from group "beingness". The individual self-identity is essentially an extended identity of the group. Citing other Nigerian researchers, Olowu reiterates the point that in traditional life, the individual did not and could not exist alone. The individual was simply an integral part of the collective unity. This collectivist world view is captured in Olowu's statement "I am because we are, and because we are, therefore I am" (Personal communication, August 7, 1997). Olowu (1985) warns of the erosion of the African view of self with Western contact, with ensuing problem behavior.

Michael Durojaiye's (1993) study of the meaning of intelligence for male/female, urban/rural Baganda (East Africa) and Yoruba (West Africa) samples augments our understanding of the concept for these cultural groups. Durojaiye seems surprised at the similarity of views about intelligence, across the two African peoples geographically so separated. This emic view of intelligence stresses knowledge, thinking, inventiveness, practice, and harmony. The linkage of practice and harmony with intelligence defines unique meaning for these cultures. "Harmony" is especially important in resolving local disputes. Durojaiye cites Jomo Kenyatta, first Prime Minister of Kenya as follows: "To the Europeans, individuality is the ideal of life; to the Africans, the ideal is the right relations with, and behavior to, other people,"(p.219). African psychologists assert that knowledge about African cultures is inaccessible to conventional research methods because such knowledge is "locked in" African folklore, rituals, proverbs, maxims, and non-verbal cues (Ojiaku, 1974). Innovation, readjustment of existing methods, flexibility, careful thought and systematic procedure are called for in designing methodology and ensuring replicability (Nsmamenang, 1995a).

Thus, Nsamenang finds the contextualist paradigm (1997) and the eco-cultural model (1995a) especially insightful. He claims that contextualist approaches are suited to the study of African cultures because of three interrelated factors. The first is the hybrid nature of Africa's politico-economic systems, and the second, African world views that sanction harmony with nature. The third factor, a territorial imperative or psycho-social attachment of identity to a place, arises from the fact that many traditional settings in Africa prescribe distinctive patterns of behavior.

Using the contextual/eco-cultural framework in his developmental research, Nsamenang (1995b;1993, respectively) makes some interesting observations about the place of the child in African society. For example, the child as a source of prestige (more children, more prestige), the child as the parents' "walking stick" (parental social security system), and the child as an agent of national development because African children are part of the economic life of their societies.

In Nigeria, Alfred Awaritife (1997) has developed the so-called "meseron technique" for use in psychotherapy in that country. The technique is based on the observation that many ethnic groups in Nigeria believe in the power of the spoken word and hence in the power of thought. The "meseron" (Urhobo expression) literally means "I refuse" but has deeper connotations. In using the "meseron" the individual both detaches him/herself from negative aspects of life and actively associates with the positive. Alternatively, the negative state may be attributed to an inanimate object. For example, a person may say: "I was very sick" followed by the "meseron" or the person may say: "my tree in the bush was sick." Rejecting illness and adopting a positive attitude towards life and living has obvious therapeutic value for the individual.

Gilbert suggests addressing the tension between global and local realities by adopting pragmatic approaches to socio-psychological problems in their local settings, e.g., rural development (Gilbert, 1997), primary health care (Seedat & Nell, 1992). Other cross-cultural psychologists also suggest a problem-oriented approach (Sinha, 1983). However, in general, the applied value of research findings has not been of central concern to cross-cultural psychology.

In one particularly, interesting study in Ghana, Puplampu (1997) examined the meaning of work for male and female, senior and junior staff in the service and manufacturing sectors of two organizations in the Accra-Tema metropolis. Puplampu found significant statistical support for his proposition that the meaning of work is understood by Ghanian workers in terms of a cosmic-spiritual-religious conceptualization. Two beliefs about the concept of work are crucial,"Work is central to human life; work derives from God", (p.8).

Urban Ghanian workers are reportedly poor performers in work settings, according to Puplampu. If these profound religious work values could be incorporated into their work ethic, motivation and work behavior may well improve.

Summary: Challenges from African Psychologists

The theories, measures, and views of the world developed in the West may have only limited utility for the study of African cultures. African psychologists challenge Euro-centered psychology by examining the status of psychology in Sub-Saharan Africa and by debating what constitutes cross-cultural psychology in an African context. African psychologists' views of the world, psychological theory, methodology, and applied issues find support through empirical studies conducted in diverse countries of Africa.

Progress in the recognition and establishment of the discipline of psychology in Afrique Noire has become increasingly visible since 1962, led by impressive developments in Nigeria and South Africa. However, political and economic instability, poor infrastructure, widespread Eurocentric attitudes, and lack of tangible support from Western cross-cultural psychologists hinder the advancement of the discipline.

South African psychologist Andrew Gilbert ponders questions of what delineates cross-cultural psychology in Africa as compared to the West. He considers the goals, methods, professional affiliations and orientation of cross-cultural psychologists to obtain understanding of when and how the contentions of African psychologists deviate from psychologists in the West. The most fundamental issue revolves around the place of indigenous psychology within mainstream Euro-American psychology. Despite some 20 years of criticism of mainstream psychology and a rising body of indigenous (emic) studies deriving from Africa and Asia, little recognition has been given to the indigenous movement. We have numerous examples of indigenous studies, conducted by Western-trained African psychologists rooted in African cultures. Noteworthy are African psychologists Cecil Bodibe, Egwu Egwu, Akinsola Olowu, Michael Durojaiye, Bame Nsamenang, and Alfred Awaritife, among others. These studies offer unique insights into African views about their world, work, the self, intelligence, children, and illness. Two assertions consistently emerge in the literature derived from African sources: (1) the need to resist over dependence on foreign psychological models of human behavior; and (2) the need for innovative methodologies to probe African spiritual beliefs, myths, ritual and world views.

Towards a Balanced Perspective

The literature clearly resonates the call by African, Asian, and increasing numbers of mainstream psychologists for the empowerment of indigenous viewpoints and unique insights provided by studies of indigenous cultures. Pumla Gobodo of the

University of Transkei in South Africa says "Because human and cultural diversity is at the core of psychology, it is psychologists who should be comfortable with celebrating cultural diversity rather than being threatened by it" (cited by Bodibe p.57).

Interestingly, it is in the political arena that indigenous concepts have been welcomed and utilized more readily than in the discipline of psychology. Two examples come to mind. First, the Truth and Reconciliation Commission in South Africa has focused on *reparative* justice rather than punitive justice in dealing with perpetrators of violations of human rights during the Apartheid era (Gobodo-Madikizela, 1997). National healing is aspired after through seeking the truth. Second, Botswana in Southern Africa has gone back to its indigenous roots of the system of *kgotlas*, in which chiefs and councillors meet to reach consensus on important matters. Present day government draws on this indigenous institution of participatory democracy (Ayittey, 1998).

Nsamenang (1995a, p. 737) observes that not only will indigenous psychology enhance understanding of local phenomena, but it will also expand our vision of what forms psychological functioning may take in diverse cultures. This may call to question models derived primarily from studies of Western populations. However, while noting the importance of indigenous studies and the development of an "African psychology", African psychologists (Bodibe, 1993; Durojaiye, 1993; Nsamenang, 1995a) also voice concern that indigenous psychology could become narrow and ethnocentric, as they claim has occurred in mainstream psychology. They generally agree that locally developed psychologies should be integrated into mainstream psychology to evolve a universal science of psychology. Indigenous psychology accounts only for cultural patterning, in that " All human beings, by virtue of being *Homo sapiens* will have similar psychological processes" (M. Durojaiye (1993; p.219). Berry and Kim's framework for pursuing a universal psychology offers promise for achieving this goal (Berry & Kim, 1993). A future Congress of the International Association for Cross-Cultural Psychology could create a forum for examining indigenous African research and mainstream psychology, promoting linkages between North-South and South-South cross-cultural psychologists. It would also provide encouragement for the initiative and progress of African psychologists laboring under very challenging political and economic conditions in most of Sub-Saharan Africa.

References

Awaritife, A. (1997). The body-mind problem in an African context. *Ife PsychologiA: An International Journal*, *5*(1), 140-149.

Ayittey, G.B.N. (1998). Democracy is Africa's only choice. *The Record*, Kitchener, Ontario, Canada, July 31, A17 (reprinted from the Los Angeles Times.)

Berry, J.W., Poortinga,Y.H., Segall, M.H., & Dasen, P.R. (1992). *Cross-Cultural Psychology: Theory, method and applications.* Cambridge, Cambridge University Press.

Berry, J.W. (1993). Psychology in and of Canada: One small step toward a universal psychology. In U. Kim & J. W. Berry (Eds.), *Indigenous psychologies: Research and experience in cultural context*, pp. 260-276. Newbury Park, CA: Sage Publications.

Berry, J.W. & Kim, U. (1993). The way ahead: From indigenous psychology to a universal psychology. In U.Kim & J.W. Berry (Eds.), *Indigenous psychologies: Research and experience in cultural context*, pp. 277-280. Newbury Park, CA: Sage Publications.

Biko, S. (1978). *I write what I like*. London: Heinemann.Bodibe, R.C. (1993). What is the truth? Being more than just a jesting Pilate in South African psychology. *South African Journal of Psychology, 23*(2), 53-58.

Durojaiye , M.O.A. (1993). Indigenous psychology in Africa: The search for meaning. In U. Kim & J.W. Berry (Eds.), *Indigenous psychologies: Research and experience in cultural context*, pp. 211-220. Newbury Park, CA: Sage Publications.

Egwu, E.U. (1996). Metaphors in aid of indigenous organizational theorising and form in Nigeria.*Ife PsychologIA: An International Journal, 4*(2), 130-155.

Gilbert, A.J. (1997). What constitutes cross-cultural psychology in the African context? Personal communication, e-mail, August 22 (Rhodes University, South Africa).

Gobodo-Madikizela, P. (1997). Healing the racial divide? Personal reflections on the Truth and Reconciliation Commission. *South African Journal of Psychology, 27*(4) 271-272.

International Association for Cross-Cultural Psychology (IACCP) membership list (1998). Personal Communication, e-mail May 14, 1998, W. K. Gabrenya Jr., Editor, *Cross-Cultural Psychology Bulletin*.

Kashima, Y. (1994). Cultural metaphors of the mind and the organization. In Anne-Marie Bouvy et al. (Eds.): *Journey into Cross-Cultural Psychology*, pp. 351-363. Lisse: The Netherlands: Swets and Zeitlinger

Moghaddam, F.M., & Taylor, D.M. (1986). What constitutes an “appropriate” psychology for the developing world? *International Journal of Psychology, 21*, 253-267.

Mpofu, E. (March, 1998). Africa contributions: Good intentions are not enough. Letters to the Editor, *Cross-Cultural Psychology Bulletin:, Vol. 32*, #1, p.4.

Naidoo, J.C. (1997). Franz Fanon: Black skin, white mask (A review). United Kingdom: A Normal Films Production for the Arts Council of England & BBC television. Video, 1995.

Nsamenang, A.B. (1993). The ecology of child development: Research considerations. Special edition: Child development in Cameroon. *Journal of Psychology in Africa, Vol. 1* (5), 81-89.

Nsamenang, A.B. (1995a). Factors influencing the development of psychology in sub-Saharan Africa. *International Journal of Psychology, 30*(6), 729-739.

Nsamenang, A.B. (1995b). Theories of developmental psychology for a cultural perspective: A view from Africa. *Psychology and Developing Societies, Vol 7* (1), 1 -19.

Nsamenang, A.B. (1997). Towards an Afrocentric perspective in developmental psychology. *Ife Psychologia: An International Journal, 5*(1), 127-139.

Ojiaku, M.O. (1974). Traditional African social thought and western scholarship. *Presence Africain, 2*, 2nd Quarterly.

Olowu, A. (1985). Adolescents in traditional societies: Implications for counselling in Nigeria. *Ife Psychologia, Vol. 28*, 144-149.

Olowu, A. (1997). A statement of our exploration into the person at Ife Centre for Psychological Studies (ICPS). Personal communication, e-mail, August 7 (Obafemi Awolowo University, Nigeria).

Puplampu, B.B. (1997). Some preliminary findings on the meaning of work in Ghana: A research note. *Ife Psychologia: An International Journal, 5*(2), 1-11.

Seedat, M. & Nell, V. (1992). Authoritarianism and autonomy.1. Conflicting value systems in the introduction of psychological services in a South African Primary Health Care System. *South African Journal of Psychology, 22 (*4), 185-193.

Sinha, D. (1983). Cross-cultural psychology: A view from the third world. In J.B. Deregowski, S. Dziurawiec & R.C. Annis (Eds.), *Expiscations in Cross-Cultural Psychology*, pp. 2-17, Lisse, Amsterdam: Swets and Zeitlinger.

Sinha, D. (1990). Applied cross-cultural psychology and the developing world. *International Journal of Psychology, 25*(3), 381-386.

Sinha , D. (1993). Indigenization of psychology in India and its relevance. In U.Kim & J.W. Berry (Eds.), *Indigenous psychologies: Research and experience in cultural context*, pp. 30-43. Newbury Park, CA: Sage Publications.

Sinha, D. (1994). Indigenous psychology: Need and potentiality. *Journal of Indian Psychology, 12*(1-2), 1-7.

The World of Learning (1998). 48th edition. London: Europa Publications Ltd.

Cognitive, Intellectual, and Assessment Perspectives

Multicultural Assessment for the Twenty-First Century

Ronald J. Samuda and John E. Lewis
Center for Psychological Studies
Nova Southeastern University
Fort Lauderdale, Florida

ABSTRACT

This paper evaluates major trends, theories and practices in assessing the culturally different. The theme is that traditional standardized tests of cognitive ability are appropriate for middle-class mainstream individuals regardless of color or ethnicity. Those who benefit from the middle-class curriculum of the typical school can be validly and reliably assessed by tests constructed by middle-class psychometricians using situations that match the background and environmental circumstances of the middle-class individual. Where there are deficiencies or fundamental differences in the rearing and environmental background and circumstances of the individual, the traditional objective standardized tests are neither valid nor reliable in measuring the cognitive performance level of mental development. Such anomalies lie not only in the content and procedural methods of the test, but also in the very approach to assessment that cannot capture the true capacity of the atypical individual. Three approaches developed by Feuerstein, Kaufman and Sternberg are discussed as viable models of assessment for the 21st Century.

The fundamental question that has occupied the last quarter of a century is whether or not tests are fair in assessing individuals who are culturally or socioeconomically different from the middle-class mainstream. Over and over it has been asked: Can we depend on test results to make responsible decisions when allocating students to streams or tracks within the school system? Can test results be trusted to select appropriate candidates for entry into college courses? Do test results discriminate fairly in choosing who will enter graduate and professional programs leading to certification as practicing physicians, lawyers, engineers, accountants, or teachers?

Test results have dire social and economic consequences for they are also employed in the workplace where they exert a powerful sorting influence with economic repercussions for those who are allocated to the lower echelon of the system. The debate has been longstanding and many arguments have been raised on both sides of the issue, but one thing is certain: test results can have disastrous effects on the lives and aspirations of minorities in any society. The purpose of this paper is to evaluate 20th century attempts to measure intellectual ability with a view to illuminating three contemporary approaches that will likely continue to be significant in the 21st century.

In 1977, the first author was one of thirteen presenters at the National Conference on Testing at the Center for Advanced Study in Education inaugurated under the auspices of the City University of New York. The focus of that conference was on why, why not, and how to test. Some of the participants favored the elimination of testing minorities; others looked towards culturally relative measures that would discard mean group differences. Leaders of the testing establishment warned that such changes would lead to subjective and potentially more biased assessments. They pointed to the fact that tests have equal predictive validity for all groups. Scoring low on a test of mental aptitude will, in all probability, indicate low performance in school. A low score on the SAT will generally predict a low grade point average in college.

The use of standardized ability and achievement tests in schools was primarily motivated by views of equal opportunity which translated as identical treatment regardless of initial differences in preparation. But, as Professor Sandra Scarr has so cogently contended, equal opportunity does not always ensue from identical treatment. In fact, equality of opportunity is more likely to result from different strokes for different folks' where the individual is treated according to the advantages or idiosyncrasies of his/her environmental, linguistic, cultural and ethnic background (Scarr, 1977, p.73.).

As we all know, Binet's purpose in devising the first test of mental ability was to help in the instructional process. At no time did he believe that what he was measuring was pure intelligence; nor did he concern himself with the probabilities of inherited genetic potential and with the nature-nurture controversy. Rather, Binet was concerned with the provision of optimum learning conditions for those who experienced learning difficulties.

The issue of color and ethnicity is irrelevant and misleading. Minority children who do well on IQ tests as a whole are those who come from homes that have similar values, similar aspirations, similar environmental circumstances, and similar attitudes as the majority white middle-class in America. The children of people like General Colin Powell and Reverend Jesse Jackson may do just as well on the *standard* traditional tests of mental aptitude as any white middle class child for they will have a similar cognitive style.

Those who would abandon psychological tests were, in the opinion of Roger Lennon (1964) guilty of trying to burn the barn to catch the mouse. In other words, let's not throw out the baby with the bath water. The fact is that psychological testing began in an effort to help rather than limit the prospects for those who were different and especially for those children who had difficulty in learning in the normal classroom. That was Binet's original purpose in devising the first set of items that were expanded into the Stanford-Binet test of intelligence. We must remember that without some kind of objective measure, we cannot calibrate an individual's level or rate of learning nor can we discover the reasons why the individual does not achieve. Psychological testing does have a vital role to play in education and in establishing the level of developed abilities in various spheres of training and on-the-job expertise.

However, if testing does have a purpose in the educational preparation of minorities, it should be geared in such a way that it will inform instruction. The procedures should help in initiating and fostering pedagogically sound programs and settings that will optimize the learning potential of the individual to help in reaching what Lev Vygotsky has called "the zone of proximal development."

The fundamental question concerns a choice of alternatives: Will testing continue to buttress institutional and structural racism in the schools in general and society at large or can assessment become the means of opening up opportunity for all individuals regardless of their ethnic and socioeconomic backgrounds? Assessment if it is to be educationally and ethically viable must adhere to the principle that it serves the good of individuals by augmenting the effectiveness of the teaching-learning process. And, on the other hand, where it necessarily abrogates the principle of social justice it contributes to the violation of civil rights of individual citizens.

Although intelligence, as a concept, has never been adequately and uniformly defined, it is still regarded by the public at large and, indeed, by many practicing teachers, counselors and professionals in the area of social work, as an important entity. More importantly, confusion is widespread concerning its definition and many still misconstrue IQ with the concept of intelligence.

What is the reason for such widespread bedlam in the use of the term? Briefly, the first initiative to define intelligence was due to the work of Sir Francis Galton who based his concept on the belief that mental tests measure, to some extent, one basic intellectual ability, which Spearman called 'g'. The concept of fixed mental aptitude, compressed in the concept of an intelligence quotient (IQ) became a dominant axiom until far into the twentieth century. Besides this general capacity, believed to be pure intelligence, was added the notion of specific factors 's' for an array of minor types of abilities. Such theories evolved into the hierarchical pyramid advanced in the models of Burt and Vernon (Guilford, 1967, pp. 5 8-59). Spearman's 'g' stood at the top of a pyramid with various levels of subdivisions or special abilities below, but it was the general capacity that determined the level of intelligence that would later be compressed in the form of the IQ.

Changes in the conceptualization of intelligence have inspired new approaches to cognitive assessment. Cattell (1963) proposed a departure from the notion of a fixed and unitary 'g' factor or general intelligence. Instead, he proposed a theory of fluid and crystallized intelligence. Cattell's theory regards fluid intelligence as a basic capacity to adapt to new situations. It is also an inherent capacity for learning and problem-solving that is independent of both education and cultural influences. In order to adapt to novel situations, fluid intelligence must encompass flexible inductive skills. Crystallized intelligence emerges from a person's use of fluid intelligence to interact with society. It is therefore a product of formal education. Thus, the way crystallized intelligence organizes knowledge and concepts reflects how the members of a given society process information and solve problems. These are "developed abilities" that can be quantified and assembled to make up tests for general mental ability. The outcome of such measures is necessarily static.

In Cattell's formulation, intelligence is the product of an active mind that is malleable and responsive to instruction. Intelligent behavior is seen in the processing of information and also in the anticipation of new situations and planning for effective solutions based on past experience. Given such a perspective, it follows that any adequate assessment of intelligence must address both these fluid and crystallized characteristics.

Traditional standardized tests of intelligence have been focused principally on assessing "global" intellectual abilities. The original Binet tests were geared to the prediction of Parisian children to learn within the "normal" school classroom. The Stanford-Binet test developed by Lewis Terman and Maude Merrill was based on Binet's model and similarly related to correlation between performance on samples of behavior and achievement within the school system. Similarly, the Wechsler Intelligence Scales were based on David Wechsler's notion that intelligence is a "global capacity of the individual to act purposefully, to think rationally, and to deal effectively with the environment" (1958, p.7.).

These individually-administered tests, originally standardized on norming populations that tended to focus on white middle-class individuals, have been subjected to heated debate and criticism precisely because of the initial homogeneous nature of the standardization samples that excluded minorities. Those two tests have since been restandardized in the form of the Stanford-Binet (SB-LM and SB-R) and the Wechsler Scales, WAIS-R and WISC-R to include minorities. However, the restandardized models are still subjected to critical scrutiny because of the paucity of sociodemographic variables in sampling procedures. Thus as Dana (1993) demonstrates "these tests apparently measure the construct of intelligence somewhat differently across groups" (Dana, 1993, p. 186). In other words, they lack cross-cultural construct validity. Despite limitations, the standardized tests can be useful when used with the care and the protocol that Jerome Sattler (1992) recommended is followed.

The work of three outstanding pioneers in the field, Feuerstein, Kaufman, and Sternberg represent the future of testing. Robert Sternberg would probably agree that the restandardized form of the Stanford-Binet and Wechsler Scales do assess some aspects of intelligence. He would also contend that the results from such tests do not describe the individual's real capacity because they do not take into account the entire spectrum of intelligent behavior. Thus, he has incorporated in his Triarchic Theory the view that any comprehensive consideration of the nature of intelligence must take into account three essential facets. These are (1) the internal world of the individual or the mental mechanisms that underlie intelligent behavior, (2) the individual's experience, and (3) the relationship of the individual to the external world. These aspects of intelligence Sternberg has labeled the componential, the experiential and the contextual subtheories.

Sternberg's triarchic theory of intelligence has had a profound impact on the psychometric enterprise. In a provocative chapter in Advances in Cross-cultural Assessment (Samuda et al, 1998), he speculates on the performance of inhabitants of a mythical planet Velda and demonstrates why it is so important to see the function of intelligence as situational and why it is significant for us to define intelligent behavior within a cultural context.

The Kaufman Assessment Battery for Children (K-ABC) represents one of the three central methodologies with which I am concerned. It is of prime importance in the advance of innovations in cross-cultural assessment. Like Sternberg, the Kaufmans were interested in the assessment of fluid intelligence and achievement. The Kaufman ABC was originally developed for psychological and clinical assessment. However, it is particularly appropriate for the educational evaluation of exceptional children including the learning-disabled. It is a landmark system of testing for educational planning and placement and, as I have implied for cross-cultural research, it is especially important for minority group assessment, for preschool assessment, and for limited neuropsychological assessment (Kaufman and Kaufman, 1985; Merz, 1984).

The K-ABC is not limited to the measurement of intellectual potential. It combines an achievement element which is separate from mental processing or problem solving in novel situations from that which is factual, school-related knowledge. The sixteen sub-tests include mental processing assessment that yields aggregated global scores for Sequential Processing, Simultaneous Processing, and Mental Processing composites. These tests of mental processes tap fluid intelligence in the form of adaptable and flexible behavior in response to unfamiliar situations and problems. There is also a Nonverbal Scale that is a shortened form of the Mental Processing Scale where pantomime is employed with motoric responses.

The system developed by the Kaufmans represents a pivotal leap in cross-cultural assessment. The testing program has been thoroughly researched with regard to relevance in cross-cultural situations. The reliability data compared favorably with the Wechsler tests and in 43 studies emphasis was placed on construct and criterion related validity. In general, the K-ABC is especially important in testing children who have limited English language proficiency or who speak a nonstandard English dialect. Research with children who speak different languages such as Spanish and French indicate that it is equally useful as a diagnostic and placement tool that can have important clues for remedial procedures in the school systems.

The fact that the K-ABC battery separates the mental processing scores from achievement scores may explain why it is more useful in assessing minority children than are the conventional tests like the WISC-R or even the System of Multicutural Pluralistic Assessment (SOMPA) which depend on traditional test results as a base. In fact, the research done on Hispanic children would indicate that the K-ABC is more appropriate and more useful than the WISC in establishing the intellectual potential and functioning level of minority children. Moreover, the flexibility in interpretation of the K-ABC tends to provide richer information with which to design effective post-test intervention strategies. The results of the K-ABC can clearly indicate characteristics of the testee's cognitive performance and verbal achievement.

The third system of assessment to examine is the Feuerstein methodology, and particularly the Learning Potential Assessment Device (LPAD) with its programmatic follow-up in Instrumental Enrichment. Feuerstein's methodology epitomizes a departure from the conventional views of intelligence. In sharp contrast to Spearman's view that tended to imply an immutable IQ fixed by genetic endowment at the moment of birth, Feuerstein derives his definition of intelligence from Vygotsky who perceives intelligence as a dynamic process that changes with development and learning. Although genetic factors have some relevance, other significant factors in the development of intelligence emanate from cultural environment, home influences, and conditioning within the school and social environment. As the learner interacts with other people, his or her learning stimulates cognitive development. As cognitive development proceeds, "a zone of proximal development" can be depicted to reflect the gap between the learner's actual development and the learner's developmental potential. It is this potential that enables the counselor, psychologist or teacher to help in the remedial and reconditioning process to raise the learner's ability to function. Testing is intentionally dynamic and geared to a remedial program whereby cognitive gaps are identified and instructional procedures are designed to enhance cognitive functioning.

Feuerstein's major concern has been to assess the untapped cognitive potential of individuals, particularly those who need to remedy any deficiencies through an active intervention process that helps the individual build a new and effective cognitive structure. The process of assessment rests on a fundamental tenet of modifiability of the cognitive structure. Linked with this is the conviction in the efficacy of mediated learning experience to enhance and condition intellectual functioning. Feuerstein's methodology deserves time and space because he deals with a related but separate phase of the procedure. One aspect is concerned with the Learning Potential Device. This dynamic method begins with a clear delineation of psychometric goals as follows.

1. To assess students' cognitive modifiability by observing their functions in situations designed to produce a change.
2. To assess the extent of modifiability in terms of cognitive functioning and how significant students' attained functioning is in the hierarchy of universal cognitive operations ranging from perception to abstract thinking.
3. To determine the transfer value of what is learned in one area to other areas.
4. To identify the student's preferred modalities for learning and the problem-solving strategies that work best.

Feuerstein's method engages both the student and assessor or counselor in an active modification procedure. When the client performs the task, the counselor's role is to intervene wherever necessary to present alternative ways of perceiving, interpreting, and problem solving. Change in the client's approach to the task is noted as well as the amount of intervention necessary to produce that change. The assessment process is therefore transformed from one of the neutral examiner to that of the active and involved appraiser. Assessment takes on new meaning and becomes part of the educational process. Further, the test items must be clear and well sequenced to permit a starting point at the individual's level of cognitive functioning. The assessment strategies focus on the process of intellectual reasoning rather than on its product and the emphasis is placed on change in cognitive skill. The LPAD thus provides the means to tap acquisition components and performance components of intelligence. It enables the appraiser to identify cognitive deficits, and is designed to help fashion a program of remediation and cognitive conditioning so the very structure of cognitive functioning can be permanently modified.

Instrumental enrichment describes Feuerstein's program for remediation of impairments that occur frequently in persons who are educationally deprived. Narrol (1978) has demonstrated that an individual is amenable to remedial help if he or she exhibits certain cognitive deficits. Some writers maintain that Feuerstein's basic assumption that everyone is modifiable may be an over generalization. Nevertheless, researchers like Sundberg and Gonzales (1981) have shown that this dynamic approach contributes significantly towards clarifying the special needs of minority individuals and groups.

The Feuerstein methodology is now in operation in various countries throughout the world. It has shifted the focus away from quantitative product scores to qualitative observations and interpretations of the process of mental ability functioning based on the assumption that intelligence is a multifaceted, multidimensional and fluid construct that continually undergoes change. This approach attempts to determine not only the characteristics of the various components of intelligence but also how they function.

Conclusion

We could not cover all the variables and issues associated with the business

The world is increasingly becoming one global village. More and more, the industrial nations of the world will face the need to absorb immigrants into the economic, social and industrial fabric. If we are to optimize the potential of all individuals, we must find the ways and means to identify and cultivate the capabilities of all individuals regardless of their origin or background. Equally important, from a moral and ethical standpoint, we must be conscious of the enormous power of assessment to impact those who are from different cultural and/or socioeconomic circumstances. Educators and social scientists of all persuasions have a moral and ethical duty to ensure that the tests they use are relevant and useful. In particular, test results and especially interpretations of those results must be fair and do no harm.

Let us recall the caveats of Ernest Hemingway who reminded his fellow writers that their fundamental purpose and moral duty was to discover what is true and to use truth in ways that are useful. In a very similar way, those of us who work in the area of psychometrics and the application of test results must bear in mind Hemingway's caveats. The psychometric enterprise must be devoted to discovering what is true and using it for the betterment of those who are subjected to our assessment devices.

References

Binet, A., & Simon, T. (1916). *The development of intelligence in children* (E. S. Kite, Trans.). Baltimore, MD: Williams and Wilkins.

Cattell, R. B. (1963). Theory of fluid and crystallized intelligence: A critical experiment. *Journal of Educational Psychology, 18*, 165-244.

Dana, R. H. (1993). *Multicultural assessment perspectives for professional psychology.* Needham Heights, MA: Allyn & Bacon.

Feuerstein, R. (1979). *The dynamic assessment of retarded performers: The Learning Potential Assessment Device, theory, instruments, and techniques.* Baltimore, NM: University Press.Feuerstein, R.,

Falik, L. H., and Feuerstein, R. (1998). The Learning Potential Assessment Device: an alternative approach to the assessment of learning potential. In R. J. Samuda, *et al* (pp.100-159) *Advances in cross-cultural assessment.* Thousand Oaks, CA: Sage.

Flaugher, R. L. (1978). The many definitions of test bias. *American Psychologist. 33*, 671-679.

Kamin, L. (1976). Heredity, intelligence, politics, and psychology: 11. In N. Block & G. Dworkin (Eds.). *The IQ controversy* (pp.374-382). New York: Pantheon Books.

Lewis, J. E. (1998). Non traditional uses of traditional aptitude tests. In R. Samuda, *et al* (pp. 218-239). *Advances in cross-cultural assessment.* Thousand Oaks, CA: Sage.

Lichtenberger, E. O., Kaufman, A. S. and Kaufman, N. L. (1998). Kaufman assessment battery for children: theory and application. In R. Samuda, *et al, Advances in cross-cultural assessment.* (pp.20-39). Thousand Oaks, CA: Sage.

Narroll, H., Silverman, H., & Waksman, M. (1982). Developing cognitive potential in vocational high school students. *Journal of Educational Research.*

Samuda, R. J. (1998). *Psychological testing of American minorities* (2 nd edition). Thousand Oaks, CA. Sage.

Samuda, R. J., Kong, S. L., Cummins, J., Pascual-Leone, J., & Lewis, J. (1989). *Assessment and placement of minority students.* Lewiston, NY: Hogrefe/ISSP.

Sattler, J. M. (1992). *Assessment of children* (revised and updated 3rd ed.). San Diego, CA: Author.

Cross-Cultural Differences on Cognitive Task Performance: The Influence of Stimulus Familiarity

Corine J. Sonke
Tilburg University
Department of Psychology

Ype H. Poortinga
Tilburg University
Department of Psychology

Jan H. J. de Kuijer
Tilburg University
Department of Psychology

ABSTRACT

Effects of differential stimulus familiarity on simple cognitive tasks were investigated. Reaction time tasks of varying cognitive complexity were administered on three subsequent days to samples of Iranian and Dutch subjects. For three tasks a set of geometric patterns was used for stimulus materials. To investigate the effects of experience one of these tasks was trained. An isomorphic task with Arabic letters as stimuli was also administered. With the geometric figures very similar patterns of results were found for the two samples across tasks and across days. The Dutch subjects responded faster on all the tasks. With the Arabic letters also similar patterns were found over the three days, but the Iranian subjects were consistently faster. It is argued that the systematic manipulation of stimulus familiarity in an experimental design obviates the need for diffuse and subjective explanatory concepts.

For reaction time (RT) tasks with a single stimulus average, response times are approximately equal in samples from widely different cultural populations (Jensen, 1982, 1985; Poortinga, 1971). Therefore, invariance across populations at an elementary level of information processing can be assumed. On slightly more complex choice reaction time tasks (CRTs) that require only a small number of transformations from stimulus to response, cross-cultural differences already emerge (Jensen, 1982, 1985; Poortinga, 1971; Van de Langenberg, 1989; Verster, 1991).

One way to explain this finding is in terms of an overall capacity in speed of processing (Eysenck 1982; Jensen, 1985). Another way is to point to cultural bias. For colored lights as well as for sounds, Poortinga (1971) found an interaction between culture and stimuli. This was interpreted as evidence that the domains from which the stimuli were sampled were not identical for the cultural populations concerned, thereby precluding any meaningful comparison of score levels (Poortinga, 1971, 1989). However, showing the presence of bias does not resolve the question of **why** it occurs.

Despite observed differences in absolute score levels, it should be noted that patterns of CRTs are very much the same cross-culturally. For example, an increase in the number of stimuli leads to longer RTs as predicted by Hick's law (1952), and training on the task to shorter RTs (Poortinga, 1971; Van de Langenberg, 1989). This makes it implausible to argue that different cognitive processes are involved in CRT tasks cross-culturally. Therefore, it appears that cross-cultural differences have to be explained in a way that leaves the cross-cultural invariance of cognitive processing unchallenged.

One factor that can be used to explain differences across cultures on any cognitive task is prior exposure and experience (Poortinga, 1985; Posner, 1985). In RT-type tasks this entails familiarity with the stimulus material, the content of the task, and the response procedures. In a quasi-experimental study, Serpell (1979) explicitly aimed at the identification of bias in response procedures. He gave paper and pencil, as well as steel wire, to children as materials for reproducing geometric forms. English school children performed better with paper and pencil, while Zambian boys were superior in the reproduction task with wire. To the best of our knowledge the presumed influence of prior experience with stimuli has often been mentioned post hoc, but never has been investigated explicitly. The present study was meant to do this.

Background Considerations

Support for the influence of stimulus and task-specific factors on CRT is provided by (intracultural) research on stimulus-response compatibility (Fitts & Posner, 1967; Kornblum, Hasbroucq & Osman, 1990; Alluisi & Warm, 1990). In CRT tasks a set of stimuli, called an "alphabet," has to be matched to an alphabet of responses. The ease with which an association is established between the two alphabets is dependent on specific characteristics of the stimulus and response configurations. For example, a task is more compatible when of a row of stimulus lights each light is coupled with a response button directly underneath than when the arrangement of the response buttons is reversed. When there is no natural connection between stimuli and responses (i.e., when stimulus-response compatibility is low), experience and familiarity with the stimuli are the most important determinants of associations. The extent of time over which experience or practice can have an effect is easily underestimated. For example, in an experimental setting Shiffrin and Schneider (1977) showed that for a memory-search CRT task it takes thousands of trials to reach a level at which performance no longer improves.

A concept that captures the relevance of the research on stimulus-response compatibility for cross-cultural comparison is "population stereotypes" (Fitts & Posner, 1967; Alluisi & Warm, 1990), i.e., the preferred assignment of response symbols to stimulus symbols shared by a particular group or cultural population. Frequency of exposure is an important determinant of such stereotypes and, as shown by the above mentioned research of Shiffrin and Schneider (1977), the effects of practice can continue for a long time, even under conditions of (controlled) frequent exposure[1].

In the present study a series of CRT tasks of varying cognitive complexity was administered to two samples of subjects of different cultural background, i.e., Iranian and Dutch. For three tasks a set of geometric patterns were used, which was likely to be more familiar to the western sample, although this was not certain. For one additional task a set of stimuli was used that was clearly more familiar to the non-western sample. The response procedure was the same for all tasks.

To show the persistence of stimulus familiarity effects, subjects were trained on one of the tasks. From previous studies with CRT tasks (Poortinga, 1971; Van de Langenberg, 1989; Helms-Lorenz & Van de Vijver, 1995; Sonke, in preparation) two findings have emerged. First, the effects of training (in msec) are larger as the complexity of tasks increases. Second, within a training period of a few days (as is usual in laboratory studies with larger samples) performance curves of different groups show little tendency to converge to a single point. It was expected that these effects would be replicated in the present investigation.

Hypotheses

The design allowed testing of hypotheses addressing three issues: (a) replication of previous results, (b) effects of experience and training, and (c) manipulation of stimulus familiarity. The first hypothesis stipulates a replication of the pattern of results of CRT tasks reported in earlier cross-cultural studies, mentioned before.

We could not assess the prior familiarity of the Iranian subjects with the geometric stimuli and with the kind of procedure used in the experiments. However, if differences would be found they should conform to the following pattern:

1a. In the case of differences between the two samples on the tasks with geometric patterns, performance is expected to be better (i.e., faster mean CRT in msec) for the Western sample.

1b. A cognitively more complex task will show a larger difference in CRT.

1c. Effects of experience (repeated administration) will be larger as a task is more complex.

---

[1] In view of this state of affairs it is hard to think of any type of S-R association in choice reaction time tasks that can be assumed to be equally compatible across a wide range of cultures. This implies that there is no task for which an equal mean CRT can be expected a priori.

With respect to the effects of stimulus familiarity the following expectation was formulated:

2. On the task with the, for them, more familiar (Arabic) stimuli, the non-Western subjects will perform better than the Western subjects.

And finally it was expected that stimulus familiarity effects are persistent, thus allowing that:

3. Possible differences as mentioned in hypothesis 1a and 1b, and the difference mentioned in hypothesis 2 will not disappear within a limited period of training.

Method

Subjects

Twenty-three Iranian (19 male and 4 female; mean age = 29.3 years, sd = 2.6) and 23 Dutch subjects (8 male and 15 female; mean age = 22.1 years, sd = 5.6, university students) participated as paid volunteers. All subjects were tested on three successive days. The Iranian subjects were political refugees who had recently arrived in the Netherlands and were still living in a temporary asylum. Because they might experience it as too threatening, no standardized questionnaire concerning demographic background was administered. However, during the testing sessions it was established informally that the Iranian participants were generally well educated. All of them had at least formal education and with the exception of one all of them were bilingual (second language was either English, German or Spanish). The Dutch subjects were Tilburg University students. An Iranian sample was selected because of their thorough familiarity with the Arabic script, which none of the Dutch subjects could read.

Tasks

A Commodore 386/SX20 PC was used to administer the stimulus presentation and response registration. Hardware functions were extended by a N(uclear) M(odules) S(ystem) and a Keithly CTM05 timer-counter board. In addition to reaction times, errors were recorded. The buttons on the response board were approximately 5 cm apart.

The basic stimulus material consisted of 16 simple geometric figures, derived from the TAART battery (Tilburgse Allochtone Autochtone Reactietijd Test; Van de Vijver & Willemse, 1990). In three of the four tasks elements from this stimulus set were used. The stimuli for the other task were Arabic letters. In all tasks four stimuli were presented, arranged in a square with a centrally located fixation point (a small yellow spot). The stimulus display was presented after a random interval of 500 to 1000 msec after appearance of the fixation point. The subject had to indicate, "as quickly and as accurately as possible," at which position the target figure was presented by pressing one of four buttons, corresponding in position with the four figures. The position of the target varied randomly over the four positions. The interstimulus interval was approximately 5000 msec. If subjects responded before the maximum presentation time (which varied over tasks), the display turned gray. All tasks were administered on three consecutive days at approximately the same time of day.

Each block of 32 trials was preceded by an instruction and 16 self-paced practice trials. These practice trials are not included in the analyses. The order in which the tasks were administered was counterbalanced over the three days. On the first day the tasks were administered in the order of increasing cognitive complexity (A, B, B', C), on the two following days a randomly selected order was used.

Task A. Three black squares and one white square, the target, were presented. Task of the subject was to press the button corresponding with the position of the white square. The maximum response time was 1500 msec.

Task B. Subjects had to memorize four target figures that were a subset of the 16 geometric figures. The targets were the squares with a 1/4 white and 3/4 black surface. On each trial a target figure was presented among three other, different, non-target stimuli. The non-target stimuli were the remaining 12 figures from the basic set. In Fig. 1 an illustration of task B is presented. The maximum time at which the subject could press the button corresponding with the position of the target was 2000 msec. This task was trained on day 1 and 2. A training session consisted of 16 blocks of 32 trials. The total training consisted of 1024 training trials in two days.

Task B'. This task is identical to task B, but the targets were four letters from a subset of 16 letters from the Arabic alphabet. The remaining 12 letters from the subset were non-targets.

Task C. This task required a combination of stimulus elements. The subject had to indicate which of four figures was complementary, in terms of black and white surface, to a fifth stimulus simultaneously at the position of the fixation dot. The maximum presentation and response time was 2500 msec.

Procedure

The Dutch subjects were tested at Tilburg University whereas the Iranian subjects were tested at the asylum. At both locations testing took place in a quiet room in which, besides the testee, only the experimenter (and occasionally an interpreter) were present. Subjects were seated at approximately 1.5 meters from the screen with index and middle finger of both hands resting on the response buttons. On the first two days the experimental session, containing all tasks, was followed by a training session for task B.

Figure 1. An example of a stimulus display of Task B (bottom) and of the memory set (top)

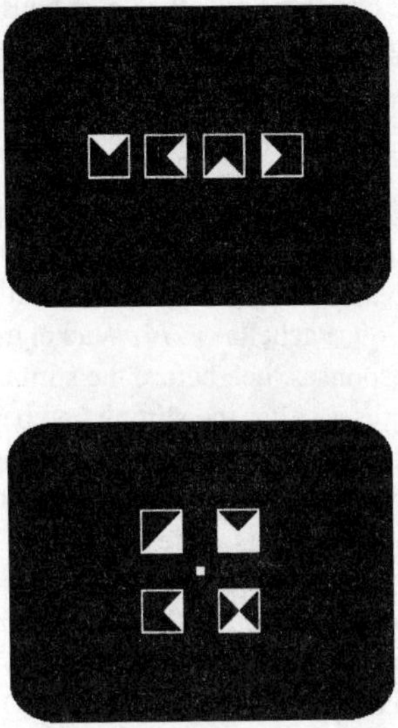

Table 1. Mean reaction times and standard deviations in milliseconds for the Dutch and Iranian subjects on all tasks and days.

	Dutch		Iranian	
	Mean	*SD*	*Mean*	*SD*
Geometric				
A1	403	45.70	462	66.10
A2	354	37.10	424	70.03
A3	343	33.36	421	64.43
B1	639	104.99	736	145.78
B2	511	64.04	608	98.33
B3	473	55.16	593	93.24
C1	883	142.91	1085	169.64
C2	760	121.63	931	106.02
C3	707	100.26	865	111.36
Arabic				
B'1	920	106.77	732	76.88
B'2	811	125.89	683	89.36
B'3	741	95.72	640	72.76

Results

The main statistical analyses for the three tasks with geometric stimuli were MANOVAs with a within-subjects repeated measures design. Within-subjects effects, i.e. tasks and days, were corrected with the Greenhouse-Geisser Epsilon procedure. The unadjusted degrees of freedom and F-values are reported; p-values are adjusted.

Errors

A potential threat to the interpretation of RT data is the proportion of errors, since in CRT tasks subjects can trade off speed for accuracy. If groups differ with respect to this trade-off, a valid comparison of the reaction times becomes very complicated (e.g., Pew, 1969; Pachella, 1974; Wickelgren, 1977).

In this study (a) early responses, i.e., before the stimuli were presented, (b) late responses, i.e., button presses after the stimuli had been removed from the screen, and (c) wrong responses were labeled as errors. Statistical analysis of the numbers of errors proved to be difficult, because of the many records without any error. Averages over subjects were as low as .13 per 32 trials. Analysis with loglinear models turned out to be impossible for this reason. In a MANOVA on the number of errors for the tasks with geometric figures, no difference between the two cultural groups was found ($F(1, 44) = .93, p = .339$). For the level of complexity a main effect was found ($F(2, 88) = 9.98, p < .001$, $\epsilon = .88536$), which is not surprising given the increasing complexity of the tasks. All other effects were non-significant. Most important is the non-significant interaction between cultural group and task ($F(2, 88) = .79, p = .445$, $\epsilon = .88536$), which argues against a difference in speed-accuracy trade off between groups over tasks.

For the task with Arabic letters a difference between groups was found for the numbers of errors ($F(1, 44) = 9.94, p = .003$). Closer inspection revealed that on two of the three days the Dutch subjects made more errors (day 1: $F(1, 44) = 6.73, p = .013$; day 2: $F(1, 44) = 11.25, p = .002$; day 3: $F(1, 44) = .89, p = .349$). Although larger than on the other tasks, the proportions of errors (mean 1.4, 1.4 and 1.3 errors per 32 trials for the Dutch subjects on day 1, 2, and 3, respectively) were still small and are unlikely to have had a major effect. As will become clear later, the direction of the difference was such that it cannot have affected the outcome of the tests of the hypotheses; at most it weakened the size of the effects.

Geometric Stimuli

For both samples there was a significant difference in performance on the three tasks with geometric stimuli, $F(2, 88) = 697.62, p < .001$, $\epsilon = .90298$. A main effect for culture was found ($F(1, 44) = 33.63, p < .001$). As illustrated in Fig. 2, the mean RTs for the Dutch subjects were faster on all three tasks with geometric stimuli. This is in support of Hypothesis 1a that if a group is faster, the Western subjects are the ones who will do better on the tasks with geometric figures. In addition, the culture by task interaction effect was significant, $F(2, 88) = 9.40, p < .001, \epsilon = .90298$. As can be seen in Figure 2 the pattern of the mean reaction times is in line with the hypothesis that the differences between samples increase with task complexity. Thus, support was also found for hypothesis 1b.

A main effect was found for day of testing ($F(2, 88) = 113.80, p < .001, \epsilon = .75804$), showing an overall effect of increasing experience with the tasks. In addition a significant task by day interaction was found ($F(4,176) = 26.44, p < .01, \epsilon = .58398$). As predicted in Hypothesis 1c,

Figure 2. Reaction times in milliseconds for the Iranian (IR) and Dutch (DU) subjects on all tasks and days

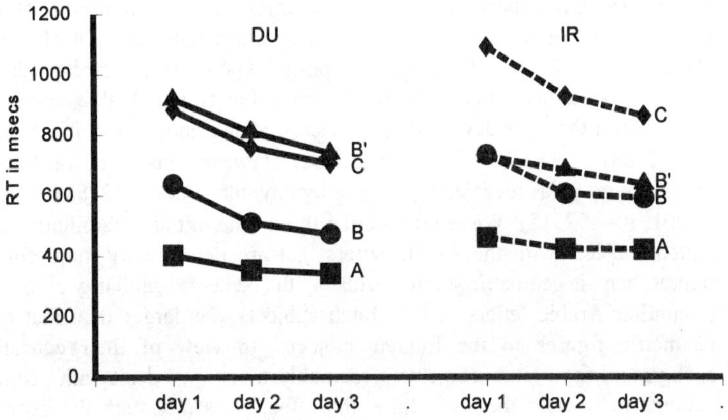

the effect of experience was largest (in terms of a decrease in reaction time in msec) for the most complex task (cf. Figure 2).

The relative differences in performance between the Iranian and Dutch subjects did not change significantly over the three testing days (the culture by day interaction was $F(2, 88) = .06, p = .895, \epsilon = .75804$). The change on the most complex task was somewhat larger in the Iranian sample, but for the two more simple tasks the change was somewhat larger in the Dutch sample (cf. Fig.

2). It is important to note that a non-significant culture by day interaction effect was also found for the task that was trained during two days (task B: $F(2,88) = .55, p = .520, \epsilon = .70923$). These two findings are in support of Hypothesis 3, which predicted that cross-cultural differences even on simple tasks do not disappear quickly.

One further way to illustrate the persistence of differential familiarity effects is an analysis of the effect size of cultural differences over testing days. For each task the mean RT of the Iranian subjects was subtracted from the mean RT of the Dutch subjects and divided by the pooled standard deviation (M_{DU}-M_{IR} / S_{pooled}) which gives a standardized expression for the size and direction of the effects. This resulted in the following values[2]: task A: -.92, -1.07, -1.22; task B: -.72, -1.01, -1.24; task B': 1.42, 1.01, 1.03 (see below) and task C: -1.09, -1.21, -1.20 on day 1, 2 and 3 respectively. It should be noted that the values are more or less equal (irrespective of direction) for all tasks and on all days.

Arabic Letters

The pattern of results was reversed when Arabic letters were used as stimulus material (see Figure 2). Iranian subjects responded faster than Dutch students ($F(1, 44) = 27.78, p < .001$). This supports Hypothesis 2, which predicted a relatively better performance for the Iranian subjects with Arabic letters.

Over the three days both groups showed an improvement in RT on task B' ($F(2, 88) = 111.87, p < .001, \epsilon = .92512$). However, this effect was larger for the Dutch group as revealed by a group by day interaction ($F(2, 88) = 11.78, p = .001, \epsilon = .92512$). We would ascribe this to the initial unfamiliarity of the Dutch subjects with the Arabic letters that are perceptually more complex figures than the geometric stimuli. Probably the perceived similarity of the rather unfamiliar Arabic letters to the Dutch subjects was larger than that of the geometric figures to the Iranian subjects. In view of their educational background the Iranian subjects presumably must have dealt with geometric patterns before. At the same time, the effect sizes (see with the geometric stimuli) for this task were of about the same magnitude as for other tasks, though in the opposite direction.

Discussion

In the present study differential familiarity with a cognitive task was emphasized as a source of variation across cultures in performance. This explanation was tested by manipulating the familiarity of the stimulus material in CRT tasks, both in terms of initial familiarity and in terms of experience or explicit training.

---

[2] Note that a negative value indicates that the Dutch subjects responded faster, whereas a negative value means that Iranian subjects were faster.

The results demonstrated the effects of familiarity unambiguously.

With simple geometric figures a pattern of results was found that has been reported previously (Jensen, 1985; Poortinga, 1971; Van de Langenberg, 1989; Verster, 1991). Specifically, it was found that the Dutch subjects responded faster and this difference in reaction times increased as tasks became more complex. A training of a few days was not sufficient to change the effects of differential stimulus familiarity of the non-western subjects with the geometric figures. However, when Arabic letters were used as stimuli for one of the tasks, the Iranian subjects who were more familiar with these stimuli outperformed the Dutch students. These results show the importance of stimulus familiarity and at the same time the persistence of its effects.

The present study was limited to relatively simple tasks. This raises the question to what extent the findings can be generalized to more complex tasks. However, it seems more than likely that familiarity effects increase rather than decrease with a further increase in task complexity; in concrete terms, it is unlikely that the divergent trend of the graphs in Fig. 2 will turn towards a convergent trend with higher complexity.

The approach of this study illustrates a "third road" between traditional comparative interpretations of cognitive differences and the so-called cultural ones (Poortinga, 1998). In the school of cultural psychology, cognitive processes are seen as culturally mediated (Vygotsky, 1978). In older studies culture-specific mental functions were postulated at a high level of generality (e.g., Luria, 1971). In Cole's sociocultural school there has been a – and in our opinion welcome -- shift to more situation-specific explanations (Laboratory of Comparative Human Cognition, 1983; Scribner & Cole, 1981). However, the concept of culturally-mediated functioning is maintained (cf. Cole 1992a, b) and this concept as such does not suggest ways to access cognitive processes directly.

The findings support the notion of identity of cognitive processes. Irrespective of the absolute value of the reaction times both groups show the same pattern of results with geometric stimuli, as is illustrated in Figure 2. At the same time, the apparent importance of familiarity with stimulus material for performance on these relatively simple tasks undermines the idea of comparativists like Jensen (1982, 1985) that some RT tasks are devoid of knowledge content. However implausible it may seem for a specific task that prior knowledge or experience plays a role, this can never be assumed. The present results show that differential familiarity with stimulus material is a sufficient reason to make cross-cultural comparison of performance levels on any cognitive task extremely questionable. The persistence of the effects over days suggests why it is so difficult to reach equal levels of performance through experience. Inferences about differences in underlying cognitive capacities between cultural populations are not warranted as long as the possibility of cultural bias due to task specific effects cannot be reasonably excluded.

Our findings point to the value of systematic analyses of cross-cultural differences that concentrate on cognitive processes per se, for example, along the lines of Sternberg's (1969; Sanders, 1980, 1993) additive factor method. Detailed analysis with mundane, well-operationalizable concepts, like "familiarity" or "experience", suggests a scope for parsimonious explanations, avoiding at the same time the use of diffuse concepts like "cognitive capacity" with its deterministic overtones and also of "cultural mediation" with its implicit suggestion of culture-specificity of psychological processes.

References

Alluisi, E. A., & Warm, J. S. (1990). Things that go together: A review of stimulus-response compatibility and related effects. In R. W. Proctor & T. G. Reeve (Eds.), *Stimulus-response compatibility* (pp. 3-30). Amsterdam: Elsevier Science Publishers.

Cole, M. (1992a). Culture in development. In M. H. Bornstein & M. Lamb (Eds.), *Developmental psychology: An advanced textbook* (3rd ed., pp. 731-789). Hillsdale, NJ: Erlbaum.

Cole, M. (1992b). Context, modularity, and the cultural constitution of development. In L. T. Winegar & J. Valsiner (Eds.), *Children's development within social context* (Vol. 2, pp. 5-31). Hillsdale, NJ: Erlbaum.

Eysenck, H. J. (1982). *A model for intelligence.* Berlin: Springer.

Fitts, P. M. , & Posner, M. I. (1967). *Human performance.* Belmont:, CA: Brooks/Cole.

Helms-Lorenz, M. & Van de Vijver, F. J. R. (1995). Cognitive assessment in a multicultural society. *European Journal of Psychological Assessment, 11*, 158-169.

Hick, W. E. (1952). On the rate of gain of information. *Quarterly Journal of Experimental Psychology, 4*, 11-26.

Jensen, A. R. (1982). Reaction time and psychometric g. In H. J. Eysenck (Ed.), *A model for intelligence* (pp. 93-132). Berlin Heidelberg: Springer-Verlag.

Jensen, A. R. (1985). The nature of the black-white difference on various psychometric tests: Spearman's hypothesis. *The Behavioral and Brain Sciences, 8*, 193-263.

Kornblum, S., Hasbroucq, Th., & Osman, A.. (1990). Dimensional overlap: Cognitive basis for stimulus-response compatibility. A model and taxonomy. *Psychological Review, 97*, 253-270.

Laboratory of Comparative Human Cognition (1983). Culture and cognitive development. In P. H. Mussen & W. Kessen (Eds.), *Handbook of child psychology* (Vol. 1, pp. 295-356). New York: Wiley.

Luria, A. R. (1971). Towards the problem of the historical nature of psychological processes. *International Journal of Psychology, 6*, 259-272.

Pachella, R. G. (1974). The interpretation of reaction time in information processing research. In B. H. Kantowitz (Ed.), *Human information processing: Tutorials in performance and cognition* (pp. 431-482), Hillsdale NJ: Erlbaum.

Pew, R. W. (1969). The speed-accuracy operating characteristic. *Acta Psychologica, 30,* 16-26.

Poortinga, Y. H. (1971). Cross-cultural comparison of maximum performance tests: Some methodological aspects and some experiments with simple auditory and visual stimuli. *Psychologia Africana,* Monograph Supplement, *No. 6.*

Poortinga, Y. H. (1985). Empirical evidence of bias in choice reaction time experiments. *The Behavioral and Brain Sciences, 8,* 236-237.

Poortinga, Y. H. (1989). Equivalence of cross-cultural data: An overview of basic issues. *International Journal of Psychology, 24,* 737-756.

Poortinga, Y.H. (1998). Cultural diversity and psychological invariance: Methodological and theoretical dilemmas of cross-cultural psychology. In J. G. Adair, D. Bélanger & K. L. Dion (Eds.), *Advances in Psychological Science* (Vol. 1, pp. 229-245). East Sussex, UK: Psychology Press.

Posner, M. I. (1985). Chronometric measures of g. *The Behavioral and Brain Sciences, 8,* 237-238.

Sanders, A. F. (1980). Stage analysis of reaction processes. In G. E. Stelmach & J. Requin (Eds.), *Tutorials in Motor Behavior* (pp. 331-354). Amsterdam: North-Holland.

Sanders, A. F. (1993). Performance theory and measurement through chronometric analysis. In D. E. Meyer & S. Kornblum (Eds.), *Attention and Performance XIV: Synergies in Experimental Psychology, Artificial Intelligence, and Cognitive Neuroscience,* (pp. 689-699).

Scribner, S. (1979). Modes of thinking and ways of speaking: Culture and logic reconsidered. In R. O. Freedle (Ed.), *New directions in discourse processing* (pp. 223-243). Norwood, NJ: Ablex.

Scribner, S., & Cole, M. (1981). *The psychology of literacy.* Cambridge, MA: Harvard University Press.

Serpell, R. (1979). How specific are perceptual skills? A cross-cultural study of pattern reproduction. *British Journal of Psychology, 70,* 365-380.

Shiffrin, R. M., & Schneider, W. (1977). Controlled and automatic human information processing: II. Perceptual learning, automatic attending, and a general theory. *Psychological Review, 84,* 127-190.

Sonke, C. J. (in preparation). *Cross-cultural differences on cognitive tasks: A psychophysiological investigation.* Ph.D. thesis, Tilburg, Tilburg University.

Sternberg, S. (1969). The discovery of processing stages: Extension's of Donders' method. *Acta Psychologica,* 30, 276-315.

Tulviste, P. (1991). *The cultural-historical development of verbal thinking* Commack, NY: Nova Science Publishers.

Van de Vijver, F. J. R., Daal, M., & Van Zonneveld, R. (1986). The trainability of formal thinking: A cross-cultural comparison. *International Journal of Psychology, 21,* 589-615.

Van de Vijver, F. J. R., & Willemse, G. R. (1990). Are reaction time tasks better suited for cultural minorities than paper-and-pencil tests? In N. Bleichrodt & P. J. D. Drenth (Eds.), *Contemporary issues in cross-cultural psychology* (pp. 450-464). Lisse, The Netherlands: Swets & Zeitlinger.

Van de Langenberg, G. (1989). *Prestatieverbeteringen op reactietijdtaken van uiteenlopende cognitieve complexiteit. Een cross-cultureel onderzoek* Master's thesis, Tilburg University, Tilburg.

Verster, J. M. (1991). Speed of cognitive processing: Cross-cultural findings on structure and relation to intelligence, tempo, temperament, and brain function. In P. L. Dann, S. H. Irvine & J. M. Collis (Eds.), *Advances in computer-based human assessment* (pp. 103-147). Dordrecht, The Netherlands: Kluwer Academic Publishers.

Vygotsky, L. S. (1978). *Mind in society: The development of higher psychological processes*. Cambridge, MA: Harvard University Press.

Wason, P. C., & Johnson-Laird, P. N. (1972). *Psychology of reasoning: Structure and content*. Cambridge, MA: Harvard University Press.

Wickelgren, W. (1977). Speed accuracy trade-off and information processing dynamics. *Acta Psychologica, 41*, 67-85.

An Indian Perspective on Understanding Intelligence

Ashok K. Srivastava
National Council of Educational Research and Training, New Delhi
Department of Educational Research/ Policy Perspectives

Girishwar Misra
University of Delhi
Department of Psychology

ABSTRACT

The study of intelligence has recently outgrown the cognitively loaded psychometric tradition of research. Explorations with the notions of social and emotional intelligence, prudence, and wisdom, as well as the emergence of social constructionist view have expanded the discourse on intelligence in different directions. Reports from diverse cultures indicate that the social representation and emphasis on aspects of intelligence vary across cultures. Against this backdrop, this study makes an effort to articulate the indigenous notion of intelligence in the Indian cultural context. The analysis of textual sources available in the form of *suktis*, proverbs in Hindi language, and laypersons' conception and use of intelligence in their day-to-day life indicates four dimensions of intelligence. In order of priority, these dimensions are: Personality and Motivation, Social Competence, Reasoning and Problem Solving, and Communication Skills. Intelligence is conceptualised mainly in terms of socio-affective characteristics of individuals. It is considered an important attribute of the individual so far as it contributes to performance, social harmony, and well-being of the people. Results have been explained in terms of the distinctive features of the Indian society.

Until recently the notion of intelligence was confined largely to individual's ability for abstract cognitive reasoning and problem solving in a relatively decontextualized framework in line with the physical scientific tradition. Thus concerted efforts were made to develop abstract theories of cognitive development and related functions among adults, and technologies for the assessment of cognitive competencies were developed. The psychometric tradition fostered the attempt at quantification of mental abilities. This position, however, is being challenged by the unfolding of research on several related concepts which indicate multiplicity in intelligence. Also, the evidence accumulating from diverse settings suggests that the notion of intelligence is culturally variable. It is realised that culture includes cognition and other intellectual functions. This paper extends the position by recognizing indigenous ideas regarding intelligence in the Indian cultural context. In particular, it examines the notion(s) of intelligence as reflected in the long and rich scholarly tradition and its social representation in a cross-section of contemporary Indian society.

In Indian philosophical treatises, intelligence, as Das (1994) has noted, refers to "waking up, noticing, recognising, understanding, and comprehending. In contrast to the western notion of intelligence, *Buddhi* (intellect) includes such things as determination, mental effort, and even feelings and opinions in addition to such intellectual processes as knowledge, discrimination, and decision making" (p.387). This literature is so rich and varied that it is difficult to summarise. For instance, in the Samkhya-Yoga model of consciousness, any act of awareness involves three levels of consciousness: *manas, ahankara,* and *buddhi*, usually translated as "lower mind", "ego", and "intellect", respectively. *Manas* picks up the input, *ahankara* sorts the input according to a continually revised scheme of classification, and *buddhi* assesses the value of the categories that *ahankara* is using. The Samkhya school construes intelligence in terms of two types of *bhavas* or the state of being, i.e., *sattvika* and *tamasika*. The *sattvika* (pure) *bhavas* constitute *dharma* (virtue), *jnana* (knowledge), *viraga* (non-attachment), and *aishvarya* (power) while *adharma* (non-virtue), *ajnana* (ignorance), *raga* (attachment), and *anaisvarya* (weakness) constitute *tamasika* (impure) *bhavas*.

Ancient Indians located intelligence in the arena of morality. They distinguished between bad and good intelligence. Good intelligence (*dharma buddhi*) leads to happiness, pleasure, prosperity, and is constructive, whereas bad intelligence (*pap buddhi*) is destructive and leads to unhappiness. This has elsewhere been referred to as *sarala* (or simple and straightforward) and *kutila* (or devious and cunning) intelligence (Badrinath, 1999). An intelligent person distinguishes between what is temporary (*nitya*) and what is permanent (*anitya*). Examining the relationship between consciousness and the physical structure, Das (1994) has noted that, according to the eastern view, pure consciousness is at the top with no material basis. From consciousness evolves discriminative intelligence or *buddhi*. The consciousness of one's own identity emerges from discriminative and evaluative intelligence.

It may even be noted that the folk or vernacular tradition in India has also been remarkable. In almost all regions there have been legendary figures and saintly poets who have articulated the folk wisdom in various languages. Also, numerous proverbs have been popular across the country throughout history.

Intelligence in the Mainstream Psychology

The conceptualisation of intelligence as a single entity or disposition is currently facing serious challenges. The concept of *mental age* as proposed by

Binet has, for several reasons such as equivocality, non-linearity, and unidimensionality, proved to be a weak link in the psychometric analysis of intelligence. Different metaphors (e.g., geographic, computational, biological, epistemological, anthropological, sociological, and systems) lead to diverse ways of conceptualising the processes of knowledge acquisition and utilisation (Sternberg, 1990a). Intelligence is now viewed as "the mental abilities necessary for adaptation to, as well as shaping and selection of, any environmental context" (Sternberg, 1997, p.1030). What is included in these processes can not be divorced from the socio-cultural milieu or ecology within which a behavior takes place (Carugati, 1990). The same set of mental processes may give rise to very different behaviors in varying environmental contexts.

Recent work on *wisdom* (Sternberg, 1990b), *prudence* (Haslam, 1991), *social intelligence* (Cantor & Harlow, 1994), *emotional intelligence* (Mayer & Salovey, 1997), and *practical intelligence* (Sternberg, Wagner, Williams, & Horvath, 1995) indicates that, to understand intelligence, it is the intermix of domains which needs exploration. The stress on socio-cultural context demands attending to the characteristics, traits or skills which are valued in everyday life of a given society. This necessitates the examination of social representation of intelligence, consisting of mixtures of precepts, images and concepts. These social representations are shared by people, passed on from one generation to the next, and imposed upon each of us without our conscious assent. Researchers have made efforts to discover the people's conceptions of intelligence in various societies (for details, Neisser *et al*, 1996; Rogoff & Chavajay; 1995, Srivastava & Misra, 1996), and have examined the definitions of intelligence in non-Western cultures.

Often these definitions differ from the definitions western researchers take for granted. For example, intelligent people are slow and conforming in Africa (Wober, 1974). In Kenya, "parents defined 'intelligence' as the ability to do what is needed to be done around the homestead *without being asked*" (Harkness, Super, & Keefer, 1992, p.105). In the African population a distinct emphasis on maintaining harmonious and stable intergroup relations is observed. The Pacific ethno-theories are also social in nature (Poole, 1985). The Japanese concept of social intelligence consists of positive social competence, receptive social competence, task efficiency, originality, and reading and writing (Azuma & Kashiwagi, 1987). Greenfield (1997) advocates using local definitions of intelligence when it is assessed in new cultural contexts.

Intelligence Testing in India

The measurement of intelligence in India has largely been confined to the psychometric tradition. Intelligence tests developed in the West were translated into Indian languages and are used extensively for selection, training, evaluation, and diagnostic purposes in various settings. However, critical appraisals of these tests have found that a majority of them are seriously limited (Misra, Sahoo, & Puhan, 1997; Sinha, 1983; Srivastava, Tripathi & Misra, 1996). Most of the tests adopt a factorial approach and include categories of abstract reasoning of various kinds. Barring a few exceptions (e.g., Das, 1994; Srivastava & Misra, 1999; Srivastava, Tripathi, & Misra, 1995), India's vast traditional treasures have largely remained unexplored by psychological scholarship.

The Present Study

This study analyzes the indigenous Indian conception of intelligence. It has two interrelated goals. First, it analzes the nature of intelligence and ways it influences behavior as guided by the *Sanskrit Suktis*, and in the proverbs in Hindi language. Second, layperson's conceptions of intelligence are examined to see the continuity and change between ancient and the contemporary notions of intelligence.

The ancient scholarly texts, written in Sanskrit, contain wisdom in the form of *suktis* or *subhasitas* (good words). The *suktis* may be comprised of only one or two sentences, but are believed to be close to ultimate reality, and reflect the essence of experiences of foresighted saints. As a small lamp lightens the entire house, these *suktis* reveal secrets of the living and non-living world. Also, the proverbs (or maxims) are used extensively to effectively express socially shared ideals. The use of these expressions in day-to-day writing and conversation makes language more precise, lively, and loaded with meanings. It is believed that proverbs represent well-known truths, social norms or moral actions. Rooted in the social traditions of a community, they often summarize the essence of folk wisdom in the form of shared experiences. Though a few proverbs and *suktis* may loose their relevance over time, a majority of them continue to serve as valuable guides (Tandon, 1995).

Traditionally, life in the Indian culture was perceived as a source of fulfilment, both spiritual and material. The four *purusharthas* (life goals) - *dharma* (virtue), *artha* (wealth), *kama* (desire) and *moksha* (salvation) clearly reflected these concerns. The fact that Indian economy has primarily been agricultural led to the development of common characteristics including deep loyalty to the family or clan. Social interdependence, sharing, and harmony were basic values. In recent years, however, it is increasingly realised that the traditional Indian culture has undergone transformation under the impact of Western education, urbanisation and industrialisation (Srivastava, 1995). To Srinivas (1966), some of these changes are: Sanskritization or a lower caste person behaving like a higher (*brahman*) caste; secularisation (or less importance to religious beliefs); modernisation, industrialisation, and urbanisation (movement of large numbers of people from rural to urban centres); and westernization (change in behavior patterns resulting due to Western cultural ethos). In these contexts, it becomes imperative to understand contemporary notions of intelligence among lay persons who have diverse backgrounds.

Method

Three lay persons, having competence for Sanskrit language and with no formal training in psychology, scanned about 20,000 *suktis* contained in Sagar's (1990) *Vishwa Sanskrit Sukti Kosh*, and Verma and Verma's (1985) *Vishwa Sukti Kosh*. They were told to indicate whether a *sukti* was in any way related to 'intelligence' as found in the everyday usage. We examined the suktis thus identified and, in case of ambiguity, clarifications were sought. In this way 254 *suktis* having reference to intelligence, were finally identified. Likewise, 214 proverbs were identified after scanning four dictionaries of Hindi proverbs: Madhav and Misra's (1965) *Kahawat Kosh*, Sharma's (1983) *Vargikrit Hindi Lokokti Kosh*, Shukla and Sharma's (1986) *Hindi Lokokti Kosh*, and Kaushik, Shastri, Shastri, and Gupta's (1990) *Muhawara Lokokti Kosh*. These volumes report about 25,500 proverbs in Hindi. Since the volumes are not mutually exclusive, a large number of proverbs are common in these volumes. It may be noted that while the volumes by Kaushik *et al* (1990), and Sharma (1983) include proverbs spoken in standard Hindi language, Madhav and Misra (1965) cover proverbs spoken in the regional languages of the state of Bihar. Shukla and Sharma (1986) report the proverbs spoken in the region of central India. Thus these volumes contain the majority of the proverbs spoken in the Hindi language.

Each *sukti* and proverb was read independently by at least two investigators proficient in these languages, and having knowledge of the historical and spiritual traditions. Based on the meaning contained in the *suktis* and proverbs a conceptual category was assigned. These categories were further grouped into a few broad categories on the basis of their conceptual configuration. There was high agreement between investigators regarding the meaning and grouping of *suktis* and proverbs.

Results

The analysis revealed four dimensions of intelligence, namely, S*ocial Competence, Reasoning and Problem Solving, Communication Skills, and Personality and Motivation*. Among Sanskrit *Suktis*, highest priority (52%) was given to personality and motivational characteristics, which was followed by social competence (34%), and reasoning and problem solving (10%). In contrast, Hindi proverbs accorded maximum weightage to social competence

(38%), which was followed by reasoning and problem solving (29%), and personality and motivational characteristics (27%). Least importance was granted to communication skills by both *suktis* (4%) and proverbs (6%).

The characteristics of an intelligent person were arranged in order of frequency of their occurrence in *suktis* and proverbs from high (rank 1) to low (rank 22). In the following description, rank is shown against each characteristic in the parenthesis.

Under the category of social competence, the analysis indicated that an intelligent person displays sensitivity to the context (1), exhibits practical thinking (2) and respect for elders (15), is not affected by criticism and adverse circumstances (15), follows *dharma* (which refers to three attributes, namely nurturing, sustaining, and securing freedom from violence) (15), and takes preventive measures (19.5). The peculiarities such as control over emotions, particularly anger (3), positive self-appreciation (4), moderation in behavior (5.5), humanitarian attitude (5.5), patience (8), speaking truth but restraining from truth that may be harmful to the society (11), willingness to learn (12.5), and vigilance (19.5) are reported under personality and motivational characteristics of an intelligent person. Six reasoning and problem-solving abilities like reflective thinking (7), ability to draw inference (9.5), future planning (9.5), learning from past experiences (12.5), dealing with problems resourcefully (19.5), and ability to translate small opportunities into big successes (19.5) emerged from the analysis. Also, an intelligent person communicates effectively (17) and gives statements that are loaded with meaning (22).

Images of the Lay People

The results of the interview conducted to obtain lay persons' understanding and use of intelligence representing different walks of life are reported in this section.

Method

A total of 200 participants volunteered for the study, all residents of New Delhi, India. An equal number of participants varying along the dimensions of schooling (schooled and unschooled), and age (12-14 years, 16-18 years, 20-25 years, 45-50 years, and 60+ years), of both sexes, were approached by the investigator either at their places of work/study or at home. The mean educational level for schooled and unschooled participants was 12 and 2 years of schooling, respectively. Persons having completed primary education (at least 5 years of schooling) were considered as schooled. Care was taken to ensure the representation of participants from diverse occupational backgrounds. The participants were asked to respond to the following open-ended question:

> In our day-to-day experience we find some people to be very intelligent while others behave in an unintelligent way. In your opinion, what are the attributes/ characteristics/ behaviors of an intelligent person?

The investigator approached the participants and, after establishing proper rapport, asked the question. The responses were recorded verbatim by the investigator in the form of written notes. Each response was read independently by two investigators and its meaning was determined.

Results

In response to the open ended question, the participants reported numerous characteristics (N=1514) of an intelligent person. A large portion (35%) of these responses were reported by unschooled females, which was followed by unschooled males (31%), schooled males (18%), and schooled females (16%). An age-wise analysis showed that it was the youth (in the age group of 20-25 years) who contributed maximum number of attributes (26%), followed by the respondents in the age group of 60+years (21%), 16-18 years (19%), 45-50 years (18%), and 12-14 years (16%).

Table 1 shows that, irrespective of schooling, age, and gender, the participants bestowed highest priority to personality and motivational characteristics, followed by social competence, reasoning and problem solving abilities, and least importance was accorded to communication skills. The only exception was the population in the age group of 20-25 years, who rated social competence higher than the personality and motivational characteristics.

Table 1. Characteristics of an Intelligent Person as Contained in Suktis and Proverbs (Percent Frequencies)

Categories	*Suktis* (N=254)	Hindi Proverbs (N=214)
1. Social Competence	34	38
2. Reasoning and Problem Solving	10	29
3. Communication Skills	4	6
4. Personality and Motivation	52	27

Tables 2 and 3 contain rankings for the most frequently reported characteristics identified by the lay people. Under the category of social competence, like *suktis* and proverbs, all respondents, irrespective of their background, reported an intelligent person as context-sensitive. The participants in the age group of 20-25 years described an intelligent person as one who is effective in interpersonal relationships. The unschooled respondents gave primacy to the quality of service to elders. Elderly unschooled females also projected an intelligent person as one who keeps the family united. To elderly males, both schooled and unschooled, the following social profile described the attributes of an intelligent person. All elderly participants described an intelligent person as one who shows respect for guests and respect for others' feelings.

Table 2. Most Frequently Noted Characteristics of an Intelligent Person (Ranks)

Characterisitcs	*Suktis*	Proverbs
Social Competence		
1. Behaves according to place, time and person	1	1
2. Is practical	8	2
3. Follows *dharma*	8	-
4. Is not affected by criticism and adverse circumstances	9	12
5. Shows respect for elders	8	-
Reasoning and Problem Solving		
6. Is able to draw inferences	12	4
7. Is reflective	5	11
8. Plans ahead	10	6
9. Learns from past experiences	-	4
10. Can discriminate between right and wrong	6	7
Communication Skills		
11. Communicates effectively	10	11
12. Gives statements with surplus meanings	-	9
Personality and Motivation		
13. Shows moderation in behaviour	3	10
14. Shows positive self-appreciation	7	3
15. Speaks truth (in context)	6	-
16. Is hardworking	5	5
17. Has control over emotions	2	-
18. Shows patience	8	9
19. Shows humanitarian attitude	4	-
20. Is vigilant	-	8
21. Shows willingness to learn	11	7

Table 3. Laypersons Conception of Intelligence and Intelligent Behavior (Percent Frequencies; N=1514 Attributes)

Groups	Social Competence	Reasoning and Problem Solving	Communication Skills	Personality and Motivation
Schooling and Sex				
1. Schooled Male	31	33	4	32
2. Schooled Female	34	18	4	44
3. Unschooled Male	33	18	5	44
4. Unschooled Female	35	14	4	47
Age Groups				
5. 12-14 years	24	20	3	53
6. 16-18 years	28	23	6	43
7. 20-25 years	41	23	3	33
8. 45-50 years	35	17	6	42
9. 60+ years	37	11	3	49

Participants agreed that an intelligent person is obedient, helpful, moderate, and has control over emotions (except by 16-18 years age group). Characteristics like honesty and hard work were reported only by young schooled females and unschooled males. Elderly people (60+ age group) described an intelligent person as friendly, religious, and the one who maintains cleanliness.

Different groups of participants in different degrees endorsed reasoning and problem solving abilities. Very few elders regarded them important. The remaining participants reported that an intelligent person is characterised by reflective thinking, and scientific orientation (except schooled females). Schooled participants were also of the opinion that an intelligent person is able to discriminate between right and wrong. Schooled males thought an intelligent person has the ability to solve problems and show independence in thought.

Barring 12-14 year olds, there was a consensus that an intelligent person is able to communicate effectively. Unschooled males and participants in the age group of 45-50 years placed a relatively greater stress on this attribute.

Discussion

The ancient and contemporary Indian construals of intelligence are in contrast to the Western notions of intelligence which, until recently, placed great emphasis on reasoning and problem solving abilities. In the Indian view, a person is judged intelligent if competent in social problem solving and is generally pro-social.

The study indicated that sensitivity to context is important. Sensitivity to context refers to the beliefs about the significance of person (*patra*), time (*kala*), and ecology (*desh*). A behavior that is judged intelligent for a given place, time and person may or may not be intelligent for other times, places and persons. This leads to the development of associative thinking, rather than abstract thinking used in problem solving and reasoning. Intelligent people handle inter-personal relationships in an effective manner. They weigh and evaluate various alternatives (reflective thinking) and choose appropriate behavior in a given context. Here, *dharma* plays an important role.

Another feature of an intelligent person is showing respect for and service to parents, elders, and guests. It may be noted that Indian child rearing practices make a special effort to inculcate in the child a regard for elders (Krishnan, 1998). The economic value of children (such as extending the family tree, service to elders, and material contribution received from them) are given primacy by the Indian parents (Srivastava, 1997). The unschooled elderly females saw intelligence localised in the activity of keeping the families united. This reflects current concern regarding the break down of the traditional family system .

The personality and motivational characteristics received prime importance in the traditional and in the lay people's conception of intelligence. These characteristics are related to three sub-groups: work ethic, dependability, and sensitivity to others. An intelligent person shows willingness to learn and moderation in behavior, remains vigilant, works hard, and shows positive self-appreciation. His/her confidence and ability to win others' trust as well as his/her honest and responsible behavior portrays him/her as a dependable person in the society. His/her control over unpleasant emotions, obedient behavior, speaking of restrained truth, and friendly and humanitarian outlook make him/her sensitive to others.

While the ancient tradition places relatively greater emphasis on work ethics, the contemporary view projects the other sensitive behaviors of an intelligent person. This is evident on two counts. First, the majority of lay people were of the opinion that an intelligent person is obedient and of a helping nature. Second, in contrast to the ancient view, only young participants talked about honesty and hard work. Willingness to learn was not included in the lay people's responses. This indicates the erosion of the work ethic from contemporary Indian society.

Instead of valuing mere possession of reasoning and problem solving abilities, the application of these abilities in real life situations is glorified in the Indian view of intelligence. The qualities like reflective thinking, drawing inference, discrimination between good and bad, future planning, translating small opportunities into big success, and learning from past experiences require the transfer and use of abilities in different contexts. The elderly people also did not visualise intelligence in terms of cognitive abilities. Rather, they have emphasised the use of abilities in different social contexts like helping the needy ones, serving the elders, and behaving according to the context.

The Indian view does not attach significance to communication alone. Rather, in order to be considered intelligent, one needs to communicate effectively. This is expected in a country like India, which had a rich oral tradition, where *jnana* (knowledge) was never written down but was handed down orally from the *Guru* (teacher) to the *Shishya* (disciple). This oral tradition emphasised the excellence of *Priyamvada* (felicitous speech). A person showing the excellence of *priyamvada* has no eye for obstinate argumentation, though in reasoned discourse (s) he is as readily eloquent as the god of speech. (S) he has a meticulous sense of place and time. (S) he descries through the people at a glance and yet behaves properly towards them. Never does (s) he utter a foul word. And to cap it all, (s) he is as acutely conscious of his or her failings as (s) he is of others.

Conciusion

The notion of intelligence as prevalent and practised in the Indian tradition stands at a distance from the prevalent Western conceptualisation of intelligence. In the Western society, intelligence is viewed in terms of one's ability to express himself/herself, communicate clearly, and succeed in society, and do it in a manner that will make a fast, positive impression among a variety of groups. A very different picture emerges in the Indian context where intelligence is conceptualised in terms of social competence, humanitarian stance and control over negative emotions. Here social competence has been viewed in terms of maintaining associations, harmony, and stability within in-groups. In other words, intelligence is not limited to the success of the individual alone. Rather, it aims at achieving common good. These trends are quite similar to the analysis of the characteristics of the wise people given by Maciel, Sowarka, Smith and Baltes (1992). They find that exceptional knowledge (e.g., procedural knowledge, functional knowledge, contextualism, uncertainty) and exceptional personality (e.g., social intelligence, open mindedness, reflexivity, humility) form part of the wise people.

According to the Indian view, intelligence stands for an adaptive potentiality of a person across different domains of life. Not restricted to cognitive domain alone, this adaptive potentiality consists of a range of skills that equip one to overcome life problems, to grow and become what one wants to achieve in personal as well as social domains. These skills are not uniformly distributed in the society and people internalise them, operate with them, and in that process move to higher levels of competence in those skills. A seer, for example, after having realized the lower order truth, aims at the attainment of a higher level. Thus transcending oneself is a continuous demand on an intellectual being. On the whole the present findings suggest a functional or pragmatic view of intelligence which operates at different levels allowing flexible multifaceted transaction between self and context. This position broadens our perspective on intelligence and invites further work to identify and assess many of the competencies which have been neglected for a long time.

References

Azuma, H., & Kashiwagi, K. (1987). Descriptions for an intelligent person: A Japanese study. *Japanese Psychological Research, 29*, 17-26.

Badrinath, C. (1999, February 5). Dharma and governance: Upholding the laws of rule. *The Times of India* (New Delhi), 12.

Cantor, N., & Harlow, R. (1994). Social intelligence and personality: Flexible life-task pursuit. In R.J. Sternberg & P. Ruzgis (Eds.), *Personality and intelligence* (pp.137-168). Cambridge: Cambridge University Press.

Carugati, F.F. (1990). Everyday ideas, theoretical models and social representations: The case of intelligence and its development. In G.R. Semin & K.J. Gergen (Eds.), *Everyday understanding: Social and scientific explanations* (pp.130-150). London: Sage Publications.

Das, J.P. (1994). Eastern views of intelligence. In R.J. Sternberg (Ed.), *Encyclopaedia of human intelligence* (pp.387-391). New York: Macmillan Publishing Company.

Geenfield, P.M. (1997). You can't take it with you: Why ability assessments don't cross cultures? *American Psychologist, 52*, 1115-1124.

Harkness, S., Super, C., & Keefer, C. (1992). Culture and ethnicity. In M.D. Levine, W.B. Carey, & A.C. Crocker (Eds.), *Developmental-behavioral paediatrics* (2nd ed., pp.103-108). Philadelphia: Sounders.

Haslam, N. (1991). Prudence: Aristotelian perspectives on practical reason. *Journal for the Theory of Social Behavior, 21*, 151-169.

Kaushik, A., Shastri, G.S., Shastri, S., & Gupta, T. (1990). *Muhawara-Lokokti-Kosh*. Delhi: Hindi Pustak Bhawan.

Krishnan, L. (1998). Child rearing: The Indian perspective. In A.K. Srivastava (Ed.), *Child development: The Indian perspective* (pp. 25-55). New Delhi: National Council of Educational Research and Training.

Maciel, A.G., Sowarka, D., Smith, J., & Baltes, P.B. (July, 1992). *Essential attributes of wise people*. Paper presented at the 25th International Congress of Psychology. Brussels, Belgium.

Madhav, B.N.M., & Misra, V. (Eds.) (1965). *Kahawat Kosh*. Patna: Bihar Rashtrabhasha Parishad.

Mayer, J.D., & Salovey, P. (1997). What is emotional intelligence? In P. Salovey & D. Sluyter (Eds.), *Emotional development and emotional intelligence: Implications for educators* (pp.3-31). New York: Basic Books.

Misra, G., Sahoo, F.M., & Puhan, B.N. (1997).Cultural bias in testing: India. *European Review of Applied Psychology, 47*, 309-316.

Neisser, U., Boodoo, G., Bouchard, Jr., T.J., Boykin, A.W., Brody, N., Ceei, C.J., Halpern, O.F., Loehlin, J.C., Perloff, R., Sternberg. R.J., & Urbina, S. (1996). Intelligence : Known and unknown. *American Psychologist, 51*, 77-101.

Poole, F.J.P. (1985). Coming into social being: Cultural images of infants in Bimin-Kuskusmin folk psychology. In G.M. White & J. Kirkpatrick (Eds.), *Person, self, and experience: Exploring Pacific ethnopsychologies* (pp. 183-244). Barkeley: University of California Press.

Rogoff, B., & Chavajay, P. (1995). What's become of research on the cultural basis of cognitive development? *American Psychologist, 50*, 859-877.

Sagar, L. (Ed.) (1990). *Vishwa sanskrit sukti kosh* (3 vols.). Jodhpur: Ramanand Garg & Co.

Sharma, S.R. (1983). *Vargikrit Hindi lokokti kosh*. New Delhi: Takshashila Prakashan.

Shukla, H.L., & Sharma, R.N. (1986). *Hindi lokokti kosh*. Delhi: Rajesh Prakashan.

Sinha, D. (1983). Human assessment in the Indian context. In S.H. Irvine & J.W. Berry (Eds.), *Human assessment and cultural factors* (pp.17-34). New York: Plenum Press

Srinivas, M.N. (1966). *Social change in modern India*. Bombay: Allied Publishers.

Srivastava, A.K. (1995). Extent of acculturation of the Indian society. *Social Change, 25*, 121-131.

Srivastava, A.K. (1997). The changing place of child in Indian families: A cross-generational study. *Trends in Social Science Research, 4*, 191-200.

Srivastava, A.K., & Misra, G. (1996). Changing perspectives on understanding intelligence: An appraisal. *Indian Psychological Abstracts and Reviews, 3*, 3-34.

Srivastava, A.K., & Misra, G. (1999). Social representation of intelligence in the Indian folk tradition: An analysis of Hindi proverbs. *Journal of Indian Psychology*, in press.

Srivastava, A.K., Tripathi, A.M., & Misra, G. (1995). Western and Indian perspectives on intelligence: Some reflections. *Indian Educational Review, 30*, 30-45.

Srivastava, A.K., Tripathi, A.M., & Misra, G. (1996). The status of intelligence testing in India: A preliminary analysis. *Indian Educational Review, 31*, 1-11.

Sternberg, R.J. (1990a). *Metaphors of mind: Conceptions of the nature of intelligence*. Cambridge: Cambridge University Press.

Sternberg, R.J. (Ed.) (1990b). *Wisdom: Its nature, origins, and development*. Cambridge: Cambridge University Press.

Sternberg, R.J. (1997). The concept of intelligence and its role in lifelong learning and success. *American Psychologist, 52*, 1030-1037.

Sternberg, R.J., Wagner, R.K., Williams, W.M., & Horvath, J.A. (1995). Testing Common sense. *American Psychologist, 50*, 912-927.

Tandon, P.C. (1995). Saidhantik aayamon ke pariprekshya mein muhaware awam lokoktiya. *Bhasa, 34*, 38-48.

Verma, S.B., & Verma, M. (Ed.) (1985). *Vishwa sukti kosh* (3 vols.). Delhi: Prabhat Prakashan.

Wober, M. (1974). Towards an understanding of the Ugandan concept of intelligence. In J.W. Berry & P.R. Dasen (Eds.), *Culture and cognition* (pp.261-280). London: Methuen.

Intellectual Development of Children in Gypsy Families in Romania

Tatiana Dumitrascu
Institute of Public Health
Timisoara, Romania

ABSTRACT

In this study, we analyzed the relationship between parental child-rearing style and child intellectual development in the Romanian and Gypsy cultures. We also performed qualitative analyses on the intelligence data of Gypsy children because they provided unique culturally-specific answers and behaviors during testing sessions. Two samples of 50 Gypsy families and 50 Romanian families (parents and 9-10-year old children) were investigated with Wechsler's Intelligence Scales. All parents completed Varga's questionnaire on parental educative attitudes. There was no relationship between these attitudes and children's IQ for either Romanian mothers or fathers or for Gypsy mothers. For Gypsy fathers, "Symbiosis is related to firstborn daughters IQ and "Authoritarianism" is related to both first- and second-born IQ. A comparison between Gypsies and Romanians shows they have different IQ profiles. The non-verbal IQ score of Gypsy children and parents is significantly lower than the verbal IQ score, whereas the reverse pattern occurs in the Romanian sample. The specific intellectual profile and characteristics such as verbal poverty, lack of common elementary knowledge are comparable to "abandoned children" rather than persons identified as mentally retarded. From this perspective, we discuss the implications for educating Gypsy children and families.

In many studies devoted to child cognitive development, certain family configuration characteristics, e.g., family size, are considered as influences on development. The family size effect actually means that the level of intellectual development of children in the family decreases as the number of children increases. This effect has been found to be highly stable, no matter which IQ tests are applied (Blake, 1989; Breland, 1977; Storfer, 1990; Zajonc, 1983).

There are a number of possible mediators of this family size effect. For example, innate parental intellectual potential could be related in the following manner: low parental IQ > high fertility > low child IQ. Limited parental schooling could constitute an environmental component of intellectual potential that determines the educative style, motivational and emotional characteristics of the family. The reduced child IQ could reflect the deterioration of parental educational resources as a consequence of increasing family size (in particular, deterioration of the quality of verbal communication). Other relevant factors are related to possible means of controlling the family size effect, such as child spacing, parental age and low socioeconomic status (Storfer, 1990). Of these, the socioeconomic status has the closest relationship with family size. A combination of large family size and low socioeconomic status is especially unfavorable for mental development of children.

Based on our review of the research on family size effect, we find consistent and efficient theory is Zajonc's confluence model (1980; 1983). Zajonc's approach is based on the concept of intellectual environment, particularly, a family environment. The intellectual environment is made up of each family member's individual contribution (including children). It is assumed that the level of family intellectual environment is diminished because the young children's contribution to the family intellectual environment is very small. With multi-cultural data, Zajonc (1983) asserts that the family size effect is strongly culture dependent. Although family size effect is present in all cultures, there is a different intensity in each of these cultures. Thus a cross-cultural analysis of child intellectual development in extended family may contribute to a better understanding of the psychological mechanisms of family size effect.

To date, the family size effect has been studied with an interfamilial (between-families) methodology but there is increasing support for intra-familial (within-family) studies. It has become apparent that the effects of family size are quite transparent in large samples (to which one can hardly apply intra-familial methodology) and quite uncertain in small samples (Ravich-Scherbo, 1988; Stocker, Dunn & Plomin, 1989). Within-family analysis shows that even in families with equal socioeconomic status and other formal characteristics (like race, religion etc.) the manifestation of family size effect may vary. So, it appears that the influence of family size on child development depends on the interaction with other environmental within-family factors, shared and unshared.

Among these "other factors", structural characteristics of family environment, e.g., gender birth order, as well as individual ones, e.g., parental educative attitudes, may be fundamental. Parental educative attitudes appear to have more pervasive influence on the child's intellectual development because parental child-rearing style may be characterized as both shared (common) and unshared (unique). First, in that the parents apply the same style to all children, it remains a common factor. Alternatively, if the parents use different attitudes toward different children, e.g., towards firstborns/lastborns children or girls/boys, it is a unique factor.

Another aspect of parenting style is that both parents may show the same general type of behavior but differ in some particular attitude. For example, both parents are authoritarian, but one is also symbiotic whereas the other is rejecting. Thus, a common "authoritarian" environment for all children in a family may be "authoritarian-rejecting" in dyads, for instance, father-child and "authoritarian-symbiotic" in dyads mother-child. Or an "authoritarian-rejecting" father may be more rejecting in his relationship with the son and less rejecting with daughter etc. Further, the overall influence of mother's and father's authoritarian style on the intellectual development of children may not be equal, as found in a study of Russian large families (Dumitrascu, 1996; 1998).

Consequently, we should take birth order and gender of the children into account in our analyses of dyadic interactions (parent-child) in extended families. Attending to these variables may help avoid confounds between family size effect and effects of other characteristics of family environment, such as parental educative attitudes.

Finally, we plan to examine structural environmental factors such as low socioeconomic status and belonging to a culture in which a large family is typical. These factors in combination with parenting style and family size represent a cluster of negative influences on child intellectual development. The present study is designed to examine families in a culture that is typified by the above negative cluster, in this case, Gypsy families.

Gypsies are a minority in Romania, their community lives in relative isolation from the Romanians and other minorities, like Germans or Hungarians. From the majority culture's perspective, Gypsies differ from others in lifestyle that appears to be a mixture of modern and archaic elements. Since their arrival in Europe, the Gypsies developed a unique strategy of survival within the hosting populations, by using all legal or illegal opportunities to earn a living (for example, re-selling second hand cars, clothes etc.). It is traditionally considered that the Gypsy population lives in poverty. However, not all Gypsies families are poor. There are families with low, middle, and high income. In part because of their life-style, the source of income of the Gypsies, (the very wealthy as well as the poor) is usually impossible to figure out.

Traditional Gypsy families are extended, with a large number of children. At present, the average number of children in Gypsy families is at least twice the number of children in families of the host country. The more traditional their way of life, the more children they have. This leads to a low level of education, lack of intellectual skills, and poverty. Moreover, Gypsy families often consist of 3-4 generations, include distant blood relatives and even biologically unrelated persons. This traditional pattern of family configuration seems to enhance survival through mutual assistance. Statistics show that the unemployed Gypsy men have the largest and most extended families.

The schooling of adult Gypsies is precarious. Most are illiterate and women receive less schooling than men. The women tend to marry young, give birth to many children and, traditionally, remain housewives. The parents show a contradictory attitude to their children's scholarship. On the one hand, they are afraid the school may alienate the children from them. There is a history of generations of Gypsy parents who educated their children at home. Consequently, parents do not strive to send their children to school. This is not to imply that Gypsy children never attend school. Most Gypsy parents and children are undoubtedly conscious about the crucial importance of literacy, the need to attain a higher cultural level, and the advantages of assimilating into the Western and Romanian culture. However, we know that certain factors do predict greater school attendance such as maternal schooling, professional qualification of father, residence (in cities more children go to school), and family income.

Thus, in addition to the negative effect of family size and low socioeconomic and status, one might expect a more negative attitude of Gypsy parents toward formal education. This composite of negative factors renders the process of social adaptation of Gypsy children more difficult. With their unique family and parenting style, standard quantitative procedures may not fully present the intellectual development of Gypsy children. Thus, it appears that qualitative descriptions of their intellectual development, may suggest ways to educate them (e.g. whether there is a need for special textbooks). Therefore, we also present a qualitative analysis of intellectual characteristics of Gypsy parents and children.

It is valid to question the relevance of standard IQ tests with a culture like the Gypsies. But consider IQ tests to have a valid place in our assessment. At the moment, the Gypsies are considered part of the Romanian people; their first language is Romanian, and the schools they and their parents have attended are Romanian. So, formally there is no reason to test Gypsy children with tests other than the accepted standardized tests in Romanian. We have evidence that German and Hungarian children (whose families live in Romania) go to Romanian schools, much like the Gypsies, and have no problems with these tests. We consider one problem is that Gypsies do not value literacy like Romanians or others. However, this attitude is changing with the conviction there is no chance to survive without adequate education.

The Wechsler intelligence tests offer a number of advantages for this study. The sub-tests do not require writing or reading skills. Thus, literacy is not a requirement for completion of the WAIS or WISC. Further, the standardized scores of the verbal and non-verbal subscales permit group comparison. At the same time, the descriptive features of the test results permit a qualitative analysis of an individual intellectual profile.

Thus, the present study compares Gypsy and Romanian parents and children on standardized IQ scales and seeks to place the results in cultural context. Further, parental educative attitudes are examined for their influence on child cognitive development.

Method

Participants

The Gypsy sample consisted of 50 4-5-child families of Gypsies. In most families, parental schooling was limited to the first 4 grades with some parents having attended secondary school. However, during the introductory interview, most parents, (fathers and mothers) manifested interest in the schooling of their children and encouraged their children's school attendance. None of the parents had a permanent job. Actually, in many families one of the parents was a seasonal worker and then the second had no job, or both had no job. In this case, parents earned a living by reselling second-hand clothes, sunflower seeds and the like. Almost all families had a low socioeconomic status, although there was no way to estimate their real income. Thus, we based our determination of socio-economic status on indirect criteria such as how the house (the apartment) looked, how the parents appraised their own living standard or even what the children's teachers thought of the living standard of their pupils.

The average age of Gypsy parents was 28.5 (26-31 years), the average age of firstborn children was 9.5 (9-10 years), and the spacing between children was less than 2 years. All participant children attended school. Among the firstborns, 28 were males and 22 females; among the secondborns, 30 were males and 20 females. Between the parents and two oldest children, 200 persons were involved in the study.

The Romanian sample consisted of 50 1-child families, all of them members of the major Romanian population. The average parent age was 31 (29-33) years. Both parents had graduated from high school or vocational school. Both parents were qualified workers and had permanent jobs. All families were of middle socioeconomic status. The average child age was 9.5 (9-10 years) with 21 males and 29 females. In each family, both parents and the child were involved in the experiment, 150 persons in all. All participant families, Romanians and Gypsies, reside in the city of Timisoara.

Measures

In correspondence to the main purposes of our study, we employed two kinds of tests: to evaluate 1) the degree of intellectual development, and 2) parental educative attitudes.

Wechsler Intelligence Scales

The degree of intellectual development was measured with two versions of Wechsler's scales (Wechsler, 1970; 1974): Wechsler Adult Intelligence Scale (WAIS) and Wechsler Intelligence Scale for Children (WISC R). Both versions were translated and adapted for Romanian speakers at the Institute of Education Science (Bucharest, 1991). We chose Wechler's methodology because it is the most widely used tool for investigation of intelligence.

The (Performance) Verbal scale of intelligence consisted of the following tests: "General Information", "Comprehension", "Arithmetic", "Similarities", "Digit Span", and "Vocabulary". The non-verbal (Performance) scale of intelligence consisted of the following tests: "Digit Symbol", "Picture Completion", "Block Design", "Picture Arrangement", and "Object Assembly". The test-retest reliability for the measures is quite high: 0.96 for WAIS Verbal IQ; 0.93-0.94 for WAIS Performance IQ; 0.97 for WAIS total IQ; 0.93-0.94 for WISC R Verbal IQ; .90 for WISC R Performance IQ; 0.95-0.96 for WISC R total IQ (Burlachuk, 1989).

Parental Educative Attitudes

To evaluate parental educative attitudes, an inventory by Varga (Varga, 1988) was used. We translated it from Russian into Romanian, then back-translated it to prove the validity of the Romanian version. This inventory includes 5 scales described below.

Scale 1, "Acceptance-Rejection", measures the general emotional attitude towards the child. The first pole ("acceptance") of the scale corresponds to the following characteristics: 1) the child is liked by his parent as he or she is; 2) the parent respects the child's individuality and sympathizes with the child; 3) the parent likes spending his or her time with the child; 4) the parent approves the child's interests and plans. The other pole ("rejection") is characterized as follows: 1) the parent feels the child is unsuccessful, unlucky, unaccepted; 2) the parent thinks the child will never succeed in his/her life due to silliness, predisposition, lack of ability; 3) the parent feels constantly angry, annoyed with and even offended by the child; 4) the parent does not trust and does not respect the child.

Scale 2, "Cooperation", is the socially desired model of parental attitude. The parent is interested in the child's concerns and plans, tries to help the child with everything and sympathizes with the child. The parent appreciates the child's intellectual and creative aptitudes, is proud of the child. The parent encourages the child's initiative and self-reliance, tends to construct a parity relationship with the child. The parent trusts the child and likes joining the child's opinion in controversial questions.

Scale 3, "Symbiosis", measures the interpersonal distance in the parent-child relationship. High scores mean the parent identifies himself or herself with the child. Subsequently, the parent tends to fulfill all the child's needs and protect him/her against hardship and disappointment. The parent is constantly anxious about the child. The child looks too small and helpless to the parent. The parent's anxiety increases as the process of the child's emancipation begins. If it were up to the parent, he or she would never give independence to the child.

Scale 4, "Authoritarian (hypersocialization)", demonstrates the way the parent controls the child's behavior. High scores mean the parental attitude is distinctly authoritarian. The parent demands that the child to obey him/her unconditionally. The parent is unable to understand the child's viewpoint and manifests dictatorial tendencies. At the same time, the parent knows very well the child's character, thoughts, and feelings. The child is severely punished for any manifestation of autonomy. The parent carefully follows the child's social achievements and demands the child to do his or her best to accomplish social success.

Scale 5, "Infantilization", measures parental perception and appraisal of the child. A high score means the parent shows a tendency to infantilize his child, to believe him incapable of personal or social achievement. The parent sees the child as if the child were younger than he or she really is. The child's interests, preferences, thoughts and feelings look immature, and not of consequence to the parent. The child is considered as inexperienced, unsuccessful, and susceptible to bad influences. The parent does not trust the child and is annoyed with the child's lack of skill and accomplishments. Consequently, the parent tends to protect the child against hardship and strictly controls the child's actions.

The inventory consists of 61 questions. To evaluate the educative attitudes, the scores are summed within each of the five groups. High scores mean respectively: high rejection, high cooperation, high symbiosis, high authoritarianism, and high infantilization. The raw test scores are substituted by percentage, according to a special scale. Respectively, a percentage greater than 50 indicates a high score.

We analyzed all data with standard statistical procedures. Quantitative relations between parameters have been evaluated with Pearson correlation. Mean differences have been calculated with the t-test analyses.

Procedure

The research project involved three stages. In the first stage, we validated the measures on a few families that belonged to the same social environment and had other characteristics were similar to those of the intended sample. In addition, this preliminary stage helped acquaint us with many of difficulties associated with testing the intelligence of Gypsy persons (see Section 1 in Results for more details). The second task was to identify and select the two samples of families, Gypsy then Romanian.

The third stage was the actual data collection. Each individual was contacted twice: first, to present brief information on the research purpose, to gather additional data about parental qualification, profession, income etc. and to determine parental educative attitudes, and second, to conduct the intelligence testing. Both the conversation and testing were accomplished in the participant's home.

Results

IQ comparisons between Romanian and Gypsy children and parents. If we categorized the IQs of the Gypsy parents and children based on comparison with the standardized sample, we would draw the conclusion that Gypsy parents and children belong to "mental deficiency" category. Similarly, we would place the Romanians in the "average intelligence" category (Wechsler's original classification: score < 69 – "mentally retarded"; 70-79 –"borderline retarded"; 80-89 – "low-average"; 90-100 – "average" intelligence). Yet, common sense says that such a global categorization is too simplistic and does not accurately reflect the intellectual strengths and weaknesses of Gypsy parents or their children.

One option might be to give up Wechsler's test and search for a more suitable IQ measure. However, the following reasons prevented us from doing so. First, our goal was to analyze special features of intellectual profile, rather than simply measure the degree of intellectual development. Second, there was variability in the scores of Gypsy individuals, similar to the range of scores in the Romanian parents and children. Third, we found that the verbal and reasoning abilities were consistent with the IQ scores. Thus, we determined that the IQ scores for Gypsy parents and children were reliable.

Table 1. Mean parental IQ across Gypsy and Romanian samples (WAIS)

	Gypsies		Romanians	
	Mothers	Fathers	Mothers	Fathers
Verbal IQ	64.8* ±9.7	68.5* ±10.3	89.1* ±10.5	91.8** ±11.3
Non-verbal IQ	60.1* ±11.2	65.6* ±13.0	96.8* ±14.6	104.5** ±15.1
General IQ	60.6 ±10.3	65.4 ±11.7	91.6 ±11.9	97.1 ± 12.7

Marked with * and ** are mean values that differ at significant level (p < .05 and p < .01) when verbal and non-verbal IQ scores are compared

Table 2. Mean IQ of children across Gypsy and Romanian samples (WISC R)

	Gypsies	Romanians
Verbal IQ	64.3* ±11.5	81.6** ±10.2
Non-verbal IQ	56.1* ±11.9	115.7** ±15.4
General IQ	57.1 ±11.1	97.3 ±13.0

Marked with * and ** are the mean values that differ at significant level ($p < .05$ and $p < .01$) when the verbal and non-verbal IQ scores are compared

Culturally-Specific Responses on IQ Tests

We subjected the answers of Gypsy parents and children to a qualitative analysis of intellectual traits. We identified some typical "inappropriate" answers to questions belonging to different subtests and named them, respectively: "Echo answer", "Synchretic answer", "Certifying answer", "Guessed answer", and "Missing answer". In the Romanian sample there were no answers of the sort. The Romanians either answered "I don't know" or there was no problem in classifying their answers and scoring them according to standard answers given in the test.

A. "Echo answer": The individual gives no answer but repeats the last word of the question or other word in the question.

B. "Synchretic answer": The individual tells a story about some objects or events occasionally related to the subject of the question, or some phrases concerning the emotions the question caused to him or her.

C. "Certifying answer": The individual does not answer the question but either adds to it some content he or she considers necessary ("Picture completion") or just tells a story about what one can see, what happens here and there, without any concern to make the story logically consistent ("Picture arrangement").

D. "Guessed answer": Basically, a combination of models A – C, accompanied by a specific behavior. For example, the individual gives an answer of type A, B or C, and then immediately looks at the experimenter in an attempt to determine whether the answer is correct or not.

E. "Missing answer": The individual answers "I don't know". Alternatively, if asked "In what ways are these two objects alike?" or "What is missing in this picture?", the individual responds, "They are not alike" or "Nothing is missing."

Based on a thorough quantitative and qualitative analysis of individual responses from the Gypsy sample, we compile the following intellectual profile. The participants demonstrated concerns about secondary details, possibly a sign of a serious anxiety. They had an impoverished vocabulary, a limited common knowledge in literature, arts, and science, with a tendency toward concrete thinking and poor spatial-perception problem-solving. Gypsy parents and children were more action- than reflective-oriented, demonstrated poor attention to tasks that appear useless to them. Overall they had low scholastic achievement, and lived in a culturally deficient environment.

Cultural comparisons of child-rearing style

The mean values that characterize child-rearing styles of parents in Romanian and Gypsy samples are presented in Table 3.

Table 3. Mean values of the educational attitudes of Romanian and Gypsy parents (%, Varga's inventory)

Educative Attitudes	Romanians		Gypsies	
	Mother	Father	Mother	Father
Rejection	77,2*	80,7	84,6*	82,1
Cooperation	34,8*	30,0*	43,8*	38,4*
Symbiosis	78,6*	75,0	84,3*	73,3
Authoritarianism	79,1	81,9	79,1	80,5
Infantilism	79,2*	76,3	86,1*	77,7
Marked with * are the mean values that differ at significant level ($p < .05$) when the Romanian and Gypsy mothers and, respectively, fathers scores are compared				

In the Romanian population, "Rejection" positively correlates with "Authoritarianism" (.30, $p < .05$) and "Infantilization" (.33, $p < .05$) for mothers alone. "Symbiosis" scores of both parents correlate significantly with "Authoritarianism" and "Infantilization" scores (for mothers - .39 and .45; for fathers - .48 and .52; $p < .05$). In addition, "Authoritarianism " correlates with "Infantilization" (.33 for mothers and .55 for fathers; $p < .05$). Hence we find two maternal and one paternal child-rearing style patterns. For the mothers, one pattern is "Authoritarianism + Infantilization + Rejection", and the other is "Authoritarianism + Infantilization + Symbiosis". For the fathers, the pattern involves "Authoritarianism + Infantilization + Symbiosis". Of all the correlative analyses between the intellectual characteristics of parents and their educative attitude, only one is significant: maternal verbal intelligence positively correlates with maternal "Cooperation" (.33, $p < .05$).

In the Gypsy population the predominant type of educative style, for both parents, is "Authoritarianism" + "Infantilization" + "Symbiosis". Maternal scores correlated (.48 between "Authoritarianism" and

"Infantilization"; .55 between "Infantilization" and "Symbiosis"; .48 between "Authoritarianism" and "Symbiosis"; $p < .05$) and paternal correlations were .39 between "Authoritarianism" and "Infantilization"; .35 between "Infantilization" and "Symbiosis" $p < .05$. Hence only the Romanian mothers show alternatively two types of behavior, whereas the Romanian fathers and both Gypsy parents behave the same way. No intellectual characteristics of Gypsy parents are correlated with their educative attitudes. Similar to the Romanian parents, the majority of the correlations between child-rearing styles and child general IQ are insignificant. In the Gypsy sample, only father's "Authoritarian hypersocialization", is related to child IQ (.29; $p < .05$).

With respect to child gender and/or birth order, there are few effects. In the Gypsy population, the firstborn daughters' intellectual score correlates with the father's "Symbiotic" style (.65, $p < .05$). The authoritative style of fathers correlates to the firstborns' intelligence (.47, $p < .05$) as well as the secondborns' (.35, $p < .05$). We found no relationship between maternal parenting style and child IQ for either gender or birth order.

Discussion

In accordance with the main purposes of our study, we have analyzed specific IQ characteristics of the Gypsies in our sample and investigated the relationship between parenting child-rearing style and child intellectual development.

Culturally-Specific Intellectual Development of Gypsies

There are some IQ findings unique to the Gypsy population. For example, the non-verbal IQ scores of Gypsy children and parents are significantly lower than the verbal IQ score. This does not match the results of similar studies carried out on other populations in which the reverse is found (as demonstrated by the scores pattern in our Romanian sample). This pattern suggests that the intelligence structure of Gypsy children is basically molded within family, rather than the school and mass media as the main intelligence shaping factors. Moreover, the above mentioned disproportionality manifests stronger with children than parents, in each of the two populations. This specific IQ structure may explain to some extent why the Gypsy students encounter difficulties at school.

The decidedly low scores of the Gypsies on intelligence tests, especially in non-verbal tests, may have been caused by a total lack of an intellectual life. In no family of our sample was there a single book in evidence, and the children had practically no toys. A slightly more developed verbal intelligence may be explained with the way the Gypsies usually earn a living: all the day they spend in crowded places, e.g., in markets, selling any imaginable sort of new and second hand stuff - a business that requires a fluid speech. At the same time, their everyday language remains quite primitive and one can easily distinguish in it the word patterns they use while doing their job.

Parallel Populations

The development of children educated in boarding schools and orphanages is similarly discrepant from average children in the culture. This discrepant IQ pattern differs from that of intellectually backward children. A number of investigations utilizing the WISC-R with children diagnosed as "mentally backward" showed that verbal intelligence is much lower than that of non-verbal intelligence. In contrast, abandoned children (who inhabit the boarding schools and orphanages) prove to have a low non-verbal IQ but a verbal IQ may be even medium degree. The abandoned children usually resolve successfully the subtests that rely on practical manipulation and action abilities ("Block Design") and fail solving the tasks which require advanced logical reasoning ("Picture Arrangement").

The abandoned children follow thus a specific type of intellectual development, which can be by no means characterized as "retardation". Consequently, to deal with this kind of specific disorders, some quite different methods are needed to improve performance intelligence. To improve these children's functioning, they should be involved with various concrete social situations and informal relations and encouraged for free activities with people of all ages (children and adults). Finally, we need to enhance the affective experience of these children.

The similarity founded between the intellectual development of abandoned children and the Gypsies permit speculation that the unique characteristics of intellectual development of the Gypsies are actually the result of life conditions much similar to "hospitalism". This analogy is by no means exaggerated but has historical precedent. Since their migration to Europe, the Gypsies have become isolated from their national roots and experience only a meager social support. "It is impossible to find a job: we are rejected everywhere. Only underpaid occasional jobs are available," the Gypsies say. The hardship strengthens and coarsens the character and leaves no room for sentiments. This leads to another similarity one may notice between abandoned children and this "abandoned people". Both have similar affective reactions to the unfair and discriminating social establishment to which they are bound.

We apply the term "abandoned people" as suitable for the Gypsy population. It is used here not merely to disparage the intellectual and personality development of Gypsies (children and adults) and abandoned children. Rather, there are parallels in these two populations in social behavior and social portrait: self-isolation, disbelief in everybody who does not belong to the community, aggressiveness with little respect for the social norms of the broader culture. The general difficulties the Gypsies have in making productive contact with the rest of society have a further parallel at the micro-social level, due to large family size. Namely, in a large family, the children have to interact just with each other because the parents spend all of their time and energy seeking basic survival.

On the other hand, at the macro-social level, the Gypsies mostly communicate with each other and very little with the rest of society. This keeps their information level constantly out-of-date. Thus, in order to function in the Gypsy culture, children do not need to improve their speech and enlarge their knowledge about the world they live in. This may explain the lack of investment in school for Gypsy children. Quite frequently, Gypsy children do not go to the kindergarten. Those who do go to school usually leave it long before the 8th grade. At the school, they are passive and never do their homework. According to teachers interviewed, Gypsy children typically attend school only long enough to learn to write a little. Or, they may, attend a driving school, again long enough to learn to set up some form of second hand car business. Therefore, in terms of Zajonc's confluence theory (1980, 1983), the parental encouragement of child intellectual development is minimal. Consequently, the degree of intellectual development, even the structure of intelligence is roughly limited in the same pattern for all family members.

With respect to formal psychological characteristics, the research data clearly demonstrate the family size effect in the Gypsy population. The substantive differences in mean IQ between the Gypsy and Romanian samples is consistent with the results of other studies, in which the family size effect is stronger at a lower socioeconomic level. We assume that, in the Gypsy population, this effect is even more emphasized due the socio-cultural isolation. In this study, we confirmed that the parents' style of child rearing relates to the family configuration. In large families, the parental behavior is more uniform across children. In small families, in the Romanian sample, there is more variability and child-specific parenting styles.

We propose certain interventions as the most direct and most efficient way to address the problem of lower IQ. First, we must put maximum effort to enrolling as many Gypsy children as possible in kindergartens. This is important because in early childhood the children are more likely to be open to the school experience (have few stereotypical antipathies and prejudices) and derive greater benefit from the educational experience. We have greatest hope that teachers, who are trained in maximizing positive interactions within a group of children, will be key contributors to an eventual resolution of the "abandoned people" problem.

Culturally – Specific Child-Rearing Style and Child Intellectual Development

Our study confirmed that the parents' style of child rearing relate to the traditions of the particular culture to which the family belongs. Parental behavior varied greatly in the two samples. The Gypsy mothers made more frequent complaints about their children than Romanian mothers. Yet, at the same time, the Gypsy mothers also encouraged their children's initiative and supported the children's concerns and plans. Not surprisingly, the Gypsy mothers spoke more of the necessity to protect and supervise their children outside the Gypsy community, and told about real dangers their children were likely to encounter anytime they left their home (e.g. when they go to school). Consistent with this view of the world, the Gypsy mothers see their children as younger and more helpless than the children objectively are. The Romanian mothers are eager to help their child when they feel he/she need it and have a tendency to supervise and protect their children. Yet the Romanian mothers' approach is consistent with general developmental principles.

Across both groups, all parents show a highly "authoritarian" attitude but the authoritarian-ness is manifested differently in each culture. The educative behavior of the Gypsy parents may be characterized as "indulgently observant" (they do not interfere with the problems of children unless there is an emergency; real emergencies cases are solved by parents in a very authoritarian way).. Conversely, the Romanian parents are rather "indulgently hyperprotective" (they interfere every now and then in their child's life and feel fully responsible for the outcome).

We expected that different parental child-rearing practices would affect child intellectual development, but found no support for this hypothesis in our correlative analyses between child-rearing style and child intellectual development However, the correlations that do occur enable us to posit a few conclusions. Because all selected families were matched on specific parameters, each depicted difference may reflect an actual population difference, related to cultural traditions. For the Gypsies, only two types of attitude positively correlate with others), namely, "Symbiosis" and "Authoritarianism", and only for fathers. The maternal attitude does not relate directly to the child's measured IQ. This result was also found in the Romanian sample. Because there is a substantive literature identifying mothers' influence on child IQ, further study with more complex statistical procedures is warranted. Yet we are intrigued with the differential effects of Gypsy paternal symbiosis or authoritarianism on child IQ as a function of birth order or gender.

Our first attempt to evaluate the psychological and intellectual functioning of the Gypsy population in Romania has raised more questions than answers or solutions. Despite the limitations of this first effort, we hope it may provide a starting point for future studies of the Gypsy people.

References

Blake, J. (1989). Number of siblings and educational attainment. *Science, 245,* 32-36.

Breland, H. (1977). Family configuration and intellectual development. *Journal of Individual Psychology, 33*, 86-96.

Burlachuk, L. (1989). *Handbook in psychological diagnostics*. Kiev: Naukova dumka.

Dumitrascu, T. (1996). Family structure and child cognitive development. *Voprosy Psihologii, 2,* 104-113.

Dumitrascu, T. (1998). *Family factors of child development. A comparative psychological study of three populations*. Timisoara: Eurobit.

Ravich-Scherbo, I.V. (1988). *The role of environment and inheritance in human individuality formation*. Moscow: Pedagogika.

Stocker, C., Dunn, J., & Plomin, R. (1989). Sibling relationships: links with child temperament, maternal behavior, and family structure. *Child Development, 6,* 715-727.

Storfer, M. (1990). *Intelligence and giftedness*. Jossey-Bass Publication.

Varga, A., Stolin, V. (1988). A questionnaire on parental attitude. In V. Stolin (Ed), *Practikum po psihodiagnostike* (pp. 107-113). Moscow: Editions of Moscow State University.

Wechsler, D. (1970). *Manuel – Echelle d'intelligence de Wechsler pour adults, W.A.I.S., adaptation et traduction.* Paris: Centre de Psychologie Appligue.

Wechsler, D. (1974). *Manual for the Wechsler Intelligence Scale for Children Revised.* New York: Psychological Corporation.

Zajonc, R., Bargh, J. (1980). The confluence model: Parameter estimation for six divergent data sets on family factors and intelligence. *Intelligence, 4*, 349-361.

Zajonc, R. (1983). Validating the confluence model. *Psychological Bulletin,93,* 457-480.

Author Note

This work was partly supported by the Research Support Scheme of the OSI/HESP, grant No 1138/1996. The author is especially grateful to Dr.Deborah Forgays for her help in preparation of this paper.

On the Cultural Relativity of Problem-Solving Styles: Explorations in India and Germany [1]

Stefan Strohschneider
Otto-Friedrich-Universität Bamberg
Lehrstuhl Psychologie II

ABSTRACT

The interaction of culture and problem-solving using a computer-simulated complex and dynamic problem was explored. The ways in which people try to tackle such problems are shaped by their learning experiences as well as the functional constraints within which they have to operate. An experiment was conducted with university students from India and Germany as participants. They had to work on one of two different versions of the ***MORO***-problem. *MORO* is a computer-simulated interactive complex problem where participants have to take the role of a developmental administrator and try to improve the living conditions of a small tribe of semi-nomads in Africa. The protocols of the problem-solving processes were analyzed with a focus on the strategic aspects of problem-solving. Indian and German problem solvers differed in their approach regardless of the version with which they worked.. German students used a more active and control-oriented strategy and committed fewer errors in the course of problem-solving, whereas Indian students used a more feedback-oriented strategy and sought more contextual information.

Cross-cultural research on thinking and problem-solving has largely been restricted to the analysis of formal tasks (van de Vijver & Willemsen, 1993). Since such tasks are of limited complexity, it is unclear whether they allow for conclusions generalizable to more realistic contexts which can often be described as complex, dynamic, intransparent or opaque to the problem solver and thus having no well defined problem-space. Over the last two decades, this kind of complex problem-solving has been at the focus of cognitive psychologists mainly in Europe (see Dörner, 1996; Frensch & Funke, 1995). Within this research tradition it is generally accepted that major psychological insights come from analyzing the problem-solving processes themselves, not the outcomes of these processes. This shifts the focus towards the problem-solving strategies or patterns of decision making. Whereas the role of individual-level factors like domain-specific knowledge, strategic competence, or intelligence is comparatively well studied (Jansson, 1995; Ramnarayan & Kumar, 1996; Ramnarayan, Strohschneider & Schaub, 1997), the cultural embeddedness of complex problem-solving remains largely unexplored and a kind of "implicit absolutism" (Lonner, 1993) prevails.

This paper reports on an experiment which is based on the assumption that the strategies which we apply in dealing with novel and complex problems are dependent on our cultural background. Participants in the experiment came from India and Germany. In the following section, the cultural dimensions that can be considered important for the development of problem-solving styles will be analyzed. Following that will be a discussion of some relevant differences between India and Germany.

Complex Problem-solving and Culture: The Case of India and Germany

If one takes a strictly functional perspective on problem-solving, there are basically five (probably interrelated) aspects of culture that contribute to the development of specific problem-solving patterns:

1. **Predictability and "planability" of the environment:**
   The stability of the environment is influential in the development of problem-solving styles. If an environment is completely predictable, there is not much problem-solving required on the part of the individual because there will be routinized solutions available for all kinds of tasks. Only in dynamic environments is some sort of problem-solving necessary. Slow and predictable rates of change may allow for knowledge-based, analytic and long-term-oriented strategies to develop (e.g., Agarwal, Tripathi, & Srivastava, 1983). An environment in a constant state of flux (like in situations of social unrest or rapid economical change) requires ad hoc and short term oriented strategies (Lindblom, 1959).
2. **Exposure, that is, the degree to which a culture requires and promotes experiences in different areas of problem-solving:**
   Exposure may be related to the accountability of the environment but it may also be a function of dominant value systems or the availability of resources necessary to promote exposure. It has been shown in intracultural studies (Schaub & Strohschneider, 1992) that the amount of problem-solving experience is a crucial factor in the development of strategic competencies. The greater the range of problems from different domains the individual has to tackle, the more he/she is likely to develop heuristic competence necessary to successfully deal with novel problems.
3. **Legitimacy of norms and value system:**
   Value Systems or philosophies of life are means to reduce uncertainties and define proper goals as well as ways to reach these goals (Rokeach, 1973). If value systems have a high degree of legitimacy and therefore assume the status of behavioral norms, this again reduces the necessity of problem-solving. In contrast, if the value systems governing different domains of life are only loosely integrated, the individual has a constant choice of different strategic possibilities.

4. **Power distance and social hierarchy:**
   Attempts to solve a problem only make sense when one is given sufficient leeway not only to find a solution but also to bring it to work. High power distance cultures are more likely to limit the control span of individuals not on top of the hierarchy and thus hamper individual problem-solving rather than promoting it. This is not to mean that high power distance necessarily results in poor strategies, however, problem-solving will pay greater attention to possibly adverse social implications of decisions and will therefore be rather conservative, or risk-avoidant (Nair, 1997).
5. **Individualism versus collectivism:**
   There should be differences between individualist and collectivist cultures as to the degree to which the social environment is taken into account. It has often been described how individualist cultures reinforce individualistic problem-solving, aimed at increasing personal benefits even at the cost of others (cf., Yu & Yank, 1994). In collectivist cultures personal benefits are less valued if other members of relevant groups suffer or if group oriented values (group harmony) are endangered. Therefore, individualist cultures should require short-term, problem focused strategies as compared to collectivist cultures where problem solvers should take a wider problem space and an extended time perspective into consideration.

We have no measures to compare cultures on these dimensions directly. However, there are indicators available that support the assumption that the German and the Indian culture indeed do differ. For instance, with respect to *predictability*, there are widely shared national stereotypes that attribute to Germans' high efficiency and planfulness (Krueger, 1996), whereas public life in India poses more frictions and barriers, and certainly runs less smoothly (see e.g., Ruback, Pandey, & Begum, 1997). With respect to *exposure*, the German schooling system often follows a pattern of "heuristic didactic" which means that in school problems, not solutions, are presented and the pupils are expected to find these solutions themselves (Strohschneider, 1996). In contrast, schooling in India in many instances consists of learning solutions by heart (PROBE, 1997). Individual approaches are not reinforced, sometimes they are even punished. Outside school, life is - at least for children and adolescents - highly regulated by family members and superiors (Joshi & MacLean, 1997) and individual decision making is not encouraged (J.B.P. Sinha, 1984). Similar differences are to be found on the other dimensions. Especially with respect to p*ower distance* and *social hierarchy*, the Indian culture is often considered an extreme case (Hofstede, 1993). Germany is characterized by less power distance and "flatter" social hierarchies.

Earlier work, designed to explore into the relationship between culture and problem-solving, supported the idea of culture-specific problem-solving behavior (see Badke-Schaub & Strohschneider, 1998): German problem solvers tended to be more active and decisive in their actions, and were more willing to take risks. Indian participants tended to avoid risks and to resort to much more fine-grained analyses of the problem context (see also Das & Khurana, 1988; Miller, Bersoff, & Harwood, 1990; D. Sinha, 1991).

Obviously, these descriptions are coarse overgeneralizations which are only justifiable for reasons of clarity and each of these points deserve a much more detailed discussion. Nevertheless, the discussion may serve the purpose of demonstrating that these cultural differences are interesting enough to motivate a more detailed study of problem-solving styles within the two cultures.

Method

MORO Simulation: Description and Evaluation

In this research, a complex, dynamic and interactive computer simulation called MORO was used (see Badke-Schaub & Strohschneider, 1998; Brehmer & Dörner, 1993 for a methodological discussion of the use of computer simulations). MORO simulates the living conditions of a small tribe of semi-nomads, living at the southern rim of the Sahara desert. Participants are given a three-page Introductory Note which describes the situation on a general level. It is their task to take the role of a developmental aide and to sustainably improve the living conditions of the tribe over a period of 20 simulated years (see Dörner, Stäudel & Strohschneider, 1986; Jansson, 1994). Participants can ask the facilitator (who serves as the participants′ interface with the system running on the computer) for any information they think is important. They can inquire, for instance, about the number of cattle, infant birth rates, millet yields, cash in the bank, intensity of the Tsetse-plague, ground water level, rain fall, and so on. All in all there are 45 numerical variables that can be assessed in this way. If the participants require more general information about, for instance, the social structure of the tribe, or inquire about details of cattle breeding, the simulation program has access to a number of text files that contain the necessary information which is then read to the participants. Such questions are coded as background questions. There is but one exception to the "information-upon-demand" rule. If an aspect of the situation deteriorates dramatically or if the Moros have severe complaints, either "alarm messages" or "complaints" appear on the computer screen which are also related to the participant.

To complete their task, participants can decide to implement a number of different measures like sinking bore wells, setting up a field hospital, buying and selling cattle and millet, purchasing fertilizers and even tractors to improve the millet condition. It is, however, expected that the participants not only spend but also earn money by selling excess food items. There are 25 possible measures in the scenario. The participants are not provided with a list of possible decisions. Rather, they must come up with their own ideas and suggestions. Of course, those decisions influence the further development of the situation.

Since MORO is a "typical" complex and dynamic problem, not all of the aspects of the situation are obvious and decisions can have unintended long term- or side-effects. Participants therefore have to make decisions under uncertainty, accept risks and even cope with the emotional strains of failure.

The analysis is based on the computer-generated protocols of each individual session. Using insights generated from earlier work (e.g., Schaub & Strohschneider, 1992) as well as ideas from Jansson (1994), an analysis scheme was developed which consists of three groups of variables, namely (1) problem-solving results, (2) global measures of activity and control, and (3) conspicuous strategic and tactical patterns.

1. Two variables describe the problem-solving results:

1a: Population after 20 years. The simulation starts with a population of 550 and regardless of all other considerations saving or even increasing the population is certainly the most important thing to do in this scenario. The interpretation, however, can be difficult. Whereas a loss in population (due to a famine) indicates a poor performance, extremely high population figures are also dangerous because they indicate a severe overpopulation which is likely to also result in a catastrophe. Therefore we also calculate

1b: Number of alarm messages. As has been mentioned above, the program automatically generates alarm messages if important variables deteriorate rapidly. The number of alarm messages therefore roughly captures the overall control of the system.

2. The following variables are global measures of activity and control:

2a: Number of decisions. This variable indicates the amount of control a participant wants to exert over the system. Large numbers of decisions can - *ceteris paribus* - be taken to indicate an active or even risky, control-oriented approach, whereas small numbers of decisions indicate passivity or cautiousness.

2b: Number of questions. The number of questions in the first three years is indicating the amount of information needed to gain an overview and therefore a measure of exploration, whereas the total number of questions reflects the permanent data necessary for controlling the state of the system. In counting the number of questions, "numerical information" and "background information" are differentiated.

3. The following strategic and tactical behavior patterns or peculiarities, which can occur in the course of dealing with a complex problem, could be precisely defined:

3a Incomplete exploration. The MORO scenario can be subdivided into a number of different problem areas . The variable is a simple count of how many of these areas were not covered by at least one question or decision during the first 45 minutes of simulation time.

3b Feedback-strategy. As opposed to a feedforward strategy, a feedback strategy only reacts to signals emanating from the system. The variable represents the number of years with feedback strategy.

3c: Insufficient adaptation of interventions. This pattern occurs when a decision (e.g., the annual sale of 20 tons of millet) that is appropriate under certain circumstances (high yields, sufficient cattle) is not changed or adapted if these circumstances change (insufficient cattle).

3d Decisions without information. It is problematic in most circumstances to decide on measures without having sufficient information about their preconditions (e.g. deciding to have 75 wells dug without knowing the price). For a number of different decisions it was possible to define precisely whether critical information about the decision was available in advance or not.

3e Lack of effect control: Meticulous effect control is one of the important prerequisites for successfully handling a complex system. For several measures (like introducing medical services) it can be safely decided whether effects (e.g., population figures, birth rates, death rates) had been controlled or not.

Hypotheses and Design

Based on the descriptions of "typical" Indian and German problem-solving styles, two versions of the MORO problem were developed. These versions were constructed by changes in internal parameters of the simulation program while still producing an identical starting situation. The first version, which was labelled CATAMORO should be better suited for an active, "feedforward" approach whereas the second version, STABMORO, should be easier to handle with a cautious, status-quo oriented strategy. The differences between these two versions are as follows:

StabMoro: This version is characterized by a large degree of stability; if one doesn´t intervene, there are no catastrophes. However, the balance is fragile and "strong" decisions can easily disturb it and then famines are relatively likely because the resources (in financial as well as ecological terms) are scarce and it is difficult to counteract accelerating negative trends.

CataMoro: In a sense, this version has just the opposite characteristics. The system has built in negative trends which, without further action, quickly lead to threatening developments. However, these developments can be reversed relatively easily because resources (money, water, food) are plentiful and one has good levers to "turn the system around".

An optimal strategy would differ between both versions. In **StabMoro**, one would be well advised to explore the system thoroughly, think about possible longterm- and side effects of decisions and act very carefully and with low dosages. In **CataMoro**, quick and decisive actions would be necessary to deal with dangerous signals and disturbing trends.

The study, then, becomes a 2 x 2 - design with factor 1 ("Culture") being quasi-experimental and factor 2 ("**Moro**-version") being truly experimental. The 68 participants in this experiment were evenly divided between each of the four cells. There were four basic research questions:

A. Adaptivity (main-effect **Moro**-version): Do participants adjust their problem-solving behavior to the requirements of the two versions, that is, do they use different strategies in both cases?

B. Behavioral flexibility differences (interaction I) : Are there any cultural differences as to the flexibility with which problem-solving behavior is adjusted to the requirements of the situation?

C. Problem-solving outcome differences (interaction II): If the participants fail to adjust their behavior and instead rely on well-learned strategies, then Indian participants should be more successful with the **StabMoro**-version and German participants should be more succesful with the **CataMoro**-version because in both cases a successful strategy is similar to the descriptions from the literature.

D. Strategic differences (main-effect culture): Are the strategies used by Indian participants different than those used by the German participants? More specifically, do they resemble the descriptions referred to above? If this were the case, Indian participants should be less active in exploring the scenario than German participants, more feedback- than feedforward-oriented and operate on a less planned basis as indicated by the different strategic indices.

Participants

The Indian participants (n=34) were students at the University of Thiruvanthapuram, Kerala and the German participants (n=34) were students at the University of Bamberg, Bavaria. The sex ratio in the Indian group was 18 males to 16 females and in the German group it was 12 males to 22 females. The mean age was 22.8 years (Indian group) and 22.4 years (German group). Among the Indian students, 11 were majoring in Psychology and the remainder were spread across Business Administration, Demography, German, Medicine, Law, Physics, and Engineering. In Germany, the largest group (n=12) came from Business Administration, the remainder from Languages, Psychology, Geography, and others.

In terms of religion, German participants belonged to Christian denominations or considered themselves without religion. In India, the majority were Hindus, but there were also Muslims and (Catholic) Christians. In Germany, students usually live either in their own apartment or share a flat with friends. Living with the parents or in a student dormitory is the exception. This pattern is true also for our group of participants. In India, most participants lived with their parents or in one of the (strictly regimented) student hostels. None of the participants was married.

Procedure

The experiment was conducted in individual sessions at the two universities mentioned above. In both settings, participation was voluntary. After welcoming the participants, the purpose of the study and the procedure was explained to them and any questions answered. Next, they filled in a broad demographic questionnaire. In order to control for possible differences in domain-specific knowledge, participants had to complete a brief test on the ecology and geography of the Sahel region which was specifically developed for this study.

When participants had completed the questionnaire, they were given the Introductory Note to the MORO problem. The simulation itself was limited to two hours. During this time participants were required to complete twenty simulated years. They were, however, free with respect to the distribution of time. The procedure was explained to all participants in great detail in order to assure that they all understood the formal format of their task. After completing the simulation, participants were asked to rate their impressions of the problem on a number of rating scales.

All instruments had originally been developed in the German language and were later translated into English using a backtranslation-forwardtranslation procedure with bilingual experts. In India, the experiments were conducted in English language. Although for most of the students Malayalam was their mother tongue, since profound mastery of English is prerequisite for university education in most universities in India, all students were fluent in English and there were no language problems whatsoever.

All MORO sessions were conducted by two German facilitators who were highly familiar with the simulation. It could be argued that using foreigners as facilitators in the Indian context but not in the German context would cause problems. In planning the experiment, a decision had to be made between sources of error that would come from introducing new facilitators and sources of error that would come from Germans acting as facilitators in India and the second option was selected as being probably less disturbing. Indeed, observations during the sessions supported this decision: Most of the participants were quickly caught by their roles and worked enthusiastically without paying much attention to the person of the facilitator.

Results

Equivalence of Problem Perception and Interpretation

Attempts were made to check for the comparability of problem perception and interpretation by the participants from both cultures as well as for the comparability of data structures. Because of space limitations these attempts will only be briefly skectched:

1. Problem perception:
   After finishing the MORO-game, participants were asked to rate their impressions about the simulation with respect to *personal experiences* with that kind of problem, perceived *realism* of the scenario, *imaginability* of the scenario, *importance* of finding a good solution, and *feeling of competence*. Two-by-two (**culture, MOROversion**) ANOVAs on these data yielded no significant effects for **MOROversion** and no significant interaction. Significant effects for **culture** were found for the *perceived realism* of the scenario (inverted scale) which was higher for the Indian participants ($M_I = 2{,}47$ as compared to $M_G = 3{,}47$, $F_{(1,68)} = 9{,}54$, $p < .01$), whereas the German participants could *imagine* the scenario to a higher extent ($M_G = 5{,}53$ as compared to $M_I = 4{,}79$, $F_{(1,68)} = 7{,}10$, $p = .01$). Judging from these data it seems at least plausible to assume that participants from both cultures were able to develop a mental model of the simulation and worked on it with personal involvement.
2. Background Knowledge:
   As has been mentioned above, participants were given a knowledge test before the start of the experiment. Given the range of this instrument (0 through 17 points), *Background Knowledge* appeared to be poor in both groups (the means were $M_I = 3{,}15$, $M_G = 4.15$), however, in the ANOVA it proved to be a little less poor for German participants

($F_{(1,68)}$ = 4,334, $p < .05$; maineffect **MOROversion** and interaction *ns*). As a next step, correlations were calculated between *Background Knowledge* and the **MORO**-outcome variables and behavioral descriptors. Correlations were in the (-.25 < r < +.25) - range and only few of them were significant. In these cases, *Background-Knowledge* was introduced as a covariate in all further analyses.

3. Internal structure of simulation data:
Next, the correlational structure of the data in the two samples was compared. If these structures are similar between the two cultures, this can be interpreted as an indication of similar "functioning" of the computer simulation in both cultures. The two outcome variables (*population after 20 years, number of alarm messages*) intercorrelated with r = -.5077 ($p < .01$) in the Indian sample and r = -.3179 ($p < .10$) in the German sample.

For the variables that describe the participants' overall activity and control, the correlational pattern with the outcome variables was generally similar between the two cultures: *Number of decisions* tended to correlate positively with *population* and negatively with *number of alarms*. For the *number of questions*, the correlations were weaker for the German participants and even reversed in sign for the *number of background questions*. Therefore, the function of questions, especially background questions, apparently was different between the two cultures. This point will be discussed later.

For those variables that represent strategic and tactical behavior patterns, again the overall picture was similar: They correlated negatively with *population* and positively with *number of alarms* which indicates that the decisions and omissions which were cautiously labelled "behavior patterns" were in fact errors. Again, the correlations were weaker for the German group which can be attributed to the low frequencies of some of these errors in the German sample. In summary, the data show that the simulation was relatively robust and "worked" with participants from both cultures in comparable ways. On this basis, the problem-solving behaviors and outcomes can be compared between both groups.

Cross-Cultural Differences in Problem-Solving Behavior and Success

The first group of results concerns the global measures of activity and control. According to the design, the 2-way ANOVA is used as the main inferential tool. Table 1 presents the results for this first group of variables.

The test of the effects of the experimental variation showed that within these data all main effects **MOROversion** were *ns* - that is, participants did not behave differently when dealing with the different versions of the

MORO problem. Also, there was only one significant interaction, indicating that Indian participants made fewer decisions during the first 3 years of the simulation

Table 1. Global activity measures; means and standard deviations for each of the four conditions (n = 17)

Dependent variable:	STAB	MORO	CATA	MORO
	M	*SD*	*M*	*SD*
Number of decisions, years 1-3				
Indian students	13.00	4.85	8.18	3.57
German students	11.12	4.03	12.00	3.62
Number of decisions, total				
Indian students	44.35	15.16	39.00	18.73
German students	61.00	15.97	58.76	16.47
Number of questions, years 1-3				
Indian students	18.35	10.48	13.41	11.18
German students	19.35	9.41	23.76	12.23
Number of questions, total				
Indian students	56.12	38.00	53.47	39.22
German students	102.82	53.70	101.18	37.93
Background questions (relative frequencies)				
Indian students				
German students	0.21	0.18	0.22	0.18
	0.08	0.06	0.08	0.05

in the **CATAMORO**-version than in the **STABMORO**-version and vice versa for the German participants ($F = 8.16, p < .01$).

There were, however, differences between the two cultural groups, regardless of **MOROversion**. Although the number of decisions was not different for the first 3 years ($F = 0.79$, *ns*), the German participants overall implemented more measures ($F = 17.49$, $p < .01$) and asked far more questions ($F = 20.75$, $p < .01$) than the Indian participants: In terms of number of interactions with the simulation program, the German participants were more active. In terms of the nature of the decisions made, there were no big differences. All participants drilled wells to get additional water, almost all participants made attempts to fight the Tsetse-fly and took steps to improve the medical situation.

Interestingly, although the Indian participants asked only about half as many questions as the German participants, the number of background questions was higher, both in absolute and relative frequencies ($F = 15.88$, p

< .01). This means that the Indian participants sought more information about both the general context and specific semantic aspects of the problem.

Table 2 presents the data concerning the second group of variables, the strategic and tactical behavior patterns:

Table 2. Strategical and tactical particularities; means and standard deviations for each of the four conditions (n = 17)

	STAB	MORO	CATA	MORO
Dependent variable:	*M*	*SD*	*M*	*SD*
Incompete exploration				
Indian students	1.24	1.44	2.06	1.95
German students	0.24	0.56	0.24	0.44
Years with feedback-strategy				
Indian students	2.41	3.54	3.88	4.23
German students	1.12	2.20	0.47	0.87
Insufficient adaptation of decisions				
Indian students	6.65	5.51	5.88	6.06
German students	1.29	2.05	1.63	1.93
Decisions without informations				
Indian students	6.65	8.22	7.76	5.36
German students	3.12	3.92	1.35	2.67
Lack of effect-control				
Indian students	1.88	1.05	1.88	1.17
German students	1.25	2.20	1.18	1.24

Again, the frequency of committing strategic or tactical errors was not dependent on the different versions of the **MORO** problem (all main effects **MOROversion** *ns*), nor were there any interactions between **MOROversion** and **culture**. However, Indian participants explored the scenario less completely (*Exploration*: $F = 17.76$, $p < .01$) they had more years with a reactive *feedback-strategy* ($F = 10.02$, $p < .01$), they were less likely to *adapt decision making* to changing circumstances ($F = 20.34$, $p < .01$), they made more *decisions without the necessary information* ($F = 14.14$, $p < .01$), and they forgot about *effect control* more frequently ($F = 4.08$, $p < .05$).

Finally, problem-solving outcomes were analyzed. On the average, participants managed to increase the tribe´s *population* considerably. For **CATAMORO** the means were $M_I = 665.0$, and $M_D = 834.2$; for **STABMORO** the means were $M_I = 699.5$, and $M_D = 765.8$, respectively. Overall, 15 participants (10 Indian, 5 German) caused a famine to happen; 8 of these resulted in a final population below 550, the minimum value being 273. After 20 years, 7 participants (2 Indian, 5 German) had a population of over 900, the maximum being 1629 people. Although the data seem to indicate the expected interaction between **MORO-version** and **culture**, this interaction was not significant ($F_{(1, 68)} = 0{,}89$, *ns*). As for the two main effects, there was no effect of **MORO-version** ($F_{(1,68)} = 0{,}10$, *ns*), whereas the effect of **culture** was significant ($F_{(1,68)} = 4{,}67$, $p < .05$). This means, that the German participants overall had a larger population after 20 years.

Since a huge population increase is dangerous, one also has to look at the *number of alarm messages* as second indication of success. The main effect **MOROversion** was not significant ($F_{(1,68)} = 1{,}94$, *ns*) and there was no interaction ($F_{(1,68)} = 0{,}05$, *ns*), while the main effect **culture** was large ($F_{(1,68)} = 32{,}72$, $p < .01$): German participants had fewer alarm messages ($M_G = 10{,}52$ as compared to $M_I = 21{,}89$) and were therefore able to better balance the system and avoid catastrophic tendencies.

Summary and Discussion

The results of this study can be summarized under different aspects. One important aspect is certainly the use of computer simulations of complex and dynamic problems in cross-cultural research on thinking and problem-solving. Since these are comparatively new instruments, different checks were made to ensure applicability and comparability. From these data it appears as if the task indeed was perceived in comparable ways in both cultural contexts.

A second aspect is the differences in problem-solving styles. Overall, participants were able to deal effectively with the problem. There were, however, a number of interesting behavioral differences: German participants dealt with the problem in a more active way in that they collected more pieces of information and decided on more interventions. Indian participants sought more background information about the tribe´s ways of living and the general context of the scenario. In the course of problem-solving, Indian participants committed more strategic and tactical errors. They were more likely to ignore key aspects of the scenario during the initial phases of problem exploration, to rely on a purely feedback-controlled strategy, to make decisions without having the necessary information available, to fail to adapt their interventions to changing circumstances, and to forget about effect control.

The experimental variation, the construction of two **MORO** versions, had only minor effects on the participants´ actual behavior and there were practically no interactions between type of problem and culture.

There were four research questions that guided the layout of this study. As for the first two questions, the results are quite clear. Participants did not adjust their behavior to the different requirements of the two **MORO**-versions and there were no cultural differences with respect to this lack of adaptation. Apparently, the participants′ problem-solving behavior was guided more by the content of the problem, by their perception of the tribe′s misery and the different interventions that were open for them to improve the situation than by abstract reasoning about the problem structure and the dangerous developmental trends.

In contrast to the third hypothesis, which expected an interaction between "type of problem" and "cultural group", Indian participants fared worse with both **MORO**-versions. This finding can be attributed to the large number of strategic and tactical errors commited by the Indian participants regardless of the version they were dealing with. This underlines the important function of strategic competence in handling complex and dynamic problems.

The fourth question focussed on the relationship between observed problem-solving behavior and more general descriptions of problem-solving styles that were drawn from earlier work. There appear to be several points of convergence. Variables that describe activity and control-orientation in problem-solving indicate that Indian problem solvers were more passive than German problem solvers. The difference in feedback versus feedforward strategy seems to be especially interesting in this context because a feedback strategy is clearly passive and "obedient": The problem solver reacts to what is demanded from him by the system. The difference in background questions can be interpreted as supporting the notion of Indian problem solvers preferring context-sensitive solutions because background questions are attempts to go beyond "hard" data about the immediate situation and find out about the context in which a specific decision is embedded. However, contrary to earlier studies, there were no clear indications for risk-avoidance or refusal of responsibility: The actual decisions implemented were comparable.

This pattern of differences can be related to the cultural dimensions discussed in the introduction. With respect to power distance and individualism/collectivism problem-solving behavior of participants from both groups seems to reflect the requirements of the respective cultural context; recognition of individual responsibility and attempts for personal control on one side, need for contextualisation and a tendency to expect "guidance" from the system on the other.

With respect to exposure, the data on the different errors clearly indicate that German participants possessed more of the strategic and tactical competences necessary for successfully dealing with the given task. We have not directly tested for "exposure", however, if one looks at the general pattern in both cultures for people of the age group we have been studying, there seem to be clear differences. Both cultures differ in the extent to which they require students to solve problems by themselves and in the amount of parental guidance that is expected towards adolescents. Indian students, in their cultural context, therefore are exposed to *other* kinds of learning experiences which promote *other* skills than those necessary for the MORO task. This has several implications. One is the important role of functional adaptation for the development of problem-solving styles. Functional adaptation to the requirements of the cultural context seems to be more crucial for the execution of "higher" cognitive processes than has been recognized by many theorists of problem-solving. Another implication is that studies of complex problem-solving that are conducted only in one culture artificially keep the *expertise*-factor constant. Doing research in a mono-cultural fashion makes it impossible to differentiate culture-bound strategic competence from the underlying processes and leads to theories of problem-solving that are highly specific for the single culture.

References

Agarwal, A., Tripathi, K. K., & Srivastava, M. (1983). Social roots and psychological implications of time perspective. *International Journal of Psychology, 18,* 367-380.

Badke-Schaub, P., & Strohschneider, S. (1998). Complex problem solving in the cultural context. *Le travail humain, 61,* 1-28.

Brehmer, B. & Dörner, D. (1993). Experiments with computer-simulated microworlds: Escaping both the narrow straits of the laboratory and the deep blue sea of the field study. *Computers in Human Behavior, 9,* 171-184.

Das, J. P., & Khurana, A. K. S. (1988). Caste and cognitive processes. In S. H. Irvine, & J. W. Berry (Eds.), *Human abilities in cultural context* (pp. 487-508). Cambridge, MA: Cambridge University Press.

Dörner, D. (1996): *The logic of failure.* New York: Holt.

Dörner, D., Stäudel, T., & Strohschneider, S. (1986). *Moro: Programmdokumentation* [Moro: Program documentation]. University of Bamberg: Unpublished manuscript (Memorandum No. 23).

Frensch, P. & Funke, J. (Eds.) (1995). *Complex problem solving: The European perspective.* Hillsdale, NJ: Erlbaum.

Hofstede, G. (1983). The cultural relativity of organizational practices and theories. *Journal of International Business Studies, 14,* 75-89.

Jansson, A. (1994). Pathologies in dynamic decision making: Consequences or precursors of failure? *Sprache & Kognition, 13,* 160-173.

Jansson, A. (1995). Strategies in dynamic decision making: Does teaching heuristic strategies by instructions affect performance? In J. P. Caverni, M. Bar-Hillel, F. H. Barron, & H. Jungermann (Eds.), *Contributions to decision making* (pp. 213-232). Amsterdam: Elsevier.

Joshi, M. S. & MacLean, M. (1997). Maternal expectations of child development in India, Japan, and England. *Journal of Cross-Cultural Psychology, 28,* 219-234.

Krueger, J. (1996). Probabilistic national stereotypes. *European Journal of Social Psychology, 26,* 961-980.

Lindblom, C. E. (1959). The science of "muddling through". *Public Administration Review, 19,* 79-88.

Lonner, W. J. (1993). Foreword. In J. Altarriba (Ed.), *Cognition and culture: A cross-cultural approach to Cognitive Psychology* (pp. V-VIII). Amsterdam: North-Holland.

Miller, J. G., Bersoff, D. M. & Harwood, R. L. (1990). Perceptions of social responsibilities in India and the United States: Moral imperatives or personal decisions? *Journal of Personality and Social Psychology, 58,* 33-47.

Nair, U. (1997). *Managerial cognition and action in complex problem solving.* Ahmedabad, In.: Unpublished Doctoral Dissertation.

PROBE (Public Report on Primary Education) (1997). Primary Education: Class Struggle. *India Today, 22 (13.10.1997),* 68-73.

Ramnarayan, S. & Kumar, E. S. (1996). Coping with SCUDs: An empirical investigation. *The TMTC Journal of Management, 6,* 40-58.

Ramnarayan, S., Strohschneider, S., & Schaub, H. (1997). Trappings of expertise and the pursuit of failure. *Simulation & Gaming, 28,* 28-43.

Rokeach, M. (1973). *The nature of human values.* New York, NY: Free Press.

Ruback, R. B., Pandey, J., & Begum, H. A. (1997). Urban stressors in South Asia: Impact on male and female pedestrians in Delhi and Dhaka. *Journal of Cross-Cultural Psychology, 28,* 23-43.

Schaub, H. & Strohschneider, S. (1992). Die Auswirkungen unterschiedlicher Problemlöseerfahrung auf den Umgang mit einem unbekannten komplexen Problem [The effects of differences in problem-solving experience on handling an unknown complex problem]. *Zeitschrift für Arbeits- und Organisationspsychologie, 36,* 117-126.

Sinha, D. (1991). Values and work behaviour. *Abhigyan, Spring 91,* 1-14.

Sinha, J. B. P. (1984). A model of effective leadership styles in India. *International Studies of Man and Organizations, 14,* 86-98.

Strohschneider, S. (1996). Eine Nation - zweierlei Denken? Versuch einer Zusammenfassung und Integration der Ergebnisse [One nation - two ways of thinking? An attempt to summarize and integrate the findings]. In S. Strohschneider (Ed.), *Denken in Deutschland: Vergleichende Untersuchungen in Ost und West* [Thinking in Germany: Comparative Studies in East and West] (pp. 175-189). Bern: Huber.

van de Vijver, F. J. R. & Willemsen, M. E. (1993). Abstract thinking. In J. Altarriba (Ed.), *Cognition and Culture: A cross-cultural approach to Cognitive Psychology* (pp. 317-342). Amsterdam: North-Holland.

Yu, A.-B. & Yank, K. S. (1994). The nature of achievement motivation in collectivistic societies. In U. Kim, H. C. Triandis, C. Kagitcibasi, S.-C. Choi, & G. Yoon (Eds.), *Individualism and collectivism: Theory, method, and applications* (pp. 239-250). Thousand Oaks, CA: Sage.

---

1 Author´s note: The research reported in this paper has been supported by the Deutsche Forschungsgemeinschaft (DFG). Dominik Güss and Alice Edrissi assisted in collecting and analyzing the data. Many thanks to S. Ramnarayan, D. Halcour and G. Hofinger for their thoughful comments on earlier versions of this paper and to Prof. Dharmangadan, Head of the Department of Psychology, University of Kerala in Thiruvananthapuram, for his support in organizing the research in India.

Applying Cognitive-Affective Processing System (CAPS) Theory to Cultural Differences in Social Behavior

Rodolfo Mendoza-Denton
Columbia University
Psychology Department

Yuichi Shoda
University of Washington
Psychology Department

Ozlem Ayduk
Columbia University
Psychology Department

Walter Mischel
Columbia University
Psychology Department

ABSTRACT

A network theory was proposed in which members of a culture or group engage in similar behavior to the extent that particular situations activate a shared network of cognitive-affective mediating units (e.g., constructs, values, beliefs, goals, expectancies) within the group members. This culturally shared network theory extends to the group level the CAPS (Cognitive-Affective Processing System) model that has been shown to have heuristic value at the individual level (Mischel & Shoda, 1995). The theory was illustrated in an analysis of people's cognitive-affective reactions to the O.J. Simpson criminal trial verdict (Mendoza-Denton, Ayduk, Shoda, & Mischel, 1997). Participants (33 White, 38 Black, 11 Latino, 25 Asian/Asian-American and 6 other) provided open-ended reactions to the verdict. In contrast to widely shared assumptions at the time, content analyses revealed that participants' race did not have a direct effect on their reactions. Instead, and consistent with the proposed theory, differences in the accessibility of cognitive-affective units and their subsequent activation pathways characterized respondents' reactions. The results help clarify how members of cultural groups can behave similarly in specific psychological situations in spite of the heterogeneity and individual differences that characterize them, creating diversity as well as commonality among group members.

Understanding the relationship between person and culture has been one of the fundamental tasks of cross-cultural psychology since the inception of the field (Triandis, 1997). Early culture and personality researchers addressed this challenge by attempting to identify and describe the dimensions along which members of one cultural group differed from members of another. For the most part, these researchers sought to describe personality "types" that were prevalent in one culture or another, and that were characterized by stable, cross-situational, dispositions or traits (Kitayama & Markus, in press; Shweder, 1991). Benedict (1934), for example, describes two personality types of the Southwest Pueblos, the Appolonian and the Dionysian, evident from the behavior of the Pueblo people across a diverse variety of domains, including the political, military, economic, and religious. Based on a distinction described by Nietzche in his studies of Greek tragedy, she characterized the Dionysian pueblos as having a generalized love for excess, and the Appolonian pueblos as sober and mistrustful of excessive behavior. The assumption that cultural groups could be characterized in terms of traits that were expressed cross-situationally also drove much of the research on the "national character" or "dominant personality" of cultural groups (e.g., Kardiner, 1945; Linton, 1945)

Despite the intuitive appeal of the culture and personality approach, however, by the 1970's the field faced the task of reconciling its basic theoretical assumptions with two emerging lines of empirical evidence (see Bruner, 1974). The first is that there is large within-group variability in behavior in any given culture (Kaplan, 1954; Minturn & Lambert, 1964). The second, stemming from the field of personality psychology itself, is that cross-situational consistency in behavior for any given individual is typically quite low (Mischel, 1968; Shweder, 1991). The "Appolonian" pueblos, for example, have been documented to at times engage in typically Dionysian behavior, as well as vice versa (Barnouw, 1973). The challenge remains of how to understand cultural differences in social behavior while still recognizing within group inter- and intra-individual variability in such behavior.

Toward a Process View of Intra-Cultural Homogeneity in Behavior

Over the past twenty years, the social-cognitive approach (see Cervone, 1991; Mischel & Shoda, 1998; Pervin, 1990) to understanding social behavior generation at the level of the individual has focused on understanding the social and cognitive mediating processes that underlie and motivate behavior (Bandura, 1986; Cantor & Kihlstrom, 1987; Dodge, 1993; Dweck & Leggett, 1988; Mischel, 1973; Read & Miller, 1989). Rather than attempting to categorize individuals in terms of stable, cross-situational dispositions, this approach emphasizes the ways in which a person's important construals, beliefs and expectations, goals pursued, strategies used, and affects experienced--all in relation to relevant features of situations--influence his or her behavior.

In a similar spirit, both classical and modern descriptions of culture in anthropology, psychological anthropology, and cross-cultural psychology emphasize the idea that what binds cultural group members together are the beliefs, customs, practices, habits, meaning systems, values, attributions, and attitudes that cultural group members share and transmit from one generation to the next (Geertz, 1973; Gordon, 1982; Obeyesekere, 1981; Triandis, 1997; Tylor, 1871). Definitions of culture based on such process variables that mediate behavior at the nomothetic level (Mischel & Shoda, 1995) provide a natural bridge to the study of culture and personality by encouraging attempts not to categorize individuals in terms of static descriptors, but rather to understand the *process* through which individuals from a given cultural group experience, negotiate, and function in their social world (e.g., Cole, 1996; Feldman, in press; Kitayama & Markus, in press; Markus & Kitayama, 1991, 1998; Shweder, 1991; Nisbett & Cohen, 1996).

Without a scheme for understanding the *interrelationships* between features of situations, mediating units, and behavioral expressions, however, even meaningful individual differences such as holding an entity vs. an incremental theory (Levy & Dweck, 1998), or cultural differences such as having an independent vs. an interdependent model of the self (Markus & Kitayama, 1991), run the risk of becoming typologies much like "Appolonian" vs. "Dyonisian." To go from a mere list of types of mediating units to a full representation of cultural and personal experience requires a dynamic framework for thinking about how these units function as a coherent whole within the individual. Such a framework provides a key to understanding the complexity and coherence of behavior organization- both for an individual's idiosyncratic responses in a given situation, as well as the same individual's congruent responses with those of other members of his or her cultural group in other situations.

In this vein, we present one such dynamic model--Mischel and Shoda's (1995) Cognitive-Affective Processing System (CAPS) Theory--as a general framework for gaining access into the world of the "other". We emphasize how the processing dynamics proposed in the theory become activated in relation to the relevant features of situations, generating diverse behaviors, some of which are characteristic of the individual's cultural group and some of which are idiosyncratic behavioral expressions. We then apply this model to a real world example from the U.S. socio-political arena--the 1995 O.J. Simpson criminal trial verdict--to demonstrate how the framework is able to account for the observed culturally shared reactions of elation and dismay to the verdict, as well as those reactions of ambivalence that defy easy categorization (Mendoza-Denton, Ayduk, Shoda, & Mischel, 1997). Our hope is not only to promote a deeper understanding and appreciation of reactions to the verdict that goes beyond racial and ethnic divisions, but in a larger sense to provide an example of how one can talk meaningfully about cultural convergences in social behavior without compromising the individuality and diversity inherent within a cultural group.

Representing Worlds: The Cognitive-Affective Processing System (CAPS)

Mischel and Shoda's (1995) Cognitive-Affective Processing System (CAPS) theory is an approach to personality which integrates insights from connectionism with recent theories of cognitive and social information processing (e.g., Anderson, 1983; Bandura, 1986; Cantor & Kihlstrom, 1987; Hinton, McClelland, & Rumelhart, 1986) within a comprehensive theoretical framework. It proposes that behavior is mediated by a set of *cognitive-affective units* (CAUs)--a person's encodings, expectations and beliefs, affects, goals, and competencies as well as self-regulatory plans- which are organized within a stable activation network that reflects the learning history of the individual. The organization of relations within the person's processing network may remain relatively stable and invariant across situations. However, as the individual moves from one situation to another, different mediating units and their characteristic interrelationships become activated in relation to different situational features. Thus, the model predicts that behavioral stability lies in the meaningfully patterned expression of behavior in relationship to situations--if A, then a person reliably does X, but if B, then she or he does Y. The stability of these *if...then* patterns of situation-behavior relations has been supported through extensive observational studies (e.g., Shoda, Mischel, & Wright, 1994; Mischel & Shoda, 1995).

The model postulates that cross-situational consistency of behavior is likely to be found not in *nominally* similar situations (e.g., "at parties") but rather in *psychologically* similar ones (e.g., "situations in which I might embarrass myself in front of strangers"). Thus, it might seem initially perplexing that Mary is sociable and engaging in intimate parties, but withdrawn and reserved at large cocktail gatherings. However, if we can understand the psychological meaning of the large cocktail party for Mary, we can immediately reconcile her seemingly contradictory behavior at parties, and even predict other nominally different situations in which she might behave similarly (e.g., shy and reserved on a blind date).

The Culturally-Shared CAPS Network

As the individual grows, learns, and gains life experience, an increasingly rich and complex network of CAUs develops. Some CAUs are acquired through the unique experience of the individual. In addition, as reviewed earlier, other CAUs seem to be shared and transmitted among members of cultural groups. Such values, goals, beliefs, and encodings can be shared through direct, intentional transmission, as when a parent teaches a child a given set of values or goals (see Triandis, 1997). Other CAUs can come to be shared as a result of having similar experiences specific to one's cultural group, as when experiences of previous discrimination lead to an expectation that one will be rejected on the basis of one's race (Purdie, Mendoza-Denton, & Downey, 1997). In this way, life experiences shared by members of a group--the teachings of elders, the experiences shared with others, the values imposed by society--are likely to generate a *culturally shared* CAPS (C-CAPS) network embedded within an individual's processing system. If features of a situation activate this culturally shared network, individuals may generate similar reactions to that situation.

A Real-World Example from the United States: The O.J. Simpson Criminal Trial Verdict

An example of the C-CAPS framework comes from the highly publicized 1995 criminal trial of former American football star O.J. Simpson. The Simpson criminal trial verdict has perhaps been the strongest reminder in recent history that Blacks and Whites in the United States live in different worlds. Images of cheering Black faces next to dismayed White faces across the front pages of newspapers and the covers of magazines illustrated how people who live in the same world can understand it and experience it differently. The same case, the same evidence, and the same trial led to two virtually opposite reactions.

The CAPS model allows us to understand reactions to socio-political information in terms of the cognitions and affects that such information activates within individuals. Guided by this model, our aim was to explore reactions to the verdict not as the thoughtless, irrational responses portrayed by opposing sides, but rather as a result of the thoughts and feelings that the case evoked for different people (Mendoza-Denton et al., 1997).

We began with the assumption that as a result of their different socio-political histories, African-Americans and European-Americans form two sub-cultures co-existing within the larger multi-cultural US context. We hypothesized that although Blacks and Whites who followed the O.J. Simpson criminal trial were faced with the same nominal situation (i.e., the same trial & the same verdict), the meaning of the situation took on different psychological connotations and activated distinct culturally-shared networks in the two sub-cultures, which in turn led to divergent reactions. We hypothesized that the CAUs that became differentially activated in Blacks vs. Whites in response to the case mediated the apparent relationship between race and opinion of the verdict. In other words, we did not expect racial background to determine people's reactions to the verdict above and beyond the mediating CAUs that became activated.

In order to test these hypotheses, we conducted a study approximately a year following the conclusion of the criminal trial in which participants were asked to describe their reactions to the verdict. We chose to have participants write their responses in a free-form essay format because that would allow us to detect the kinds of cognitions and affects that participants spontaneously generated, as well as to examine the relations among CAUs that people would mention. Specifically, we investigated i) the accessibility of a set of cognitive-affective mediating units, ii) the inter-connections between these units, and iii) the relationships between the accessible units and the people's agreement/disagreement with the verdict. We briefly review the method and results of this study, which is published in detail elsewhere (Mendoza-Denton et al., 1997).

Method

Participants of this study were 113 people (49 females and 64 males) who were either taking classes or working at Columbia University during the summer of 1996. Thirty-three participants identified themselves as White, 38 as Black, 11 as Latino, and 25 as Asian/Asian-American. Six of our participants did not identify themselves as belonging to any of these groups. The mean age was 21.7 (range: 14 to 49). Educational levels were 36.3% high school students, 37.2% college students and 24.8% graduate students, while 1.7% were not currently students.

Participants were shown eighteen movie and sound clips related to the O.J. Simpson trial, downloaded from the *CNN* (http://www.cnn.com) and *Court TV* (http://www.courttv.com) World Wide Web sites onto a Macintosh computer. The clips were specifically selected to recreate as vividly as possible the most dramatic aspects of the trial in rough temporal sequence. Having watched all the clips, participants were then asked to write down their reactions to the verdict, with specific instructions to specify whether they agreed, disagreed, or were somehow ambivalent about the verdict.

In order to identify the cognitive-affective units that were spontaneously generated by the participants, their essays were subjected to content analysis following the procedure outlined by Lampert and Ervin-Tripp (1993). In this procedure, meaningful thought units that seem to recur within the pool of responses are identified from the essays themselves and subsequently used for the content analysis. Twenty-two representative cognitive- affective units (e.g., "Mark Fuhrman is racist"; "there is a mountain of evidence"), as well as 7 emotional reactions specific to the verdict (e.g., happiness, sadness), were identified. Two independent judges coded each essay according to whether or not each of the cognitive-affective units and/ or emotional reactions were mentioned. Each essay was also coded for agreement, disagreement, or ambivalence toward the verdict (median Cohen's kappa for inter-judge reliability = .84, range = .49 to 1.00).

The links between these constructs were identified by way of correlations computed among all the constructs that were coded for using the whole sample, based on the assumption that relevant pathways were societally shared given the larger socio-political context. A positive correlation between two items was interpreted as an excitatory link, meaning that the activation of one construct led to the activation of another. A negative correlation, by contrast, was interpreted as an inhibitory link; that is, the activation of one construct led to the inhibition of another. In the two sections that follow, representative CAUs from our analysis appear in quotations.

Accessibility of CAUs and Emotional Reactions to the Verdict

Accessibility of thoughts and affects was conceptualized in our analysis as the frequency with which each CAU was mentioned among those who agreed ($\underline{N}$ = 45), disagreed ($\underline{N}$ = 46) or felt ambivalent towards the verdict ($\underline{N}$ = 22). Only those cognitive-affective units that were differentially accessible to one group over the others, as revealed by chi-square analyses, were thought of as belonging to that group.

Chi-square analyses revealed that those who agreed with the verdict accessed the cognitions "the court system has long biased against Blacks," "O.J. was assumed to be guilty because he was Black," and "Mark Fuhrman was racist" significantly more frequently than those who disagreed. By contrast, those who disagreed accessed "racism is no excuse for murder" and "the defense played the race card," and “there is a mountain of evidence” significantly more frequently than those who agreed. With respect to domestic abuse, "O.J. was aggressive and abusive" was more accessible to those who disagreed than those who agreed, whereas "abuse doesn't mean murder" was more accessible to those who agreed than those who disagreed. "The evidence is questionable" was highly accessible to people whom agreed, yet entirely non-existent among those who disagreed. People who agreed greeted the verdict with a combination of happiness and relief, while people who disagreed were mostly upset.

The ambivalent recognized both that the evidence overwhelmingly pointed at O.J. as well as the long-standing bias of the court system against Blacks. Moreover, the ambivalent felt that the evidence was questionable less than people who disagreed, but more than people who agreed. The apparent conflict that existed between the accessible cognitions of the ambivalent mirrored itself in their emotional reactions to the verdict. Happiness was more common for the ambivalent than those who disagreed, whereas sadness was more accessible to them than it was to those who agreed.

Network Relationships Among CAUs

A series of regression analyses on opinion towards the verdict revealed that agreement with the verdict was significantly predicted by the CAUs "the evidence is questionable" and "O.J. was pre-judged because of his race." Disagreement with the verdict, in contrast, was predicted by thinking, "the evidence against O.J. was overwhelming," that "O.J.'s behavior was suspicious," that "his celebrity status blinded people to his guilt," and "the jury was stupid." Finally, analyses indicated that ambivalence was predicted both by the CAUs "there is a mountain of evidence" and "the court system has been biased against Blacks for years."

Further analyses were conducted to investigate the links different emotional reactions to the verdict had with CAUs. Results revealed that being upset by the verdict was solely predicted by disagreement itself. Relief was predicted by the cognition that "O.J. was acquitted despite his being a Black man." On the other hand, happiness in response to the verdict was predicted by perceiving the verdict as fulfillment of "justice and a victory for Blacks." Finally, sadness as a reaction to the verdict was related to the empathy the cognition "the victims and their families suffered."

Race and Opinions of the Verdict

Correlations between race and opinion of the verdict confirmed the popular view that being Black was significantly related to agreement ($\underline{r}$ = .54), whereas being White significantly associated with disagreement ($\underline{r}$ = .50). In our sample, being Black was also significantly related to ambivalence toward the verdict ($\underline{r}$ = .28). To investigate whether race (specifically, being Black or White) had an effect over and above the accessible CAUs in determining one's opinion to the verdict, the regressions reported above were also conducted including race as an independent variable. It was found that when controlling for all CAUs, the relationship between race itself and opinion to the verdict was no longer statistically reliable (agreement: ß = .15; disagreement: ß = - .05; ambivalence: ß = .24).

Implications

Our results demonstrate how, in particular situations that activate culturally shared cognitions and affects, members of cultural groups can behave in similar ways. Consistent with the popular perception that opinions to the verdict divided along racial (cultural) lines, our results indicated that being Black was correlated with agreement to the verdict and being White was correlated with disagreement. Importantly, however, the relationship between race and responses to the verdict were *mediated* by particular networks of cognitions and affects that were differentially activated in response to the trial.

Thus, if a person has been the victim of prejudice at the hands of the law, or has been warned by members of his or her cultural group that the police force is racist, it is understandable that Mark Fuhrman would be perceived as "another example of a racist LAPD." For someone who has not experienced such discrimination, however, the cognition "one can't judge the whole police force by this one bad apple" may be more readily accessible. Such differential encodings of stimuli can in turn lead to diverging interpretations and increasingly polarized opinions of the same events. Not surprisingly, then, our results indicated that race was not related to opinions to the verdict above and beyond the C-CAPS that became activated in response to the trial. These results in particular help us understand that one's response to a given situation is influenced, but not necessarily dictated, by the cultural group one belongs to or identifies with. The framework thus provides a window to the processing dynamics of those who were elated, those who were dismayed as well as those who were ambivalent, allowing us to take our explanation out of the Black vs. White dichotomy.

Understanding Cultural Cohesion and Within-Culture Variability Through the CAPS Approach

The C-CAPS approach allows us to reconcile within-culture variability with between-group differences within a single framework. We propose that culture and shared experience can influence the psychological meaning that specific situations will have for members of a given cultural group, and in this way may yield commonalities in the sub-networks that become activated. Thus, the model predicts that members of a cultural group may behave similarly only in situations that activate the culturally shared sub-network, as was the case with the Simpson verdict. To the extent that not all situations activate this culturally shared network, the model expects within-group variability in behavior. For example, prior to the verdict, within-group similarities, as well as between-group differences, were not visible to the same extent. Similarly, now that the case is no longer prevalent in people's minds, it is easy to see individual differences in how cultural group members deal with everyday situations.

Nevertheless, it is important to note that even in situations that activate a culturally shared sub-network, we would not expect a uniform response from all group members. This is because the cultural sub-network does not function independently of the larger, idiosyncratic CAPS network that each individual develops over the course of a lifetime (Shoda, in press). The C-CAPS is not cut off from the rest of a person's processing system; its flow is constrained by the interconnections it has with other more unique cognitions and affects. Thus, two individuals who were equally dismayed with the verdict and who shared the underlying sub-network may have dealt with their dismay in very different ways--one may have taken to publicly protesting the verdict to anyone who would listen, while another may have internalized his or her feelings, gone home, and avoided all social contact for a few days.

Conclusions

One of the major criticisms of the culture and personality approach has been its inability to account for within-culture, inter- and intra-individual variability in social behavior. The cognitive-social approach in general attempts to account for individual and cultural differences by focusing on the psychological process through which a person's unique as well as culturally-shared goals, values, beliefs, encodings, and meaning systems can influence behavior. In order to go from description to understanding the dynamics of how culture and person interpenetrate each other (Shweder & Sullivan, 1990), it is proposed that an appreciation of the interrelationships among mediating units and the psychological features of situations that trigger their activation is required. Mischel and Shoda's (1995) CAPS theory is presented as one approach towards such understanding.

Based on this framework, we have proposed that 1) similar life experiences of individuals within a culture may lead to the development of a culturally-shared CAPS (C-CAPS) sub-network; 2) in specific situations in which this sub-network becomes activated, individuals from the same culture may behave similarly; and 3) within-group individual differences will be readily observed in situations in which the shared sub-network is not relevant, and thus, not activated. We have attempted to demonstrate the model's applicability to understanding the elated and dismayed reactions displayed by many following the verdict of the O.J. Simpson criminal trial verdict, as well as the reactions of those who experienced ambivalence toward the verdict.

One limitation of the present analysis is that it does not directly address the third prediction of the model, namely, that members from the same cultural group can behave differently when the C-CAPS is not activated. While this notion seems intuitive, it remains a central aspect of the theory that must be addressed empirically in order to complement any discussion of intra-group similarity. Future work is needed to draw a more complete picture of the situational specificity of within-group homogeneity and heterogeneity in social behavior. Nevertheless, we believe our approach provides a promising framework for the investigation of cultural differences without compromising the individuality of members of cultural groups.

References

Anderson, J. R. (1983). *The architecture of cognition*. Cambridge, MA: Harvard University Press.

Bandura, A. (1986). *Social foundations of thought and action: A social cognitive theory*. Englewood Cliffs, NJ: Prentice-Hall.

Barnouw, V. (1973). *Culture and personality*. Homewood, IL: Dorsey Press.

Benedict, R. (1934). *Patterns of culture*. Boston. Houghton Mifflin.

Bruner, J. S. (1974). Concluding comments and summary of conference. In J. L. Dawson & W. Lonner (Eds.), *Readings in cultural psychology*. Hong Kong: University of Hong-Kong Press.

Cantor, N., & Kihlstrom, J. F. (1987). *Personality and social intelligence*. Englewood Cliffs, NJ: Erlbaum.

Cervone, D. (1991). The two disciplines of personality psychology. *Psychological Science, 2*, 371-377.

Cole, M. (1996). *Cultural Psychology*. Cambridge, MA: Harvard University Press.

Dodge, K. A. (1993). New wrinkles in the person-versus-situation debate. *Psychological Inquiry, 4*, 284-286.

Dweck, C. & Leggett, E. L. (1988). A social-cognitive approach to personality and motivation. *Psychological Review, 95*, 256-273.

Feldman, J.M. (in press). Four questions about human social behavior. In J. Adamopoulous, & Y. Kashima (Eds.), *Social Psychology and Cultural Context: Essays in Honor of Harry C. Triandis.*

Geertz, C. (1973). *The interpretation of cultures: Selected essays.* New York: Basic Books

Gordon, E. (1982). Culture and Ethnicity. In M.D.Levine, W.B. Cavey, A.C. Crocker, and R. Gross (Eds.), *Textbook of behavioral and developmental pediatrics.* Philadelphia, PA: W.B. Sanders.

Hinton, G. E., McClelland, J. L., & Rumelhart, D. E. (1986). Distributed representations. In D. E. Rumelhart & J. L. McClelland (Eds.), *Parallel distributed processing: Explorations in the microstructures of cognition, Vol I., Foundations* (pp. 77-109). Cambridge, MA: MIT Press/Bradford Books..

Kaplan, B. (1954). A study of Rorschach responses in four cultures. *Papers of the Peabody Museum of American Archaelogy and Ethnology, Harvard University* 42:2.

Kardiner, A. (1945). *Psychological frontiers of society.* New York: Columbia University Press.

Kitayama, S. & Markus, H. R. (in press). Yin and yang of the Japanese self: The cultural psychology of personality coherence. In D. Cervone & Y. Shoda (Eds.), *The coherence of personality: Social cognitive basis of personality consistency, variability, and organization.* New York: Guilford Press.

Lampert, M.D., & Ervin-Tripp, S.M. (1993). Structured coding for the study of language and social interaction. In J.A. Edwards & M.D. Lampert (Eds.), *Talking data: Transcription and coding in discourse research* (pp. 169-206). Hillsdale, NJ: Erlbaum

Levy, S. R. & Dweck, C. S. (1998). Trait- versus process-focused social judgment. *Social Cognition, 16*, 151-172.

Linton, R. (1945). *The cultural background of personality.* New York: Appleton.

Markus, H. R. & Kitayama, S. (1991). Culture and the self: Implications for cognition, emotion, and motivation. *Psychological Review, 98*, 224-253.

Markus, H. R. & Kitayama, S. (1998). The cultural psychology of personality. *Journal of Cross-Cultural Psychology, 29*, 32-61.

Mendoza-Denton, R., Ayduk, O. N., Shoda, Y., & Mischel, W. (1997). Cognitive-affective processing system analyses of reactions to the O.J. Simpson Criminal Trial Verdict. *Journal of Social Issues, 53*, 563-581.

Minturn, L. & Lambert, W. W. (1964). *A scientific theory of culture.* Chapel Hill, NC: University of North Carolina Press.

Mischel, W. (1968). *Personality and assessment.* New York: Wiley.

Mischel, W. (1973). Toward a Cognitive Social Learning Reconceptualization of Personality. *Psychological Review, 80* (4), 252-283.

Mischel, W. & Shoda, Y. (1995). A cognitive-affective system theory of personality: Reconceptualizing situations, dispositions, dynamics and invariance in personality structure. *Psychological Review, 102*, 246-268.

Mischel, W. & Shoda, Y. (1998). Reconciling processing dynamics and personality dispositions. *Annual Review of Psychology, 49*, 229-258.

Nisbett, R. & Cohen, D. (1996). *Culture of honor: The psychology of violence in the south.* Boulder, CO: Westview.

Obeyeskere, G. (1981). *Medusa's hair: An essay on personal symbols and religious experience.* Chicago, IL: University of Chicago Press.

Pervin, L. A. (1990). *Handbook of personality: Theory and research.* New York: Guilford Press.

Purdie, V.J., Mendoza-Denton, R., & Downey, G. (1997). Sensitivity to racially-based rejection. Invited paper presentation, 105th annual convention of the American Psychological Association, Chicago, Illinois.

Read, S. J. & Miller, L. C. (1989). The importance of goals in personality: Toward a coherent mode of persons. In R.S. Wyer, & T.K. Srull (Eds.), *Social intelligence and cognitive assessments of personality. Advances in socialcognition* (2: pp. 163-174). HIllsdale, N.J.: Erlbaum.

Shoda, Y. (in press). Behavioral expressions of a personality system: generation and perception of behavioral signatures. In D. Cervone & Y. Shoda (Eds.), *The coherence of personality: Social cognitive basis of personality consistency, variability, and organization.* New York: Guilford Press.

Shoda, Y., Mischel, W., & Wright, J. C. (1994). Intra-individual stability in the organization and patterning of behavior: Incorporating psychological situations into the idiographic analysis of personality. *Journal of Personality and Social Psychology, 67*, 674-687.

Shweder, R. A. (1991). *Thinking through cultures: Expeditions in cultural psychology.* Cambridge, MA: Harvard University Press

Shweder, R. A. & Sullivan, M. (1990). The semiotic subject of cultural psychology. In L. Pervin (Ed.), *Handbook of personality: Theory and research* (pp. 399-416). New York: Guilford Press.

Triandis, H. C. (1997). Cross-cultural perspectives on personality. In R. Hogan, J. Johnson, & S. Briggs (Eds.), *Handbook of personality* (pp.440-459). San Diego: Academic Press.

Tylor, E. B. (1871). *The origins of culture*. Glouchester, MA: Peter Smith

Acculturation, Individualism-Collectivism, and Ethnic Identity

Models and Measurements of Acculturation

Colleen Ward
National University of Singapore
Department of Social Work and Psychology

ABSTRACT

The paper reviews models and measurements of acculturation and describes the development and use of the Acculturation Index (AI) in a series of studies on sojourner adaptation. The AI is based on an orthogonal model of cultural identity and relies upon two subscales that independently assess perceived similarity to co-national and host national groups. When employed in conjunction with bipartite splits, the AI subscales can also be used to assign sojourners to one of Berry's four acculturation categories: integration, separation, assimilation and marginalization. AI data are presented from five samples: 1) 104 multinational aid workers in Nepal, 2) 100 Singaporeans in the United States, 3) 139 Americans in Singapore, 4) 113 Britons in Singapore and 5) 150 Chinese in Singapore. Across these samples, data indicate that the AI's two subscales are reliable, independent and relate in different ways to psychological and sociocultural adaptation in sojourners.

Acculturation refers to changes that take place as a result of continuous firsthand contact between individuals of different cultural origins (Redfield, Linton & Herskovits, 1936). While changes may occur in attitudes, values, and behaviors, one important component of acculturation relates to changes in cultural identity. Three models exist for describing and explaining these changes. First is an assimilation model whereby cross-cultural travelers are seen to relinquish identification with culture of origin and "progress" towards identification with the culture of contact by adopting the cultural traits, values, attitudes and behaviors of the host society (Olmeda, 1979). This unidimensional and unidirectional model is embodied in a range of self-report measurements designed for the assessment of acculturation. These include the Acculturation Rating Scale for Mexican Americans-I (ARMSA; Cuéllar, Harris & Jesso, 1980), the Greek Immigrant Acculturation Scale (Madianos, 1980, cited in Mavreas, Bebbington & Der, 1989) and the acculturation scale devised by Ghuman (1994) for Asian adolescents in Canada and the United Kingdom.

The second model offers a bicultural perspective whereby identification with home and host cultures are seen as counterbalancing, rather than opposing, forces in shaping the social identification of members of immigrant groups. Biculturalism is viewed as the middle ground between assimilation and separatism; however, as measurement scales typically position biculturalism as the midpoint between identification with heritage and contact cultures, the two referent identities are still viewed as somewhat interdependent, counteracting forces. Measurements that rely upon this approach include: the Multicultural Acculturation Scale (Wong-Rieger & Quintana, 1987), the ARMSA-II (Cuéllar, Arnold & Maldonado, 1995), the adult and youth versions of the Short Acculturation Scale for Hispanics (Barona & Miller, 1994; Marín, Sabogal, Marín, Otero-Sabogal & Perez-Stable, 1987); the Behavioral Acculturation Scale for Hispanics (Szapocznik, Scopetta, Kurtines & Aranalde, 1978), the Suinn-Lew Asian Self-Identity Acculturation Scale (Suinn, Rickard-Figueroa, Lew & Vigil, 1987), the Acculturation Scale for Southeast Asians (Anderson, Moeschberger, Chen, Kunn, Wewers & Guthrie, 1993), the Acculturation Scale for Asian Americans (Lai & Linden, 1993) and the International Relations Scale for International Students (Sodowsky, Lai & Plake, 1991).

The third model recognizes the orthogonal nature of the relationship between home and host culture identification (e.g., Cortés, Rogler & Malgady, 1994; Szapocnik, Kurtines & Fernandez, 1980) and adopts a categorical approach to describing and explaining acculturation (e.g., Hutnik, 1986; Lasry & Sayegh, 1992). Berry's (1974, 1984, 1994) work on acculturation is perhaps the best known example of the categorical approach. Berry has argued that sojourners, immigrants and refugees are faced with two basic questions: "Is it of value to maintain my cultural heritage?" and "Is it of value to maintain relations with other groups?" If the evaluative responses to these two dimensions are dichotomized, four acculturation attitudes or strategies may be distinguished: integration, separation, assimilation and marginalization. Various measurement techniques have been employed in connection with categorical models of acculturation. Some instruments allow the independent assessment of both home and host culture identity and the combination of the two scales for categorical assignment (e.g., Felix-Ortiz, Newcomb and Meyers' (1994) Cultural Identity Scale). Berry and colleagues, however, have generally preferred the independent assessment of marginalization, assimilation, separation and integration via parallel scales as found in their work with Portuguese, Hungarian and Korean immigrants to Canada (Berry, Kim, Young, Power & Bujaki, 1989).

This paper describes the development and use of the Acculturation Index (AI) in studies of international sojourners. The AI adopts an orthogonal model of cultural identification, tapping both host national and co-national identity as independent domains. In addition, the AI subscales may be used in combination with bipartite splits to identify Berry's four modes of acculturation. The original work with the Acculturation Index was published by Ward and Kennedy (1994) in their study of New Zealand civil servants on overseas postings. This paper presents data from five additional samples.

Method

Samples

The samples are described in Table 1 and include: 1) 104 (predominantly North American and European) multinational aid workers in Nepal, 2) 100 Singaporeans in the United States, 3) 139 Americans in Singapore, 4) 113 Britons in Singapore and 5) 150 Chinese (from Hong Kong, People's Republic of China and Taiwan) in Singapore. Mean length of residence in the host country ranged from 29.7 to 100.2 months ($M = 49.9$) across the five samples. These data were taken from larger studies on the prediction of psychological and sociocultural adjustment of sojourners.

Instruments

Acculturation Index. The AI contains 21 cognitive (e.g., in-group and out-group perceptions) and behavioral (e.g., language, food, recreational activities) items. Respondents are asked to consider two questions about their current lifestyles: 1) "Are your experiences and behaviors similar to those of people from your country of origin (co-nationals)? and 2) "Are your experiences and behaviors similar to those of members of the host culture?" Similarity is rated for both co-nationals and host nationals on 7-point rating scales (endpoints: *not at all/ very much*). This approach results in two independent similarity scores which are termed co-national identification and host national identification.

Psychological adjustment. The Zung Self-rating Depression Scale (ZSDS) was employed as a measurement of psychological adjustment. Subjects rely on 4-point rating scales (endpoints: *never or a little of the time/ most of the time*) in response to 20 statements that cover affective, physiological and psychological components of depression. Higher scores indicate greater depression (Zung, 1965). The scale has consistently proven reliable in sojourner research by Ward and colleagues (Searle & Ward, 1990; Ward & Kennedy, 1993, 1994).

Sociocultural adaptation. The Sociocultural Adaptation Scale (SCAS) broadly taps general adaptation to everyday life in a new culture. Subjects use 5-point rating scales (endpoints: *no /extreme*) to rate the amount of difficulty experienced in engaging in a variety of everyday activities (e.g., making friends, going shopping, understanding jokes and humor). Higher scores represent greater difficulty or more sociocultural adaptation problems. The SCAS typically includes 20-23 items. It is a flexible instrument and can be easily modified according to the characteristics of the sojourner sample.

The development of the scale, including its reliability and validity, is discussed in Ward and Kennedy (in press).

Results and Discussion

Psychometric Properties of the AI

Tests of internal consistency via Cronbach alphas are presented in Table 1. As can be seen, both host and co-national identification scales are highly reliable with alphas ranging from .87 to .97. In addition, the subscales are clearly independent as evidenced by intercorrelations ranging from -.03 to .12. The one exception to this is a significant positive correlation (r = .32, p<.001) between host and co-national identity in Chinese sojourners in Singapore. This pattern of correlations suggests that while host and co-national identification are essentially orthogonal, the relationship may be affected by the situational context. When sojourners share similar ethnic and linguistic backgrounds with hosts, the relationship between co-national and host national identification may be increased.

Host and Co-national Identification

Table 1 also reports the means and SD's for co-national and host national identification in five sojourning samples. *T*-tests reveal that sojourners uniformly report greater similarity to members of their own cultural group than members of the contact culture. This is not to suggest that host and co-national identification remains static, even in sojourning groups. For Singaporeans resident in the United States, for example, length of stay was positively related to identification with host nationals (r =.28, p <. 004) while for Americans in Singapore, co-national identification appeared to weaken over time (r =-.19, p<.025).

Identity and Adaptation

Table 2 reports the correlations between cultural identity and sojourner adjustment. Host national identification is clearly associated with better sociocultural adaptation. A significant relationship was found in four of these five samples as well as Ward and Kennedy's (1994) previous study of New Zealand civil servants on overseas postings. There is also some evidence that identification with co-nationals can impede sociocultural adaptation, at least in cases where the recipient society may be seen as a relatively tight culture and sojourners originate from ethnically and culturally dissimilar backgrounds. This is observed, for example, in both the British and American samples in Singapore. Contrary to the outcomes suggested by culture

Table 1. Sample Characteristics and Psychometric Properties of the AI subscales

	Identity					Subscale Analyses	
	Mean length of residence (in months)	Co-national		Host national		r	t
Sample		alpha	Mean	alpha	Mean		
Multinational aid workers in Nepal (N = 104)	29.7 (24.2)	.91	81.75 (17.75)	.89	38.97 (16.15)	-.04	17.55**
Singaporeans in the United States (N = 100)	100.2 (92.2)	.94	67.14 (19.55)	.97	48.59 (31.19)	.12	5.41**
Americans in Singapore (N = 139)	30.7 (34.5)	.93	83.91 (19.59)	.87	40.89 (14.97)	.07	21.34**
Britons in Singapore (N = 113)	53.5 (88.8)	.92	78.98 (22.61)	.87	41.90 (17.76)	-.03	13.53**
Chinese in Singapore (N = 150)	35.4 (31.0)	.94	77.44 (22.52)	.93	67.34 (20.59)	.32*	4.90**

*p <.001, **p <.0005

Note. SD's are in parentheses.

learning theory, however, co-national identity was associated with *better* sociocultural adaptation in Singaporean residents in the United States.

On the whole, the data on cultural identity and psychological adjustment are somewhat less consistent. There is some suggestion that co-national identification may facilitate psychological well-being. The data from both the multinational aid workers in Nepal and the Chinese sojourners in Singapore support this relationship. These findings, in accord with Social Identity Theory (Tajfel, 1978), are also in line with Ward and Kennedy's (1994) earlier study of New Zealand expatriates in multinational settings. However, for Americans in Singapore, it is identification with host nationals that was associated with fewer symptoms of depression. This is in line with the "cultural fit" proposition (Ward & Chang, 1997) and may be more typical in relatively tight receiving societies. Altogether the data remind us that not only individual difference measures but also characteristics of

Table 2. Correlations between Identity and Adaptation Measures

Sample	ZSDS	SCAS
Co-national Identity		
Multinational aid workers in Nepal	-.26**	.08
Singaporeans in the United States	-.05	-.24*
Americans in Singapore	.04	.23**
Britons in Singapore	.05	.25**
Chinese in Singapore	-.19*	-.10
Host-national Identity		
Multinational aid workers in Nepal	-.05	-.28**
Singaporeans in the United States	-.17	-.47**
Americans in Singapore	-.31*	-.22**
Britons in Singapore	-.11	-.17
Chinese in Singapore	-.15	-.17*

*p <.05
**p <.01

home and host cultures should be considered in cross-cultural investigations of the acculturation process.

Four Modes of Acculturation

While Berry has identified two fundamental components of the acculturation process, his research on acculturation and adaptation has emphasized the significance of four acculturation attitudes or strategies and their relationship to acculturative stress. The Acculturation Index also lends itself to the investigation of integration, assimilation, separation and marginalization and their relationship to adaptive outcomes. This is accomplished by using host and co-national identification subscales in conjunction with a bipartite split and a 2 (co-national identity) x 2 (host national identity) analysis of variance with the adjustment outcome as the dependent measure. The four modes of acculturation can be identified in the interaction term. High host-high co-national identification represents integration, high host-low co-national identification indicates assimilation, low host-high co-national identification points to separation, and low host-low co-national identification signifies marginalization.

There are two approaches, however, to splitting the identification scales, and these are discussed in greater detail by Ward and Rana-Deuba (in press). Either the scalar midpoint or the median score may be selected as the cut-off criterion. The first approach was adopted in Donà and Berry's (1994) study of Central American refugees in Canada. This approach results in a "purer" classification of the acculturation strategies and affords greater cross-sample comparisons. The second approach, adopted by Ward and Kennedy (1994) in their study of New Zealand expatriates abroad, relies upon a relative within-sample classification but under some circumstances may be more suitable for distinguishing *four* acculturation modes.

Table 3 reports the frequency breakdown of four acculturation strategies across the five samples based on scalar midpoint splits. Chi square analysis indicated that acculturation modes were evenly distributed across the sample of Singaporeans in the United States ($X^2 = 3.82$, $df = 3$, *n.s.*). All other samples, however, demonstrated clear preferences for specific strategies ($X^2 > 44$, $df = 3$, $p < .001$). The separation strategy occurred as the modal choice of aid workers in Nepal and Americans in Singapore. While it was also prevalent in British sojourners in Singapore, marginalization was found to be the modal strategy in this group. Only the Chinese in Singapore evidenced a preference for integration. Although this has been identified as the acculturation strategy of choice by Berry and colleagues in their work with immigrants and refugees in Canada (Berry *et al.*, 1989), the integrated option was infrequently observed in the samples of Western sojourners in Asian countries.

What is also obvious from the data presented in Table 3 is that the distribution of subjects across the acculturation modes by scalar midpoint splits does not always permit four group comparisons. This was also recognized as a problem in Donà and Berry's (1994) study of refugees where only 4% of the sample were classified as assimilated and none as marginalized. Consequently, the subsequent 2 (host national) x 2 (co-national) analyses variance that were undertaken with psychological and sociocultural adjustment as outcome measures were based on median splits. In no cases was the interaction effect significant. In most instances Fs < 1 and in no cases greater than 3.5.[1] Contrary to Ward and Kennedy's (1994) earlier study, these data failed to substantiate a significant relationship between acculturation strategies and psychological and sociocultural adjustment in sojourners.

Table 3. Number of Sojourners Classified in each of the Acculturation Modes using the Scalar Midpoint Cut-off Criterion

Sample	Integrated	Assimilated	Separated	Marginalized	N
Multinational aid workers in Nepal	7	1	83	13	104
Singaporeans in the United States	30	20	19	28	97
Americans in Singapore	8	0	105	22	135
Britons in Singapore	1	1	43	65	110
Chinese in Singapore	67	41	18	19	145

Conclusions

The Acculturation Index clearly provides a useful psychometric approach to the measurement of identity and acculturation. The instrument includes the assessment of both host and co-national identification and when used with bipartite subscale splits also permits the distinction of four acculturation modes. The AI has evidenced good reliability and validity and has been used successfully across a variety of cross-cultural sojourning groups. Research with the instrument has supported an orthogonal model of acculturation and identity; findings have indicated that host and co-national identification are independent domains and that they relate in different ways to sojourner adaptation.

The Acculturation Index also provides an avenue to explore Berry's (1974) conceptual framework. This is accomplished by bipartite splits of the two independent subscales and the resultant classification of assimilation,

[1] The analysis was repeated for the Singaporeans in the United States and the Chinese in Singapore using the scalar midpoint splits, but this also failed to establish significant interaction effects.

integration, separation and marginalization. This approach offers some advantages over the assessment of the four acculturation attitudes by parallel measurements as is typically employed in work by Berry and colleagues (Berry *et al.*, 1989). Berry's instruments have been criticized by Rudmin (1996) on psychometric grounds, particularly the ipsative nature of the subscales. In addition, Ward and Rana-Deuba (in press) have pointed out the limitations of early cumbersome versions of these culture-specific scales which include lengthy, multiple concept statements. The AI, by comparison, unequivocally relies upon orthogonal subscales, is more compact, is easier to use, and requires little, if any, modification for cross-cultural purposes.

Although the AI studies of identity and acculturation have produced convincing results, the research reported here is not without its limitations. The most obvious shortcoming is that the investigations have been confined to sojourners. It is probable that this group, compared to immigrants and refugees, is likely to experience fewer acculturative changes. Indeed, those who view their stay in a new culture as temporary retain stronger identity with culture of origin and develop weaker identity ties with culture of contact, compared to those who plan for their stay to be more permanent (Mendoza, 1989). Minimally, this would have implications for the distribution of acculturation strategies found in these samples. Beyond that, the samples described here have been taken from a series of larger studies on sojourner adaptation. They were not systematically selected for comparative studies of identity and acculturation. Consequently, the cross-cultural conclusions that can be drawn from these data are limited.

Despite this limitation, the data do suggest directions for further investigations. The most obvious is the expansion of the research to include samples of immigrants and refugees. Secondly, it would be of interest to undertake within-culture comparisons of immigrant groups who systematically vary in cultural distance from members of the host culture. Comparisons should also be made across different receiving societies. Systematic variation of open versus closed, loose versus tight, individualist versus collectivist, and monocultural versus multicultural receiving societies merits further attention.

In conclusion, the Acculturation Index has been presented as a reliable, valid and versatile instrument for the assessment of identity and acculturation. It compares favorably with existing measurements as it permits the independent assessment of both host and co-national identification as well as the investigation of the integration, assimilation, separation and marginalization acculturation strategies. Although not yet widely used, it is hoped that the Acculturation Index will ultimately play a significant role in synthesizing theory and research on identity and acculturation.

References

Anderson, J., Moeschberger, M., Chen, M.S., Kunn, P., Wewers, M.E., & Guthrie, R. (1993). An acculturation scale for Southeast Asians. *Social Psychiatry and Psychiatric Epidemiology, 28,* 134-141.

Barona, A., & Miller, J.A. (1994). Short Acculturation Scale for Hispanic Youth (SASH-Y): A preliminary report. *Hispanic Journal of Behavioral Sciences, 16,* 155-162.

Berry, J.W. (1974). Psychological aspects of cultural pluralism. *Topics in Culture Learning, 2,* 17-22.

Berry, J.W. (1984). Cultural relations in plural societies. In N. Miller & M. Brewer (Eds.), *Groups in contact* (pp.11-27). New York: Academic Press.

Berry, J.W. (1994). Acculturation and psychological adaptation. In A.-M. Bouvy, F.J.R. van de Vijver, P. Boski, & P. Schmitz (Eds.), *Journeys into cross-cultural psychology* (pp. 129-141). Lisse: Swets & Zeitlinger.

Berry, J.W., Kim, U., Power, S., Young, M., & Bujaki, M. (1989). Acculturation attitudes in plural societies. *Applied Psychology, 38,* 185-206.

Cortés, D.E., Rogler, L.H., & Malgady, R.G. (1994). Biculturality among Puerto Rican adults in the United States. *American Journal of Community Psychology, 22,* 707-721.

Cuéllar, I., Arnold, B., & Maldonado, R. (1995). Acculturation rating scale for Mexican Americans-II: A revision of the original ARMSA scale. *Hispanic Journal of Behavioral Sciences, 17,* 275-304.

Cuéllar, I., Harris, L.C., & Jasso, R. (1980). An acculturation scale for Mexican American normal and clinical populations. *Hispanic Journal of Behavioral Sciences, 2,* 199-217.

Donà, G., & Berry, J.W. (1994). Acculturation attitudes and acculturative stress of Central American refugees. *International Journal of Psychology, 29,* 57-70.

Felix-Ortiz, C.M., Newcomb, M.D., & Meyers, H. (1994). A multidimensional measure of cultural identity for Latino and Latina adolescents. *Hispanic Journal of Behavioral Sciences, 16,* 99-115.

Ghuman, P. (1994). Canadian or Indo-Canadian: A study of South Asian adolescents. *International Journal of Adolescence and Youth, 4,* 229-243.

Hutnik, N. (1986). Patterns of ethnic minority identification and modes of social adaptation. *Ethnic and Racial Studies, 9,* 150-167.

Lai, J., & Linden, W. (1993). The smile of Asia: Acculturation effects on symptom reporting. *Canadian Journal of Behavioral Science, 25,* 303-313.

Lasry, J.C., & Sayegh, L. (1992). Developing an acculturation scale: A bidimensional model. In N. Grizenko, L. Sayegh, & P. Migneault (Eds.), *Transcultural issues in child psychiatry* (pp. 67-86). Montreal: Editions Douglas.

Marín, G., Sabogal, F., Marín, B., Otero-Sabogal, R., & Perez-Stable, E.J. (1987). Development of a short acculturation scale for Hispanics. *Hispanic Journal of Behavioral Science, 2,* 21-34.

Mavreas, V., Bebbington, P., & Der, G. (1989). The structure and validity of acculturation: Analysis of an acculturation scale. *Social Psychiatry and Psychiatric Epidemiology, 24,* 233-240.

Mendoza, R.H. (1989). An empirical scale to measure type and degree of acculturation in Mexican-American adolescents and adults. *Journal of Cross-cultural Psychology, 20,* 372-385.

Olmeda, E.L. (1979). Acculturation: A psychometric perspective. *American Psychologist, 34,* 1061-1070.

Redfield, R., Linton, R., & Herskovits, M.J. (1936). Memorandum for the study of acculturation. *American Anthropologist, 38,* 149-152.

Rudmin, F.W. (1996, August). *Critical review of acculturation.* Paper presented at the XIII International Congress of the International Association for Cross-cultural Psychology, Montreal, Canada.

Searle, W., & Ward, C. (1990). The prediction of psychological and sociocultural adjustment during cross-cultural transitions. *International Journal of Intercultural Relations, 14,* 449-464.

Sodowsky, G.R., Lai, J., & Plake, B.S. (1991). Psychometric properties of the American-International Relations Scale. *Educational and Psychological Measurement, 51,* 207-216.

Suinn, R.M., Rickard-Figueroa, K., Lew, S., & Vigil, P. (1987). The Suinn-Lew Asian Self-Identity Acculturation Scale: An initial report. *Educational and Psychological Measurement, 47,* 401-402.

Szapocznik, J., Kurtines, W.M., & Fernandez, T. (1980). Bicultural involvement and adjustment in Hispanic-American youths. *International Journal of Intercultural Relations, 4,* 353-365.

Szapocznik, J., Scopetta, M.A., Kurtines, W.M., & Aranalde, M.A. (1978). Theory and measurement of acculturation. *Interamerican Journal of Psychology, 12,* 113-130.

Tajfel, H. (1978). *Differentiation between social groups: Studies in the psychology of intergroup relations.* London: Academic Press.

Ward, C., & Chang, W.C. (1997). "Cultural fit:" A new perspective on personality and sojourner adjustment. *International Journal of Intercultural Relations, 21,* 525-533.

Ward, C., & Kennedy, A. (1993). Where's the culture in cross-cultural transition? Comparative studies of sojourner adjustment. *Journal of Cross-cultural Psychology, 24,* 221-249.

Ward, C., & Kennedy, A. (1994). Acculturation strategies, psychological adjustment and sociocultural competence during cross-cultural transitions. *International Journal of Intercultural Relations, 18,* 329-343.

Ward, C., & Kennedy, A. (in press). The measurement of sociocultural adaptation. *International Journal of Intercultural Relations.*

Ward, C., & Rana-Deuba, A. (in press). Acculturation and adaptation revisited. *Journal of Cross-cultural Psychology.*

Wong-Rieger, D., & Quintana, D. (1987). Comparative acculturation of Southeast Asian and Hispanic immigrants and sojourners. *Journal of Cross-cultural Psychology, 18,* 345-362.

Zung, W.W.K. (1965). A self-rating depression scale. *Archives of General Psychiatry, 12,* 63-70.

Acculturation and Delinquency among Cambodian Male Adolescents in California

Kaine Vierachai Lim
University of Hawaii at Manoa
Clinical Psychology Program, Department of Psychology & The East-West Center

Michael Levenson
University of California at Davis
Department of Human and Community Development

Charles G. Go
University of California at Davis
Department of Human and Community Development

ABSTRACT

Adolescence is a time of stressful transitions. For minority adolescents, this problem is compounded by problems of acculturation (Berry, 1986). Using Cambodian refugees as participants, this study examined whether there is a relationship between the difference in the degree of parental vs. adolescent acculturation and adolescent delinquent behavior. Twenty-nine adult-adolescent pairs were gathered from San Francisco and Stockton, California. The hypothesis that parent-child difference in acculturation would be related to delinquency was not supported by the data. However, regression analyses showed that adolescents' acculturation score, age of the adolescents at time of entry to the U.S., and the presence of both parents were all negatively associated with delinquency. This suggests that adolescents who were less acculturated, despite their earlier age of entry, tended to have delinquent behaviors. Possible explanations for delinquency among Cambodian adolescents were explored.

Cambodians in America

As refugees to the United States, Cambodians bring with them their traditions, values, beliefs, and ways of life. Although some have established themselves in their new homeland, many others still face a number of problems. In trying to better understand some of these problems and their underlying processes, this study examines the problems of acculturation and delinquency among Cambodian adolescents.

Delinquency

Adolescent delinquency has been the focus of many research studies. In general, cross-sectional studies have reported a higher level of delinquency during adolescence, especially for boys (see reviews by Emler & Reicher, 1995; Moffitt, 1993; Patterson & Yoerger, 1993).

However, very little work has been done with Asian American delinquents, especially Southeast Asians. The California Youth Authority (1996) reported that Southeast Asian youth represent 67% of all incarcerated Asian youth (Vietnamese, 30%, Laotians, 17%, Cambodians, 10%, Thai, 9%). In comparison, Southeast Asians comprise about 17% of the total Asian population in California (1990 Census Data). Therefore, Southeast Asian youth, which includes Cambodians, are over-represented in the California youth correctional system.

The general patterns of delinquent behavior can be affected by individual, family and community factors. Tonry, Ohlin and Farrington (1991), in a review of longitudinal studies, found that families of delinquents were marked by economic adversity, marital instability, and erratic, harsh discipline. At the community level, higher delinquency rates occurred in socially disorganized communities where human services were often inadequate to meet the needs of families and young children, which may be evident in living conditions of immigrant and minority populations in the U.S. Thus, acculturation difficulties may be one factor in the delinquency patterns of Southeast Asian youth.

Acculturation and Delinquency

There are very few studies on the effect of acculturation on delinquency. Those that examine the effects of acculturation on delinquency have measured this relationship in two ways. One approach determines the correlation between adolescent acculturation and adolescent delinquency while another assesses the acculturation differences between the adolescent and his/ or her parents and relates these differences to delinquency. An example of the first type is Sommers, Fagan, and Baskin's (1993) study of Puerto Rican youth in New York. They gathered 1,007 self-report questionnaires completed by male adolescents who ranged from 12 to 19 years of age. Adolescents who reported being the least acculturated were more likely to report certain types of delinquent behaviors such as drug use and theft. Thus, immigrant groups were found to be more at risk for delinquent behaviors.

An example of the second type of study was conducted by Vega, Gil, Warheit, and Zimmerman (1993). Differences in acculturation levels between the adolescent and the parent have been linked to delinquent behaviors in the acculturation of Cuban adolescents in Miami (Vega et al., 1993). In this study, family pride, family cohesion, and parental support were found to be negatively linked to acculturation differences in adolescents. Acculturation differences were also found to be significantly correlated with delinquent behaviors of adolescents. However, these data were gathered by a questionnaire in English and did not take language problems into account. In addition, Vega et al. did not differentiate generation effects. Selection for inclusion in the study merely required one to be of Cuban descent. Whether these findings generalize to other populations, such as Southeast Asian ones, is unknown.

Cambodian Context

Cambodians represent an important Southeast Asian immigrant population, especially in California. There were approximately 149,000 documented Cambodian immigrants in 1990. Now there are undoubtedly many more. Between 1990 and 1994, 190,192 refugees and asylum seekers immigrated to California (California Department of Finance, 1996). While most are concentrated in the Los Angeles area, a significant number of Cambodians are found in other cities, including communities in the Central Valley. Among Asian immigrant groups, there is tremendous diversity in three factors that affect their adjustment to the U.S.: Educational status, residential background, and reason for immigrating (Min, 1995). Between 1985 to 1990, 41 percent of Asian immigrants who entered the U.S. were college graduates as compared to 20 percent of the U.S. population. However, when Asian immigrants are divided into sub-groups according to regional origin, one exception stands out: Only 7 percent of the recent Vietnamese immigrants were college graduates.

Diversity further exists between the Southeast Asian refugee groups. The majority of Southeast Asian refugees that came to the United States before 1979 were predominantly Vietnamese. As a group, this early waves of refugees were highly educated and skilled, and more affluent compared to those that arrived after 1979 (Kelly, 1986; Meinhardt, 1990; Rumbaut, 1985, 1991). In addition to the demographic differences between different waves of refugees, 92 percent of the Hmongs and 53 percent of the Cambodians came from rural backgrounds while 95 percent of the Chinese-Vietnamese and Vietnamese came from urban areas. With an average of 10.5 year of education in their home country, compared with 5.9 year for Cambodians and 7.2 year for Laotians, the Vietnamese were also the most highly educated.

In spite of some diversities between the different Southeast Asian refugees, virtually all of them migrated to the U.S. because of well-founded fear of political persecution. Thus they are refugees according to the United States Immigration and Nationality Act (1980). They did not choose to immigrate to the U.S. to search for better economic opportunity. Thus, taken together, of the Asian immigrants, Southeast Asian immigrants were the least prepared for life in the U.S.

These factors may affect the acculturation process of Cambodian adolescents. In addition to the "normal" crisis of adolescence, the acculturation process has also been seen as a common source of stress for refugees (Ascher, 1985; Berry, 1986; Tobin & Friedman, 1984; Westermeyer, 1989a, 1989b; Williams & Berry, 1991; Yu, 1984). For example, Cambodian adolescents had to attend school and learn to associate with their American peers. As a result, these adolescents became more accustomed to the host culture than their parents. At the same time, they also wanted to retain the values of their original culture, due in part to the insistence of their parents and their own loyalty to their old culture. However, in the U.S., the predominant culture, with an emphasis on individuality, socializes adolescents to develop an independent sense of self, whereas most Southeast Asian cultures emphasize the development of a self that is interlaced with others (Phinney, 1990). Thus, the incompatibility of the two cultures is very likely to result in stress for these adolescents. Furthermore, they may feel the isolation expressed by Lee (1988, p.173), "The greatest threat to identity is not the feeling of belonging to two cultures but the feeling of belonging to none." Berry (1986) also reported that those who were from a culture that was most different from the host culture were most likely to have the highest acculturative stress.

Most Cambodian refugee parents, however, came to the U.S. when their values had already been firmly established. They were rural inhabitants and had little education and exposure to Western society (Ouk, Huffman, & Lewis, 1988). Thus, added to their lack of English skills, the acculturation process was also potentially very stressful for the parents (Waters, 1990). Furthermore, concordance of acculturation levels between the adolescent and the parent may affect the stress experienced. Szapocznik, Scopetta, and Kurtines (1978) found that the development of inter-generational acculturation differences between the children and their parents led to family disruptions. Likewise, Ascher (1985) also found that the bigger the gap in acculturation between Southeast Asian parents and their children, the more likely conflicts were to arise.

To make the acculturation process even more challenging, many Cambodian refugees experienced significant amount of premigration traumas (e.g., during the Khmer Rouge regime or during the refugee camp stay) and are still preoccupied with and affected by these experiences. In a study of 2180 Southeast Asian refugees (890 Cambodians), Chung and Kagawa-Singer, (1993) found that the number of traumas experienced during the premigration phase and the length of time spent in a refugee camp were significant premigration predictors of psychological distress for these refugees with Cambodians reporting the highest levels of distress. Chung and Kagawa-Singer also found Cambodian refugees to still be primarily concerned with premigration issues. In studying 209 Cambodian adolescents and their parents, Sack et al. (1994) found that one fifth of the adolescents, over one half of the mothers, and about one third of the fathers met the DSM-III-R criteria for PTSD. Furthermore, Sack and colleagues found that 34.9 percent of the youths, 23.4 percent of the mothers, and 14.1 percent of the fathers met criteria for clinical depression.

Added to the acculturative stress and premigration trauma, many Cambodian parents have often been observed to feel out of control because their ways of disciplining their children (e.g., corporal punishment) conflict with the local child protection laws in the U.S. Furthermore, they are not familiar with the child disciplining techniques (e.g., time out) more appropriate in the American culture (Ratliff, 1997). In addition, Cambodian parents may have inadequate understanding of the social and school environment in which their adolescent children interact (e.g., their children's peers, activities, academic and extra curricula, and hang out places).

Present Study

To examine the relationship between immigration, acculturation and delinquency, we used a sample of Cambodian adolescent males and their parents. This study contrasts two approaches: (a) the relationship between adolescent acculturation level and its relation to adolescent delinquency, and (b) the relationship between acculturation differences of the adolescent and his parents and the corresponding delinquent behavior. Thus, we hypothesized that adolescents who reported the least acculturation would also report the most delinquency. Alternatively, the greater the difference in the degree of reported acculturation between the parents and their sons, the more delinquent behaviors the sons would report.

Method

Participants

With the help of social workers, bilingual school counselors, and personal contacts of the first author, a total of 58 participants were recruited from Stockton and San Francisco, California. The participants from Stockton were from two apartment complexes, both of which have over 90% Cambodian residents, while the participants from San Francisco were spread throughout the city. Twenty-nine of the participants were male adolescents from 13 to 18 years old, and 29 were the adult parents—one parent for each adolescent. In cases where both parents were present, either the father or the mother was selected, on voluntary basis, to participate in the study. Of the 29 adult participants, two subsequently failed to complete the acculturation questionnaires. To compensate for this, the missing parental scores were estimated based on the regression slope of the pairs with complete data and the adolescent delinquency scores.

The average age of adolescent respondents was approximately 15 years old. Most of them entered the U.S. at age 5, and had spent about 10 years in the U.S. As a group, they were behind in the number years of schooling since the average was 9 years -- at least one year less than the average U.S. born child of the same age. In addition, the average delinquency score was 12, although it ranged from 0 to 69.

There were 11 male parents and 18 female parents in our sample. The average age of entry of the parents was 34 years with a minimum age of 24 and a maximum age of 49 years. This group of adults can be characterized as having low educational experience since the average Cambodian schooling was 1 year and the average U.S. schooling was 3 years -- a total of only 4 years. This is reflected in the low average family income which was $12,500.

When acculturation scores were compared, Cambodian adolescents' mean scores were found to be 10 points higher than those of their parents on the acculturation scale (35.86 vs. 25.03, respectively). Interestingly, the standard deviations and the differences between the highest and the lowest scores were similar for adolescents and adults. Thus, acculturation mean differences do exist between Cambodian parents and adolescents despite the similar range in variation.

Measures

The measures used were two sets of questionnaires, one assessing acculturation and the other assessing delinquency. The acculturation scale used was a modified version of the Suinn-Lew Asian Self-Identity Acculturation Scale (SL-ASIA) (Suinn, Rickard-Figueroa, Lew, & Vigil, 1987). Although most of the items on the SL-ASIA were retained, changes were made to take into account a recent factorial validation (Suinn, Ahuna, & Khoo, 1992). Furthermore, some changes were made to make questions more relevant to Cambodian participants. For example, the term "Cambodian" was added to choice 1 of question 9, "Only Asian music (for example, *Cambodian*). . ."

We used the same modified acculturation questionnaire for the adolescents and the parents. Only the English version of the adolescent acculturation questionnaire was available since these adolescents have limited Khmer skills. The parental acculturation questionnaire was translated from English into Khmer (language of Cambodia) following a back-translation procedure recommended by Brislin (1970). The questionnaire items were first translated into Khmer, and then back-translated into English. This version was then compared to the original version, revised, and edited for compatibility. The original English questionnaire was also revised and edited for compatibility with the translated version. The parental acculturation questionnaire was made available in both English and Khmer; however, because of limited English skills, most parent participants took the Khmer version of the acculturation questionnaire.

Both versions of acculturation questionnaire utilize a five point Likert-like scale (only Asian, mostly Asian, equally Asian-American, mostly American, only American). Acculturation level was computed by adding the total number of points on the questionnaire. Individuals with the most number were equated as the most acculturated or American vs. the least acculturated as the most Asian.

The other questionnaire, the Adolescent Behavior Questionnaire (ABQ), was a modified general delinquency scale, modeled after the Seattle Self-report Instrument (Hindelang, Hirschi, & Weis, 1981), and the National Youth Survey questionnaire (Brennan, Huizinga, & Elliott, 1978). Both of these scales contained a large pool of questions and covered a wide range of topics. They were combined and rephrased to make them more appropriate for the target participants. Since delinquent behaviors are those that are minor offenses, whether criminal or status, questions on armed robbery, murder, and other felony-type are excluded from the ABQ.

Each question on the ABQ has a six point Likert-like scale (never, 2 or less, 2-5 times, 5-7 times, 7-9 times, 10 or more) and asks how many times the participant engaged in the delinquent behavior within the last three years. The delinquency score was computed by adding the total number of points on the questionnaire. Adolescents with the most number of points were viewed as the most delinquent vs. the least number of points as the least delinquent.

Since we modified the acculturation and delinquency questionnaires, we performed the Cronbach's Alpha reliability tests on the adolescent acculturation scale (ACC1), adult acculturation scale (ACC2), and the ABQ. Several items in the acculturation scales loaded negatively and thus, these items were deleted. The final acculturation scale was comprised of 9 items measuring spoken language(s); ethnic origin of friends at age 6; ethnic origin of friends between 6-18; current associations in the community; chosen associations in the community; type of music listened to; type of movie watched; food preference at home; and type of food eaten at restaurants.

Because each of the questionnaires was believed to represent a construct (acculturation or delinquency), the standardized alpha score was derived for each. The alpha for the ACC1 was .72, and .79 for the ACC2. Moreover, all 36 items in the ABQ loaded positively. The alpha score for the ABQ was .91. The final delinquency questionnaire focused on vandalism and property damage, drugs, theft, assault, gang fights, weapon possession, traffic violation, trespassing, and school delinquency and family delinquency.

Procedure

Prior to participation, parental consent forms were obtained. After receiving a referral, the primary investigator contacted the family and scheduled an appointment to visit the family. All questionnaires were individually administered at participants' homes or within the vicinity of their residences. Sometimes, the son and parent would be administered the questionnaires in the same room, and sometimes in different rooms. If the parent and son were to be in the same room, it was not possible for the parent to know how the son answered because of parental limited English language skills. Furthermore, we directed the son and parent to be far enough away from one another that one could not hear how the other was answering, and did not allow completed questionnaires to be viewed by anyone other than themselves. Sometimes parent/son participants would complete the questionnaires at different times. Whenever the participants could not read English or Khmer proficiently, the first author served as a translator.

Most parents who participated in this study used the translated version of the acculturation questionnaire or resort to using the translator. The parents received only the acculturation questionnaire, while the sons received both the acculturation and the delinquency questionnaires. The administration time for the acculturation questionnaires was 15-35 minutes depending on the degree of familiarity the participants had with completing survey instruments and their comprehension level of such questions. Those who were more literate completed the questionnaire faster than those who were not. The delinquency questionnaire took 20-30 minutes to complete. The order in which the questionnaires were given to the sons was random.

Results

Bivariate Statistics

We found that adolescent acculturation scores were significantly correlated to adult acculturation and the difference between the adolescent and parental acculturation scores. The more the parents were acculturated, the more likely their adolescent sons were also acculturated ($r = .65$, $p < .001$). However, adolescents sons' acculturation scores were also found to be related to differences between their acculturation scores and their parents' acculturation scores ($r = .68$, $p < .001$). There was no significant relationship between parental acculturation scores and the difference between the adolescent and parental acculturation scores ($r = -.12$, $p = .55$).

Contrary to our hypotheses, we found no significant relationship between all the acculturation measures and adolescent delinquent behavior.

Specifically, we found a non-significant correlation between adolescent acculturation and adolescent delinquency ($r = -.14$, $p = .47$). Similarly, the correlation between delinquency and the difference between the acculturation of adolescents and adult participants was found to be non-significant ($r = -.05$, $p = .81$). Interestingly, only parental marital status was significantly correlated with delinquency. Specifically, we found that two parent households tended to have adolescent sons who were less delinquent ($r = -.39$, $p < .05$). We also found a trend whereby the adolescents who entered the U.S. at a younger age engaged in fewer delinquent behaviors ($r = -.35$, $p = .07$).

Multivariate Statistics

A regression analysis was performed to ascertain which variables accounted most for adolescent delinquent behaviors. The adolescent delinquency scores were regressed on all other variables using a backward elimination procedure (Note: This procedure was used to control for the small sample size). The resulting regression equation accounted for 42% of the variance, $F(2, 29) = 9.25$, $p < .001$, with the following variables remaining in the equation: Adolescent's age upon entry to the U.S. and adult marital status. We found that adolescents who had a younger age of entry to the U.S. ($\beta = -.54$) and who came from single parent households ($\beta = -.58$) were associated with higher delinquent behaviors.

Discussion

We proposed two hypotheses: a) adolescents who reported the least acculturation would also report the most delinquency, and b) the greater the difference in the degree of reported acculturation between the parents and their sons, the more delinquent behaviors the sons would report. Our data did not supported either of the hypotheses. We found no significant correlations between the acculturation measures and adolescent delinquent behaviors. This could indicate that adolescent and parental acculturation levels are not related to adolescent delinquency leaving the possibility of the existence of mediating variables. Higher family conflict (Patterson et al., 1993, Vega et al., 1993), and poor parenting (Haapasalo & Tremblay, 1994; Simons, Wu, Conger, & Lorenz, 1994) have been found to be linked to higher reported rates of delinquency. Thus, we suggest that future studies include mediating factors between acculturation measures and adolescent delinquency.

Alternatively, the lack of support could be due to a lack of more appropriate acculturation measure for Cambodians in the U.S. While the SL-ASIA is a psychometrically sound instrument and was the most appropriate instrument available for our study, it was validated on 82 unspecified Asian participants from the University of California at Los Angeles and Colorado

State University. A more culture-specific acculturation instrument, as recommended in a recent conference (Latino Acculturation Conference, University of San Francisco, 1998) may have yielded a more significant result. Furthermore, the SL-ASIA measures acculturation on a linear scale. Thus, the complexity of acculturation involved in this study may not have been fully captured.

However, we did find a positive relationship between adolescent acculturation and adult acculturation. Thus, Cambodian parents seem to have a role in their adolescents sons' acculturation. Perhaps Cambodian parents who are trying to be more acculturated and are supportive of "Americanization" tend to have adolescents sons who are more acculturated. This could explain why we also found that the more acculturated adolescents tended to have higher differences with their parents.

Furthermore, in our effort to better understand the relationship between immigration, acculturation and delinquency, we performed a regression analysis of all the variables on adolescent delinquency. We found that single parent households and younger adolescent age of entry to the U.S. were both positively associated with adolescent delinquent behaviors. These results point to the importance of single parent households in increased risk for juvenile delinquency. Single parenting has been previously linked to increased risk for delinquent behavior. For example, African American adolescent drug use has been linked to single parenting and low income (Farrell, Danish, & Howard, 1992). Moreover, using a Mexican and Caucasian sample, Fridrich and Flannery (1995) found that parental monitoring was a better predictor of early adolescent delinquent behavior rather than ethnicity or level of acculturation. To the extent that immigrant single parents are facing adjustment to an unfamiliar culture and lacking knowledge of English, their parenting resources maybe stretched very thin and prove to be inadequate support for their male adolescents.

Further, the results seems to suggest a link between cultural isolation and increased risk for delinquent behavior. Cambodian adolescents' who entered the U.S. at a younger age would be expected to be more acculturated than those who arrived when they were older. However, in our study, some of these adolescents were also found to be less acculturated and more delinquent. This could indicate a conflict in the parent and adolescent relationship. For instance, many Cambodian parents do not approve of their children's participation in after-school activities, such as school sports. This may prove frustrating to Cambodian American adolescents. Thus, conflicting messages from family and the larger culture could lead adolescents to the feeling of belonging to none (Lee, 1988) since they are neither fully Americanized nor Cambodianized. This kind of conflict has been linked to delinquent behaviors (Vega et al., 1993).

Several limitations of our study should be noted. First, the sample size (29 pairs) was unavoidably small and thus compromised statistical power and further age distribution analyses. A replication of our study, with a larger sample would give us greater confidence in our findings and might uncover other important variables contributing to delinquency in immigrant populations. In addition, we caution the readers in terms of generalizing the findings from our study. This study was not a random sample design and sampled only from Cambodian populations in San Francisco and Stockton. Second, only adolescent males were included in this study. Third, since this is a preliminary study, there could be problems in our measures. As discussed above, this study did not measure family conflict, or quality of parenting which might have a mediating effect on the outcome of adolescent delinquency. Fourth, the questions used in the questionnaires, although modified to fit the Cambodian population, could be inadequately tapping the issue of delinquency and acculturation. For example, in the acculturation questionnaires, participants were not given the option of saying that they identified with neither the American nor Asian culture. Furthermore, the delinquency questionnaire lacks some items of contemporary relevance such as whether the adolescent has sold or tried to sell guns. Thus, an updated instrument might better document adolescent delinquent behaviors. Finally, this study assumed an American family model of single or two parent families. Other reports (Ling & Nguyen, 1993) have documented reconstituted family structures (i.e., adolescents living with aunts and uncles, living with adopted parents, living with a friend's parents) that have varying impacts on the child's delinquency.

Delinquency is a complex issue. The past and present circumstances of Cambodian refugees add to this complexity. However, our initial investigation indicates that more focus should be placed on low income single parents and on adolescent males who were isolated. Specifically, we suggest more studies on the linkage between the social relationships (family, peer, teachers, etc.) of adolescent immigrants and their acculturation process.

References

Ascher, C. (1985). The social and psychological adjustment of Southeast Asian refugees. *The Urban Review, 17*(2), 147-52.

Berry, J. W. (1990). Acculturation and adaptation: A general framework. In W. H. Holtzman, T. H. Bornemann (Eds.), *Mental health of immigrants and refugees* (pp. 90-102). Austin, TX: Hogg Foundation for Mental Health.

Berry, J. W. (1986). The acculturation process and refugee behavior. In J. Westermeyer & C. L. Williams (Eds.), *Refugee mental health in resettlement countries* (Chap. 2). Washington, DC: Hemisphere Publishing Corp.

Brennan, T., Huizinga, D., & Elliott, D. (1978). *The social psychology of runaways*. Lexington, MA: D.C. Heath.

Brislin, R. W. (1970). Back-translation for cross-cultural research. *Journal of Cross-Cultural Psychology, 1*(3), 185-216.

Census of Population and Housing (1990). Summary of social, economic, and housing characteristics. Washington , DC: U.S. Dept. of Commerce, Bureau of the Census.

Chung, R. & Kagawa-Singer, M (1993). Predictors of psychological distress among Southeast Asian refugees. *Social Science Medicine, 36*(5), 631-639.

Farrell, A. D., Danish, S. J., & Howard, C. W. (1992). Risk factors for drug use in urban adolescents: Identification and cross-validation. *American Journal of Community Psychology, 20*(3), 263-86.

Fridrich, A. H., & Flannery, D. J. (1995). The effects of ethnicity and acculturation on early adolescent delinquency. *Journal of Child and Family Studies, 4*(1), 69-87.

Haapasalo, J. & Tremblay, R. E. (1994). Physically aggressive boys from ages 6 to 12: Family background, parenting behavior, and prediction of delinquency. *Journal of Consulting and Clinical Psychology, 62*(5), 1044-1052.

Hindelang, M. J., Hirschi, T., & Weis, J. (1982). Reply to "On the use of self-report data to determine the class distribution of criminal and delinquent behavior". *American Sociological Review, 47*(3), 433-35.

Kelly, G. (1986). Coping with America: Refugees from Vietnam, Cambodia, and Laos in the 1970s and 1980s. *The Annals of the American Academy, Political and Social Science, 487*, 138-149.

Lee, E. (1988). Cultural factors in working with Southeast Asian refugee adolescents. *Journal of Adolescence, 11*, 167-79.

Ling, C. W., & Nguyen, Y. H. (1993). *The parenting problems of the Vietnamese and ethnic Chinese-Vietnamese communities in Sacramento county*. Unpublished Thesis, California State University, Sacramento.

Meinhardt, K. (1990). Contribution of epidemiological surveys to planning and evaluating clinical services. In Wayne H. Holtzman & Thomas H. Bornemann (Eds.), *Mental Health of Immigrants and Refugees*. Austin, TX: Hogg Foundation for Mental Health.

Ouk, M., Huffman, F. E., & Lewis, J. (1988). *Handbook for teaching Khmer-speaking students*. Folsom, CA: Folsom Cordova Unified School District.

Patterson, G. & Yoerger, K. (1993). Developmental models for delinquent behavior. In S. Hodgins (Ed.), *Mental disorder and crime* (pp. 140-172). Newbury Park, CA: Sage Publications, Inc.

Ratliff, S. K. (1997). *Caring for Cambodian Americans: A multidisciplinary resource for the helping professions*. New York: Garland Publishing, Inc.

Rumbaut, R G. (1991). The agony of exile: A study of the migration and adaptation of Indochinese refugee adults and children. In F. L. Ahearn, Jr., & J. L. Athey (Eds.), *Refugee children: Theory, research, and services*. Baltimore, MA: Johns Hopkins University Press.

Rumbaut, R. G. & Ima, K. (1987). *Southeast Asian Refugee Youth Study. The adaptation of Southeast Asian refugee youth: A comparative study.* Department of Sociology, San Diego State University.

Rumbaut, R. G. (1985). Mental health and the refugee experience: A comparative study of Southeast Asian refugees. In Tom C. Owan, Bruce Bliatout, Keh-Ming Lin, William Liu, Tuan Nguyen, & Herbert Wong (Eds.) *Southeast Asian mental health: Treatment, prevention, services, training, and research.* Washington, DC: U.S. Department of Health and Human Services.

Sack, W. H., McSharry, S., Clarke, G., Kinney, R., Seeley, J., & Lewinsohn, P. (1994). The Khmer adolescent project I. Epidemiologic findings in two generations of Cambodian refugees. *Journal of Nervous and Mental Disease, 182*, 387-395.

Simons, R. L., Wu, C., Conger, R. D., & Lorenz, F. O. (1994). Two routes to delinquency: Differences between early and late starters in the impact of parenting and deviant peers. *Criminology, 32*(2), 247-276.

Sommers, I., Fagan, J., & Baskin, D., (1993). Sociocultural influences on the explanation of delinquency for Puerto Rican youths. *Hispanic Journal of Behavioral Sciences, 15*(1), 36-62.

Suinn, R. M., Rickard-Figueroa, K., Lew, S., & Vigil, P. (1987). The Suinn-Lew Asian Self-Identity Acculturation Scale: An initial report. *Educational and Psychological Measurement, 47*, 401-07.

Suinn, R. M., Ahuna, C., & Khoo, G. (1992). The Suinn-Lew Asian Self-Identity Acculturation Scale: Concurrent and factorial validation. *Educational and Psychological Measurement, 52*, 1041-46.

Szapocznik, J., Scopetta, M. A., Kurtines, W., & Aranalde, M. A. (1978). Theory and measurement of acculturation. *Interamerican Journal of Psychology, 12*, 113-30.

Tobin, J. J., & Friedman, J. (1984). Intercultural and developmental stresses confronting Southeast Asian refugee adolescents. *Journal of Operational Psychiatry, 15*, 39-45.

Tonry, M., Ohlin, L. E., & Farrington, D. P. (1991). Human development and criminal behavior: New ways of advancing knowledge. *Contemporary Sociology, 20*(6), 920-938.

U.S. Immigration and Nationality Act of 1980, 8 U.S.C. 1158.

Vega, W. A., Gil, A. G., Warheit, G. J., Zimmerman, R. S. (1993). Acculturation and delinquent behavior among Cuban American adolescents: Toward an empirical model. *American Journal of Community Psychology, 21*(1), 113-25.

Waters, T. (1990). *Migration as process: Youthful crime in immigrant communities*. Unpublished Dissertation. University of California, Davis.

Westermeyer, J. (1989a). Causes and precipitants. In J. Westermeyer (Ed.), *Mental health for refugees and other migrants: Social and preventive approaches* (pp. 99-130). Springfield, IL: Charles C. Thomas.

Westermeyer, J. (1989b). Distribution of mental disorders among migrants. In J. Westermeyer (Ed.), *Mental health for refugees and other migrants: Social and preventive approaches*. (pp. 65-98). Springfield, IL: Charles C. Thomas.

Williams, C. L., & Berry, J. W. (1991). Primary prevention of acculturative stress among refugees: Application of psychological theory and practice. *American Psychologist, 46* (6), 632-41.

Wong, M. (1986). Post-1965 Asian immigrants: Where do they come from, where are they now, and where are they going? *Annals of the American Academy of Political and Social Science, 487*, 150-168.

Yu, L. C. (1984). Acculturation and stress within Chinese American families. *Journal of Comparative Family Studies, 15*(1), 77-94.

Individualism-Collectivism Revisited: Some Consequences for Group Decision-Making

Asoke K. Saha
Department of Psychology
University of Allahabad

Emmanuel S. K. Ghosh
Department of Psychology
University of Allahabad

ABSTRACT

Following developments in individualism and collectivism theory, the current study was designed to investigate the effects of self-orientations, as opposed to Group orientations, in a Group decision-making task, in both India and Bangladesh. Fifty high self-oriented participants and 50 high group oriented participants were taken from India and Bangladesh. The sample was divided into small groups of five participants each and examined for pre-group decision making and consensual group decision making rating on risk taking items. Results indicated that in both India and Bangladesh high group oriented participants showed more group polarization and took riskier consensual decision as compared to the self oriented participants. The findings are discussed in the context of collectivistic orientation, which characterizes both India and Bangladesh and the subsequent moderation by individualistic versus collective orientations as group effects salient to group decision making and group polarization.

In recent years the dimension of individualism-collectivism has been used as an explanatory variable in several research studies. Hofstede (1991) defined individualism-collectivism as follows: "Individualism pertains to societies in which the ties between individuals are loose: Everyone is expected to look after himself or herself and his or her immediate family. Collectivism as its opposite pertains to societies in which people birth onwards are integrated into strong, cohesive ingroups, which throughout people's life time continue to protect them in exchange for unquestioning loyalty." (p. 51). According to Triandis (1994) individualism entails giving priority to personal goals over the goals of the ingroup, whereas collectivism entails giving priority to ingroup goals over personal goals. With the recent development of psychology of the self, important theoretical contributions have been made by several researchers (e.g., Crocker & Luhtanen, 1990; Markus & Kitayama, 1991; Triandis, 1989). Markus and Kitayama (1991) assume that people in different cultures differ in their understanding of themselves, others, and the relationships among people. They propose that degrees of separation or connectedness among individuals vary across cultures. The understanding that individuals are not separate but connected to each other is called the interdependent construal of the self and is supposed to be shared by the

Indian subcontinent culture as well as other Asian cultures. Sinha and Tripathi (1994), however, conceptualized the coexistence of individualism in India along with collectivism and emphasized the contextual nature of values and behavior. It may be noted that Triandis (1989) has also argued that people differ in the probability that they will sample different aspects of self (i.e., the private, public, and collective self). He asserts that people in collectivist cultures sample the collective aspects of the self more often than the other aspects. If the collective self is sampled more frequently, more elements of the collective self become salient (Triandis, 1989).

Hence as the individual's membership in the group becomes more salient, it would in turn lead him or her to behave differently in ingroup and outgroup situations. Researchers have found significant differences between ingroup and outgroup behavior in collectivist cultures compared with individualist cultures (e.g., Gudykunst, Yoon, & Nishida, 1987; Leung & Bond, 1984). Such results indicate that a person's self-definition as a member of a group determines how he or she acts in social situations. Crocker and Luhtanen (1990) propose the existence of collective self-esteem in individuals, which is differentiated from personal self-esteem. Collective self-esteem is defined as the motivation to maintain a positive social identity, which is an aspect of the individual's self-concept deriving from one's membership in social group(s). Crocker and Luhtanen's formulation is an extension of social identity theory (Tajfel, 1982; Turner, 1982) which posits that a person is motivated to maintain a positive social identity, or what Crocker and Luhtanen call collective self-esteem. With the assumption that collective self-esteem functions like personal self-esteem, they predicted that high collective self-esteem participants would engage in ingroup enhancing biases or distortions when faced with a threat to their collective self-esteem.

The present study favors the framework of the social identity theory (Tajfel, 1972; Turner, 1975) in relation to group decision making processes and individualism-collectivism orientation. The group decision-making situation seems to have been tailor made for testing the cultural dimension of individualism-collectivism as representing personal identity processes as opposed to socially derived group based identity processes. Group decision making involves group interaction as an essential process that creates effective bonds between the members and greater group saliency (Kogan & Wallach, 1967). While individualistically-oriented group members may display greater accentuation of personal self-esteem and may not share the collective self-esteem of the groups, the collectively oriented participant would engage differently with the group. Thus, it was expected that the cultural dimension of individualism-collectivism would be expressed in the group decision making task as a continuum from individualism, where persons are considered as distinct units clearly separable from their social context, to collectivism, where people think of themselves not so much as separate entities but rather as members of the groups to which they currently belong. The relevant research question was to specify the conditions under which the collective self (social identity) is sampled more frequently than the personal self.

In addition, the present study has used ratings of adjectives as stereotypes for self- definitions and group definitions. The use of stereotypes as "scripts" for self and own group definition perhaps constitutes an indirect but possibly a more stable measure of individualistic and collectivistic orientations since stereotypes generally display stability over time. The decision to use stereotypes in the present study was taken also because popularly used I/C measures (e.g., Cha, 1994; Kwan & Chan, 1994; Yamaguchi, 1994) designed for the present investigation failed to show statistically significant relationship in an earlier pilot study with group decision making (Saha, 1997). It was felt that the use of stereotypes as social cognition indicators of individualism and collectivism offer a distinct advantage to behavioral items generally used by Individualism/Collectivism (I/C) inventories. Stereotypes fulfill a three fold social function; social causal explanations, social justifications and social differentiation (Tajfel, 1981). From the social identity perspective, the crucial feature of the stereotypes is that they are shared. They are not merely idiosyncratic generalizations, which are coincidentally, or by chance, made by a number of people. This sharedness is due to a social process of social influence that causes conformity to group norms, called referent informational influence (Hogg & Abrams, 1988). Therefore, in the present research an attempt was made to use stereotypes as social cognition indicators of individualistic and collectivistic orientations. The details of the procedure used for deriving the stereotype technique of social identity are described at length in the method section.

Objectives

The present study is designed to investigate the effects of self-orientations as contrasted with group orientations in a risk decision-making task in both India and Bangladesh. Two majority ethnic groups (i.e., Hindus in India and Muslims in Bangladesh were selected for characterizing ethnic differences in their self/group orientations in risk decision making.).

The study involved a 2 x 2 factorial design consisting two levels of social identity (High Group Orientation (HGO)/ collectivism and High Self-Orientation (HSO)/ individualism) and two levels of ethnicity (Hindus in India and Muslims in Bangladesh) as the two independent variables. The effects of the independent variables of ethnicity and social identity were observed for group decision-making change scores from pre-group individual decision making scores as the dependent variable.

Since both India and Bangladesh share a common cultural heritage fostering collectivistic orientations, it was predicted that irrespective of ethnicity in India and Bangladesh, Hindus and Muslims would not show differences in their pattern of decision-making scores. No effects of ethnicity would be found. Following the social identity theory (Tajfel, 1982; Turner, 1982) and referent informational hypothesis (Hogg & Abrams, 1988), it was predicted that collectively (group) oriented participants will show more shift in judgment for riskier group decision than individually (self) oriented participants. Thus, effects for social identity difference in group decision-making would be significant. Finally, in view of the above predictions, there would be no interaction between ethnicity and social identity effects (i.e., Hindus and Muslims in India and Bangladesh combined would show similar pattern of group decision scores.).

Method

Participants

A total of 200 Hindu undergraduate male students from India and 200 Muslim undergraduate male students from Bangladesh were initially considered in the first phase of the study. Both the India and Bangladesh sample consisted of 200 students between the ages of 18 to 26 years. The median age of the participants from Bangladesh was 22 years and for India was 21 years. The Bangladeshi sample was drawn from the M.M. College of Jessore district in the Eastern part of Bangladesh and the Indian sample was drawn from the D.L. Roy Commerce College of Krishnanagar city, the district headquarters of Nodia at West Bengal in India. Jessore district in Bangladesh is the region most comparable with Nodia district of West Bengal in India, as far as social, economic, and educational standards are concerned. The colleges selected were randomly chosen from the other similar colleges in the respective cities.

Materials

Social Identity Scale. Based on the research of Majeed and Ghosh (1982), 22 items from an adjective checklist were used as stereotype "scripts" for self and own group definitions. Participants rated each adjective on a five point scale (1 = "Totally True", to 5 = "Totally False") for applicability to self/own group. Eleven adjectives were positive attributes and eleven adjectives reflected negative attributes. These two adjectives were selected after pilot testing for familiarity and applicability for the participants. Positive adjectives used were loyal, affectionate, friendly, charitable, competitive, cooperative, honest, laborious, patriotic, progressive and cooperative. Negative adjectives used were cruel, inimical, miserly, narrow minded, dull, dishonest, unfaithful, dirty, irresponsible, pessimistic and selfish. Split-half reliability was computed and the Spearman's r was .49. When Spearman Brown prophecy formula was applied, the correlation increased from .49 and .66 indicating high reliability of the measure.

Risk Decision Measure. A risk decision measure was constructed for individual and group decision making. Ten risk taking items, representing need based and equality based situations, were used for rating on an 11 point scale, ranging from zero to hundred, using the end points. The risk decision measure was adapted from Kogan and Wallach's (1964) Choice-Dilemma Questionnaire. In this questionnaire the respondent is confronted with two alternative course of actions, one safe but less rewarding and the other risky but more rewarding. The probability of choosing one or the other option was measured on a rating scale. A similar version of the Risk Decision Measure showed a reliability coefficient of .84 in an earlier study (Sharma, 1982). The decision-making choices in situations used for the study pertained to social justice as reflected in need and equality concepts. The choice for using need based and equality based social justice related items were determined earlier through pilot testing due to heightened interest expressed and relevance of these situations for the respondents over other types of situations. The mean ratings from the pilot study for the two types of items in India and Bangladesh are as follows (Need Type: India, 2.75; Bangladesh, 3.60. Equality Type: India, 4.60; Bangladesh, 5.90). While the scale used these two types of items (need and equality based type) a single summated score has been derived for each participant separately for all the 10 items comprising the scale including both type of items.

Need was defined as allocation of something because the receiver is in need of it. For example: "A devastating cyclone has taken place in the coastal region. Your organization has undertaken a relief programme for the people of the affected area. A minority group member (outgroup) has suffered great damage to his house in the cyclone. You have a relative also who has suffered damage to his house in the cyclone. You have limited funds. You can help only one person. If you help the minority group member (outgroup) your organization can go against you and ask you to leave the organization. What are the chances that you will help the out group minority member?"

Equality was defined as allocating the same to everyone belonging to a specific category. For example: " In a tribal area in your country there are many illiterate people who are not able to read or write. For this purpose, a literacy programme has been launched with a view to bring these people in the national mainstream as equal citizens. For this volunteers are required, but volunteers are under threat by the powerful local leaders who are against this literacy programme. To what extent would you like to join as volunteer to work in this literacy programme?"

Procedure

In the first phase of the study participants were divided into high Self or Group oriented categories on the basis of scores obtained on the Social Identity Scale of 22 items. Extreme groups of 50 participants each were selected both in India and Bangladesh, which indicated the maximum difference score between self and group rating as High Group Oriented

(HGO) and High Self Oriented (HSO) participants. Scoring for the Social Identity Scale may be described as follows. The 22 adjectives of the Social Identity Scale were administered to 200 participants who rated the adjectives on a five-point scale, under two sets of instructions (i.e., self-ratings/adjectives that applied to one's own self and group ratings/adjectives that applied to one's own ethnic group).

The following instructions were used for the administration under self and own group rating conditions: "You will see a list of adjectives that are usually used for evaluating a person or a group. Please read these adjectives carefully and say how far each adjective is true or false for your OWN SELF/ OWN GROUP by giving a tick mark (/) on the blank space given against each adjective ranging from totally true to totally false. Remember there are no right or wrong answers."

From the summated ratings for Self and Own group, a difference score was derived by subtracting Group ratings from Self-ratings for each participant separately. The difference score thus derived for each participant indicated a higher self-orientation (HSO) if the difference score derived was positive and a higher group orientation (HGO) if the difference score derived was negative. Fifty participants from each country who formed the upper quartile on the difference score comprised the High Self-Oriented (HSO) group, whereas the 50 participants from each country formed the lower quartile which comprised the High Group Oriented (HGO) group. In essence, within each group, individuals who scored high on individualism relative to the sample and individuals who scored high on collectivism relative to the sample were selected to participate further in the decision making task.

An independent sample t-test between the two groups (HSO and HGO) on social identity score for India and Bangladesh was calculated. The results indicated that in both India and Bangladesh HGO and HSO groups were significantly different for social identity scores (HGO: $M = 4.59$, $SD = 0.19$; HSO: $M = 5.42$, $SD = 0.23$, $t(98) = 20.50$, $p < .001$). An independent sample t-test was also done for the two countries for HSO and HGO group differences on social identity scores separately. (HSO: India $M = 5.42$, SD = 0.23; Bangladesh $M = 5.40$, $SD = 0.22$, $t(48) = 0.40$ and HGO: India $M = 4.59$, $SD = 0.19$; Bangladesh $M = 4.59$, $SD = 0.20$, $t(48) = 0$). No significant differences were obtained.

In the second phase of the study, 50 High Group Oriented (HGO) participants and 50 High Self Oriented (HSO) participants were divided into small groups of 5 participants each in both India and Bangladesh for individual and group decision judgment on the Risk Decision Measure.

The following instructions were given for the individual condition: "Various situations are given below. Such situations frequently occur in our lives when we have to choose between two alternatives, one is risky but advantageous to the needs or equality and justice for the larger society. The other alternative is not risky but more advantageous to the individual making decision. You are required to give your choice for each item on a scale ranging from 0% to 100% (Zero to Cent percent) when faced with such situations. Below each problem is given the following percentage scale. You have to remember there are no right or wrong answers whatever answer you decide is correct answer. You have to indicate the chances in percentage probability of choosing the alternative given for each situation. By placing a tick (/) mark on the scale below, you indicate approximately how sure you are that you will accept the more risky alternative in each situation. Do not leave any items unanswered."

Additionally, the following instructions were given for the group decision making condition: "This questionnaire contains similar situations that you have completed earlier. Now we are interested in having you discuss each of the situations in a group to arrive at a consensus decision. You have to find the majority decision. For group discussion you will be given 50 minutes time, approximately 5 minutes for each situations. When you have decided one situation, then proceed to consensus decision for the next situation."

Pre-group individual decision making ratings were collected followed by group decision- making ratings after one-month duration for safeguarding against carry over memory effects. Consensual Group decision was required from the participants. The difference scores between pre-group individual and group decision making score were calculated for both Self and Group oriented participants separately, by subtracting pre-group individual scores from post group consensual scores.

It may be noted that the decision to use substantive time gap of 4 weeks between the two ratings was intentional since it ensured that the latter group decision judgments were sufficiently independent from the first set of individual situation judgments. The specific objective was to measure shifts in scores from individual to group conditions of risk taking ratings across each participant separately. Thus, effects, if any, of the small group processes as moderated by the more stable personality orientation of either High Self Orientations or High Group Orientations would be indicated by the change scores.

Results

The data was analyzed using a 2 x 2 factorial ANOVA with independent variables of social identity (high self oriented vs. high group oriented) and a dependent variable of change in risk decision (group consensus minus pre-group individual scores). There were no significant differences in risk change scores as a function of ethnicity $F(1, 196) < 1$, and the interaction of social identity and ethnicity $F(1, 196) < 1$. However, a significant difference in risk change was demonstrated for social identity $F(1, 196) = 16.65$, $p = .001$, $MSE = 27{,}594.60$; HGO participants demonstrated riskier consensual decisions

(India, $M = 23.40$, $SD = 175.08$; Bangladesh, $M = 11.20$, $SD = 164.12$) than HSO participants (India, $M = - 78.40$, $SD = 174.11$; Bangladesh, $M =$ -84.40, $SD = 142.37$). Negative scores indicate lower risk decision within group consensus conditions and positive scores indicate a higher or risky decision within group consensus conditions compared to individual decisions.

Discussion

These results supported fully the three hypotheses formulated. First, no differences in risk decision change were obtained for ethnicity. Second, social identity differences between HGO and HSO participants were obtained for risk decision change scores. Third, no interaction effect between ethnicity and social identity was noted. The results of the study tend to further support the contention that both individualism and collectivism can be sampled as different aspects of the self, the individual personal self versus a socially determined identity.

In both India and Bangladesh the results indicated that participants high on the articulation of their own self (HSO) tended to show lower level of risk change in their decision making score in a group decision making situation, when a collective goal of consensual decision was required from them. By contrast, the participants high on group articulation (HGO) tended to display greater ingroup effect in enhancing individual decisions and when faced with the collective self-esteem situation in risk taking. It is therefore suggested that the individual self and the collective self perhaps function at different levels of social and personal relevance. It may also be observed that while no effort was made in the present study to elicit ingroup/outgroup comparison enhancing group based identities, the mere requirement of a collective consensual group decision was sufficient to elicit group saliency and group orientations resulting in a risky shift in decision making.

These findings thus lend strong support to the social categorization and social identity approaches that assert that mere categorization is sufficient to trigger off group identity processes and preferences (Tajfel, 1981, 1982). According to Turner et al. (1987), people form self-categorizations at different levels of abstraction, ranging from an abstract conception of the self as a human being, to the intermediate level of ingroup/outgroup representations, to the subordinate level of personal self-categorizations as a unique individual. The self is thus simultaneously part of several levels: human kind, groups, individuality. At each level, the individual is motivated to evaluate the self-categories positively. Depending on which level of comparison is salient, the individual will try to establish a positive distinctiveness either between the self and other ingroup members, or between ingroup and outgroup. The principle determining the category's "goodness of fit" is what most closely corresponds to the data in their specific context, the normative fit, and that which maximizes the differences between categories while minimizing the differences within categories, the comparative fit (Oakes, 1987; Turner et al., 1987). This latter aspect is also defined as the metacontrast principle.

It could be asserted that participants predisposed to individualistic orientation do not evaluate themselves as a member of a group and evaluated themselves as a distinctive "Self" in comparison to other ingroup members. While as per the "goodness of fit" the high group oriented (HGO) participants minimize their self differences and maximize the group identity leading to, a risk decision change score for higher risk in the group consensus condition, demonstrating the metacontrast principle of contextual saliency. In fact, High Self Oriented (HSO) participants tended to show negative risk decision change score indicating a "cautiousness" against risk taking when placed in a group discussion/consensus decision situation. This finding seems to be more robust and requires further investigation in the future. That group processes should polarize risky decisions to high or low risk changes in relation to I/C, also needs to be examined further through more carefully planned and precise experimental studies.

It should also be noted that in both India and Bangladesh similar findings were obtained indicating similar processes of individualistic and collectivistic orientations characterizing both India and Bangladesh. Though India and Bangladesh are designated as more traditional collectivistic societies, individualistic and collectivistic orientations appear to co-exist and are expressed contextually. These conclusions have found support in the studies of several Asian researchers in the area (Mishra, 1994; Sinha & Tripathi, 1994; Yamaguchi, 1994). The relevant boundary condition for the salience of Self (individualism) or Group (collectivism) could be merely the function of the immediate context within which the behavior is to be engaged. In risk taking situations, it seems personal relevance and group enhancing biases differentially influence decision making in interaction with prior individualistic and collectivistic orientations.

Finally, it should be stated that the study has the following limitations. Cultures other than collectivistic societies and gender differences need to be included for a comparative understanding of the moderating role of social identity processes in group decision making studies. Recently in a nine culture study of individualism-collectivism and gender differences in self concepts Watkins et al. (1998) found that considerable variation was found within both individualistic and collectivistic groups and strong culture by gender interactions was also noted. The hypothesis that females would provide less idiosyncratic but more large group, small group, and allocentric self descriptions was found only for the more individualistic cultures. Thus, the need of studying gender differences across cultures in determining individualistic and collectivistic identities can scarcely be over emphasized.

In conclusion, it may be emphasized that most small group decision making studies focus only on the "here and now" ongoing group processes. The self/group identities that are brought into play in these groups as pre-existing moderating variables (in the present case individualistic versus collectivistic orientation) have not been given due attention. Since High Group Oriented participants and High Self Oriented participants polarized and changed their earlier individual risk decisions to a more risky or cautious decision in a group discussion, there is a need to examine antecedent variables derived from the social context of the participants, which in turn may also reflect wider cultural variations. It may also be speculated, that societies like India and Bangladesh which are undergoing rapid social change in the process of economic development and modernization perhaps reflect a more fluid state of individualistic and collectivistic orientations. Thus the need to revisit individualism-collectivism theory, as consisting of normative versus non-normative social cognition derived from a matrix of personal self and ingroup saliency, are clearly implicated by the findings of the present study.

References

Cha, J.H. (1994). Aspects of individualism and collectivism in Korea. In U. Kim, H. Triandis, C. Kagitcibasi, S. Choi, & G. Yoon (Eds.), *Individualism and collectivism: Theory, method and applications* (pp. 157-174). London: Sage Publications.

Crocker, J., & Luhtanen, R. (1990). Collective self-esteem and ingroup bias. *Journal of Personality and Social Psychology, 58,* 60-67.

Gudykunst, W., Yoon, Y.C., & Nishida, T. (1987). The influence of individualism-collectivism on perceptions of communication in ingroup and outgroup relationships. *Communication Monographs, 54,* 295-306.

Hofstede, G. (1991). *Cultures and organizations: Software of the mind.* London: McGraw Hill.

Hogg, M.A., & Abrams, D. (1988). *Social identification: A social psychology of intergroup relations and group processes.* London: Routledge.

Kogan, N., & Wallach, M.A. (1964). *Risk taking: A study in cognition and personality.* New York: Holt.

Kogan, N., & Wallach, M.A. (1967). *Risk taking as a function of the situation, the person and the group. New directions of psychology.* New York: Holt, Rinehart and Winston.

Kwan, D., & Chan, S. (1994). COLINDEX: A refinement of three collectivism measures. In U. Kim, H. Triandis, C. Kagitcibasi, S. Choi, & G. Yoon (Eds.), *Individualism and collectivism: Theory, method and applications* (pp. 200-210). London: Sage Publications.

Leung, K., & Bond, M.H. (1984). The impact of cultural collectivism on reward allocation. *Journal of Personality and Social Psychology, 47,* 793-804.

Majeed, A., & Ghosh, E.S.K. (1982). A study of social identity in three ethnic groups in India. *International Journal of Psychology, 17,* 455-463.

Markus, H., & Kitayama, S. (1991). Culture and self: Implications for cognition, emotion and motivation. *Psychological Review, 98,* 224-253.

Mishra, R.C. (1994). Individualist and collectivist orientations across generations. In U. Kim, H. Triandis, C. Kagitcibasi, S. Choi, & G. Yoon (Eds.), *Individualism and collectivism: Theory, method and applications* (pp. 225-238). London: Sage Publications.

Oakes, P.J. (1987). The salience of social categories. In J.C., Turner, M.A., Hogg, P.J., Oakes, S.D., Reicher, & M., Wetherell (Eds.), *Rediscovering the social group: A self- categorization theory* (pp. 117-171). Oxford: Blackwell.

Saha, A.K. (1997). *Theory of social identity, individualism-collectivism and group decision making.* Unpublished manuscript, Department of Psychology, University of Allahabad, Allahabad, India.

Sharma, G. (1982). *Risky shift as a function of group structure and personal relevance.* An unpublished dissertation, Department of Psychology, University of Allahabad, Allahabad. India.

Sinha, D., & Tripathi, R.C. (1994). Individualism in a collectivist culture: A case of coexistence of opposites. In U. Kim, H. Triandis, C. Kagitcibasi, S. Choi, & G. Yoon (Eds.), *Individualism and collectivism: Theory, method and applications* (pp. 123-136). London: Sage Publications.

Tajfel, H. (1972). La Categorisation Sociale. In S. Moscovici (Ed.), *Introduction a la psychologiesociale* (pp. 272-302). London: Larousse.

Tajfel, H. (1981). *Human groups and social categories.* Cambridge University Press.

Tajfel, H. (1982). Social psychology of intergroup relations. *Annual Review of Psychology, 33,* 1-39.

Triandis, H.C. (1989). Self and social behavior in differing cultural contexts. *Psychological eview, 96,* 269-289.

Triandis, H.C. (1994). Theoretical and methodological approaches to the study of collectivism and individualism. In U. Kim, H. Triandis, C. Kagitcibasi, S. Choi, & G. Yoon (Eds.), *Individualism and collectivism: Theory, method and applications* (pp. 41-51). London: Sage Publications.

Turner, J.C. (1975). Social comparison and social identity: Some prospects for intergroup behavior. *European Journal of Social Psychology, 5,* 5-34.

Turner, J.C. (1982). Towards a cognitive redefinition of the social group. In H. Tajfel (Ed.), *Social identity and intergroup relations* (pp. 15-40). Cambridge: Cambridge University Press.

Turner, J.C., Hogg, M.A., Oakes, P.J., Reicher, S.D., & Wetherell, M. (1987). *Rediscovering the social roup: A self-categorization theory.* Oxford: Blackwell.

Watkins, D., Adair, J., Akande, A., Gerong, A., Mcinerney, D., Sunar, D., Watson, S., Wen, F., & Wondimu, H. (1998). Individualism-collectivism, gender and the self-concept: A nine culture investigation. *Psychologia, 41,* 259-271.

Yamaguchi, S. (1994). Collectivism among the Japanese: A perspective from the self. In U. Kim, H. Triandis, C. Kagitcibasi, S. Choi, & G. Yoon (Eds.), *Individualism and collectivism: Theory, method and applications* (pp. 175-188). London: Sage Publications.

The Measurement of Collectivism in India

Jyoti Verma
University of Patna
Department of Psychology

Harry C. Triandis
University of Illinois
Department of Psychology

ABSTRACT

It was hypothesized that India would be a vertical collectivist culture. We used 16 scenarios to measure tendencies toward horizontal or vertical, individualism or collectivism with a sample of 180 Indian students of Patna University, Patna. The hypothesis was confirmed as the Indian fist choice on vertical collectivism was consistently more popular across the scenarios when compared with that of the students of University of Illinois, (Champaign-Urbana), USA. However, when the results are examined exclusively for the Indian profile, it was observed that the Indian students gave highest percentage of emphasis to horizontal collectivism, usually choosing this category as descriptive of their values and beliefs.

Kagiticibasi and Berry (1989) identified individualism and collectivism as one of the major themes of cross-cultural psychology in the 1980's. The 1990's proved to be an even more fertile ground for the development of theory and method centered around these constructs (see Bond & Smith, 1996; Berry, Segall & Kagitcibasi, 1997; Landis & Bhagat, 1996; Triandis, Dunnette & Hough, 1994). Furthermore, there are several reviews of the literature that are relevant to these constructs (Kagitcibasi, 1997; Kim, Triandis, Kagitcibasi, Choi, & Yoon,1994). Triandis (1995) has argued that individualism and collectivism can be identified by examining the following four elements: **(a) The definition of the self** which can emphasize personal or collective aspects or can be independent or interdependent (Triandis, 1989; Mardus & Kitayama, 1991). **(b) Personal goals** which can have priority over-in-group or vice versa (Triandis, 1990; Yamaguchi, 1982), or **rationality rather than relatedness** (Kim, Triandis, Kagitcibasi, Choi, & Yoon, 1994). **(d) The importance of attitude and norms as determinant of social behavior** (Davidson, Jaccard, Triandis, Morales & Diaz-Guerrero, 1976).

While there are a number of ways to assess collectivism and individualism, there are correlations (Triandis, McCusker & Hui, 1990) among the various measurements suggesting the existence of a "cultural syndrome" (Triandis, 1993). Cultural syndrome is defined as shared attitudes, beliefs, norms, role and self definition, and values, centered around a theme found among those who speak a language dialect, and live in the same historical period and geographic region. The theme for collectivism is the centrality of the in-group. The theme for individualism is the focus on the individual.

The Different Kinds of Individualism-Collectivism

Triandis (1990, 1995) suggested that the most important attributes that distinguish among the different kinds of individualism-collectivism, refer to the emphases on horizontal and vertical social relationships. In **Horizontal Individualism (HI)**, people want to be unique, but they are not especially interested in becoming distinguished or having high status. **Vertical Individualism (VI)** allows people to compete with others for distinction and status. In **Horizontal Collectivism (VC)**, people want to be as similar as possible, and emphasize common goals. In **Vertical Collectivism (VC)** people sacrifice their personal goals for the sake of in-group goals, and support competition of their in-groups with out-groups.

There are costs associated with each cultural pattern. The **HI** pattern can result in social isolation. The **VI** pattern can result in extreme stress. The **HC** pattern could absorb much of the individual's energy in social relationships, while the vertical collectivist pattern could result in authoritarian regimes. Rokeach (1973) discussed political systems that reflect the patterns cited above. For example, an Israeli Kibbutz may represent a horizontal collectivist society. In India, members of communities often adhere to principles of vertical collectivism.

Measurement of the Individualism-Collectivism Constructs

The literature includes references to many measures of the individualist-collectivist tendencies. The concept of self, **(a)**, can be assessed using responses to 20 statements that begin with "I am…" (Triandis, McCuster & Hui, 1990). Some scales measure an independent versus interdependent self (Singelis, 1994; Gudykunst, Matsumoto, Ting-Toomey, Nishida & Karimi, 1994). Personal goals, **(b)**, can be measured with a scale developed by Yamaguchi (1994), or by examining individual preferences for individualist or collectivist goals and values (Schwartz, 1994; Triandis, McCusker & Hui, 1990). The tendencies described under **(c)** can be measured by scales developed by Clark, Ouellette, Powell & Milberg (1987), and those that reflect **(d)** by using Fishbein & Ajzen (1975) model of attitudes and behavior, which separate factors for attitude and norms.

Nevertheless, measurement of individualism and collectivism has been difficult. The appendix in Triandis (1995) describes many relevant methods, but none capture the very broad constructs satisfactorily. Therefore, any measurement samples part of the "elephant". Singelis et al. (1995) developed 32 attitude items, 8 for each of the four kinds of collectivism and individualism (i.e., HI, VI, HC, and VC). While these items have alphas in the range of .69 to .75, they seem to be quite susceptible to the social desirability factor.

Triandis and Gelfand (in press) developed a series of scenarios that are less susceptible to social desirability. Since the participants are confronted with the social desirability of 4 aspects of the scenarios which they rank order, they are forced to choose among four socially desirable responses. This reduces the influence of social desirability. The researchers reported that the responses to the scenarios were correlated with responses to the attitude items, thus suggesting they have convergent validity.

Objectives

The example of the cultural syndromes discussed by Triandis (1996) included the expectation that India would be higher in vertical collectivism than many other cultures. Therefore, the objectives of the study were to confirm this hypothesis, and to develop a greater insight into the nature of Indian collectivism.

Method

Participants

A total of 180 students (112 males, 68 females, between 19 to 25 years of age) of Patna University, belonging to both science and social sciences faculties, responded to the 16 scenarios in English.

Procedure

The students were approached individually or in small groups of three to four in their leisure time. They were requested to go through the scenarios carefully and select the most preferred and the second most preferred options among the 4 alternatives for each scenario. The rationale behind asking for a second choice was to find out the second most preferred cultural pattern of the respondents. We also wanted to see whether there was any consistency in the two choices the students made.

Treatment of the Data

For each scenario, we noted the percentage of the total sample that selected each of the four responses as their first and second choice. We averaged the percentages of the first choices, and separately averaged the percentages of the second choices. Then we gave a weight of 2 to the first choice percentages and a weight of 1 to the second choice percentages, resulting in a profile of the endorsement of the HI, VI, HC and VC responses.

Results

In the case of the Indian sample we obtained, **HI of 24%, VI of 23%, HC of 29% and VC of 25%.** Since these percentages are based on 16 times 180 responses, even a small difference in the percentages is statistically significant. The present Indian profile appears to be fairly evenly distributed across the four cultural patterns with collectivist responses somewhat more preferred than the individualistic ones.

To assess the stability of these results we compared responses to the 8 odd and the 8 even numbered scenarios. The results were as follows.

Odd numbered scenarios were HI of 17%, VI of 21%, HC of 35% and VC of 27%.

Even numbered scenarios were HI of 30%, VI of 25%, HC of 23% and VC of 22%. Thus, while the vertical scenarios are reasonably reliable, with smaller percentage of differences (e.g., 4 or 5 points), the horizontal scenarios resulted in larger differences of 12 to 13 points. It appears that the students may have had difficulty interpreting the horizontal aspects of the scenarios. For comparative purposes, data from a similar study by Triandis et al. (in press), presented in Table 2, indicated that Indians were low on HC, average on VI and HC, and quite high on VC.

Table 1. Percentages Agreeing with Responses to Scenarios in Illinois, USA (N=123) and Patna, India (N=180). (Under each choice we show on the left the percentages of the first choices in Illinois and Patna, and on the right the same percentages for the second choice).

1. You and your friend decided spontaneously to go out to dinner at a restaurant. What do you think is the best way to handle the bill?

	US (IL)	Patna	US (IL)	Patna
	First Choice		Second Choice	
HC Split it equally, without regards to who ordered what.	15%	32%	57%	31%
VI Spilt it according to how much each person makes.	2%	12%	7%	23%
VC The group leader pays the bill or decides how to split it	3%	30%	16%	25%
HI Compute each person's charge according to what that person ordered.	78%	27%	17%	21%

2. You are buying a piece of art for your office. Which one factor is most important in deciding whether to buy it?

	US (IL)	Patna	US (IL)	Patna
	First Choice		Second Choice	
VI It is a good investment.	18%	18%	48%	21%
HC Your coworkers will like it.	5%	29%	25%	28%
HI You just like it.	75%	38%	12%	21%
VC Your supervisor will approve of it.	2%	14%	11%	30%

3. Suppose you had to use on word to describe your self. Which one would you use?

	US (IL)	Patna	US (IL)	Patna
	First Choice		Second Choice	
HI Unique.	41%	16%	26%	13%
VI Competitive.	22%	26%	31%	21%
HC Cooperative.	28%	40%	20%	28%
VC Dutiful.	9%	18%	17%	38%

4. Happiness is attained by

	US (IL)	Patna	US (IL)	Patna
	First Choice		Second Choice	
VC Gaining a lot of status in the community.	9%	20%	27%	21%
HC Linking with a lot of friendly people.	60%	38%	16%	30%
HI Keeping one's privacy.	12%	4%	25%	128%
VI Winning in competitions.	11%	37%	18%	28%

5. You are planning to take a major trip which is likely to inconvenience a lot of people at your work place during your absence. With whom will you discuss it, before deciding whether or not to take it?

	US (IL)	Patna	US (IL)	Patna
	First Choice		Second Choice	
HI No one.	9%	7%	13%	10%
VC My parents.	16%	21%	28%	30%
HC My spouse or close friend.	54%	28%	29%	37%
VI Experts about the place I plan to travel to, so that I can decide if I want to go.	21%	43%	22%	24%

6. Which one of these four books appears to you to be the most interesting?

	US (IL)	Patna	US (IL)	Patna
	First Choice		Second Choice	
HC How to make friends.	6%	15%	17%	22%
VI How to succeed in business.	27%	29%	26%	29%
HI How to enjoy yourself inexpensively.	42%	25%	25%	27%
VC How to make sure you are meeting your obligations.	21%	31%	21%	22%

7. Which is the most important factor in an employee's promotion, assuming that all other factors such as tenure and performance are equal? Employ is or has

	US (IL)	Patna	US (IL)	Patna
	First Choice		Second Choice	
HC Loyal to the corporation.	16%	32%	26%	30%
VC Obedient to the instructions from the manager.	6%	34%	13%	37%
HI Able to think for him/herself.	42%	8%	21%	8%
VI Contributed to the corporation much in the past.	35%	26%	34%	24%

8. When you buy clothing for a major social event you would be most satisfied if

	US (IL)	Patna	US (IL)	Patna
	First Choice		Second Choice	
HI you like it.	80%	47%	13%	26%
VC your parents like it.	0%	6%	6%	24%
HC your friends like it.	8%	13%	35%	27%
VI It is so elegant that it will dazzle everyone.	12%	34%	34%	23%

9. In your opinion an ideal society's national budget will be determined so that

	US (IL)	Patna	US (IL)	Patna
	First Choice		Second Choice	
HC All people have equal income to meet basic needs.	37%	59%	17%	17%
VI Some people will be rewarded for making brilliant contributions.	15%	11%	20%	21%
VC There will be maximal stability, law and order.	18%	21%	30%	40%
HI People can feel unique and self actualized.	27%	9%	20%	22%

10. When people ask me about myself, I

	US (IL)	Patna	US (IL)	Patna
	First Choice		Second Choice	
VC Talk about my ancestors and their traditions.	2%	20%	9%	21%
HC Talk about my friends and what we like to do.	21%	22%	31%	27%
VI Talk about my accomplishments.	25%	33%	30%	27%
HI Talk about what makes me unique.	48%	25%	20%	25%

11. Suppose your wife and your parents do not get along very well. What would you do?

	US (IL)	Patna	US (IL)	Patna
	First Choice		Second Choice	
HI Nothing.	38%	8%	16%	8%
VI Tell my wife that I need my parent's financial support and she should learn to handle the politics.	6%	14%	16%	20%
HC Tell my wife that she should make a greater effort to "fit in with the family.	28%	42%	25%	34%
VC Remind my wife that my parents and family are very important to me and she should submit to their wishes.	17%	36%	17%	38%

12. Teams of five people entered a science project contest. Your team won first place and a prize of $ 100. You and another person did 95% of the work on this project. How should the money be distributed?

	US (IL)	Patna	US (IL)	Patna
	First Choice		Second Choice	
HC Split it equally, without regards to who did what.	41%	52%	23%	22%
VI The other person and I get 95% of the money and the rest goes to the group.	35%	11%	20%	13%
VC The group leader decides how to split the money.	12%	20%	24%	42%
HI Divide the money the way that gives me the most satisfaction.	14%	17%	21%	23%

13. Imagine you are selecting a band for a fund raising event given by your organization. Which are the most important factors in making your decision?

	US (IL)	Patna	US (IL)	Patna
	First Choice		Second Choice	
HI I really like the band.	16%	30%	28%	18%
HC My friends approve of this band.	1%	7%	15%	35%
VC The administration of my organization approves of the band.	11%	30%	31%	27%
VI The band will draw a large crowd.	71%	33%	18%	19%

14. You need to choose one more class for next semester. Which one will you select?

	US (IL)	Patna	US (IL)	Patna
	First Choice		Second Choice	
VI The one that will help me get ahead of everyone else.	27%	36%	46%	45%
VC The one my parents said to take.	0%	8%	3%	10%
HC The one my friends plan to take.	0%	4%	20%	12%
HI The one that seems most interesting to me.	73%	52%	23%	33%

15. You are at a pizza restaurant with a group of friends. How should you decide what kind of pizza to order?

	US (IL)	Patna	US (IL)	Patna
	First Choice		Second Choice	
VC The leader of the group orders for everyone.	1%	10%	24%	31%
HI I order what I like.	14%	34%	40%	33%
HC We select the pizza that most people prefer.	84%	54%	13%	24%
VI We order the most extravagant pizza.	1%	2%	10%	12%

16. Which candidate will you vote for in the election for President of the Student Union?

	US (IL)	Patna	US (IL)	Patna
	First Choice		Second Choice	
HC The one that your friends are voting for.	2%	9%	10%	18%
HI The one I like best.	77%	56%	16%	32%
VI The one who rewards me personally.	7%	2%	22%	15%
VC The one who is member of an organization important to me. The status of the organization will improve if that candidate is selected.	12%	32%	38%	35%

Table 2. Percent Emphasis on Horizontal and Vertical Individualism and Collectivism among Students in Nine Countries (First choice weighted twice as much as second choices).

	HI	HC	VI	VC
USA	38	26	23	13
AUSTRALIA	39	29	18	14
NETHERLANDS	43	27	20	10
GERMANY	39	32	17	12
JAPAN	35	26	24	16
GREECE	32	31	22	14
HONG KONG	25	36	20	19
KOREA	31	31	22	15
INDIA	24	29	23	25

Discussion

Triandis (1995) found that Indian subjects were high on vertical collectivism, and hypothesized that results of this study would be similar. The data obtained suggested this was accurate. For all 16 scenarios, the VC response were chosen by Indian more often than by US students (see Table 1).

Furthermore, the present measurement of collectivism and individualism among Indian students when compared with similar data from eight countries, showed a relatively low score on horizontal individualism, and a relatively high score on vertical collectivism (see Table 2). Thus, the Indian student sample was not especially interested in being unique and independent of its groups.

Triandis (1995) emphasized that all humans have both individualist and collectivist values and response tendencies, but that the situations in which they find themselves determine the tendencies they will emphasize. Apparently, in collectivistic cultures people express more collectivistic tendencies and in individualistic cultures they express more individualistic tendencies. Thus, in the given scenarios that represent a variety of situations, responses are likely to reflect both the basic tendencies of the culture, and the effects of the situations.

In this study it was observed that in 16 out of 16 scenarios, the Indian students' first choice on VC responses was significantly more frequent than the VC responses among the US students. The Indian sample showed preference for tendencies such as strong family orientation, embeddedness with the primary in-group, belief in hierarchy and concept of a happy life that is consistent with what has been reported in some Indian studies (see J.B.P. Sinha & D. Sinha, 1990; Kakar, 1971; Mishra & Tiwari, 1980; Roy & Srivastava, 1986; S.K.Sinha, 1986; Sinha & Verma, 1987; Verma, 1992).

The Indian Case: A Summary

The results of this study confirmed the hypothesis that Indian students were more collectivistic than students in the United States. Indians showed a higher emphasis (25%) on the VC dimension which was greater than the responses from subjects sampled in other countries (see table 2).

However, a look at the Indian profile exclusively, (e.g., **HI of 24%, VI of 23%, HC of 29% and VC of 25%),** shows highest percentage of emphasis on the HC dimension. Indians also choose **HC as their first choice most frequently,** (e.g., in 7 out of 16 scenarios, range of percentage emphasis, 59-32%) while VC is their first choice only twice. It was concluded that the that the Patna sample preferred the collectivism dimension. The HC cultural pattern is their first choice, and VC is a preferred second choice.

References

Berry, J.W., Segall, M.H., & Kagitcibasi, C. (1997). *Handbook of cross-cultural psychology,* Volume 3. Boston: Allyn and Bacon.

Bond, R. & Smith, P.B. (1996). Culture and conformity: A meta-analysis of studies using Asch's (1952b, 1956) line judgment task. *Psychological Bulletin,* 119, 111-137.

Clark, M., Ouelette, R., Powell, M.C., & Milberg, S. (1987). Recipient's mood, relationship type and helping. *Journal of Personality and Social Personality, 53, 94-103.*

Davidson, A.R. Jaccard, J.J., Triandis, H.C., Morales, M.L., & Diaz-Guerrero, R. (1976). Cross- culture model testing: Towards a solution of the etic-emic dilemma. *International Journal of Psychology, 11,* 1-13.

Fishbein, M., & Ajzen, I. (1975). *Belief, attitude, intention, and behavior: An introduction to theory and research.* Reading, MA: Addition-Wesley.

Gudykunst, W.B., Matsumoto, Y., Ting-Toomey, S., Nishida, T. & Karma, H. (1994). Measuring self-construals across cultures: A derived etic analysis. Paper presented at the International Communication Association Convention. Sydney, Australia, July.

Kagitcibasi, C. (1997). Individualism and collectivism. In J.W. Berry, M.H. Segall, & C. Kagitcibasi (Eds.), *Handbook of cross-cultural psychology* (2nd ed.). pp. 1-50. Boston, Mass. Allyn & Bacon.

Kagitcibasi, C., Berry, J.W., (1989). Cross-cultural psychology: Current research and trends. In *Annual Review of Psychology, 40,* 493-531.

Kakar, S. (1971). Authority pattern and subordinate behavior in Indian organizations. *Administrative Science Quarterly, 16,* 298-307.

Kim, U., Triandis, H.C., Kagitcibasi, C., Choi, S.C., & Yoon, G. (Eds.), (1994). *Individualism and collectivism: Theory, method, and application.* Newbury Park, CA: Sage.

Landis, D. & Bhagat, R. (1996). *Handbook of intercultural training* (2nd ed.). Thousand Oaks, CA: Sage.

Markus, H. & Kitayama, S. (1991). Culture and self: Implications for cognition, emotion, and motivation. *Psychological Review,* 98, 224-253.

Mills, J. & Clark, M.S. (1982). Exchange and communal relationships. In L. Wheeler (Ed.), *Review of personality and social psychology.* Volume 3. Beverly Hills, CA: Sage.

Mishra, R.C. & Tiwari, B.B. (1980). *Dialogues on development.* New Delhi: Sage.

Rokeach, M. (1973). *The nature of human values.* New York: Free press.

Roland, A. (1991). The psychological and psychosocial in Indian organizational relationships. Mimeographed manuscript obtained from American Institute of Indian Studies.

Roy, S. & Srivastava, R.K. (1986). *Dialogues on development.* New Delhi: Sage.

Schwartz, S.H. (1994). Beyond individualism and collectivism: New cultural dimension of values. In U. Kim, H.C. Triandis, C. Kagitcibasi, S.C. Choi, & G. Yoon (Eds.), *Individualism and collectivism: Theory, method, and application* (pp. 85-122). Newbury Park, CA: Sage.

Singelis, T.M. (1994). the measurement of independent and interdependent self-construals. *Personality and Social Psychology Bulletin, 20,* 580-591.

Singelis, T.M., Triandis, H.C., Bhawuk, D., & Gelfand, M. (1995). Horizontal and vertical dimensions of individualism and collectivism: A theoretical and measurement refinement, *Cross-Cultural Research, 29,* 240-275.

Singh, S.K. (1986). Social groups within a work organization. Doctoral Dissertation Patna University.Sinha, J.B.P. & Verma, J. (1987). Structure of collectivism. In C. Kagitcibasi (Ed.), *Growth and progress in cross-cultural psychology* (pp. 123-129). The Netherlands: Swets & Zeitlinger.

Sinha, J.B.P. & Sinha, D. (1990). Role of social values in Indian organizations. *international Journal of Psychology*, 25, 705-714.

Triandis, H.C. (1989). The self and social behavior in differing cultural context. *Psychological Review*, 96, 506-520.

Triandis, H.C. (1990). *Cross-cultural studies of individualism and collectivism.* In J. Berman (Ed.), Nebrask Symposium on Motivation, 1989 (pp. 41-133). Lincoln, Nebraska: University of Nebraska Press.

Triandis, H.C. (1993). Collectivism and individualism as cultural syndromes. *Cross-Cultural Research*, 27, 155-180.

Triandis, H.C. (1995). *Individualism and collectivism.* Boulder, CO: Westview Press.

Triandis, H.C. (1996). The psychological measurement of cultural syndromes. *American Psychologist*, 51, 407-415.

Triandis, H.C. & Gelfand, M. (in press). Converging measurement of horizontal and vertical individualism and collectivism. *Journal of Personality and Social Psychology.*

Triandis, H.C., Dunnette, M. & Hough, L. (1994). *Handbood of industrial and organizational psychology* (2nd ed. Volume 4). Palo Alto, CA: Consulting Psychologists Press.

Triandis, H.C., McCusker, C. & Hui, C.H. (1990). Multimethod probes of individualism and collectivism. *Journal of Personality and Social Psychology*, 59, 1006-1020.

Verma, J. (1992). Allocentrism and relationship orientation. In S. Iwawaki, Y. & Leung (Eds.) *Innovation in cross-cultural psychology* (pp. 152-163). The Netherlands: Swets & Zeitlinger.

Verma, J. & Sinha, J.B.P. (1992). Self referents and the concept of a happy life. *Psychological Studies*, 38, 45-54.

Yamaguchi, S. (1994). Empirical evidence on collectivism among the Japanese. In U. Kim, H.C. Triandis, C. Kagiticibasi, S.C. Choi, & G. Yoon (Eds.), *Individualism and collectivism: Theory, method, and application* (pp. 175-188). Newbury Park, CA: Sage.

Coping with the "Syndrome of Imposed Ethnicity" among Ethnic Russians

Nadezhda Lebedeva
Institute of Ethnology and Anthropology
Russian Academy of Sciences
Department of Ethnic Ecology

ABSTRACT

The "acculturative stress" of ethnic Russians in the post-Soviet states is considered in the spectrum of the crisis of social (ethnic) identity. Correlation analysis of the results obtained in the study of changed identity of two samples of respondents (N = 700) opting for strategies of Integration and Separation revealed the core problem. It lies in the separationists' disturbed relationship between positive ethnic identity and ethnic tolerance. It is assumed that a cluster of features that can be called the syndrome of imposed ethnicity causes the disturbance. The syndrome is characterized by a high valency of ethnic belonging combined with the negative valency of ethnic identity. The finding was obtained through principal components factor analyses of items related to ethnic identity and ethnic tolerance across the two groups of respondents. Correlation analysis revealed acculturation and personal characteristics influencing the valency of ethnic identity. Strategies of coping with the syndrome of imposed ethnicity are also described. Maintaining positive ethnic identity can be viewed as a basic condition of successful acculturation. On a broader scale, the maintenance of positive ethnic identity should be seen as a socio-psychological mechanism for maintaining a given cultural whole.

Berry (1970) conceived of acculturation as involving the two essential issues: (a) *cultural maintenance* (To what extent do individuals maintain and strive to maintain their cultural identity and its characteristics?) and (b) *contact and participation* (To what extent do they come to be involved in cultural groups other than their own or prefer to remain within their own group?). Depending on various combinations of reactions to the issues, the four basic strategies of acculturation are defined as integration, assimilation, separation and marginalization (Berry et al., 1989).

Studies of immigrants' acculturation strategies have inevitably led to the conclusion that integration is the strategy most widely preferred (Berry, Kim, Power, Young, Y Bujaki, 1989; Krishnan & Berry, 1992; Partridge, 1988; Sam, 1995). In many studies it has been revealed that Separation is the second preferable strategy (Partridge, 1988; Sam, 1995). The general preference given to integration and separation suggests that many immigrants desire, in fact, to maintain a substantial part of their cultural heritage and identity in the society of settlement (Berry & Sam, 1977).

It is well known that an individual's or group's preferred acculturation strategy may or may not be permitted by the dominant group. For example, in societies that are explicitly assimilationist, the adoption of integration may be constrained because of a national ideology that promotes a single culture and single identity in the nation state. When national policies are assimilationist, the notion of 'minorities' is commonly embodied. In this case the process of 'minorization' usually accompanies the process of acculturation and this itself may be a risk factor (Berry & Sam, 1997).

In the domain of cross-cultural psychology of migration and acculturation, very few studies have been conducted thus far on these problems in Russia and other post-soviet states. It should be stressed, moreover, that the disintegration of the USSR and the rise of new nation-states in the region have generated a whole new web of issues related to the acculturation of 'ethnically alien' residents. To use some of the formulations of Kolstoe's (1995) research, while the political dissolution of the super- and multi-ethnic Soviet State happened to be a peaceful process, ethnic harmony could not be durable in the post-Soviet States. After political independence was achieved, the authorities in the newly formulated states embarked on policies of building their nations. The newly built national structures embody principles and elements of the civil nation-state pattern as well as of the ethnic one. Insofar as the ethnic conceptions prevail, the authorities begin striving to achieve some kind of maximum possible conformity between the concept of a political nation and that of a cultural one. The ideal, then, is that all the inhabitants within a state should belong to one dominant (titular) ethnic group. The existence of national-ethnic minorities is seen as a problem to be overcome sooner or later and/or to be marginalized--culturally, politically, demographically (Kolstoe, 1995).

The processes became a typical commonplace in the recent history of the newly independent post-soviet states. Such issues as civil rights, property rights and employment rights were often directly related to ethnic realities. The office of the UN High Commissioner for refugees estimates that over 60 million people became residents of foreign countries as a consequence of the USSR's disintegration. In almost all those states Russians make up the largest minority group, sometimes accounting for more than 70% of the non-titular population. By early 1996, over 3.5 million forced 'repatriates' had to leave places of their long-standing residence for reasons of the so-called *ethnic discomfort*.

For the last five years I have studied the acculturation of ethnic Russians in such newly-independent states as Kazakhstan, Uzbekistan, Armenia, Azerbaijan, Georgia, Ukrain, Lithuania and Estonia--in the framework of the individual research project The New Russian Diaspora: Prospects for Development supported by the MacArthur Foundation (1994-95, 1997). The research focused on a personal view of the problems of ethnic Russians in their *newly-found homes abroad,* not in the spectrum of any political interests (those of the authorities of the Russian Federation or any other post-Soviet States), but by revealing how the overall societal crisis resulting from the disintegration of the Soviet Super-Ethnic State is reflected and reinterpreted at the level of individuals-- those 'simple and humble people' who are involved superficially in it.

The 'Syndrome of Imposed Ethnicity'

Initially, the research was conducted within the theoretical framework of the model of social identity (Tajfel & Turner, 1979). Conforming to the model, the radical societal changes and shock experienced by the ethnic Russians led to what was defined as a 'crisis of social identity.' The main characteristic of the experience is the loss of positive evaluation of one's social identity, both ethnic and civil. At the level of personality structure, the following more specific manifestations of the crisis were revealed (Lebedeva, 1997): *radical growth/reduction of an ethnic component of one's social identity; negative feelings towards one's ethnic identity (shame, guilt, frustration, humiliation); dissatisfaction with one's changed civil identity (lack of new citizenship); negative or super-positive (defensive) attitude towards one's ethnic identity; ethnic intolerance towards titular-indigenous ethnic groups; generally negative evaluation of one's social situation (one's changed and low status, encroachment on one's rights, etc.).*

In later research the above-described crisis came to be termed in a different and, I believe, more accurate way; '*the syndrome of imposed ethnicity.*' The term refers to a person's changed societal situation where his or her ethnic identity, against his or her will and desire, comes to be an *overimportant* characteristic of one's realities and awareness of life, determining one's social position, rights, and responsibilities as well as becoming an important factor in one's self-identity. The human condition is well illustrated by the phrase uttered by one of our respondents in Kazakhstan (who was leaving Kazakhstan for Russia): "I am sick and tired of having to remember that I am Russian all the time."

In 1997, the results of the research I had conducted in 1994 and 1995 were reinterpreted within Berry's paradigm of '*acculturative stress*' (Berry et al., 1989). Research into acculturation of various groups (immigrants, refugees, aboriginal peoples, ethnic minorities) may be based on a variety of factors influencing attitudes to acculturation: voluntary or forced nature of migration, the fact of migration to a foreign culture, time-span of adaptation, etc. (Berry, 1990). It must be stressed that with ethnic Russians in the post-

Soviet States the paradigmatic picture of acculturation is complicated by a number of additional factors that should be taken into account: a) One's immigration to a foreign culture does not involve one's physical displacement or travel (the ethnic Russians involved may be residing in the same place and within the boundaries of the same country of their birth - the former USSR); b) The present-day ethnic Russians' awareness of their own *Russian ethnic identity* (cultural, religious) is often very limited. (Among other ethnic groups of the former Soviet Union, the 'Russian people' happen to be the only ethnic group who have come to associate their national identity with the super- and multi-ethnic Soviet Union to a significant degree (Kolstoe, 1995); and c) The fact that the USSR disintegrated very quickly and unexpectedly for most of the people involved, the problem of new acculturation took many of them unawares and was not only forced on them, but forced quite suddenly.

Since the Russian diaspora on the territories of the present-day post-Soviet States has been developing for centuries, one can find Russian residents of different historical record there--those whose ancestors came there in the times immemorial (northern Kazakhstan, Ukraine, Eastern Estonia) to 'old inhabitants' (with the length of record of up to six or seven generations) or to much more recent residents (the record of residence from five to forty years). Accordingly, their types of acculturation can vary a lot ranging from 'ethnocultural groups' to immigrants and refugees (taking into account the fact that some of them are forced to remain in the post-Soviet States because they cannot return to Russia for economic reasons).

A considerable amount of research has addressed the issue of ethnic and cultural identity of ethnocultural group members (Camilleri & Malewska-Peyre, 1997; Liebkind, 1984; Phinney, 1990). Berry and Sam (1997) pointed to a clear link (both theoretical and empirical) between identity choices and acculturation strategies. One recent empirical study showed that having a positive sense of oneself is linked to having an identity with particular ethnic groups, but not (except for whites) with an American identification (Phinney et al., 1994). On the other hand, there is empirical evidence that positive group identity leads to tolerance, and threats to that identity to intolerance (Berry & Pleasants, 1984).

Studying ethnic Russians in the post-Soviet States, we assumed that the disintegration of the USSR and the development of the newly-founded nation-states with their strategies of rapid acculturation made the Russian residents face an acute need for self-determination in a changed social and cultural environment. The indicators of a chosen acculturation strategy were the respondents' valency of ethnic identity (positive or negative ethnic autostereotypes and feelings related to their ethnicity) and their tolerance/intolerance towards the society of settlement (positive or negative ethnic heterostereotypes).

The valency of ethnic identity and ethnic tolerance/intolerance can be seen as indicators of successful acculturation. These indicators are related to the generally accepted acculturation patterns (Berry, 1990): integration, then, corresponds to the combination of positive ethnic identity and ethnic tolerance, assimilation corresponds to negative ethnic identity and ethnic tolerance, separation corresponds to positive ethnic identity and intolerance, marginalization corresponds to negative ethnic identity and intolerance.

My working hypothesis was that there should exist a close internal relationship between positive group ethnic identity and inter-ethnic tolerance. In unfavourable social conditions, however, the above direct relationship can disintegrate or turn into an inverse one. Inasmuch as ethnic intolerance arises, the mechanisms of social perception are enacted whose function is to restore positive ethnic identity. Thus, ethnic intolerance can be seen as a signal of certain trouble, while the principal target of the ensuing re-balancing is a newly restored group ethnic identity.

Objective

The object of the paper is to show how ethnic Russians in the post-Soviet States choose various strategies of acculturation to cope with the 'syndrome of imposed ethnicity.'

Method

Participants

The respondents chosen for the research were ethnic Russians--100 respondents in each of the States, their total number being 700. The respondents belonged to one of the two most salient types of acculturation strategy--separation or integration. To determine strategic type used by each respondent, interviews were carried out at the two different sites: 1) the Consulate sections of the Embassies of the Russian Federation on the day a respondent was submitting his or her application for Russian citizenship; or 2) Russian cultural centers and other social institutions of the Russian diaspora such as cultural societies, political parties, etc. The attitudes of those individuals who were actually participating in the activities of such centers of Russian diaspora (cultural maintenance) and wanted to remain permanent residents in the 'newly found home abroad' (contact and participation) were considered to be typical of integration-oriented individuals. The strategic attitudes of those that were applying for Russian citizenship (cultural maintenance) and were thinking of leaving for Russia (avoidance of contact and participation) were defined as separation-oriented individuals. Some of the latter might later be *forced* to implement, in effect, not the strategy of separation, but the strategy of assimilation or marginalization. They would not be able to leave for Russia for a number of reasons determined by factors outside their control. I, however, have chosen to consider only those respondents whose choice of strategies of acculturation was *voluntary.* Among such respondents *'separationists'* made up approximately 59%, whereas *'integrationists'* comprised 41%. The percentage of men and women among the respondents was 46% and 54%, respectively. The respondents' ages varied from 24 to 62, the average age being 46.7 years (75% were in the 30-55 age category). Most of the respondents (92%) belonged to the category of economically active population. As to their educational background, 73% had higher education, whereas 27% had secondary education. The average length of formal education was 13.2 years. The respondents' records of residence in the countries of settlement varied considerably. Eighteen per cent lived in these countries concerned since birth (10% among them had parents and/or grandparents who had lived in these countries), 60% lived in these countries for 20-30 years; 15% live in these countries 10-20 years, and 7% live in these countries for less than 10.

Instruments

The respondents were asked questions from a questionnaire that focused on several aspects of their experiences. The components of the questionnaire are listed below.

Russian ethnic identity and its transformation in the environment of the different culture (15 questions): *ethnic stereotypes (open-form questions); attitudes to Russia and to the country of residence (a scale with options from 'true homeland' to 'country where I am not being waited for'); M. Kuhn's and T. McPartand's test Who am I; positive/negative feelings about one's ethnic belonging (a scale with options from 'feeling proud' to 'feeling humiliated'); culture learning and culture shedding (open-form questions);participation in the diaspora's social and cultural institutions; needs and strivings of those who participate in the activities of such social and cultural institutions; evaluation of felt cultural distance toward Russian culture (5-point scale from 1-very close to 5 – very far)* and others.

Contact and participation (8 questions): *ethnic heterostereotypes; frequency of contacts with Russians and with people of the titular-dominant ethnic group in one's working and leisure time; having or not having friends among people of the titular- dominant ethnic group; evaluation of felt cultural distance towards titular-group culture; pro-migration or counter-migration attitudes* and others.

Perceived discrimination (15 questions): *how relations between titular-dominant group and the Russians have changed since the country of settlement gained independence (become better or worsened); one's experience of encroachment on one's rights because of one's ethnic belonging; specific kinds of discrimination (if any) one has had to come across* and others.

Social change: *one's attitude to the Russians' changed status as an 'ethnic minority' social changes in one's life after the disintegration of the USSR; one's evaluation of how acute the 'Russian question' is in the country of settlement and how it should be solved.*

Personal characteristics: *locus of control (Rotter, 1966); level of satisfaction as to the realization of a meaningful life (Crumboudht, 1968).*

The total number of questions in the questionnaire was 52. Open-form as well as closed-form questions were used. In the latter I used continuum scales based on the results of the pilot study conducted in 1993 and 1994. The validity of the scales was examined and checked with the aid of twelve expert psychologists.

Procedure

The research was conducted in the capital cities of the countries concerned where the Russian population make up a considerable minority and where the governments and legislative bodies responsible for national-ethnic policies are seated. The questionnaires were completed in the presence of an interviewer. The respondents were given the following instruction, "The object of the present research are the problems of acculturation and adaptation of the Russian residents in the newly independent states and the study of prospect of development of the new Russian diaspora. We ask you to answer the questions of the questionnaire as fully and sincerely as possible. The questionnaire is anonymous and the results of the research will be used for scientific purposes only. It usually took a respondent from 20 to 30 minutes to complete the questionnaire. The percentage of returned questionnaires was 98.5. The results were subjected to correlational and factor analyses using SPSS.

Results

Correlation analysis

The Pearson correlational analysis of the data revealed a significant correlation between positive ethnic autostereotypes and positive ethnic heterostereotypes with the respondents favouring Integration ($r = .28$, $p < .001$). With those favouring segregation the said correlation was absent.

Since the valency of ethnic identity is one of the most important indicators in determining a person's choice of acculturation strategy, characteristics related to it were studied too. The analysis of the data in both samples revealed the following characteristics influencing the valency of ethnic identity. For the degree of acculturation in the country of settlement, the variables length-of-settlement status, knowledge of the language and culture of the titular ethnic group were significantly correlated such that the higher the degree of acculturation, the more positive ethnic autostereotypes. For availability of social support, the stronger social support, the more positive ethnic autostereotypes. For perceived discrimination, the higher perceived discrimination, the more negative feelings related to ethnic belonging.

It is worth noting that the salience of ethnic identity ('over-emphatic' attitude towards ethnicity, ethnic values, and motivations) was one of the most influential characteristics related to the valency of ethnic identity. The more salient or pronounced ethnic identity, the more negative are feelings associated with it and the more negative ethnic autostereotypes.

I then analyze the relationship between personality characteristics and ethnic identity. The correlation analysis pointed to the importance of two relationships. For internal locus of control, the higher the internality, the more positive ethnic autostereotypes and feelings related to ethnic belonging. For level of satisfaction with one's life as meaningful, the higher the level of such satisfaction, the more positive ethnic autostereotypes and feelings related to one's ethnic belonging. The results of correlation analysis are shown in Table 1.

Further, we tried to define which strategies of social perception of behaviour can help to preserve or restore positive ethnic identity. The correlation analysis has revealed a number of socio-psychological mechanisms or coping strategies that may neutralise the *syndrome of imposed ethnicity* and restore positive ethnic identity and tolerance. Those mechanisms are the formation of positive local ethnic identity, the predominance of personal identity over group identity, increased cultural distance of Russia and Russians, decreased cultural distance to the country of residence, and the creation of local Russian community centers.

Since social-perceptive and behavioural strategies are important in terms of acculturation and maintaining/restoring positive ethnic identity, I believe they can help individuals cope with the stress of acculturation. The results of the analysis of correlation between various coping strategies and their acculturation effects are shown in Table 2.

Principal Components Factor Analyses

It is assumed that disturbances in the relationship between positive ethnic identity and ethnic tolerance are caused by a cluster of features that I have termed the syndrome of imposed ethnicity. *The latter was obtained through the principal components factor analyses (followed by varimax rotation) of*

Table 1. Characteristics of Acculturation and Personality Correlated with Valency of Ethnic Identity

Characteristics of acculturation and personality	Positive ethnic autostereotypes	Positive feelings related to ethnic belonging
Degree of acculturation	.38***	
Social support	.35**	
Perceived discrimination		-.40***
Salience of ethnic identity	-.35**	-.34**
Internal locus of control	.23*	.32**
Satisfaction with one's life as meaningful	.23*	.34**

* p < .05., **p < .01., *** p < .001

Table 2. Coping Strategies and their Acculturation Effects

Coping strategies (behavioral And social-perceptive)	Effects on acculturation and ethnic identity	Coefficient of correlation
Positive local identity formation	Desire to return to Russia	-.24*
	Perceived discrimination	-.36**
Predominance of personal identity Over group identity	Positive ethnic autostereotypes	.25*
'Closer' cultural distance to the dominant culture	Perception of country of residence as 'true homeland'	.23*
'Farther' cultural distance off Russia	Positive ethnic autostereotypes	.27*
	Need for social support at Russian community centers	.24*
Creation of Russian Community centers	Positive ethnic autostereotypes	.33**
	Positive ethnic heterostereotypes	.26*

*p < .05, **p < .01

items related to ethnic identity and ethnic tolerance across the groups of 'integrationists' and 'separationists' independently. Five factors with eigenvalues greater than 1 in both analyses resulted from the analysis. The variance explained by those five factors for the groups of integrationists and separationists were 46.6% and 44.9%, respectively.

From both analyses the same first factor with eigenvalues greater than 3.9 emerged for each group. The minimum loading used to identify items to factors was .40. Labelled i*mposed ethnicity*, the factor was comprised of the following items: ethnically relevant markers in self-identification, negative feelings related to one's ethnicity, perceived discrimination, negative ethnic heterostereotypes, growing cultural distance off the 'titular' ethnic group, and attitudes favouring migration to Russia.

Among the second factors substantial differences emerged between the two groups. The second factor for the sample of Integrationists was labeled *positive ethnic identity* (eigenvalue 2.29, variance .09) and consisted of the items: positive ethnic autostereotypes, positive ethnic heterostereotypes, closer cultural distance to titular-dominant culture, and participation in activities of Russian cultural centres. The second factor for the separationists was labeled *negative ethnic identity* (eigenvalue 2.19; variance - .09) and was comprised of the following items: negative ethnic autostereotypes, striving for Russian citizenship, lack of knowledge of the local state language, and non-attendance of Russian cultural centres.

The third factors were labeled *voluntary acceptance of new status* (eigenvalue 2.02; variance .08) for the integrationists and *involuntary acceptance of new status* (eigenvalue 1.54; variance .06) for the separationists. Between these two groups, there were differences in such items as positive/negative feelings related to one's ethnicity (respectively in the two samples), and positive/negative evaluation of one's minority status (respectively in the two samples).

The fourth factors were *positive local identity* (eigenvalue 1.56; variance .06) for the integrationists and *negative local identity* (eigenvalue 1.53; variance .05) for the separationists. For the integrationists, items such as positive feelings related to one's ethnicity, striving to stay in the country of residence, closer cultural distance to the titular-dominant culture, and attendance of Russian cultural centers comprised the factor. For the separationists, the items that comprised the factor were striving to migrate to Russia, negative feelings related to one's ethnicity, farther cultural distance off the titular-dominant culture, and non-attendance of Russian cultural centers.

The fifth factor was *biculturalism* for the integrationists (eigenvalue 1.35; variance .05) comprised of the items striving for citizenship in the country of residence, positive ethnic autostereotypes, positive ethnic heterostereotypes, closer cultural distance to the titular-dominant culture, attendance of Russian cultural centres, and satisfaction with one's life as meaningful. For the sample of separationists the fifth factor was *refusal of ethnic identity (assimilation)* with the items striving for citizenship in the country of residence, negative ethnic autostereotypes, negative feelings related to one's ethnicity, positive ethnic heterostereotypes, and acceptance of minority status comprising the factor.

Discussion

In the present study, I investigated 'acculturative stress' of ethnic Russians in the post-Soviet States in the spectrum of the crisis of their social (ethnic) identity. In my opinion, the crisis manifests itself in a disturbed relationship between positive ethnic identity and ethnic tolerance with those Russians who have opted for the strategy of separation, not integration. I hypothesized that there should normally exist a close internal relationship between positive ingroup (ethnic) identity and outgroup (inter-ethnic) tolerance in ingroup ethnic consciousness. In unfavourable social conditions the above direct relationship can disintegrate or turn into an inverse relationship.

As was noted, there is empirical evidence that confidence in one's own individual identity leads to ethnic tolerance (Berry & Pleasants, 1984). Later, Berry (1991) distinguished the two forms of 'confidence in one's identity.' The first is that of 'own group glorification' or 'strongly positive ingroup attitudes' following ethnocentric patterns (Brewer & Campbell, 1976) and is usually negatively correlated with ethnic tolerance. The other form, based on a 'sense of security' or 'self-esteem,' has a positive correlation with ethnic tolerance (Aboud & Scerry, 1984; Bagley, 1979; Berry et al., 1977). I agree that this distinction between forms of positive identity may be, to a certain extent useful, yet I do not think the ethnocentric pattern is of universal value. Within my model, the existence of a relationship between 'strongly positive ingroup attitudes' and ethnic intolerance is seen as a manifestation of the ethnic-identity crisis and a product of the enacted mechanism put into operation to restore positive identity. In my research the ethnocentric pattern was revealed only in Kazakhstan. The relationship between positive ethnic identity and ethnic tolerance appears to be a more universal pattern pointing to the absence of acculturative stress, as was shown in the research of British-Canadians and French-Canadians in Canada (Berry et al., 1977).

The results of correlation analysis, conducted independently for the groups of Integrationists and Separationists, pointed to a significant correlation between positive ethnic identity (positive ethnic autostereotypes) and ethnic tolerance (positive ethnic heterostereotypes) in the first of the two groups, while it turned to be nonsignificant in the second group. Conforming to my hypothesis, the results thus point to a crisis of social (ethnic) identity with those respondents whose strategy is separation.

I assumed that the crisis was caused by the assimilationist policies of some of the post-Soviet States, on the one hand, and by lack of any clear positive ethnic identity with many Russians who had had 'soviet-people' identity before the disintegration of the USSR. Using correlation analysis, I found that *salience of ethnic identity, perceived discrimination, degree of acculturation in a host country, the availability of social support* influence significantly the valency of ethnic identity.

The research has shown that the degree of acculturation in a host country and the availability of social support are important factors to maintain positive ethnic identity. The degree of acculturation (generational status, knowledge of language and culture of a dominant society, etc.) influence positively the experience of acculturative stress (Berry, 1990; Berry & Sam, 1997). The positive influence of social-support characteristics (the presence of social and cultural institutions that support the acculturating individual: ethnic associations, residential enclaves, extended families, contacts and links with host societies, etc.) on the process of acculturation has been stressed by many researchers (Beiser, Turner & Ganesan, 1989; Berry & Sam, 1997; Furnham & Shiekh, 1993; Golding & Burnam, 1990; Shisana & Celentano, 1985).

The influence of perceived discrimination or, in a broader context, the influence of the attitudes of a dominant society on various ethnic groups has been analysed in many research studies (Berry, 1990; Berry, Kalin, & Taylor, 1977; Berry & Sam, 1997; Murphy, 1965). In my research, the perceived discrimination and the salience of ethnic identity were significantly related to the negative valency of ethnic identity. In this case, I believe, the specific nature of acculturative stress of the post-Soviet Russians as an ethnic group manifests itself particularly well. The growing salience of ethnic identification processes of Russians in the 'new abroad' leads to the growth of negative ethnic autostereotypes and negative feelings related to one's ethnic belonging (shame, guilt, offence, and humiliation). The negative valency of ethnic identity and ethnic intolerance can thus be seen as the by-products of the overstressed importance of human ethnic belonging in the newly independent ethnocratic states. That may be the main factor in the emerged reality of the so-called 'imposed ethnicity' ('imposed negative ethnicity', to be more exact).

To understand the above reality better, one should consider the results of the factor analyses of ethnic Russians in the groups of integrationists and separationists. The factor analyses made for the two groups point to the existence of two distinctly different processes--that of coping with the syndrome of imposed ethnicity and that of a psychological defence against it. In both cases, the first and foremost factor for both groups is the same, the imposed ethnicity, which comprises such items as the growing salience of one's ethnic identity, negative feelings associated with one's ethnic identity, sharply perceived ethnic discrimination, ethnic intolerance and other negative aspects of the acculturative stress.

Starting with the second factor, substantial differences appear. Separationists tend to have a negative ethnic identity (general as well as local) and accept their new status involuntarily, whereas the integrationists tend to have a positive ethnic identity and accept their new status voluntarily.

The influence of changed status on the success of acculturation was noted in a number of studies relative loss of status may result in stress and poor mental health (Berry, 1990; Berry & Sam, 1997). In factors 4 and 5 demonstrate how negative ethnic identity may lead the separationists to the refusal of ethnicity and even to the acceptance of assimilation. However, the integrationists's positive ethnic identity led them to biculturalism and integration. As Berry and Sam (1997) noted, the term 'bicultural' is employed to refer to acculturation that involves the individual simultaneously in the two cultures that are in contact (LaFromboise, Coleman & Gerton, 1993; Padilla, 1994; Szaposhnik & Kurtines, 1993), a concept corresponding closely to the strategy of integration.

It is also important to consider the latent attitudes for assimilation revealed by the factor analysis in the group of separationists. The fact that such attitudes exist shows that under the influence of assimilationist policies assimilation may become a more successful acculturation strategy than separation. Berry and Sam (1997)assert that in assimilationist societies, acculturation may be easiest by adopting the assimilation strategy. Thus, preferences for one acculturation strategy over others are known to vary, depending on context and time period (Berry & Sam, 1997).

The basic difference between the two groups seems to be that the integrationists are those who have been able to keep up positive ethnic identity and strive to maintain it in the institutions of Russian diaspora, whereas the separationists did not have any initially given positive ethnic identity as a result of the acculturative stress their ethnic identity gained negative valency. Moreover, members in the Integrationist group did not strive to maintain ethnic identity in the centres of Russian diaspora, making it easier for some of them to float towards assimilation. It is also possible that in the given conditions a considerable number of ethnic Russians may have to gravitate toward the marginalization strategy of acculturation.

The results of correlation analysis show that individual (personal) characteristics may contribute to or impede the maintenance of positive ethnic identity--particularly, such characteristics as the internal locus of control and satisfaction with one's life as meaningful. The influence of personal factors on successful acculturation was noted in a number of works (Berry & Sam, 1997; Ghuman, 1991; Sam, 1995; Schmitz, 1994). The results of my research allow me to assume that on the whole an individual may be able to resist negative change insofar as he or she has the internal locus of control and believes that his or her life is meaningful.

One of the tasks of my research has been to reveal strategies of coping with the acculturative stress, in our case with the *syndrome of imposed ethnicity*. I have revealed that such behavioral and social-perceptive strategies as the formation of local ethnic identity, the preference of personal identity over group identity, the creation of Russian community centers, farther cultural distance from Russia and Russians, closer cultural distance to the culture of a host country may help to overcome the syndrome of imposed ethnicity-- to maintain positive ethnic identity and ethnic tolerance. The importance of active coping strategies to overcome acculturative stress is emphasized by other researchers (e.g., Berry & Sam, 1997). The strategies revealed in our research are directly oriented towards the maintenance of positive ethnic identity and ethnic tolerance.

In previous research I have studied another active coping strategy among ethnic Russians--that of implemented migration (repatriation) to Russia. The research conducted in 1996 focused on the adaptation of Russian migrants from Estonia, Uzbekistan, and Kazakhstan--people with outspokenly negative heterostereotypes and negative feelings associated with their ethnic belonging. From the results of this study I found that a year after the implemented migration the respondents revealed growing positive ethnic heterostereotypes (towards their former 'titular' ethnic group) as well as growth in their own positive ethnocultural identity, which made them different from other local ethnic Russians (Lebedeva, 1997).

Ethnic intolerance can thus be seen as a signal of certain trouble, while the principal objective of the ensuing re-balancing process is to restore positive group (ethnic) identity. Inasmuch as ethnic intolerance arises, the mechanisms of social perception are enacted for the purpose of restoring positive ethnic identity. The use of such strategies promotes growing positive ethnic identity and ethnic tolerance, helping to restore a balance in individual and group consciousness. All those socio-psychological strategies may, to a large extent, be unconscious. Yet, I believe, they serve to preserve positive ethnic identity and a given culture as a whole, ensuring its super-organic character (Kroeber, 1917).

Conclusion

The analysis of the research data has revealed some major peculiarities of acculturation of ethnic Russians in the post-Soviet newly independent countries. The major psychological feature of 'acculturation stress' (Berry, 1990) among the ethnic Russians can be seen as the *crisis of social identity*, *civic* as well as *ethnic* (Tajfel & Turner, 1986). The internal psychological core of the crisis lies in the destruction of a strong link between positive ethnic identity and ethnic tolerance, the link being the basis of a balanced and integral social-ethnic identity. One characteristic aspect of the crisis is what I termed the *syndrome of imposed identity* (Lebedeva, 1996). In the process of acculturation, this syndrome stimulates the psychological changes leading to the re-generation of positive ethnic identity and helps to overcome 'ethnic depersonalization.' Maintaining positive ethnic identity can be seen as the main condition of successful acculturation. In a broader context, the maintenance of positive ethnic identity is a socio-psychological mechanism working to maintain a given culture as a whole. One's degree of acculturation in the country of residence, one's perceived discrimination and one's valency of ethnic identity can be seen as factors determining how the crisis of social identity will be resolved and successful acculturation attained.

The results of my research show that the role of the syndrome of imposed identity is ambivalent. On the one hand, it promotes attitudes favouring the separation strategy or the assimilation strategy. On the other hand, it may stimulate search for positive ethnic identity and biculturalism that is characteristic of the Integration strategy. In any case, it forces an individual to solve problems of his or her cultural and ethnic self-identification in search of an adequate and positive identity in the changing world.

It should be noted that although many findings in my research correspond to the findings of many other studies, the process of acculturation of Russians in the post-soviet countries has certain specific features of its own. One peculiarity of the situation is the ethnocratic mode of many of the post-Soviet States. The other peculiarity lies in the fact that many Russians lack clear positive ethnic identity (the phenomenon of 'ethnic depersonalization'). Those peculiarities caused the emergence of the above-described *syndrome of imposed ethnicity* and forced me to focus attention in the research on the problem of ethnic identity and its connection with ethnic tolerance.

Despite the considerations enumerated above, the research has shown quite convincingly that among Russians in the post-Soviet countries, integration is the most preferred and successful acculturation strategy, as was shown in many other studies of various groups in various countries (e.g., Berry & Sam, 1997). From the specific point of view of my study, integration is the shortest and best way to restore positive ethnic identity and ethnic tolerance, which is important for an individual as well as for a state. At the individual level, to the extent that a bicultural identity (combining a heritage identity and a national identity) is associated with the integration strategy, evidence generally suggests that this identity would be the most supportive of good adaptation (Berry et al., 1987; Berry & Sam, 1997). At the societal level, the evidence is similar, holding that ethnic (i.e., heritage culture) or dual identity does not diminish one's sense of attachment or commitment to a unified society (Kalin & Berry, 1996). Thus, Russians now being acculturated in the post-soviet states should strive to attain and maintain their own positive ethnic identity as well as to have contacts and be part of life in their host societies, while the politicians in those societies should allow them to do so.

References

Aboud, F. & Scerry S. (1984). The development of ethnic attitudes: A critical review. *Journal of Cross-Cultural Psychology, 15,* 3-34.

Bagley, C. (1979). Self-esteem as a pivotal concept in race and ethnic relations. *Research in Race and Ethnic Relations, 1,* 127-167.

Beiser, M., Tuner, R.J., & Ganesan, S. (1989). Catastrophic stress and factors affecting its consequences among Southeast Asian refugees. *Social Science and Medicine, 28,* 183-195.

Berry, J.W. (1970). Marginality, stress and ethnic identification in an acculturated Aboriginal community. *Journal of Cross-Cultural Psychology, 1,* 239-252.

Berry, J.W. (1990). Psychology of acculturation. In J. Berman (Ed.), *Cross-cultural perspectives: Nebraska symposium on motivation* (pp. 201-234). Lincoln: University of Nebraska Press.

Berry, J.W. (1991). Understanding and managing multiculturalism: Some possible implications of research in Canada. *Psychology and Developing Societies, 3,* 17-49.

Berry, J.W., Kalin, R., & Taylor, D. (1977). *Multiculturalism and ethnic attitudes in Canada.* Ottawa: Ministry of Supply and Services.

Berry, J.W., Kim U., Minde, T. & Mok, D. (1987). Comparative studies of acculturative stress. *International Migration Review, 21,* 491-511.

Berry, J.W., Kim, U., Power, S., Young, M. & Bujaki, M. (1989). Acculturation attitudes in plural societies. *Applied Psychology, 38,* 185-206.

Berry, J.W. & Pleasants, M. (1984). *Ethnic tolerance in plural societies.* Paper given at the International Conference on Authoritarianism and Dogmatism, Potsdam, NJ.

Berry J.W. & Sam, D. (1997). Acculturation and Adaptation. In J.W.Berry et al. (Eds.) *Handbook of cross-cultural psychology* (Vol.3, pp. 291-326).

Brewer, M., & Campbell, D.T. (1976). *Ethnocentrism and intergroup attitudes: East African evidence.* New York: Sage/Halsted.

Camillery, C. & Malewska- Peyre, H. (1997). Sociaization and Identity Strategies. In In J.W.Berry, Y.H. Poortinga, J.Randey, P.R. Dasen, T.S. Sarswathi, M.H. Segall, & C. Kagitcibasi (Eds.) *Handbook of cross-cultural psychology* (Vol.2, pp. 41-68).

Crambought G. (1968). Cross-validation of purpose-in-life test, based on Francl's concept. *Journal of Individual Psychology, 24,* 74-81.

Furnham, A. & Shiekh, S. (1993). Gender, generation, and social support correlates of mental health in Asian immigrants. *International Journal of Social Psychiatry, 39,* 22-33.

Ghuman, P.A.S. (1991). Best or worst of two words? A study of Asian adolescents. *Educational Review, 33,* 121-132.

Golding, J.M. & Burnam, M.A. (1990). Immigration, stress and depressive symptoms in a Mexican-American community. *Journal of Nervous and Mental Disease, 178,* 161-171.

Kalin, R. & Berry, J.W. (1996). Ethnic and civic self-identity in Canada: Analyses of 1974 and 1991 National Surveys, *Canadian Ethnic Studies, 28.*

Kolstoe, P. (1995). *Russians in the former Soviet republics.* London: Hurst & Company.

Krishnan, A. & Berry, J.W. (1992). Acculturative stress and acculturation attitudes among Indian immigrants to the United States. *Psychology and Developing Societies, 4,* 187-212.

Kroeber, A.L. (1917). The superorganic. *American Anthropologist, 19,* 163-213.

LaFromboise, T., Coleman, H., & Gerton, J. (1993). Psychological impact of biculturalism: Evidence and theory. *Psychological Bulletin, 114,* 395-412.

Lebedeva, N.M. (1997). *The new Russian diaspora: Socio-psychological analysis.* Moscow: Institute of Ethnology & Anthropology Press.

Liebkind, K. (1984). *Minority identity and identification processes.* Helsinki: Societas Scientarum Fennica.

Murphy, H.B.M. (1965). Migration and the major mental disorders. In M. Kantor (Ed.), *Mobility and mental health* (pp.221-249). Springfield, IL: Thomas.

Neto, F. (1994). *Predictors of satisfaction with life among second generation migrants.* Paper presented at 23d International Congress of the International Association of Applied Psychology. Madrid, July 17-22, 1994.

Padilla, A. (1994). Bicultural development: A theoretical and conceptual examination. In R.G. Malgady & H. Rodriguez (Eds.), *Theoretical and conceptual issues in Hispanic mental health* (pp.16-31). Malabar, India: Krieger.

Partridge, K. (1988). Acculturation attitudes and stress of Westerners living in Japan. In J.W. Berry & R.C. Annis (Eds.), *Ethnic psychology* (pp. 105-113). Amsterdam: Swets and Zeitlinger.

Phinney, J. (1990). Ethnic identity in adolescents and adults: A review of research. *Psychological Bulletin, 108,* 499-514.

Phinney, J., DuPont, E., Espinosa, C., Revill J., & Sanders, K. (1994). Ethnic Identity and American identification among ethnic minority youth. In A-M. Bouvy, F. Van de Vijver, P. Boski, & P.Schmitz (Eds.), *Journeys into cross-cultural psychology* (pp. 167-183). Lisse, Netherlands: Swets and Zeitlinger.

Rotter, J.B. (1966). Generalised expectancies for internal versus external control of reinforcement. *Psychological Monographs,* 80.

Sam, D.L. (1995). Acculturation attitudes among young immigrants as a function of perceived parental attitudes to cultural change. *Journal of Early Adolescence, 15,* 238-258.

Schmitz, P.G. (1994). Acculturation and adaptation process among immigrants in Germany. In A-M. Bouvy, F.J.R. van de Vijver, & P.Schmitz (Eds.), *Journeys into cross-cultural psychology* (pp. 142-157). Amsterdam: Swets and Zeitlinger.

Szapocznik, J. & Kurtines, W. (1993). Family psychology and cultural diversity. *American Psychologist, 48,* 400-407.

Shisana, O., & Celentano, D. (1985). Depressive symptomatology among Namibian adolescent refugees. *Social Science and Medicine, 21,* 1251-1257.

Tajfel H. & Turner, J. (1979). An integrative theory of intergroup conflict. In W. C. Austin & S. Worchel (Eds.), *The social psychology of intergroup relations,* Monterey, CA.: Brooks/Cole.

The Construction of a Supra-National Identity in Chile and Venezuela

Jose Miguel Salazar
Universidad Central de Venezuela, Caracas
Instituto de Psicología

Julio Villegas
Universidad Central, Santiago de Chile
Facultad de Psicología

ABSTRACT

Latin American identity was explored with University students from Chile (n= 102) and Venezuela (n= 145) by asking them to evaluate a) their degree of identification with different social categories, b) characteristics used to define the social categories and c) to engage in social comparison with three other national or supra-national categories. Even though a high degree of identification with the Latin American category was generalized, this was greater among Venezuelans. In the construction of the category, *culture* was frequently mentioned by both groups, as well as *positive personality characteristics. Negative political conditions* were more frequent among Chileans. The mention of *race* was related to the degree of identification in both groups. Social comparisons did not indicate generalized ethnocentrism or negative social identity, although the latter was found in relation to the Japanese. The study provides evidence about the reality and characteristics of a supra-national Latin American social identity.

Identities of origin, a term we use to include what is usually referred to as "national identities", "cultural identities", "regional identities", and so forth, continue to be very relevant in this age of globalization. Yet they are not static essences and the question of change must always be kept in mind when considering the issue of "identities" and what they are. These changes may occur at either the individual or the societal level. The paradigmatic example of such changes is the case of migrating individuals who come to participate in a different society and become assimilated or integrated into it (Berry, 1993). But changes may occur also when whole societies come in contact, be it through a process of colonization, massive immigration, or other movements, as occurred in the so-called process of "encounter of two cultures" in the Southern part of the Americas starting with the arrival of Columbus in 1492. And while the society that was in political and military control had the upper hand in establishing its language, culture and religion, it did not completely exterminate the members of the other group or isolate them geographically. Hence it could not escape penetration of the indigenous elements. Through a process of *mestizaje*, both biological and cultural, a mixed culture and identity emerged, slowly, in a period of about 500 years.

Yet this new identity has certain peculiarities. Examining studies carried out in different countries in Latin America, we see evidence of a negative "social identity"; that is, a tendency of characterizing the national group in a relatively negative way. In Venezuela we identified the widespread manifestations of an ideological phenomenon we designated as "ideology of dependence", which may be interpreted as a manifestation of a neo-colonial ideology. This is where things European or North American are considered superior, and by comparison the local country is degraded or debased; later, evidence that similar phenomena were evident in other countries of the region was obtained.

In other studies (Salazar, 1992) it was found that the tendency towards a negative social identity was diminished when the referent was Latin America as a general supra-national identity and not the specific nation. Even though the "idea" of Latin America as a unit has had a long history, and was very much present during the wars of independence in the early XIX century, the processes of "globalization" that has been sparked by the technological developments in the mass media, and accompanied by economic changes, has probably played an important role in re-launching it. Our interest is centered on describing how the supra-national (Latin American) identity is construed at the end of this century, and how the elements of this construction are interrelated.

In Social Identity Theory (Tajfel, 1981), three processes are involved: Categorization, Identification, and Comparison. These processes are obviously interrelated, and exploring them and their interrelationships could inform us about the Latin American supra-national identity, that is shared by people who live in 20 different countries. We could explore how this identity is structured if we agree that the structure of an identity implies three things: a definition of the category, a high degree of identification with the category, and positive social comparisons

In this study we started with two countries within the same general geopolitical category: Latin American. For this purpose Chile and Venezuela were selected. These two countries are geographically located at the two extremes of the Andes, and there have been contrasting developments in the recent past. Chile, even though it has experienced a very painful process of dictatorship, is at present the most solid economy of the sub-continent. On the other hand Venezuela which has experienced a sustained democracy for over forty years, has suffered a great economic crisis in recent years after experiencing a boom economy in the 1970s.

The aim of the study was to describe how Chile and Venezuela handle their identity in three respects: elements used in the construction of the supra-national category, degree of identification with it, and social comparisons with selected outgroups, as well as the relationship between these elements. Our goal was to determine how well structured the Latin American identity is and how it may help to cope with a world moving towards a cosmopolitizing identity.

Method

Participants

102 undergraduate university students from Chile (76 females, 26 males) and 145 from Venezuela (88 females, 57 males) volunteered to participate in this study. The data from Venezuela were collected in 1995 and 1996 in four different regions of the country, while the data from Chile were collected in 1997 in Santiago de Chile, the capital of the country.

Instruments

The participants were asked to complete questionnaires with open and closed items. Three techniques were used, as follows:

a. The way the social category was construed was obtained from two open questions:
    1) What differentiates Latin-Americans from inhabitants of other regions of the world?
    2) What makes Latin America different form other regions of the world?

b. The degree of identification with the social category was evaluated with two closed items (with responses using five-point scales: Completely, Very Much, Somewhat, Not Much, Not At All).
    1) To what degree do you feel Latin American?
    2) Do you consider yourself a typical Latin American?

   Two other items, equally closed (with responses: I like it immensely, I like it a lot, I like it somewhat, I do not like it much and I do not like it at all) were asked:
    1) How would you describe your feeling for Latin America?
    2) How do you feel when people identify you as a Latin American?

c. Social comparisons were obtained using six semantic differential scales (happy-sad; lazy-hardworking; socially nice ("simpatico")-not "simpatico", cultured, ignorant, spendthrifts- thrifty, irresponsible-responsible) to evaluate, besides Latin-Americans, Europeans, North Americans and Japanese.

Results

The Construction of the Social Categories

The responses to the first two questions enumerated above were grouped into 8 broad content categories, obtained by a meticulous inferential process of grouping responses in terms of similarity. In this process several intermediate sub-categories were identified.

In Table 1 the responses to these items are presented, organized in function of the overall percentage of subjects using each one.

Table 1. Percentage of participants using content categories

Content Categories	Participants			
	All (n=247)	Chile (n=102)	Ven (n=145)	p
Positive Personality characteristics.	61.5%	75.5%	51.7%	<.01
Culture (customs, ways, habits)	56.3%	56.9%	55.9%	n.s.
Geography	41.3%	38.2%	43.4%	n.s.
Negative Political	34.0%	41.2%	29.0%	<.05
Language	23.5%	9.8%	33.1%	<.01
Race	21.9%	17.6%	24.8%	n.s.
Negative Personality characteristics	17.0%	19.6%	15.2%	n.s.
Positive Political	13.0%	19.6%	8.3%	n.s.

The two content categories most frequently used were ***Positive Personality Characteristics*** (simpatico, hospitable, merry) and ***Culture*** (customs, ways, habits). Chileans use the first category significantly more than the Venezuelans do. Other differences are observed in regards to ***Negative Political Conditions*** (lack of identity, political disorganization and corruption) which Chileans were more likely to use, and ***Language*** more frequently used by Venezuelans as a defining characteristic of Latin American identity.

Degree of identification

As shown in Table 2, the results indicate substantial percentages of subjects indicating the two highest categories of identification, although there is a tendency for this to be more so in the case of the Venezuelan subjects. When a single index of identification is calculated using the four items (alpha= .79) and a t-test is calculated, there is a significant difference with a higher degree of identification amongst the Venezuelans.

Table 2. Participants in each group indicating high identification

Identification items	Participants		
	Chile (n=102)	Ven (n=145)	All (n=247)
Feel Latin American	78.4%	91.0%	85.8%
Typical Latin American	55.9%	61.4%	59.1%
Feeling towards Latin America	88.2%	91.0%	89.9%
Liking to be Identified as Latin American	82.4%	89.7%	86.6%
4 item Index	M=1.98 sd=0.57	M=1.70 sd=0.58	t=3.69 P <.001

Social comparisons

For the purposes of the social comparison, subjects evaluated three external groups: North Americans, Europeans and Japanese using Semantic Differential scales, and comparing with the evaluation of the Latin American with the same instrument. The results (see Table 3) indicated that a relatively negative evaluation was observed in both groups in relation to the Japanese. This was also true in the case of the Chileans in relation to the Europeans.

Table 3. Attitudes towards different countries or regions and social comparisons

	ACT LA	ACT EUR	ACT USA	ACT JAP	LA-EUR	LA-USA	LA-JAP
CHI	20.65	21.76	20.18	23.98	t=3.58**	t=1.31	t=12.40**
VEN	22.17	22.68	21.89	24.55	t=1.23	t=0.58	t=6.39**

The Relationship Between the Variables

Identification and Use of Content Categories

In order to compare the use of content categories, we decided to place the subjects into three groups on the basis of their overall measure of identification. Because each subject gave multiple responses, our analysis aimed at comparing the percentage of participants within each group using a particular category. The results are presented in Table 4.

Table 4. Percentages using content categories in identification groups

Content categories	Chilean participants				
	High Ident. (n=30)	Moderate (n=51)	Low Ident. (n=21)	Chi 2	p
Positive Personality characteristics.	83.3.	78.4	57.1	5.06	.08
Costumes-Culture	66.7	56.9	42.9	2.85	n.s.
Geography	56.7	29.4	33.3	6.21	<.05
Negative political	16.7	49.0	57.1	10.95	.004
Language	3	4	3	-	-
Race	30.0	9.8	19.0	5.34	.07
Negative Personality characteristics	13.3	21.6	23.8	1.11	n.s.
Positive Political	10.0	27.5	14.3	-	-
	Venezuelan participants				
	High Ident. (n=46)	Moderate (n=69)	Low Ident. (n=30)	Chi 2	P
Positive Personality characteristics.	60.9	46.4	50.0	2.37	n.s.
Costumes-Culture	50.0	59.4	56.7	1.00	n.s.
Geography	54.3	39.1	36.7	3.31	n.s.
Negative political	28.3	27.5	33.3	0.36	n.s.
Language	37.0	29.0	36.7	1.00	n.s.
Race	37.0	18.8	20.0	5.32	.07
Negative Personality characteristics	13.0	15.9	16.7	0.25	n.s.
Positive Political	10.9	8.7	3.3	-	-

The results indicated that in both groups the degree of identification was related to the perception of racial characteristics, and to a lesser degree to geographical elements and positive personality characteristics. In the Chilean case there was a marked use of negative political characteristics by those less identified with Latin America.

Identification and social comparisons

In all identification groups, except high identifiers in Venezuela, the Japanese were evaluated more positively than the Latin Americans were. The Europeans were evaluated more positively among the low identifiers in both groups, and also among the moderates in Chile. On the other hand, the North Americans were evaluated more negatively by the high identifiers in both nations; and in the Venezuelan case also the Europeans. See Table 5.

Table 5. Attitudes towards different countries or regions, and social comparisons in identification groups

	ACT LA	ACT EUR	ACT USA	ACT JAP	LA-EUR	LA-USA	LA-JAP
CHI High	21.50	21.90	20.37	23.83	t=-0.62	t=+2.03*	t=-6.44**
CHI Mod	20.65	21.82	20.00	23.90	t=-3.39**	t=1.31	t=8.60**
CHI Low	19.33	21.38	20.33	24.38	t=-2.12*	t=-0.92	t=-7.82**
VEN High	23.93	22.17	22.10	24.32	t=+2.01*	t=+2.38*	t=-0.56
VEN Mod	21.30	22.87	21.46	24.25	t=-2.56	t=-0.30	t=-5.87**
VEN Low	21.23	23.03	22.53	25.63	t=-2.19*	t=-1.59	t=-5.73**

Discussion

Our results indicate that Latin-American identity -- that is, the identification with the supra-national category -- is widely accepted by our subjects, since nearly 90% indicated high identification in three of the items used for its evaluation (exception being on an items asking them to indicate whether they consider themselves "typical Latin-Americans", where even then the majority gave highly positive responses). Nevertheless, we cannot lose sight of the fact that all our subjects were university students, making generalizations dangerous.

The category is construed around perceived cultural commonalties and positive personality characteristics. More of the subjects used these categories, in response to open questions, which as we know, produce a lower degree of agreement than other procedures. The use of positive personality characteristics is what is expected in social identity theory. The presence of perceived cultural commonalties indicates the perception of a category that goes beyond national limits, and hence the existence of a supra-national identity which is more than a mere political artifice as some would argue.

What is more, the degree of identification is somewhat related in both groups to perception of "racial" similarities. This suggests an underlying ethnonationalism. Smith (1981) has written extensively about this phenomenon, but puts emphasis on the emergence of ethnic nationalism within existing states; in this particular case a similar phenomenon may be identified at a supra-national level. There is also another peculiarity in this ethnonationalism regarding its myths of origin; the particular form of the myth has to do with the emergence of a "mixed race". Saiz et al. (1993) have documented this phenomenon in the Chilean case.

The perception of negative political aspects (lack of identity, corruption, etc.) is related to a lower degree of identification, which may explain the lower average identification of the Chileans, who are more likely to perceive negative political traits.

In terms of social comparisons, there was no evidence of a generalized negative social comparison. Relative to North America there are no differences in the evaluation scores and within some of the more identified groups in both countries there is even a more negative attitude. This is somewhat at odds with the previous finding of the minus valued image of their own country when compared with the USA among Venezuelans (Salazar, 1983), but reinforced the idea that such minus-valued perceptions are decreased when the comparisons were made with Latin America as the referent and not the particular country. What is conspicuous in these social comparisons is the presence of negative comparison relative to Japan in both groups, a perception that is shared independently of the degree of identification. The very positive Japanese image seems to be widely shared, so much so that it has been found even amongst USA students.

The main finding of this study is the description of a Latin-American identity which is widely shared by, at least, students of Venezuela and Chile conceived in cultural terms and that has elements of an emerging ethnonationalism. This identity tends towards positive use of preferred personality traits for its construction. At the same time the social category is evaluated differentially in relation to other external groups, without a generalized ethnocentrism or its opposite: minusvaluation or negative social identity.

References

Berry, J. (1993). Ethnic identities in plural societies. In M.E. Bernal & G.P. Knight (Eds). *Ethnic identities.* Albany, NY: State University of New York.

Saiz, J.L., Rehbein, L. & Pérez-Luco, R. (1993). *Identidad nacional: Mito de origen del chileno y autoatribución de estereotipos ascritos al indigena mapuche y al español pretéritos* (Informe final del proyecto No. 9221). Temuco, Chile: Universidad de la Frontera, Dirección de Investigación y desarrollo

Salazar, J.M. (1983). *Bases psicológicas del nacionalismo.* México: Trillas.

Salazar, J.M. (1992). Dos acercamientos a la identidad latinoamericana. *Boletín de Avepso, 15,* 75-86.

Smith, A.D.(1981). *The Ethnic revival in the modern world.* Cambridge: Cambridge University Press.

Tajfel, H. (1981). *Human groups and social categories.* Cambridge: Cambridge University Press.

Clinical and Mental Health Considerations

Stress, Coping and Mental Health among Immigrants to Australia

F.Sushila Niles
Northern Territory University
Psychology Discipline/School of Social Sciences

ABSTRACT

It is generally argued that immigrant populations experience acculturative stress, and the prevalent view for many years was that this resulted in a decline in mental health. However, this argument of lowered mental health is not fully supported. There seem to be many factors that moderate the effects of acculturation on mental health. A study was undertaken to examine the relationship between acculturative stress and mental health, with two immigrant groups (Greeks and Filipinos) now residing in Northern Australia. The sample, composed of 50 from each group (25 males and 25 females), were interviewed. Apart from a free-response strategy, checklists of stressors and ways of coping as well as the General Health Questionnaire were used to obtain relevant data. The results suggest that overall the mental health of members of both groups (but more especially that of the Filipinos), seem to be only minimally affected by migrant experiences. A strong sense of cultural identity, and the support from family and association with members of their own community, seem to bolster immigrants even against stressors arising from perception of racism and discrimination. Overall these immigrant groups seem to enjoy good mental health.

It is well documented that continuous and first hand contact between two distinct cultural groups results in changes in the cultural pattern of either or both groups. Such change, described as acculturation, however, tends to be largely one-sided and experienced mostly by migrating cultures. Negative consequence of acculturation is described as *acculturative stress* (Berry, Kim, Minde & Mok, 1987). The prevalent view for a long time was that acculturation inevitably brought about a decline in mental health of individuals. But this view is no longer fully supported (Berry & Kim, 1988). There seem to be many factors that mitigate acculturative experiences and consequently mental health status is unaffected or only marginally influenced.

Many factors contribute to successful acculturation. At the group level, the acceptance of diversity or pluralism by the larger society (Murphy, 1965), and the opportunity for immigrants to fully participate in the larger society, are influential, and at the individual level, the personal experience of each individual, often associated with age and gender, as well as social status indicators such as education, and employment value, previous contact with diverse cultures, familiarity with the language and culture of the host country, similarities of religious traditions, as well as personality related factors are important.

Evidence from different studies/countries support the view that a number of factors moderate the effects of stressful migration experience on mental health. For instance, a study by Cochrane (1979) in Britain suggested that country of origin was an important variable in mental health status of different acculturating groups. Studies in Canada and Australia (Kim, 1984, Lasry, 1977, Taft, 1979) suggested that different cultural groups acculturate differently and that certain factors as well the modes of acculturation are related to high or low stress (Berry & Kim, 1988).

A comprehensive model of the stress process was developed by Lazarus & Folkman, (1984). Slavin and colleagues, however, expressed concern about the Euro-centric nature of the Lazarus and Folkman model, which assumes an orientation towards individualistic goals and individual mastery, and does not take into account the social embeddedness of the individual in some cultures (Slavin, Rainer, McCreary, & Gowda, 1991). Slavin et al. therefore suggested an adaptation of this model to accommodate the cultural dimension. They asked culturally-relevant questions at every stage. The Slavin et al. (1991) cultural model of stress was adapted for this study, but contains only three stages:

STRESSORS→COPING→ADAPTATIONAL OUTCOMES.

The culturally relevant question in appraising stress is how belonging to a specific cultural group affects the nature and frequency of potentially stressful life events. Apart from the day to day stressors common to most people, there are stressors unique to the immigrant experience. Slavin et al. (1991) listed stressors such as events related to; (1) minority status, (2) discrimination, (3) socio-economic status and (4) specific customs. These potential stressors must therefore be taken into account in appraising stress factors for immigrants. Myers (1982) suggested that prolonged exposure to stressful conditions of poverty and racism can lead to overreactivity to events. Therefore, acculturative experiences can exacerbate the effect of daily stressors.

It is acknowledged that mere exposure to stressful life events does not inevitably lead to physical or psychological symptoms, because of external and internal mediators (Dohrenwend & Dohrenwend, 1974). The process of coping defined as a cognitive process that reduces the negative effects of stress, is believed to be a multivariate interaction between the individual's internal resources, the support resources available, and the actual type of stressors experienced (Cervantes & Castro, 1985). Cultural factors can have a wide-ranging effect on coping. Beliefs and attitudes as well as social resources available, such as the moderating effect of family support/belongingness, vary between cultures and are important in successful coping.

Family cohesion and external support (Brown, Harris, Adler & Bridge, 1986), are considered to be significant influences. Social support has been found to mitigate the effects of stressful life events. Many immigrant communities are from collectivist cultures and have strong family networks which may bolster them against the effects of acculturative stress. Further, Lin, Masuda and Tazuma (1979) found that the impact of stressors was negligible when community involvement was high. Cultures both prescribe some coping behaviour and proscribe others (Slavin et al., 1991). For example, religious beliefs can play an important role in some cultures. On the other hand majority cultural institutions may offer ways of coping that are not familiar to a given minority culture (e.g.: counseling and psychotherapy). Hence in examining coping, it is important to include culturally relevant factors.

Culture also informs the final stage of the model, that of physical and emotional health outcomes. Cultures may prescribe specific ways of showing distress. Sue and Sue (1990) discussed findings that Asian Americans were more likely than other people to present somatic concerns in counseling interviews. They argued this reflects the fact that physical complaints are usually perceived as legitimate and psychological complaints as shameful or unacceptable.

Research focusing on the **whole** process of acculturation of immigrants, especially the many and varied stresses of acculturating to a new and often very different way of life, as well as coping with these stresses successfully, so that psychological distress is minimal, has received only limited attention. Previous studies of the stress process have employed both quantitative and qualitative methods and instruments. This study was undertaken to examine the whole immigrant experience, adopting a qualitative, free-response strategy, and examining as many of the stressors and ways of coping as possible.

The aim of this study was to let immigrants speak for themselves, with minimum input from the researcher. Cross-cultural research often seems to be driven by existing Western paradigms and, as Slavin et al. (1991) write, tend to be Euro-centric. It is important that non-Western people are encouraged to express themselves without constraint. Therefore, this study attempted to examine the stress process in immigrant communities in Australia, without being too constrained by existing theoretical models.

Since the experiences of different immigrant groups cannot be identical, this study sampled two distinct groups in Australia. Literature suggested that ethnic identity, religion and culture influence the acculturative experience differently for different groups (Slavin et al., 1991). The two groups sampled represented these differences. Therefore, differences between them in the effects of acculturation would provide greater insight into how migration affects individuals andgroups differently. The choice of these two immigrant communities, Greeks and Filipinos, was intentional and based on perceived cultural differences between them. Since Greek migration took place many years before Filipino migration, and Greeks are an intact European culture, it was expected that they would have had more time and greater facility to develop an Australian-Greek identity. Filipinos are Asian in origin and their migration is more recent. However, Filipinos historically have been more open to Western influence and have greater facility when speaking English. Further, many Filipino women have married Anglo-Australians.

Method

Participants

The two immigrant communities chosen, Greek and Filipino, were resident in the Northern Territory, Australia. In-depth interviews were conducted with 50 subjects selected from each of the two communities. Individuals were selected on the basis of certain demographic variables such as gender, (25 males and 25 females from each community) age, education, and employment (to represent as equally as possible all age, employment and educational categories). The number of years resident in Australia was taken into account. The age range of the samples was 15-72 for the Filipinos and 20-65 for the Greeks, with a mean age at 34.44 (SD 14.62) for Filipinos and 39.36 (SD 14.9) for Greeks. Of the Filipino sample only 12% were born in Australia whereas 32% of Greeks were Australian born. The mean for schooling was 4.12 (SD=1.19) and 2.78 (SD=1.13) for Filipinos and Greeks respectively. (Schooling was coded 1= No schooling and 6=Post-graduate). There were 2% Greeks and 26% Filipinos in the unemployed category. There were no Filipinos in the professional category, and only 8% among the Greeks. Of the Greek sample 28% were single, 54% were married, 12% were divorced or separated and 6% were widowed. Of the Filipinos 38% were single, 50% were married and 12% divorced or separated. One-hundred per cent of Greeks and 98% Filipinos identified themselves as Christians.

The interviews were conducted by members of the same community. All interviews with Greeks were conducted by a Greek woman. The Filipinos were interviewed by a male (who interviewed the males) and a female (who interviewed the females). Selection of the sample was based on lists obtained from ethnic community organizations. Prospective subjects were contacted by telephone and if willing were then interviewed in their homes. The interviews took about two months to complete. Interviewers were thoroughly briefed by the researcher. Pilot interviews were also conducted and the interview schedule revised accordingly.

Instruments

The interview schedule consisted of assessment of stressors, coping strategies and demographic information. It consisted of both open-ended questions about stress and coping, as well as structured questions. The strategy was to first ask open-ended questions. (e.g.,) Have you had any worries lately? Would you like to talk about them?). If no response was forthcoming, certain prompts were used (e.g.,) Have you worried about your health (or finances etc. lately?). Finally, we adapted a checklist of ten of the most frequent hassles (Kanner, Caynes, Schaeler, & Lazarus, 1981). The interviewer ran through this checklist of common problems that individuals experience, (e.g.: health, finance, unemployment). Other stressors that were assessed included perceptions of discrimination, marginalisation, problems in social interaction outside one's community, employment history (possible loss of status), and lack of a sense of belonging. In assessing ways of coping, following free responses, a checklist of coping strategies (Mena, Padilla, & Maldonado, 1987) was used.

To estimate mental health, interviews and a shortened version (18 items) of the General Health Questionnaire (Goldberg & Williams, 1991) were used. This instrument measures both physical and psychological symptoms of distress. It has cross-cultural applicability having been used in about 38 languages and has over 50 published validity studies (GHQ Manual, p. 4). The authors claim that this instrument originally designed for use in South London is performing well in settings as diverse as Calcutta and rural Iceland. The GHQ has good psychometric properties and alphas range between .82 - .93.

There are now several shortened versions of the original 60 item test. For this study, an 18 item test was put together from results of pilot studies conducted with small samples from the two communities. Items that were retained from the 30 item version were those that seemed to be culturally appropriate and had acceptable item-total correlations. The GHQ is designed to identify specific psychological conditions such as the incidence of depression, anxiety, sleep disturbance as well as somatic symptoms,(Goldman & Williams, 1991, pp. 32-34). In this study the focus was on identifying general symptoms (psychological and somatic). Hence the shortened versions was suited to our purpose. Reliability of the shortened scale was .84 for Filipinos and .80 for the Greeks and compares well with reliabilities reported for the GHQ. The items were scored in the positive direction and a higher score indicated a higher sense of well-being.

Factor analysis of the GHQ scores, of both communities combined, was carried out. The technique used was principal components with varimax rotation, a technique used in most studies of the GHQ, (Goldberg & Williams, 1991, p. 27). Although six factors were identified, the screen plot as well as the items that loaded on each factor suggested that a two-factor solution would be the most efficient. The two factors together explained 41.32% of the variance. The first factor (eigenvalue=5.02) consisted of 11 items which described psychological symptoms such as feeling nervous and strung up, being constantly under strain, feeling scared and panicky, unhappy and depressed etc. The second factor (eigenvalue=2.42) consisting of 7 items, described physical symptoms such as tightness in the head, pain in the head, feeling run down, feeling ill etc. Regression factor scores were computed for the two factors that were labeled psychological and physical well-being.

Procedures

During the interviews respondents were encouraged to talk freely and expand on issues that evoked strong feelings. Interviewers were briefed by the researcher and the whole process was carefully monitored. A pilot study of sample interviews was carried out and the interview schedule revised accordingly. All interviews were taped and then transcribed. The GHQ was translated into Tagalog and Greek and back-translated to check for accuracy of translation. The transcribed interview material and the responses to the GHQ were returned to the researcher who then carried out the analyses.

Results

The responses to the checklists and to the GHQ scale, as well as to some open-ended questions were codified and converted to an SPSS file. In this paper the results of only the quantitative data analysed using the SPSS program will be presented. Some descriptive statistics will be reported to make comparisons between the communities as well highlight the preferred stress factors and coping strategies.

Stressors

An examination of day to day stressors revealed that Filipinos worried most about health (34%), unemployment (29.5%) and children (28.1%) and least about unfriendly neighbours, relationship problems, and physical appearance. Greeks worried most about finances (66%), health (54%), children (53.3%), too much work (50%) and unemployment (44.9%) and least about unfriendly neighbours, physical appearance and problems at work. Health related problems seemed to concern both groups. However, open-ended responses indicated that they worried mostly about family ill-health. Some Filipinos were especially concerned about ill-health of parents, especially those who were still in the Philippines. Although both groups had similar concerns, overall, day to day stressors seemed to affect Greeks more. A significantly larger percentage of Greeks endorsed the existence of many of these stressors. A composite score of daily stressors was computed and Greeks scored significantly higher (M=13.00, SD=2.00 & M=11.30, SD=1.98; t=-4.27 df= 98, p=.0001).

Other stressors (associated with the acculturative process), examined were perception of discrimination, both generally and in the work place, feeling of loneliness or isolation, not being accepted as equals by Anglo-Australians, misunderstanding with people of other ethnic communities, and being underemployed. These stressors seemed to affect the Greeks more. Fifty-four per cent of Greeks felt that they experienced difficulties because of their ethnicity and 52% believed that they were the butt end of racial jokes, and 36.2% of Greeks felt they were not treated as equals by the majority

Table 1. Differences in Stressor as a Function of Culture

Day to day stressors: Percentage Responding YES				
Stressors	Filipinos	Greeks	χ^2	p
Health	34.0	54.0	4.08	.04
Relationships	16.0	24.0	1.00	.31
Financial	28.0	66.0	14.87	.0001
Too much work	28.0	50.0	5.14	.02
About children	28.1	53.3	4.13	.04
Problems at work	20.0	21.7	1.71	.42
Unemployment	29.5	44.9	2.34	.12
Physical appearance	20.0	20.0	1.39	.49
Unfriendly neighbors	2.0	10.0	3.08	.07
Death in family/friend	20.0	26.0	0.51	.48
Stressors associated with acculturation: Percentage Responding YES				
Stressors	Filipinos	Greeks	χ^2	p
Problems due to ethnicity	30.0	54.0	5.97	.01
Butt end of racial jokes	44.0	52.0	1.89	.38
Discrimination at work	16.0 (20.0)*	16.0 (16.0)*	0.28	.86
Lonely/isolated	10.0	26.0	4.46	.03
Problems with other ethnics	16.0	04.0	4.25	.04
Not accepted as equals	24.5	36.2	2.75	.25
Educated in native language	02.1	62.0	52.76	.00000
Spoke native language only	06.0	62.0	42.71	.00000

* Figures in parentheses were 'maybe' responses.

population. In comparison, only 30% of Filipinos felt they had difficulties because of their ethnicity (a few mentioned the mail-order bride stigma) and 24.5% felt they were not treated equally. Although only 16% from both groups felt they had been discriminated against in terms of employment, 20% of Filipinos and 16% of Greeks, seemed unsure about it. Neither group seemed to feel lonely or isolated. Items of perceived discrimination were combined to get an overall score and the Greeks scored higher, (although the difference was not statistically significant). Another possible source of stress was lack of fluency in the English language. A large percentage of Greeks (62%) were educated in their native language and spoke only Greek at home.

Moderating Factors

Greeks migrated to Australia over a much longer period and hence the average years that they have been resident is 22.08 years. In comparison Filipinos have been in residence in Australia for only 11.27 years. Factors that contribute to a sense of family and social support were examined. All Filipinos sampled claimed to have several family members still in the Philippines and they claimed they visited the Philippines regularly and frequently (on the average 1.46 visits in 5 years) and called 'home' often (20% claimed to call weekly). The Greeks also had family links abroad and 82% said they had family members living in Greece, had visited on the average 1.1 times in five years. However, they did not call home as frequently (the reason for this could be either higher costs or less need). Fifty-eight percent called very infrequently. More Filipinos belong to indigenous organisations (68%) than Greeks (28%). However, more Greeks (57.4%) than Filipinos (34.7%) associated only with members of own their community. Both groups, (86% Filipinos and 84% Greeks), stated that their own traditions and customs were important to them. Neither group seemed to associate much with other immigrant groups. Fifty-nine per cent (59.2%) of Filipinos and 40.4% of Greeks said they had Anglo-Australian friends. A composite score of items measuring family ties was computed. Filipinos scored significantly higher than the Greeks on this (M=8.48, SD=1,77 and M=6.34, SD=1.71; t= 6.16 df=98, p = .0001).

Questions were also asked to determine level of satisfaction with life in Australia. Apart from asking what individuals particularly liked and disliked about living in Australia, they were also asked whether life was what they had expected it would be and if they felt they belonged. They were also asked whether they would like to return to their home country. Seventy-four per cent (74%) of the Filipinos and 78% of Greeks said that they belonged here. The majority (72% Filipinos and 54% Greeks) also said that life here was what they had expected it to be. However, 42% of the Filipinos and 40%

of the Greeks said that they would like to go back to their home country. A composite score of *feeling settled* showed that Filipinos felt more settled than the Greeks but the difference was not statistically significant (M=5.12, SD=0.98 & M=4.90 SD=1.14; t=0.96 p= .34).

Coping Strategies

Taking positive action seemed to be the most popular strategy for coping for both groups, followed *by talking to family and/or friends*, although Greeks found *doing something positive to take one's mind off the problem* more attractive. *Praying about the problem* was a popular option for both. Both groups were least likely to *seek professional help* (20% of the Greeks and 4% of Filipinos had seen a doctor for physical ailment). *Not worrying about problems* or *seeking community support* were not popular options. (See table 2 for percentages and chi-square results). An analysis of the relationship between levels of stress and ways of coping did not reveal any discernible pattern. Those who experienced more stress were not differentiated from those who experienced less in their choice of strategy for coping. In fact the choice of coping strategy did not seem to be related to the level of stress. Correlations ranged between -.08 (involve myself in other things to keep mind off problem) to .28 (seek professional help) for Filipinos and between -24 (talk to family/friends) and .24 involve myself in other things.....) for Greeks. None of the correlations were statistically significant (See Table 2).

Mental health status

The results (of the GHQ) suggest a high sense of well-being among individuals in both groups. The possible range of scores was 18 to 72[1], and the actual ranges were 40-72 (Filipinos) and 52-72 (Greeks). Mean scores for overall well-being were 62.42 for Filipinos and 63.24 for Greeks. A comparison of the mean scores of the two samples indicated that there was no statistical difference between them in their levels of physical and psychological well-being. On the whole both groups indicated a high sense of general well-being.

Factors contributing to mental health

Finally, an attempt was made to estimate the relationship between some of the independent variables and sense of well-being. Composite scores for independent variables such as the degree of involvement with family, perception of discrimination, feeling settled in Australia,

Table 2. Differences in Coping Strategies as a Function of Culture (Percentage Responding YES)

Strategies	Filipinos	Greeks	χ^2	*p*
Talk to friends/family	86.0	70.0	3.79	.05
Not worry, it will go away	32.0	38.0	0.49	.48
Take positive action	86.0	96.0	3.21	.07
Pray about it	70.0	68.0	0.05	.82
Seek professional help	04.0	20.0	6.55	.01
Do other things/take mind off	60.0	88.0	10.61	.001
Seek community support	22.0	08.0	3.97	.04

and an index of stress factors (worries) were computed. These variables as well as age and gender sex were correlated with GHQ total scores, as well as scores measuring physical and psychological well-being. On the whole relationships between well-being and the IVs were small and non-significant for Filipinos. However, a significant relationship between gender and total GHQ, as well as psychological well-being was found. Filipino women seem to have a higher sense of well-being than men. There was also a negative relationship between age as well as worry with physical well-being, which suggested that older Filipinos worried more and reported more physical distress. The younger subjects seem to experience more psychological distress.

Statistically significant correlations between several of the independent measures and physical and psychological well-being for the Greek sample seemed to suggest stronger relationships between them. Physical well-being was related to perception of discrimination, worry, and gender (with women experiencing less well-being). Psychological well-being was influenced by age, (younger Greeks having a higher sense of well-being), perception of discrimination, and worry. Those who felt more settled in their environment had a higher sense of psychological well-being. General well-being was also related to age (with the younger Greeks having a higher sense of well-being), and perception of discrimination and worry. Overall there seemed to be a more recognisable pattern of influence on mental health, especially psychological well-being for the Greeks. (see Table 3).

Table 3. Correlations between General Health Questionnaire Measures and Age, Gender, and Stressors

	Well-being					
	Physical		Psychological		General	
	F	G	F	G	F	G
Age	-.25	-.17	.27	-.48***	-.02	-.41**
Gender	.07	-.35**	.34**	.13	.29*	-.21
Home-ties	-.22	.13	-.00	.01	-.19	.11
Discrimination	-.21	-.28*	-.09	-.36**	-.22	-.42**
Settled	.17	-.23	-.19	.50**	.08	.11
Worry Index	-.35**	-.33**	.12	-.28**	-.18	-.42**

*** $p < .001$ ** $p < .01$ * $p < .05$ (all tests 2-tailed)
F=Filipino G=Greek

A standard linear multiple regression was performed between overall sense of well-being as the dependent variable and age, sex, number of years resident in Australia, ties with home, perception of discrimination, feeling settled in Australia, and an index of worries as independent variables for each of the two samples. The results suggest that only a weak and non-significant relationship exists between IVs and the DV for Filipinos. Only sex (β=.32) seemed to contribute to better mental health and together the IVs explained only 17% of the total variance.

For the Greeks however, perception of discrimination (β= -.30) as well as length of residence (β=-.34) contributed (negatively) to good mental health. Together the independent variables explained nearly 38 % of the variance (see table 4).

Discussion

The results suggest that both immigrant groups enjoy a remarkably high sense of well-being, which lends support to the argument advanced by Berry & Kim, (1988), that acculturative experiences do not inevitably bring about a decline in mental health. Although both groups seem to experience the stresses of day to day living (Greeks more than Filipinos), their sense of well-being seems positive. What seems to affect them negatively are perceptions of racism and discrimination.

The immigrant experience seems to be generally positive, for both groups, but more especially for Filipinos. To the open-ended questions about what they liked about living in Australia, the majority of respondent said that Australia provided better opportunities, a better living standard and a better future for their children. The Greeks mentioned unemployment in Greece as a factor in their decision to migrate and some of them expressed satisfaction that despite limitations of their own educational and occupational status their children had done well and some had even achieved tertiary education.

Table 4. Linear Multiple Regression analysis with GHQ as DV and age, sex, number of years resident, worry index, perception of discrimination, ties with home, & feeling settled as IVs for Greek sample only. (Method=Enter)

Multiple R	.616
R Square	.379
Adjusted R Square	.275
Standard Error	4.161

Analysis of Variance

	DF	Sum of Squares	Mean Square
Regression	7	443.84059	63.40580
Residual	42	727.27941	17.31618
F = 3.66	Sig. F = .0036		

Variables in the Equation

Variable	B	SE B	Beta	T	Sig T
AGE	-.023	.055	-.069	-.409	.684
PERDISCR	-.950	.483	-.299	-1.966	.056
SETTLED	.029	.864	.006	.033	.974
HOMETIES	-.345	.524	-.121	-.659	.514
WORRYIND	-.464	.411	-.190	-1.129	.265
YRSRESID	-.194	.095	-.338	-2.035	.048
SEX	-.026	1.276	-.003	- .020	.984
(Constant)	82.841	7.162	11.566	.000	

Therefore, although acculturative experiences seem to inevitably include certain negative aspects, better life chances in Australia seem to compensate for them to a great extent.

Most studies of acculturation seem to assume that mental health is promoted most by a strategy described as *integration*. Integration, one of the four different types of acculturative strategies (assimilation, integration, separation, and marginalisation; see Berry, Poortina, Segall, & Dasen, 1992), takes place when immigrant groups acculturate to their host culture while maintaining their own. Hence successful acculturation is assumed to take place when immigrants begin to participate in the life of the larger society (Murphy, 1965). This study however suggests that although 'integration' is the closed strategy to what seems to happen here, it does not necessarily pre-suppose full participation in the life of mainstream culture. It seems that both immigrant groups continue to maintain strong ethnic identities, and only minimally 'integrate' with the wider Australian community. The results of this study suggest that *integration* as a strategy needs re-defining or a new strategy defined.

Ideally in a multicultural society, all cultures are presumed to have equal status and are encouraged to maintain their way of life while integrating with mainstream culture. However, there is always a dominant culture and several minority cultures. It is possible that when a cultural group encounters an unfamiliar and dominant culture, it may be faced with the fear of losing it's familiar way of life and becoming swamped by the mainstream culture. This could provide the impetus to attempt to preserve familiar and valued traditions and culture. It seems that Filipinos and Greeks living in Australia continue to see themselves as primarily Filipino and Greek persons. Their own group provides a sense of community. It is said that the Greeks in Australia hold on to traditions even when people in Greece have changed them. This study certainly suggests that both groups, but especially the Greeks, seem to maintain strong ethnic identities even after many years in Australia.

The sense of cultural identity seems to be promoted by strong family/community ties (both in Australia and abroad). The Filipinos still have many close family members living in the Philippines with whom they keep in close contact and visit often. Therefore continuity of cultural identity does not seem to be threatened by immigration to a foreign country. However, stress associated with living in an alien cultural environment, especially perception of discrimination and racism as well as language difficulties, seem to have some impact on mental health for the Greeks. It must however be reiterated that day to day stressors as well as acculturative experiences do not seem to seriously jeopardise mental health. This brings us to the questions of how and why. This study suggests that close family involvement, and other means of coping (e.g., prayer) are effective means for immigrant groups.

Greek migration to Australia began many years before Filipinos were permitted to immigrate. But the Greeks seem more strongly embedded in their own culture and traditions than Filipinos. Interview data suggested that the older Greeks especially, are tradition driven. Many Greeks work for Greek employers, especially in the building trade and have social relationships mostly with each other. They have their church and cultural organisations and seem to celebrate their culture openly and proudly. Most older Greeks do not speak English fluently and seem to have a negative attitude about life in Australia. However, the younger generation of Greeks seem to have acculturated more and perhaps even assimilated with the mainstream, and seem to enjoy better mental health. Some inter-generational conflict was reported.

The acculturative experience which seems to be less stressful for the Filipinos, is perhaps related to greater exposure to Western influences

(Spanish and American) in their own country, greater competency in the English language, more education and inter-marriage with Anglo-Australians.

It seems that generally speaking migration to Australia of people of quite distinct cultures, which are different from the dominant Anglo-Saxon culture, does not necessarily impair mental health. Cultural groups have every opportunity to maintain their way of life as well as enjoy the benefits of material prosperity. They work hard and sacrifice immediate benefits for the sake of their children. The children then achieve higher status, and are more integrated. Those who experience lower sense of well-being seem to do so because of acculturative stress and not because of everyday stressors. Good mental health status seems to be related to a sense of cultural identity and sense of family.

References

Berry, J.W., & Kim, U. (1988). Acculturation and mental health. In P.Dasen, J.W. & N. Sartorius (Eds.), *Cross-cultural psychology and health: Towards applications* (pp. 207-236), London: Sage.

Berry, J.W., Kim, U., Minde,T., & Mok, D. (1977). Comparative studies of acculturative stress. *International Migration Review,* 21, 491-511.

Berry, J.W., Poortinga, Y.H., Segall, M.H., & Dasen, P.R. (1992) *Cross-cultural psychology*. Cambridge: Cambridge University Press.

Brown, G.W., Harris, A.T., Adler, Z., & Bridge, L. (1986). Social support , self-esteem and depression. *Psychological Medicine*, 16, 813-831.

Cervantes, R.C., & Castro, R.G. (1985). Stress, coping and Mexican American mental health: A systematic review. *Hispanic Journal of Behavioural Sciences, 7, 1-73.*

Cochrane, R. (1979). Psychological and behavioural disturbances in West Indian, Indian and Pakistanis in Britain: A comparison of rates among children and adults. *British Journal of Psychiatry*, 134, 210-210.

Dohrenwend, B.S., & Dohrenwend, B.P. (1974). *Stressful life events: Their nature and effects*. New York: Wiley.

Goldberg, D & Williams, P. (1991). *A user's guide to the General Health Questionnaire.* Berkshire: FER-Nelson.

Kanner,A.D., Cayne, J.C., Schaeler, C., & Lazarus, R.S. (1981). Comparison of two modes of stress measurement: Daily hassles and uplifts versus Major life events. *Journal of Behavioral Medicine*, 4 (1), 4 -39.

Kim, U. (1984). Psychological acculturation of Korean immigrants to Toronto: A study of modes of acculturation, identity, language and acculturative stress. Unpublished Master's thesis, Queens University, Canada.

Lasry, J.C. (1977) Cross cultural perspective on mental health and immigration adaptation. *Social Psychiatry*, 12, 49-55.

Lazarus, R.S. and Folkman, (1984). *Stress, appraisal and coping.* New York: Springer.

Lin, K.H., Masuda, M., & Tazuma, L. (1979). Adaptation problems of Vietnamese refugees I: Health and mental status. *Archives of General Psychiatry*. 36, 955-961.

Mena, F.J., Padilla, A.M., & Maldonado, M. (1987). Acculturative stress and specific coping strategies among immigration and later generation college students. *Hispanic Journal of Behavioral Sciences*, 9 (3), 207-225.

Murphy, H.B.M. (1965). Migration and the major mental disorders. In M. B. Kantor (Ed), Mobility and mental health (pp. 221-249). Springfield, IL: Thomas.

Murphy, H.B.M. (1973). The lower rate of mental hospitalization shown by immigrants in Canada. In Zwingmann & Pfister-Amende (Eds)., *Uprooting and after*. New York: Springer-Verlag.

Myers, H.F. (1982). Stress, ethnicity and social class: A model for research with Black populations. In. E.E. Jones & S.J. Korchin (Eds), *Minority mental health*. (Pp. 118-148). New York: Praeger.

Slavin, L.A., Rainer, K.L., McCreary, M.L., & Gowda, K.K. (1991). Towards a multicultural model of the stress process. *Journal of Counseling & Development*, 70, (Sept/Oct), 156-163.

Sue, D.W., & Sue, D. (1990). *Counseling the culturally different: Theory and practice*. New York: Wiley.

Taft, R. (1979). A comparative study of the initial adjustment of immigrant school children in Australia. *International Migration Review*, 13, 71-80.

---

[1] There are alternate methods of scoring the GHQ. The most common is the Likert scale format with scores ranging from 0-1 or the modifed version, where columns were assigned scores of 0,0,1,2 or 0,0,1,1. In this study in order to maximize differences, the items were scored from 1-4, hence the range of 18 to 72. This makes comparison with other studies of the GHQ difficult. However, in this study such comparisons were not intended. What we wanted was a useful measure of mental distress that could be correlated with stressors and coping strategies. Hence the unorthodox scoring was not considered a threat to the usefulness of the results.

Clinical Implications of Racial Identity in the Legacy of Apartheid in South Africa

Dan Hocoy
John F. Kennedy University
Graduate School of Professional Psychology
and
Pacifica Graduate Institute
Department of Psychology

ABSTRACT

Constructions of race have long played a central role in the apartheid ideology of South Africa that served to ensure White minority domination, while legitimizing the subordination of the Black majority. This chapter presents research from a 1995 nation-wide investigation, employing ethnography and phenomenological interviews, examining the impact of racial identification in the apartheid context. Content analyses of formal interviews with 15 Black South Africans revealed 14 common themes. The themes corresponded to a duality in response to racial identification, some suggesting psychological damage, while others indicating psychological resilience. When racial identification included the internalization of the myths of Black inferiority, negative psychological consequences resulted. Racial identification had a positive psychological impact when it involved the facilitation of a group consciousness, political mobilization, and acted as a source of empowerment, belongingness and pride. Racial categorizations in South Africa may be intractable given the persistence of socio-economic disparities between groups, and the positive functions racial identity serves for Blacks.

Constructions of race have long played a central role in the political psychology of South Africa. The boundaries defining racial categories have been constructed differently at different times and in different parts of the world (Birman, 1994), however, these boundaries are generally determined by the dominant or sociopolitically powerful group (Helms, 1994). In the case of South Africa, racial and ethnic boundaries were manipulated to benefit the interests of the White minority, and notions of inherited differences, which were fundamental to apartheid ideology, provided the requisite legitimation for Black exploitation.

Dommisse (1986) asserts that discrimination based on a racial categorization handed down from an external classifying authority is certain to have the direct psychological consequences of engendering insecurity and powerlessness. Apartheid has created feelings of "incompleteness" and "inferiority" among Blacks, and in general, has been "psychologically devastat(ing)" for the mental health of Black South Africans (Mohutsioa-Makhudu, 1989, p. 134). In addition, racial identity development among Black

South Africans is interrupted by the racial prejudice engendered by apartheid. South African social scientists (e.g., Dawes, 1985; Duncan & Rock, 1995; Foster, 1986; Whittaker, 1990) have long established the negative impact of racism on the psychological development of Blacks, and especially in regards to racial identity. Simpson (cited in Duncan & Rock, 1995) argues that the institutional racism of apartheid induces a host of race-related "disorders" or "conditions" among Blacks, including an extremely distorted and negative sense of self and anger towards their own group, as well as a pathological striving to be White (Simpson, cited in Duncan & Rock, 1995; Whittaker, 1990).

A Qualitative Study of the Impact of Racial Identification

The research presented here is based on a 1995 nation-wide study, employing qualitative methods, examining the impact of racial identification for the indigenous African peoples in the apartheid context. Although apartheid resulted in socio-economic and political conditions which had multiple and varied effects of their own, the focus of this study is the psychological effects and clinical implications of imposed racial classification and individual identification. The investigation consisted of formal and informal interviews, the study of census information and demographics, the examination of folklore and rituals, as well as observational study, conducted throughout the country, in townships and major cities, and in a variety of communities, representative of the socio-economic and cultural diversity of Blacks in South Africa.

Informal Interviews

Informal interviews were conducted to obtain additional information in order to supplement the formal interviews. Information regarding socio-political and economic context, history, attitudes and general lifestyles among the many diverse communities was gathered in informal interviews. These interviews were conducted in various townships (e.g., Khayalitcha, Crossroads, Gugulethu, Soweto, Sharpville), cities (e.g., Belleville, Cape Town, Knysna, Port Elizabeth, Durban, Johannesburg, Pretoria, Vanderbijlpark), as well as among the diversity of communities in South Africa, including various African ethnic communities, Coloured, British White, Afrikaner White, Indian, Greek, Italian, and Chinese communities. This qualitative research often involved living in households of the various communities, and immersing oneself in the community activities.

Informants

Informants for informal interviews generally consisted of what are termed "key informants," that is, individuals who possess special knowledge about the topic of interest, are in positions of authority or status in their community, and have the communicative skills to convey that knowledge. Key informants included local church ministers, domestic servants, national and provincial elected government officials (including a member of parliament, and a minister of local affairs), Black student leaders, owners of shabeen (i.e., illegal drinking establishments) owners, academics, newspaper hawkers (i.e., mobile street vendors), government lawyers, representatives of various political parties (e.g., African National Congress, South African Communist Party, Pan-Africanist Congress, Azanian People's Organization), etc. Informants were selected as community members through word of mouth as people "in the know" identified them. These informants were approached and information was gathered on an informal (i.e., casual conversation) and formal basis (i.e., elaborate interviews with note taking). The process of sampling and investigation involved identifying all those who have something to contribute to the question, getting their perspectives, continually recycling these perspectives among participants until some agreement is reached, then adding new participants as long as they bring new information or fresh viewpoints to the discussion. The data collected were compared and contrasted; a search for patterns was systematically conducted, and the framework was constantly adjusted to accommodate new information.

Formal Interviews

Formal interviews were conducted with individuals at Cape Technikon in Cape Town, Vaal Triangle Technikon in Vanderbijlpark, and Pretoria Technikon in Pretoria, South Africa. Technikons are tertiary education in situations that comprise a system running parallel to the university system, offering degrees in applied technology. Interviews ranged from 55 to 75 minutes in length.

Informants

The informants for the formal interviews consisted of 7 women and 8 men, aged 18 to 54, all of whom were Black (i.e., both parents were of indigenous African heritage), except in the case of one woman and one man, for whom one parent was Coloured. Informants were drawn from the technikons, and selected so as to constitute a fairly diverse cross-section of Black South African society. The sample in this study included, for instance: a library assistant, technikon lecturers, a computer salesperson, Black student leaders, a receptionist, a counselling psychologist, technikon students, and a vocational officer.

Method of Analysis (Formal Interviews)

The first step in the investigation involved the procedure of "bracketing." Bracketing is the active identification of one's own biases and expectations, as well as the sociohistorical context in which this research is taking place, and the implicit values therein which may influence the research. Extensive self-examination and an evaluation of present sociohistorical currents achieved this, and a documentation of these prejudices, desires, values and anticipations with regard to the research question. The particular phenomenological procedures used in this study conform to the phenomenological praxis (techniques) recommended by Giorgi (1983) and the systematic procedure of investigation advocated by Kruger (1982). Fifteen informants were interviewed to discern an experiential framework for the effects of racial identification on Black South Africans. The informants were interviewed in an unstandardized, open-ended manner, consistent with Kvale's (1989) recommendations regarding the primacy and importance of the initial research interview and effective interviewing.

The Interview

Informants were asked if they had experienced discrimination, and what effect it had on their lives. Informants were asked to provide a life-long retrospective on how apartheid affected them in general, and especially, with regard to their racial identity development and mental health. Each interview was audiotaped and reviewed several times until the author had an intuitive "feel" for what had been said. It is here the investigator gets a sense of the gestalt, and the spirit of what was said, which may sometimes be different from the components that comprise the experience. Each interview was transcribed and then analyzed employing the following procedure recommended by Spinelli (1989). First, "natural meaning units" relevant to the topic of study were extracted from the transcribed text. Natural meaning units are units of speech (i.e., word, phrase, or sentence) that in themselves form independent, but whole sentiments, having discrete meanings. The natural meaning units were then compared and condensed into what are called "aspects" of the phenomenon of interest, which are the themes or common meanings upon which the natural meaning units converge.

A second order profile of the original text was developed in terms of these aspects for each individual, which included the frequency with which a particular aspect was expressed. An "essential description" of the individual's experience of discrimination was then formulated; this serves to communicate the tone and spirit of the perspective particular to the individual. It also serves to elaborate on the more generic categorical descriptions found in the second order profiles. The second order profiles of all the subjects were then compared for common aspects in an aggregate analysis. The common aspects were further condensed into distinct "themes" found in the experience of discrimination. The criterion for the designation of a theme was that at least four of the fifteen protocols found description in a particular theme.

Results

Fourteen themes emerged from the aggregate analysis of informants' testimonies (N=number of informants endorsing the theme): 1) experiences heightened

Black self-perception (N=15), 2) experiences anxiety and fear (N=15), 3) possesses high Black esteem (N=15), 4) experiences challenges to self-esteem (N=14), 5) feels hatred toward Whites (N=14), 6) discovers resilience, determination, and defiance (N=13), 7) possesses symptoms of depression (N=12), 8) identifies socio-economic restrictions, racial inequities, and personal loss (N=12), 9) employs coping mechanisms (N=11), 10) receives support, heritage, and inspiration from various sources (N=10), 11) experiences physiological symptoms (N=9), 12) various attributions are made for apartheid and inferior status (N=9), 13) women experience double discrimination (N=4), and 14) feels pressures to assimilate to the dominant / White culture (N=4).

Duality

The themes discerned corresponded to a dichotomy in the psychological impact of racial identification for Black South Africans, namely damage and resilience.

Damage

Qualitative findings revealed that when racial identification included the internalization of the myths of Black inferiority, negative psychological consequences resulted, including experiencing fear and anxiety, lower self-esteem (and sense of inferiority), depression, physiological problems, desires to assimilate, and a double discrimination (i.e., race and gender) for women.

These results find substantial support in previous empirical research. For instance, Simpson (cited in Duncan & Rock, 1995) and Whittaker (1990) similarly found in Black South Africans a pathological striving for assimilation into the dominant group. This assimilationist tendency is clearly not an attempt at biculturalism or an integrationist strategy as the pursuit of the dominant culture is at the expense of one's indigenous heritage and mental health. Based on a review of clinical studies, Peters (1978) concluded that racism results in psychopathology in Blacks by depriving them of the self-esteem necessary for the maintenance of good mental health. Previous research conducted with Black South Africans has also indicated the prevalence of depression. For instance, Hickson and Kriegler (1991), in a study to identify the mental health needs of Black South Africans, found depression and suicide to be major problems and ones which were escalating. Similarly, Mkhize (1994), looking at mental health implications as a result of violent racial oppression, found 75% of respondents to be suffering from depression. Other studies consistently demonstrate the prevalence of depression and high incidence of suicide among Black South Africans (e.g., World Health Organization, 1983).

Women in the study experienced a "double discrimination," from not only Whites but other Africans as well. Women experienced greater socio-economic restrictions on their lives, as a result of strict gender roles in patriarchal African traditions, as well as greater challenges to their self-esteem.

These findings are consistent with the "double jeopardy hypothesis" (e.g., Pak & Dion, 1991) that women of Color experience the additional oppression of gender discrimination.

Data also revealed that the depression found among participants in the present study originated from many sources, many of which concerned the socio-economic situation of Blacks in South Africa as a result of apartheid. This is similar to findings in the U.S. For instance, Baker (1990), in an attempt to identify etiological factors in Black suicide in the U.S., reviewed the literature and statistics since 1950, and concluded that only psychological theories that consider racism and the effects of poverty and financial problems and family discord can adequately address the specific causes of Black suicide. Similarly, Dillihay (1989) identified racism, changing cultural values, high rates of unemployment, lack of educational opportunities, and low family income as factors that have contributed to the dramatic increase in youth suicides in African Americans over the last 30 years.

The evidence of psychological damage in the present study is consistent with Dommisse's (1986) assertion that discrimination, based on a racial categorization handed down from an external classifying authority, is certain to have the direct psychological consequences of engendering insecurity and powerlessness. Psychiatric illness has been implicated as a consequence of police repression and torture, while stress and illness have been associated with the apartheid system in urban-dwelling, Black South Africans (Turton & Chalmers, 1990). H.I. Van der Spuy and D. A. Shamley (cited in Duckitt, 1985) suggest that chronically elevated levels of neurotic symptomatology in Black South Africans can be attributed to the experience of racial discrimination and prejudice in that country.

Analysis of life-span interview data showed that one of the negative psychological consequences of apartheid and its ideological racial order is internalized inferiority. Clearly, one of the intentioned outcomes of the ideology of apartheid was to engender in Africans a sense of inferiority, which would legitimize the racial order and pre-empt any resistance to it. This powerful form of social control was effective and successful in South Africa. Other researchers have also found identification with a derogated race to create feelings of "incompleteness" and "inferiority" among Blacks, and in general, has been "psychologically devastat(ing)" for the mental health of Black South Africans (e.g., Mohutsioa-Makhudu, 1989, p. 134). Schlemmer (1976) found among 298 Black South Africans, 25% conceding some justification for apartheid by citing lack of education or skills in Blacks, or the superiority of White culture, thus exhibiting an internalization of apartheid dogma. To explain this phenomenon, Clark (1975, cited in Guishard, 1992) argued that an internalized denigration is part of a strategy of "adaptive inferiority", to survive a world in which Black people everywhere inevitably come to experience life from an inferior position

(Megwalu, 1990). Individuals who have internalized inferiority and self-hatred are described as bearing the "mark of oppression" (Kardiner & Ovesey, 1951).

The results of the present study reflect a long history of the mark of oppression in oppressed groups. Foster (1993) provides an extensive and eloquent review. Early American psychologists demonstrated the mark of oppression in Black children, evidenced by a preference for things White (Klineberg, 1944), and a preference for and identification with White rather than Black dolls (Clark & Clark, 1947). Myrdal (1944) writes that this valuation of White and denigration of Black "produces a personality problem for practically every single Negro. And few Negroes accomplish an entirely successful adjustment" (p. 699). At the same time, writings about the response of Jewish people to cultural oppression contributed to the notion of "mark of oppression." Bettelheim (1943) asserted that one defence used by Jews in Nazi concentration camps was to identify with Nazi camp commanders; Sartre (1948) and Lewin (1948) regarded Jewish self-hatred as one response to anti-Semitism. The writings of Black psychiatrists Fanon (1952/67) and Memni (1957/67), the former forwarding the concept of "Black skin, White masks" furthered notions of psychological damage from colonial oppression. In the U.S., both Black activists and White liberals had found a tool against the remnants of racial inequity. In 1954, social scientists, including Kenneth Clark and Gordon Allport, using the damage thesis, contributed to legal argument in the historic *Brown vs. Board of Education* case, the result of which was the prohibition against educational segregation in the U.S. By the mid-1960s, it was generally accepted that Blacks were "damaged," identity-conflicted, and had lower self-esteem as a result of discrimination and segregation (Foster, 1993).

Resilience

In addition to psychological damage resulting from racial identification, the results also show evidence of positive psychological consequences or responses. Themes derived from the qualitative findings indicated that racial identification also facilitated: group consciousness (and political mobilization), Black esteem, employing coping mechanisms, receiving support, heritage, and inspiration from various sources, and a sense of one's own resilience. Black racial identity was reclaimed to become a source of empowerment, belongingness, pride, and confidence. Interview data clearly indicated that Blacks were not merely passive recipients or victims of oppression, but exhibited resilience, determination, defiance, and courage as a response to their oppression. The life-span interviews revealed that the struggles inherent in apartheid allowed Black South Africans to witness their own strength, capabilities, versatility, and ultimately their own worth. Coping with and overcoming the difficulties of apartheid has engendered confidence, character, identity, and pride in themselves, other Blacks, and their African heritage. As a result, they also experienced feelings of love, responsibility, commitment to and solidarity with other Blacks. Many participants articulated that apartheid stimulated their personal "maturation" and formation of their racial identity, and that witnessing their resilience allowed for belief and pride in themselves. It seems that apartheid was the fire by which their strength, character, pride and identity was forged.

Duncan and Rock (1995) assert that South African Blacks are not passive victims of apartheid, but rather active agents in shaping their reality. Edwards and Riordan (1994) found Black South African university students to be high in resourcefulness compared to Whites and attributed this resourcefulness to a general stress-inoculation effect from the deprived conditions of apartheid. Similarly, Cain (1994) found racism to result in a strengthened sense of inner-directedness rather than a lack of control in the lives in African Americans. Also alluding to a person's basic resilience, Cross (1995) posits that "one's basic personality strengths act as a psychological cushion or relative backdrop of stability for the intense struggle taking place...successful completion of Nigrescence rides or floats on whatever are the person's extant personality strengths" (p. 69). Comparable findings are purported in acculturation studies. Berry (1992b) writes that some individuals change psychologically in an adaptive fashion rather than necessarily in a maladaptive way, and that "acculturation sometimes enhances one's life chances and mental health" (Berry, 1992a, p. 9).

The sense of unity found among participants in the study is also consistent with previous findings in South Africa, which have generally shown a "consistent trend of increased common Black identification and an erosion of tribal-based identities" (Foster & Nel, 1991, p. 156). There is considerable evidence of a collective sense of common Black identity above and beyond individual ethnic identities (e.g., Crijns, 1959; Edelstein, 1972), one which is derived from the common fate of the "(W)hite man's oppression" (Crijns, 1959, p. 127). Previous intergroup research has also found a sense of in-group solidarity with the heightened in-group identification resulting from perceived discrimination (e.g., Coser, 1956; Fiedler, 1967; Janis, 1968; Sherif, 1953).

The theme of resilience among Black South Africans was also found in conjunction with the active employment of various coping mechanisms, including cognitive strategies, such as attributing their inferior status in the country to an oppressive government, not inherent traits. The consciousness that the origin of Black problems was external was reported to be facilitated by the writings and alternative conceptualizations, of Black activists and intellectuals (e.g., Steven Biko). Other coping strategies including resorting to community, religion, humour and song. These findings have support in South African research. Finchilescu (cited in Foster, 1993) found that for South African Blacks, attributions for apartheid were a function of the perceived legitimacy of the race hierarchy. Many Black South Africans have been found to attribute their inferior status and socio-economic situation to a racist government (Geber & Newman, 1980), and South African Blacks who attributed their failures to external factors were found to have high self-esteem (Lobban, 1975). These coping strategies are consistent with the Black struggle elsewhere. Bagley and Copeland (1994), comparing the coping skills of African and African American graduate students, found no differences in coping strategies. Consistent with these findings, a factor analysis of the racial socialization of African American adolescents revealed four factors, including spiritual and religious coping, extended family caring, cultural pride reinforcement, and racism awareness teaching (Stevenson, 1994).

The theme of drawing strength and support from family, community and African heritage to withstand the oppression of apartheid from the present investigation finds support in South African and U.S. research. For instance, Orpen (1992) found social support from Black peers to moderate the effects of work stress on personal strain among Blacks in South Africa. Social support from White supervisors did not reduce work stress. Demo and Hughes (1990) found that relations with family, friends, and community were important in fostering a sense of racial and group identity among African Americans. Haw (1991) found African American women deriving self-esteem from family and friends, which allowed them to challenge the inferiorizing effects of racism. In addition to the family caring, racism awareness teaching, cultural pride reinforcement found in African American adolescent socialization, themes of protective and proactive racial socialization and cultural empowerment were also found (Stevenson, 1994). Similarly, Baldwin, Brown, and Rackley (1990) found that the development of African self-consciousness among Black college students to be dependent on the racial or cultural orientation of the home or external socialization environment. Ward (1995), examining the historical traditions of caring and interdependence in African communities, concluded that a reconnection with African communal values and traditions allows Blacks to develop racial identity and solidarity and in turn, to withstand economic and social oppression. Ford-Harris et al. (1991) and Ford, Harris, and Schuerger (1993) found role models, mentors, family and group counselling to be useful intervention strategies for counselling Black students. Similarly, Berry (1992a) identifies social support (i.e., intact communities, extended families, and cultural institutions) as a key psychological variable for the acculturating individual in coping with the stresses of (enforced) acculturation. It seems that African cultural traditions and community counter the influences of the dominant culture and facilitate a favourable resolution of the inevitable identity conflict that emerges from enforced acculturation (Peretti & Wilson, 1995). In a national survey of Black self-concept in the U.S., Hughes and Demo (1989) found all components of self-concept (i.e., racial self-esteem, personal self-esteem and personal efficacy) to be founded in the quality of interpersonal relations with friends and family.

Informants regarded African tradition and values (conveyed by family and community) as a means to dealing with the difficulties of racial identity in apartheid; this finding is also consistent with previous research. For instance, Africentric values were found to be more important than Black identity and self-esteem in drug prevention strategies for African Americans (Belgrave et al., 1994). Informants in this study remember specific events and people in their development of racial identity. Similarly, Stevenson (1995) found specific types of racial socialization corresponding to different stages of racial identity development. Participants also mentioned personal religious beliefs as sources of support (Hocoy, 1997). Religiosity has long been found to be a psychosocial resource in facing the difficulties of racism and acculturation in African Americans (e.g., Neff & Hoppe, 1993).

This finding of resilience among Black South Africans finds support in past research on Blacks. Again, Foster (1993) provides a review. Empirical research has provided substantial evidence of resilience, including: consistent findings of equal or higher self-esteem in Blacks in contexts of oppression, (e.g., Rosenberg, 1979; Stone, 1981), themes of protest, resistance to assimilation (Pettigrew, 1964), resilience and strength in overwhelming oppression (Coles, 1964), and "Black rage" against continued discrimination (Grier & Cobb, 1968). This resiliency is highlighted by the Black Power / consciousness movement of the late 1960's in reframing and bringing attention to the attributes of resistance, striving, courage, and resilience (Foster, 1993), providing an alternative to the damage thesis. More recently, Parham and Austin (1994) argue for the recognition of the concept of Nigrescence, which suggests that Blacks have not universally assimilated into European American culture. In addition, Haw (1991) has found that African Americans, rather than capitulating to dominant culture ideology, construct their own, one in which their racial heritage is affirmed.

Duality or Bidirectionality of Influence?

The findings of the present study on Black South Africans reflect that of the general literature, in its findings of both psychological "damage" and positive developments (including buffering mechanisms) that emerge from the individual as a result of racial identification in a context of apartheid. There has been consistent and substantial evidence from previous empirical research in support of the damage thesis, and equally, evidence to various positive attributes and processes that are revealed or facilitated through racial identification in racial oppression. It seems that these two tendencies are not mutually exclusive and that there appears to be a duality with regard to the effects of race identification in oppression. On the one hand, problems of racial identity, self-esteem, mental health, own-group hatred, and dominant group identification emerge as a result of racial identification in oppression. On the other hand, the resilience, coping, defiance, and solidarity similarly emerge in response, and the oppression serves as a stimulus in the development of identity, character, maturation, pride, and confidence. A resilience response suggests that the social and contextual conditions of aparthied may not impact unidirectionally on individual psychology, but rather that the environment is shaped also by the character of the oppressed individuals. The duality elaborated here is consistent with Allport's (1954/1979) intro- and extro-punitive personality dichotomy for African Americans. According to Allport, there exist a dual response to racial oppression, intropunitive Black "tends, if not actually to blame himself (for having suffered disproportionately), at least to take the responsibility upon himself for adjusting to the situation, while the extro-punitive Black blames the outer causes of his handicap" (p. 160).

The Dictate to "Unthink" Race

South Africa is a microcosm of world situations in which culture and race are used in the political psychology of political domination and social control. However, Black racial identity persists not only as a function of an imposed identity from outsiders, it is also sustained in large part by group members' own perceived needs, instrumental and symbolic (Adam, 1995). When voluntary, race identification serves essential personal identity and group affiliation needs, is fundamental to psychosocial development (e.g., McEwen et al., 1990) and a contributor to psychological health (Berry, 1994). In addition, race continues to serve important political ends for Blacks; race is an issue not to be dismissed in a color-blindness that only serves the status quo. In the same vein, race classifications also delineate claims to entitlement. As well, race also must inevitably be invoked to be able to address past and present injustices, discriminatory practices based on race. The continued importance of attention to race in redressing past wrongs will sustain inescapably sustain such categorizations. Another likely factor perpetuating racial distinctions is the natural psychological processes of perception. The salience of racial identity (e.g., skin color), combined with natural psychological tendencies to categorize in human perception (e.g., Olson & Zanna, 1993), make not seeing race exceptionally difficult. Cultural and historical factors also impinge here to make race "an ingrained collective perception" for all groups (Adam, 1995; p. 463). Language also conspires against non-racialism, as any reference to "race" only serves to reinforce these perceptions (as in the example of trying "not thinking of a pink elephant"). However, this may be unavoidable, as South Africa is discovering, since it is difficult to employ language outside the pre-existing racial terminology to refer to these collectivities.

Given these factors, the demand to "unthink" race is likely an unreasonable and unattainable one. It appears that such distinctions may be intractable and even serve some beneficial purpose. The problem may have more to do with the differential valuing of racial collectivities, rather than notions of race itself (e.g., Adam, 1995).

References

Adam, H. (1995). The politics of ethnic identity: Comparing South Africa. *Ethnic and Racial Studies, 18*, 457-475.

Allport, G. W. (1954/1979). *The nature of prejudice*. Cambridge, MA: Addison-Wesley.

Bagley, C. A., & Copeland, E. J. (1994). African and African American graduate students' racial identity and personal problem-solving strategies. *Journal of Counseling and Development, 7,* 167-171.

Baldwin, J. A., Brown, R., & Rackley, R. (1990). Some socio-behavioral correlates of African self-consciousness in African-American college students. *Journal of Black Psychology, 17*, 1-17.

Baker, F. M. (1990). Black youth suicide: Literature review with a focus on prevention. *Journal of the National Medical Association, 82,* 495-507.

Belgrave, F. Z., Cherry, V. R., Cunningham, D., & Walwyn, S. (1994). The influence of Africentric values, self-esteem, and Black identity on drug attitudes among African American fifth graders: A preliminary study. *Journal of Black Psychology, 20,* 143-156.

Berry, J. W. (1992a). *Psychological and social health of Aboriginal Peoples in Canada.* Paper prepared for the Royal Commission on Aboriginal Peoples, Ottawa.

Berry, J. W. (1992b). *Panel 3e5 - Health: Psychological impacts.* Draft report submitted to the Moose River / James Bay Coalition.

Berry, J. W. (1994). *Aboriginal cultural identity.* Report prepared for the Royal Commission on Aboriginal peoples, Urban Perspectives Research.

Bettelheim, B. (1943). Individualism and mass behavior in extreme situations. *Journal of Abnormal and Social Psychology, 38.*

Birman, D. (1994). Acculturation and human diversity in a multicultural society. In J. Trickett, R. J. Watts, and D. Birman (Eds.), *Human diversity: Perspectives on people in contex (*pp. 261-284). San Francisco: Jossey-Bass.

Cain, R. A. (1994). Perception of power/control among African Americans: A developmental approach. *Western Journal of Black Studies, 18,* 164-174.

Clark, K. B. & Clark, M. P. (1947). Racial identification and preference in Negro children. In T. M. Newcomb and E. L. Huntley (Eds.), *Readings in social psychology* (pp. 169-178). New York: Holt.

Coles, R. (1964). *Children of crisis*. Boston: Atlantic Monthly.

Coser, L. A. (1956). *The functions of social conflict.* Glencoe, IL: Free Press.

Crijns. A. G. J. (1959). *Race relations and race attitudes in South Africa.* Nijmegen: Janssen.

Cross, W. E. (1995). In search of Blackness and Afrocentricity: The psychololology of Black identity change. In H. W. Harris, H. C. Blue, and E. E. H. Griffith (Eds.), *Racial and ethnic identity* (pp. 53-72). New York: Routledge.

Dawes, A. (1985). Politics and mental health: The position of clinical psychology in South Africa. *South African Journal of Psychology, 15,* 55-61.

Demo, D. H., & Hughes, M. (1990). Socialization and racial identity among Black Americans. *Social Psychology Quarterly, 53,* 364-374.

Dillihay, T. C. (1989). Suicide in Black children. *Psychiatric Forum, 15,* 24-27.

Dommisse, J. (1986). The psychological effects of Apartheid psychoanalysis: Social, moral and political influences. *International Journal of Social Psychology, 1986; Summary Volume.*

Duckitt, J. H. (1985). Prejudice and neurotic symptomatology among White South Africans. *Journal of Psychology, 119,* 15-20.

Duncan, N. & Rock, B. (1995). *Inquiry into the effects of public violence on children (Preliminary Report).* Cape Town: Commission of Inquiry Regarding the Prevention of Public Violence and Intimidation. (GPS Publication No. 003-0198).

Edelstein, M. L. (1972). *What do young Africans think?* Johannesburg: South African Institute of Race Relations.

Edwards, D., & Riordan, S. (1994). Learned resourcefulness in Black and White South African university students. *Journal of Social Psychology, 134,* 665-675.

Fanon, F. (1952/1967). *Black skin, white masks.* New York: Grove Press. Fiedler, F. E. (1967). The effect of intergroup competition on group member adjustment. *Personnel Psychology, 20,* 33-44.

Ford, D. Y., Harris, J. J., Schuerger, J. M. (1993). Racial identity development among gifted Black students: Counseling issues and concerns. *Journal of Counseling and Development, 71,* 409-417.

Ford-Harris, D. Y., Schuerger, J. M., Harris, J. J. (1991). Meeting the psychological needs of gifted Black students: A cultural perspective. *Journal of Counseling and Development, 69,* 577-580.

Foster, D. (1986). The development of racial orientation in children: A review of South African literature. In S. Burman & P. Reynolds (Eds.), *Growing up in a divided society: The context of childhood in South Africa.* Johannesburg: Raven Press.

Foster, D. (1993). The mark of oppression: Racism and psychology reconsidered. In L. J. Nicolas (Ed.) *Psychology and oppression: Critiques and proposals.* Johannesberg: Skotaville Publishers.

Foster, D., & Nel, E. (1991). Attitudes and related concepts. In D. Foster & J. Louw-Potgieter (Eds.), *Social psychology in South Africa.* Johannesburg: Lexicon Publishers.

Geber, B. A., & Newman, S. P. (1980). *Soweto's children: The development of attitudes.* London: Academic Press.

Giorgi, A. (1983). Concerning the possibility of phenomenological research. *Journal of Phenomenological Psychology, 14,* 23-29.

Grier, W. H. & Cobb, P. M. (1968). *Black rage.* New York: Basic Books.

Guishard, J. (1992). People who live in posh houses shouldn't throw stones. *Educational and Child Psychology, 9,* 42-47.

Haw, K. F. (1991). Interactions of gender and race – A problem for teachers? A review of the emerging literature. *Educational Research, 33,* 12-21.

Helms, J. E. (1994). The conceptionalization of racial identity and other "racial" concerns. In J. Trickett, R. J. Watts, and D. Birman (Eds), *Human diversity: Perspectives on people in context.* San Francisco: Jossey-Bass, pp. 285-311.

Hickson, J. & Kriegler, S. (1991). The mission and role of psychology in a traumatised and changing society: The case of South Africa. *International Journal of Psychology, 26,* 783-793.

Hughes, M. & Demo, D. H. (1989). Self-perceptions of Black Americans: Self-esteem and personal efficacy. *American Journal of Sociology, 95,* 132-159.

Janis, I. L. (1968). Group identification under conditions of external danger. in D. Cartwright & A. Zander (Eds.) *Group dynamics* (3rd ed.). New York: Harper & Row.

Kardiner, A. & Ovesey, L. (1951). *The mark of oppression: A psychological study of the American Negro.* Cleveland: World Publishing.

Kruger, D. (1982). *An introduction into phenomenological psychology.* Pittsburg: Duquesne University Press.

Kvale, S., 1989, The primacy of the interview. *Methods* (Spring 1989 Annual Edition).

Lewin, K. (1948). *Resolving social conflicts.* New York: Harper.

Lobban, G. (1975). Self attitudes of urban Africans. In S. J. Morse &C. Orpen (Eds.), *Contemporary South Africa.* Cape Town: Juta.

McEwen, M. K., Roper, L. D., Bryant, D. R., Langa, M. J. (1990). Incorporating the development of African-American students into psychosocial theories of student development. *Journal of College Student Development, 31,* 429-436.

Megwalu, H. R. (1990). Black identity development: An international perspective. *Journal of African Psychology, 1,* 9-14.

Memmi, A. (1957/1967). *The colonizer and the colonized.* Boston: Beacon Press.

Mkhize, H. (1994). Violent oppression: Implications for mental health priorities in South Africa. *Medicine and Law, 13,* 193-203.

Mohutsioa-Makhudu, Yvonne, N. (1989). The psychological effects of apartheid on the mental health of Black South African women domestics. *Journal of Multicultural Counseling and Development, 17,* 134-142.

Myrdal, G. (1944). *An American dilemma.* New York: Harper & Brothers.

Neff, J. A., Hoppe, S. K. (1993). Race/ethnicity, acculturation, and psychological distress: Fatalism and religiosity as cultural resources. *Journal of Community Psychology, 21,* 3-20.

Olson, J. M., & Zanna, M. P. (1993). Attitudes and attitude change. *Annual Review of Psychology, 44,* 117-154.

Orpen, C. (1992). Social support as a moderator of the effect of work stress on personal strain among Black employees in South Africa. *Journal of Social Psychology, 132,* 269-270.

Parham, T. A., & Austin, N. L. (1994). Career development and African Americans: A contextual reappraisal using the nigrescence construct. *Journal of Vocational Behavior, 44,* 139-154.

Peretti, P. O., & Wilson, T. T. (1995). Unfavourable outcomes of the identity crisis among African-American adolescents influenced by enforced acculturation. *Social Behavior and Personality, 23,* 171-175.

Peters, M. (1978). Psychosocial determinants of depression among Blacks. *Transnational Mental Health Research Newsletter, 20,* 5-9.

Pettigrew, T. F. (1964). *A profile of the American Negro.* Princeton: Van Nostrand. Rosenberg, M. (1979). *Conceiving the self.* New York: Basic Books.

Sartre, J. P. (1948). *Portrait of the anti-semite.* London: Secker & Warburg.

Schlemmer, L. (1976). Political adaptation and reaction among urban Africans in South Africa. *Social Dynamics, 2,* 3-18.

Sherif, C. W. (1961). Self radius and goals of youth in different urban areas. *Southwestern Social Science Quarterly,December,* 259-270.

Sherif, M. (1953). The concept of reference groups in human relations. In M. Sherif & M. O. Wilson (Eds.) *Group relations at the crossroads.* New York: Harper.

Spinelli, E. (1989). *The interpreted world.* London: Sage.

Stevenson, H. C. (1994). Validation of the Scale of Racial Socialization for African American adolescents: Steps toward multidimensionality. *Journal of Black Psychology, 20,* 445-468.

Stevenson, H. C. (1995). Relationship of adolescent perceptions of racial socialization to racial identity. *Journal of Black Psychology, 21,* 49-70.

Stone, M. (1981). *The education of the Black child in Britain.* London: Fontana.

Turton, R. W., & Chalmers, B. E. (1990). Apartheid, stress and illness: The demographic context of distress reported by South African Africans. *Social Science and Medicine, 31,* 1191-1200.

Ward, J. V. (1995). Cultivating a morality of care in African American adolescents: A culture-based model of violence prevention. *Harvard Educational Review, 65,* 175-188.

Whittaker, S. R. (1990). Education for oppression: The case of psychology in Azania/South Africa. *Psychology Quarterly, 1,* 5-14.

World Health Organization. (1983). *Apartheid and health.* Geneva: Author.

Author Note

The author would like to thank Jenny Pretorius, George Savage, and Mariana Bothma for their invaluable assistance in this research.

Psychologists on Board South Africa's Health Care Train: Can We Offer a Service, or are We Just There for the Ride?

Sonja Goedeke
Formerly of the University of Natal Pietermaritzburg, South Africa
Department of Educational Psychology

Robin Farman
University of Natal Pietermaritzburg, South Africa
Department of Educational Psychology

ABSTRACT

A Primary Health Care Train brings health care services to historically disadvantaged rural communities in South Africa. These services are provided by university faculty and trainees in the various disciplines. For many, this provides a novel experience in living and working among people of other cultures and languages as co-workers and clients. Psychology offers psycho-education, limited counselling, resource development facilitation, support for other train personnel, and education about the potential role of psychology. The communities served have had little access to formal health care resources. Coping with child abuse, sexual abuse, depression, learning difficulties and family relationships emerged as areas of need. This paper reflects upon the experiences of faculty, trainees and community members. It asks and provides tentative answers to the question of whether westernised psychology can offer a relevant service in this setting.

The Crisis in Psychology in South Africa

Several criticisms have been directed at the profession, practice and theory of psychology in South Africa in recent years. In 1981, Holdstock described psychology as "probably the most useless endeavour in society" (Holdstock, 123). Many of his criticisms about psychology are still voiced today: psychology is (1) pathology orientated, retroactive and curative in nature (Daniels, 1994); 2) focused on an elitist client base that is predominantly white, middle class (Bassa & Schlebusch, 1984; Dawes, 1985; Lazarus, 1988; Manganyi & Louw, 1986; Swartz, Dowdall & Swartz, 1986); and 3) too individualistic and fails to take cognisance of social contexts in the origin and treatment of disorders (Foster & Louw-Potgieter, 1991). Traditional psychology has failed to adequately acknowledge that many South Africans see their mental health as inextricably linked with the political reality with which they have been forced to live (Daniels, 1994). While thousands of South Africans have been victims of violence, oppression, prejudice, abuse and neglect, these issues have remained largely unaddressed. In the past, psychology remained largely silent about the evils of apartheid (Foster & Louw-Potgieter, 1991).

Where intervention has occurred, it has been reactive, rather than proactive or health- promoting. Interventions have tended to emphasise Euro-American theories, with insufficient multicultural emphases in theory and practice and insufficient understanding of the issues facing communities and the relationship between mental health and environmental stressors. (Berger & Lazarus, 1987). Furthermore, the past tendency has been to select students mainly from the white middle class. Trainees have not received training that prepares them to deal with work in the community, and, owing to the small number of psychologists relative to the population, have little hope of reaching all those in need of services. Daniels (1994) sees problems concerning (1) who has been trained, (2) the numbers that have been trained, and (3) the client base for whom students have been trained. On a positive note, recent years have seen a gradual shift in these practices.

For a field of practice and research that claims to be concerned with mental health, this past (and some would argue, current) failure to acknowledge the influence of macro systems on the psychological health of the vast majority of the population has been quite ironic. Lazarus (1988) argues that psychology is not value free. Daniels (1994) thus argues that we need a theory and practice that overtly takes into account the influence of our past and present sociopolitical context. South African health and social services need to be transformed into a non-racial, equitable, cost-effective system which emphasises primary health care and community needs, and is relevant to the people it hopes to serve (Coovadia, 1990).

Community Psychology and Primary Health Care

Community psychology has been seen by many as providing a form of practice and theory from which to address the problems outlined above (Lazarus, 1988; Perkel, 1988). Community psychology is overtly value based or partisan (Rappaport, 1977). In contrast to traditional psychology, Community psychology emphasises (1) an understanding of the individual as part of a context; prevention and health promotion rather than treatment or remediation; (2) competency, empowerment and social action, rather than pathology; citizen participation; and (3) consultation rather than unequal power relationships. Community psychologists generally work in the community, together with the community. Thus, the assumptions about the causes of problems are different, and the levels of analysis are broader. In contrast to customary models of service delivery, the approach to planning services is more proactive. The attitude towards 'sharing' psychology and working with non-professionals is positive (Orford, 1992). The goal is to locate the practice as close as possible to people's everyday context. Thus, community psychology is not merely moving psychology out of the consulting room and into the community, but exploring alternative forms of practice routed in alternative theories of understanding human behaviour. (Orford, 1992) As yet, this is an emerging discipline, but one which can perhaps provide some of the solutions to the perceived crisis in psychological theory and practice.

In South Africa, government initiatives in the post-apartheid era have emphasised primary health care as the key to achieving a state of national wellness. The World Health Organisation (WHO) depicts health as 'a state of complete physical, mental and social wellbeing and not merely the absence of disease and infirmity" (In Ross, 1984:1). WHO views primary health care as based on community needs, relying on 'on-site' health care as far as is possible, to be undertaken in the community by general health workers under supervision of professionals. This returns responsibility to the community who are encouraged to attain, secure and promote their own health. With particular reference to mental health, the focus in primary health care is on psychological well-being and the 'quality of mental health'. Lazarus, Freeman and Rispel (1995) argue that preventative/mental health-promoting programmes could result in substantial reduction in later impairment. The WHO see psychology playing a diverse role in the provision of basic health care. These include the identification of mental disorder, education in common mental health principles, identifying at-risk individuals or groups, mobilising support groups, running elementary programmes, diagnosing and treating, consulting, liasing with other sectors to promote and raise awareness of mental health issues (WHO, 1990). Primary health care aims to reduce prevalence and incidence. In many ways, the goals of community psychology and primary health care overlap. Freeman (1991) argues however, that community psychology is more social action orientated and that the potential danger in primary health care lies in the medical model framework within which it is often embedded.

Psychology on board the Phelophepa

In 1993, Transnet, the South African rail company, joined the Rand Afrikaans University in setting up a mobile eye clinic in converted railway carriages to make eye care more readily available to the large sectors of the community that were not accessing services. The clinic was based on the example of the Lifeline Express, a hospital train travelling through and serving the rural communities of India. In 1994, Transnet assumed responsibility for the running of the train clinic and extended the services offered to provide basic dental, medical, nursing and educare services in co-operation with university training departments. The aim was to provide rural, disadvantaged, and disempowered communities with access to primary health care facilities and education, and to encourage participation of the local service community through consultation with educational, religious, business and political leadership. Minimal fees are charged for services. However, where there is particular hardship and unemployment, fees may be waived at the discretion of the train manager. Final year students work in conjunction with university faculty and a small contingent of permanent staff provide services. Thus, the train functions not only as a vehicle of service delivery, but also as a training opportunity.

Initially, Transnet had believed that traditional psychology would be unable to offer a service in such a setting – the train stops in an area for one to two weeks at a time, and the focus of intervention is mainly crisis intervention and prevention/health-promotion. However, after several requests from a group of concerned academics and psychologists, a single compartment was offered to psychology in 1994 for a period of 3 weeks in order to conduct a need analysis. Several areas of concern related to psychological health were identified. The following year, one permanent compartment was allocated to psychology, and, in 1997, psychology was allocated a second compartment. Initially, the nature and scope of psychological services on the train were not clearly specified. Psychological interventions were conducted in a fairly haphazard manner, without much consideration of available resources in the community (Lilian Cingo, Personal Communication). In response to this situation, a reference group of psychologists and academics, "Counsellors on Phelophepa" (COPE), was established to develop guidelines for psychologists' services on board the train. This group suggested that workshops and group sessions should be offered on topics identified by needs analyses. Nonetheless, psychology departments from different universities continued to adopted different, sometimes conflicting orientations in their approach to service delivery. Some focussed more on assessment and identification of psychological problems, while others emphasised research or short-term psychotherapy or psycho-education.

During 1996, the Educational Psychology and Psychology Departments of the University of Natal Pietermaritzburg agreed to commit themselves to planning for and staffing the train for a period of ten weeks during the train's journey through KwaZulu Natal. The decision to become involved was rooted in the faculty's belief that psychology in South Africa needed to be made more accessible to the community. The train venture appeared to be the ideal opportunity to put into practice the community psychology principles taught on courses and to investigate how or even whether psychology could play a role in such a primary health care setting. This paper will discuss this involvement on the train, outlining the services and interventions that were provided, the rationale for these, and evaluating their effectiveness and appropriateness.

Method

Participants

The University of Natal Pietermaritzburg provided two psychologists (faculty or students) for duty at each of the ten stations in the province. The stations fell in rural areas, with the exception of two areas, which were described as peri-urban. The communities in these areas were characterised by experiencing problems with unemployment, poverty, poor lifestyle habits (such as substance abuse), and political instability leading to violence. Staff decided to target the teachers, nurses and key community figures in each geographical area. This focus was based on the belief that equipping identified community leaders with skills and confidence would have a greater effect on residents than short term work by outsider psychologists. Orford (1992) defines this indirect intervention as an attempt to influence 'intermediaries' who have direct contact with the 'clients'. These intermediaries have ongoing relationships with 'persons-at-risk' but their work is not exclusively of a mental health nature. It was felt that this approach would offer more hope of sustaining an intervention than "simply rushing in and rushing out in an effort to achieve as much as possible in a short space of time".

Intervention - Service Delivery

University staff decided to focus mainly on two activities in their service delivery on the train: (1) psycho-education through workshopping, and (2) networking with community members/related professionals both on and off the train. It was agreed that individual counselling should be limited, and focus mainly on 'crisis intervention' rather than longer-term psychotherapy. Questionnaires and information sheets were drawn up for Transnet staff based on preliminary needs assessments. It was hoped that information from these need assessments could be used to structure workshop outlines. In many cases, Transnet was unable to carry out these assessments and a list of workshop ideas was drawn up on the basis of predicted needs in an area, considering the area's population and history, and on communication from other colleagues who had worked in these or similar areas previously. The goal was to provide a relevant service based on expressed needs, rather than come in with pre-packaged notions.

Workshops were designed around health-promotion as well as 'remedial' topics. These included child abuse, substance abuse, behaviour management, coping with violence (see graphs 1 and 2 for more detail). The workshops were structured to share information and ideas about the specified topic and to discuss ways of sharing these ideas with others that participants came into contact with. The approach was rooted in the principles of community psychology: to work collaboratively, and to assist in the identification of existing resources and coping strategies rather than presenting the psychologist role as 'expert'.

Secondly, staff aimed to network with key community figures and other professionals. Staff felt that networking with resources within the community, and establishing links among these various resources would represent a potential solution to the issue of sustainability. The staff hoped to identify resources, facilitate their development, and set up contact with other existing resources. Lists of available agencies, schools, and clinics for each region provided a starting point for this process. The intention was that the psychologists would contact these agencies and plan meetings of various key figures. Networking with professionals on board the train was also seen an opportunity to develop close working relationships with the professionals from other disciplines, and to demonstrate the importance of mental primary health care and the potential role and scope of psychology.

In several areas, Transnet had been unable to conduct a thorough need assessment. Thus, staff often conducted needs assessments upon their arrival. Despite the limited time available, needs assessments were a priority. The act of assessing a community's needs can be very empowering personally and politically as people can come to realise that they have resources and skills to address their needs. Solomon (1997, personal communication) points out that through articulating their needs, a community may come to realise that they can transform themselves into an active minority. At several stations, staff found that no community members arrived for meetings on Monday mornings (either because of a lack of clarity about the role of psychology or insufficient publicity) In these cases, the psychologists were more proactive, and went out to schools and clinics themselves. Rappaport (1977) would see this as quite an appropriate seeking mode of working rather than a reactive mode.

Data Collection

In order to enable the researchers to evaluate the services, records were kept of the services rendered (e.g., number and nature of groups, workshops, individual sessions, networking, etc.), psychology staff completed open-ended questionnaires and attended a focus group about the nature of their experiences and impressions of service delivery, and clients completed participant evaluation forms after each intervention.

Results and Discussion

In the ten-week period, 103 workshops were conducted, and 26 schools were visited. In all, 3758 people attended these workshops. Since many of the participants were teachers and nurses, it is likely that they took this information back into their everyday work contexts. Group sessions covered a wide range of topics. Those given the most frequently and believed to represent topics of greatest need concerned discipline, child abuse, substance abuse and stress management. Nine (out of a possible 10) formal need analysis meetings were held. This indicates that attempts **were** made to structure interventions according to expressed community needs. Seven resource networking meetings were held, which was in line with the principle of accessing resources available and facilitating contact. Information about the workshops provided and community attendance is presented in the graphs below.

Graph 1. Workshops Presented (This graph shows the number of workshops presented on each topic. Letters represent workshop titles. Please see the key below Table 2 for the full workshop title.)

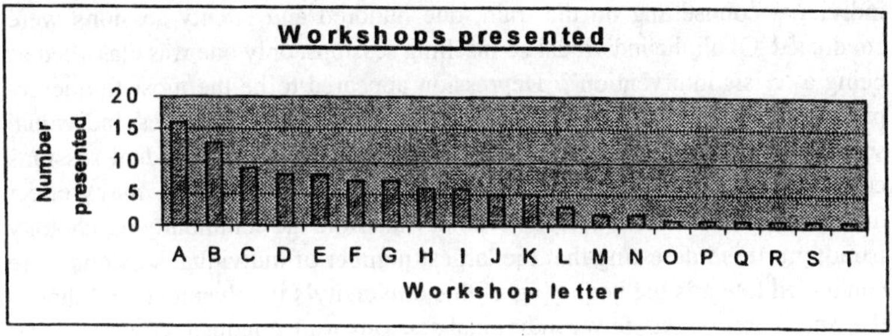

Graph 2. Number attending. (This graph shows the number of people attending the various workshops. Please see the key below.)

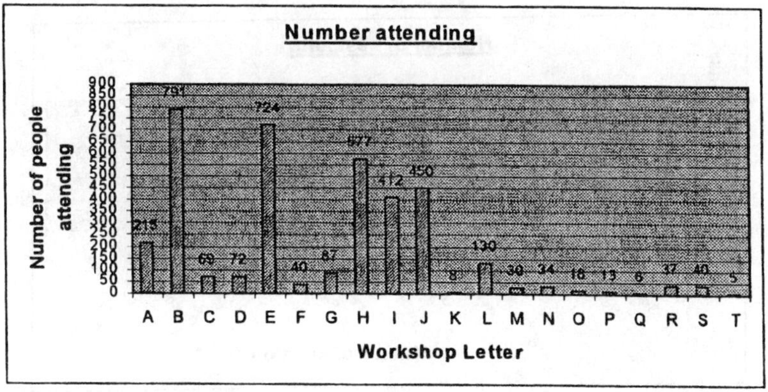

A	Discipline	F	Resource networking	K	Women's Group	P	Depression
B	Child Abuse	G	Basic Counselling Skills	L	HIV/AIDS	Q	Mental Health
C	Needs Analysis	H	Self-Concept	M	Conflict Management	R	Relationships
D	Stress Management	I	Careers	N	Learning Difficulties	S	Unemployment
E	Substance Abuse	J	Sex Education	O	Cognitive Skills	T	Violence

The emergence of discipline and child abuse as primary concerns is of particular interest. It has been suggested that political violence and conflict has to a certain extent been replaced by domestic conflict (Killian, 1994). Only three workshops were presented on HIV/AIDS. Yet, HIV infection in KZN indicates a dire need for HIV/AIDS/sex education. It appears that there is resistance to addressing this problem. The staff became acutely aware of the political dynamics surrounding the issue of HIV/AIDS and their own lack of understanding of these political intricacies. For example, in one area, a staff member was told by a school principal that AIDS was not prevalent yet a clinic sister suggested that HIV infection was a great concern.

In spite of the University of Natal's policy of offering only very limited individual counselling on the train, one hundred and twenty sessions were conducted. Of all the individual counselling sessions, only one was classified as being a 'crisis intervention'. Depression appeared to be the most frequently presented problem, followed by relationship and sexual difficulties. Individual sessions are presented in graph 3 below. The number of individual sessions conducted differed greatly from area to area. This situation may reflect individual staff members' reluctance to deviate from the community psychology paradigm. It is interesting that the largest number of individual sessions were conducted towards the beginning of this university's involvement, and that as the weeks progressed, fewer individual sessions were conducted.

Graph 3. Focus of individual counseling sessions

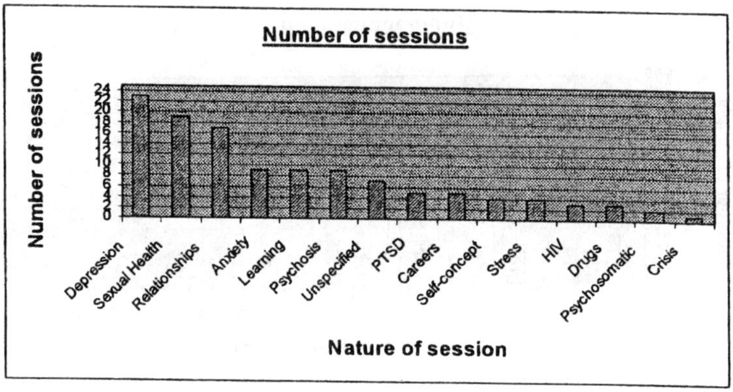

Key:
Sexual Health: includes sexual difficulties, pregnancy-related issues and rape counselling.
Learning: includes learning difficulties and disabilities
PTSD: Post-Traumatic Stress Disorder
HIV: HIV and AIDS counselling
Crisis: Crisis Intervention

For the past three years, Transnet has evaluated contributions from the various disciplines on the train by an output approach focusing on the number of clients seen. With psychological interventions where effects are 'less visible' than in some of the other disciplines, their evaluation is more problematic. Reporting the number of people seen (as above) tells us little about how effective these interventions were, whether any possible effects are lasting or whether information is transferred to others with whom clients subsequently come into contact (Orford, 1992).In an attempt to get a fuller picture of effectiveness of the interventions, content analyses of responses to client evaluation forms, facilitator evaluation forms, and the focus group interview were carried out.

Most psychologists reported difficulty in getting clients to complete the client evaluation forms. For the majority of the community, English was a second or third language. Although the questionnaire was straightforward and open-ended, clients struggled to reflect on their experiences in this way. Several staff expressed frustration at this, claiming that the verbal feedback they had received was insufficiently captured in responses on the client evaluation forms. Nonetheless, content analyses and comments noted by staff suggest largely positive feedback from clients. One staff member commented that from what she could judge, the value in the interventions lay in affording people the opportunity to work in a dramatically different way: the opportunity to be heard, the encouragement to think. Client comments included: "They've let us discuss some problems in groups", "I've realised that we are not alone in our problems. We had our problems aired and learned how to cope".

While such comments inspire optimism as to the efficacy of the interventions, the extent to which the goal of empowerment was met is debatable. This concern was expressed in the focus group and feedback forms. One psychologist pointed out that it was sometimes all too easy to slip back into the 'expert' role, especially with community members that were ready to credit them with the power of being "dokotela go kande" (Zulu for doctors of the head), believing they would know exactly what to do and provide all the answers. We are reminded here of Freeman's (1991) comments that the medical model is implicit in primary health care. Psychologists also expressed concern at their own lack of cross-cultural awareness. For example, several questioned the appropriateness of workshops on topics such as assertiveness, in communities where women are bought for "lobola" (traditionally payment in cattle).

Workshops were not always based on identified needs but rather on what the presenters had available. It was up to the individual presenter to adapt the pre-packaged workshop materials according to the context. This was not always done in collaboration with community. Hence people were not always engaged in the actions designed by the planners and thus, perhaps, not empowered.

Furthermore, it is apparent that more sessions were held with pupils, than with teachers alone. Psychologists reported difficulty in communicating to those present at needs' discussions the appropriateness of working indirectly. Many community members had been socialised to think in terms of responding to the scale of need by demanding the expansion of direct service delivery. Generally the psychologists were overwhelmed at the nature and extent of expressed needs and were unsure where to focus their attention ("Just too many issues requested"). Anxiety was expressed around the limited time available for intervention and the fact that issues had been 'opened up' but not necessarily explored. One participant commented: "I felt guilt afterwards about the patient's wellbeing - it's hard to sustain this".

The need assessment meetings were poorly attended and time-pressurised. Nonetheless, psychologists reflected that they were able to establish what resources were available and to uncover what attempts the community had already made to address their problems. They assisted the community in identifying their own resources and to strengthen their access to these and their confidence in doing so. Health, social service, nursing and teaching personnel in each area welcomed the opportunity to make contact with others, and spoke of the need to take practical steps to address their sense of professional isolation. In a few instances, the psychologists met with some resistance from local workers who were territorial in their attitude towards an area. It is possible that they feared that expectations would be raised during the brief stay of the train and that they would be confronted by disappointed local residents who would demand the provision of services beyond the resources at their disposal. It was evident that some of these workers were frustrated by their work situation and lacked awareness of the larger context and the macro issues which militated against the rapid expansion of scarce resources in remote areas. Although the university does not have the resources to promote the continuation of networking and peer support in these areas, psychologists deemed this an urgent priority. For this reason, the departments of psychology have sought research and development funding to address these issues on an ongoing basis.

The stint on the train provided psychologists with the unusual opportunity to work alongside other professionals at close quarters. These professionals are also working in an unfamiliar context, often in cramped quarters and without recourse to the full range of technological equipment and laboratory support to which they are accustomed. Most of them had little knowledge of the nature and scope of applied psychology, and some misunderstandings arose. These were reflected in the inappropriate referral of some clients and also in some glib comments comparing the relative workloads and time cost effectiveness of psychology and the other disciplines. Mealtimes and evenings gave the train staff and volunteers the chance to socialise in the dining car. At these times, psychologists were able to provide some psycho-education, to alert their colleagues to the range of services on offer and also to emphasise the shift from a medical model to a community psychology orientation. Other professions at this expressed some surprise, and it was realised that psychology is not well known or understood in health care circles.

Given the circumstances under which workers on the train function, and considering that the majority are young and inexperienced individuals nearing the completion of their own professional training, it is to be expected that some people will experience stress and discomfort. For many, it is their first experience of coming face to face with the scale and detail of disadvantage in this country. Some of the areas visited have extremely high rates of political and social violence, necessitating the provision of armed guards to ensure the safety of those living and working on the train. Students from large metropolitan areas were unaware of the day-to-day lives of people in rural areas. In addition to this, the large numbers of people presenting for service provision created pressure on these inexperienced workers. It must be emphasised that Transnet provides optimal living facilities within the constraint of a converted train. The management is sensitive to the demands that this work places upon individuals, yet from the first week of duty on the train, psychologists received referrals and self-referrals of professional colleagues. Some individual counselling sessions were convened and the psychologists were placed in a dilemma of deciding to what extent they could get involved. It was sometimes difficult to disentangle the effects of the present demanding situation from previously existing distress.

It would be naive to assume that psychologists are somehow spared these effects. The departments provided ongoing supervision for psychologists and students acknowledging that such an intense placement, in an unfamiliar context, would be potentially stressful.

Concluding Comments

Although psychologists who served on the train grappled with working under stressful conditions, the experience on the train affirmed their belief in a role for psychology. Comments included: "This is psychology. This is something that I can do, appropriate and worth doing"; "We experienced something broader than what we think a psychologist is...it will facilitate a rethinking of priorities and modes of service delivery; it will facilitate a broadening of perspective"; "Being on the train led to an expansion of my thinking". Staff were overwhelmingly positive and keen to get on board again in the following year, though it has not been easy to pinpoint what it is about the experience that proved to be so appealing. This enthusiasm does not however, provide a compelling reason for the retention of psychology on the train in the absence of evidence that the service is appropriate and cost-effective. Feedback from clients and professional colleagues affirms the value of psychological intervention, yet the effects of psychology are difficult to assess in the terms applied by Transnet and others to health care professions. Psychology as a discipline will need to identify the bases for evaluation of elusive, but clearly valued effects.

On a professional development level, the Phelophepa experience provided faculty and students the opportunity to test their assumptions and skills in an intensive hothouse situation. Faculty had believed that the professional skilling of trainee psychologists at this university was already firmly located in the models of community psychology and primary health care. They had assumed they were aware of the realities of day-to-day life for the peoples of this province. Yet, they were overwhelmed by the extent of poverty and suffering they witnessed during their time on the train. This humbling experience made them uncomfortable about some of their own insensitivities and caused them to revisit some of their assumptions. Their own reaction to the train experience alerted them to some oversights and contradictions in the courses they teach.

Community psychology aims to go beyond extending access of traditional interventions to marginalised communities. The service offered on the train was just a first step towards moving psychology out of the consulting room into the South African community and changing the mode of delivering familiar services. It remained individually orientated and failed to address the socio-economic and political context. In terms of social action, in promoting empowerment, it is debatable how much was achieved. Empowerment in remote under-resourced regions is complicated by the difficulty in engaging with structures and practices at the macro level. Individuals and groups may feel empowered after affirmation of existing skills and learning new skills, but sense of extended control is not the same thing as an extension of actual control. It is beyond the agency and authority of psychologists on the train to address larger socio-political forces but as Orford (1992) points out, interventions may be doomed to transitory or ineffective actions unless this is done.

On an educational level, the Phelophepa experience afforded faculty and staff the opportunity to explain the range and scope of psychological services to both other professionals on board the train, and to community figures visiting the train. Although psychology may not as yet, have clarified the precise nature and value of its services abroad the train, at the very least, it has been able to communicate to others that psychology can play a role. We may have made mistakes and experienced difficulties in this project, but are confident that the insights gained from this project can be applied to develop more appropriate training for this and other contexts in which psychologists work. We are encouraged by Leslie Swartz's comments of the developmental nature of change:

"I do not accept though, that raising expectations is always wrong, or even bad for people...I am sure that in our work we have raised many expectations, and that we have disappointed many people, but the only way to avoid doing this is to do nothing at all - to remain in the confines of the

consulting room. Change can't happen without expectations being raised and without mistakes being made - the challenge is to make mistakes as reflectively as possible" (Swartz, 1996:5).

References

Bassa, F.M. & Schlebusch, L. (1984). Practice preferences of clinical psychologists in South Africa. *South African Journal of Psychology, 14 (4),* 118-123.

Berger, S. & Lazarus, S. (1987). The views of community organisers on the relevance of psychological practice in South Africa. *Psychology in Society, 7*, 6-23.

Coovadia, J. (1990). Towards a new health policy for South Africa. *Critical Health, 31/32*, 24-25.

Daniels, F. (1994). *Clinical psychology trainees' perceptions of a 'relevant' clinical psychology for South Africa: An exploratory study.* Unpublished Masters thesis. University of Natal Pietermaritzburg.

Dawes, A. (1985). Politics and mental health: The position of clinical psychology in South Africa. *South African Journal of Psychology, 15(2),* 55-61.

Foster, D. & Louw-Potgieter, J. (1991). *Social Psychology in South Africa.* Johannesburg: Lexicon.

Freeman, M. (1991). Mental health for all - moving beyond rhetoric. *South African Journal of Psychology, 21 (3)*, 141-146.

Holdstock, T.L. (1981). Psychology in South Africa belongs to the colonial era: Arrogance or ignorance? *South African Journal of Psychology, 11*, 123-129.

Killian, B. (1994). *The effects of chronic violence on children living in South African townships.* Unpublished paper, University of Natal Pietermaritzburg.

Lazarus, S. (1988). *The role of the psychologist in South African society: In search of an appropriate community psychology.* University of Cape Town: Unpublished doctoral thesis.

Lazarus, S. Freeman, M., & Rispel, L. (1995). *Resources for primary health care.* Johannesburg: Wits.

Manganyi, C.N. & Louw, J. (1986). Clinical psychology in South Africa: A comparative study of emerging professional trends. *Professional Psychology: Research and Practice, 17(3),*171-178.

Orford, J. (1992). *Community Psychology: Theory and Practice.* New York: John Wiley and Sons.

Perkel, A.K. (1988). Towards a model for South African clinical psychology. *Psychology in Society, 10*, 53-75.

Rappaport, J. (1977). *Community Psychology: Values, Research and Action.* New York: Holt, Rinehart, and Winston.

Ross, S.M. (1984). *Health for all by the year 2000: Possibility or pipe dream?* Pietermaritzburg, South Africa: University of Natal Press.

Swartz, S; Dowdall, T. & Swartz, L. (1986). Clinical psychology and the 1985 crisis in Cape Town. *Psychology in Society, 5*, 131-138.

Swartz, L. (1996). Crossing or creating boundaries: Challenges in clinical psychology in the community.World Health Organisation (1990). *The introduction of a mental health component into primary health care.* Switzerland: WHO.

Later-Life Depression in Ten European Countries: A Study Using the Multilevel Approach

Pieter Van den Eeden
Vrije Universiteit Amsterdam
Department of Social Research Methods

Arjan W. Braam
Vrije Universiteit Amsterdam
Department of Gerontology

ABSTRACT

In ten European countries prevalence of later life depression has been studied using Prince's EURO-D meta-assessment scale. It is well-known that women tend to be more depressive than men, and that depression increases with age. Since there are differences in the size of the effects of age and gender between the countries, a multilevel methodology is appropriate. An attempt was made to explain those differences by referring to the national culture, especially regarding the national religious climate and Hofstede's classification of values. The countries involved were: Belgium, England, France, Germany, Iceland, Ireland, Italy, The Netherlands, Spain, and Sweden. The 16,692 respondents were elderly persons of 64 years and over. Religious climate was assessed using data of the European Value Survey, and national climate by Hofstede's classification. It turns out that the gender-depression relationship tends to be more susceptible for mitigating effects of the national religious climate, and that age-depression relationship tend to be more susceptible for their provoking effects. The mean depression score depends differently on different aspects of religious climate. Any effect of Hofstede's classification could not be detected

An abundance of studies regarding mood exists in cross-cultural research, also for everyday depressive feelings, named "minor depression". However, the theoretical interpretations remain poor. A good exception seems to be Weiss and Kleinman (1988), but also their model, which has been based on a meta-analysis, is unfortunately very imprecise.

This chapter describes the differences of the prevalence of depression in a number of countries and addresses some processes that lead to depression that vary from country to country. In particular, it pays attention to the effects of gender and age of older adults. Since the differences in the size of the effects of an individual's gender and age between countries are well-known, it is worthwhile to explain them by referring to the nation's culture [for example, being dominated by a Catholic or Protestant religion and the position of Hofstede's (1991) classification of national cultures]. Because in this analysis attention has to be given to individuals and countries as distinct types of analysis, a multilevel methodology is appropriate. Using a multilevel methodology not only the differences in the means of depression, but also the differences in the slopes regarding depression can be explained.

Expanding the evidence about the higher rate of depression in women (Wolk & Weissman, 1995), variation in the differences between men and women in the various countries has to be assessed, thus offering some insight into the gender cleavage. Another question to be addressed is whether these differences are related to a nation's religious and cultural factors. Parallel to this, taking the effect of age on depression for granted, which is generally based on a decline of physical health (Beekman et al.. 1997), this effect in each country merits study. If there are differences across the countries, the relation between the size of those effects and a nation's religious and cultural factors is worthy of investigation.

We next turn to some elaborations of the central theoretical notions. Following this, the database will be described. Then we will turn to the results of the analysis and some conclusions.

Theory

It is generally acknowledged that gender and age are related to the rate of depression. However, the mechanisms involved in this relationship are not fully clear. If in later life women do have more chronic physical and social difficulties than men, and if physical and social difficulties increase with age, then the psychological stress-centered theory (Brown & Harris, 1978) helps to explain both phenomena. Unfortunately, the design of this study did not allow a distinction about the validity of the underlying mechanisms.

If the gender- and age-related results of these mechanisms turn out to differ from country to country, it will be challenging to look for their correlates. Do religious climate and a nation's culture relate to the mean depression rate in a country? Do religious climate and a nation's culture relate to a nation's effect of gender and age on depression?

The study on the relation between religion and depression is based on two approaches (Ellison, 1994) which are in line with the queries. The *first* is the cognitive-psychological approach, in which people use religion as an aid in the cognitive structuring of their life. Religious beliefs and practices serve as a comprehensive framework of understanding, which is viewed as a coping-factor when people are confronted with the difficulties in old age (Koenig et al.1995). This fits into the stress-vulnerability model (Brown & Harris 1978). The *second* approach is of a sociological nature, and suggests that religion provides social networks within the religious community and their accompanying normative contexts. Religion then protects older adults against depression because of the availability of social support and normative frameworks (Durkheim, 1897; Pescosolido & Georgianna, 1989; Idler & Kasl 1992).

Individual approaches to the negative relationship between religion and depression are paralleled by the level of a nation, since individual religiousness is reflected in a nation's religious climate. It can be hypothesized that such a religious climate will decrease the differences in depression between men and women as well as according to age. Religious climate is a mitigating condition for the individual processes which run from depressogenic personal circumstances (indicated by gender and age). In contrast to this strand, Yap (1971) and Ellis (1980) stated that religious climate is a depression-provoking condition for individual processes. In Yap's view this is due to the fact that especially the Western monotheistic religions emphasize feelings of guilt.

The mitigation effect hypothesis, although rudimentary, can be viewed as an elaboration of Weiss and Kleinman (1987)'s "cultural informed model" for explaining cross-cultural differences in depression. It is to their credit that they distinguish the nested levels of units and that they mention some general variables. Unfortunately, they neglect to offer some helpful hypotheses. The present study, however, specifies some relevant individual and cultural variables and explains precisely how the process of affecting of religious climate a nation's depression is expected to operate. A religious climate cannot operate directly, since it occurs at a level different from the level of individual processes that give rise to depression.

It can be expected that a nation's religious climate is connected to other national cultural factors, and hence they have to be introduced in the analysis as covariates. In order to do so, Hofstede's (1991) classification of cultural traits is introduced in the analysis.

The Multilevel Model

The multilevel model is appropriate for the analysis of cross-cultural studies since these encompass units of various levels: the individual level and the cultural level (Van de Vijver & Leung, 1997). The multilevel model permits description of differences in means of individual answers per country and their relations with cultural factors (as in standard variance analysis or regression analysis) but also differences in individual level regression slopes between the countries, and even to relate those slopes to cultural factors. Since in multilevel analysis a fundamental distinction in types of units of analysis has been made, the model avoids the notorious aggregative error in country-level regressions and it also avoids the overestimation of standard errors in individual level regression. However, it assumes a multiple phase random selection procedure: individuals are chosen within their countries, and countries from a theoretical population.

The multilevel model of cross-cultural research can be described fundamentally as consisting of two equations. The first equation (regarding level 1) concerns the within-group regression where a dependent variable is explained by a number of independent variables. The erroneously neglected independent variables, measurement errors, and estimation errors are expressed in the disturbance term (e_{ij}). With respect to lower-level unit *i* and the higher-level unit *j* the equation is as follows:

$$Y_{ij} = \beta_{0j} + \beta_{1j} X_{1ij} + \beta_{2j} X_{2ij} + ... + \beta_{kj} X_{kij} + e_{ij} \qquad (1)$$

where:

i: the lower level unit (*i*= 1,...,I)
j: the higher level unit (*j* = 1,...,J)
Y_{ij}: output variable
X_{kj}: input variables (*k* = 1,...,k) for *i*
β_{0j}: intercept for *j*
β_{kj}: regression coefficient of the output variable Y_{ij} on the input X_{ki}
e_{ij}: disturbance term belonging to Y_{ij}, with variance σ^2 and mean 0

The second equation is on the level of the higher level units. It specifies the regression of the lower level coefficients β_{kj} (*k* = 0, 1,...,K) on the higher level characteristics incorporated. As a result, a new regression equation is formulated for each coefficient. It is formulated as follows:

$$\beta_{kj} = \gamma_{k0} + \gamma_{k1} Z_{1j} + ... + \gamma_{kN} Z_{Nj} + u_{kj} \qquad (2)$$

where:

Z_{in}: independent variables (*n* = 1,...,N) for *j*
γ_{k0}: tintercept of the regression
γ_{kn}: regression coefficient of the dependent variable β_{kj} on the independent higher level variable Z_{nj}.
u_{kj}: disturbance term belonging to β_{kj}, with variance σ^2_k and mean 0.

The common assumptions are valid; moreover it is supposed that ρ(z,e) =0. By substituting equation (2) into equation (1) we get the final model. It expresses the differences of the independent variables- dependent variable processes on the higher level, expressed by σ^2_k, if the higher level variables are absent. If any σ^2_k is not equal to zero, it is worthwhile to introduce the higher level variables into the analysis.

On the basis of this structure of units, the variance of a given variable can be decomposed according to each level, and the resulting types of variance can be regressed on a set of input variables on the lower level unit. There is also a covariance matrix of the disturbances on the higher level.

Figure 1a depicts the situation that there are unequal intercepts and equal slopes and Figure 1b the situation that there are equal intercepts and unequal slopes. In reality, however, a combination of both situations exists.

Figure 1a. Different intercepts and same slopes.

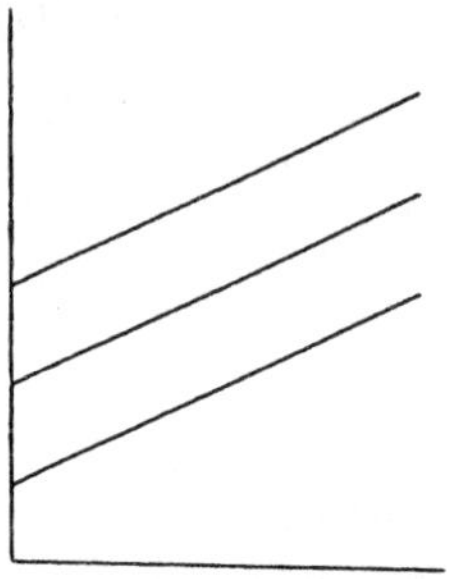

Figure 1b. Same intercepts and different slopes.

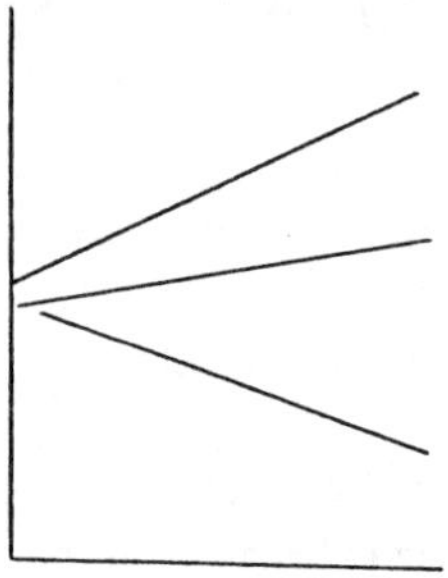

Samples and Measures

The data are adopted from the EURO-DEP-database concerning late-life depression in twelve regional areas in ten countries (Copeland et al. submitted). The regional areas and countries involved are:), Belgium (*n*=1130), France (*n*=3604), Germany (Berlin rcgion, *n*=488; Munich region n=293), Eire (*n*=914), England (Liverpool region, *n*=5222; London region, *n*=637), Iceland (*n*=772), Italy (*n*=202), The Netherlands (*n*=1944), Spain (*n*=1037), and Sweden (*n*=449). The total number of respondents is 16,692. All samples were population-based, using registrations of general practitioners, municipalities, or electoral rolls. The regional areas and countries varied with respect to the procedures of the interviews, which were administered by trained lay-interviewers, research nurses, or research psychiatrists.

Minor depression was measured by Prince's EURO-DEP scale on the basis of twelve items assessed by four instruments. Nine regional areas and countries used GMS/AGECAT (Copeland et al.1986) or the similar SHORT-CARE depression scale (Gurland *et al.* 1984). Three regional areas had used the Centre for Epidemiologic Studies Depression scale (CES-D) (Radloff 1977), one regional area the Zung Depression Scale, and one regional area the Comprehensive Psychopathological Rating Scale (CPRS) (Asberg et al. 1978). EURO-D shows a rather good reliability (α =.71).

The independent variables on the individual-level *gender* and *age* were assessed in all regional areas and countries. Gender was coded as 1 (man) and 2 (woman) and age ranges from 64 to 108 years. Several variables, such as church membership, church attendance and marital status could not be included in the analysis because they were measured in all regional areas.

To characterize the regional areas, measures were adopted from the national level from the European Value Study (Ester et al. 1994) to indicate *national religious climate*. The following estimates were used: (1) the percentage of Roman Catholics, (2) percentage of Protestants, (3) the percentage of people attending church at least once a week, (4) the mean score on the orthodoxy scale, using the items about traditional Christian beliefs in ‘life after death’, ‘a soul’, ‘the devil’, ‘hell’, ‘heaven’, and ‘sin’, according to the factor-analysis discussed by Harding et al. (1986), and (5) the mean score on the religious devotion index. Religious devotion mirrors intrinsic religious motivation. The items are descriptions of the self as a religious person, belief in God, getting comfort and strength from religion, taking moments of prayer and meditation, and believing in the importance of God. The scale is increasing, which means that the higher the score, the higher the motivation.

In the analysis, the places of the countries in Hofstede's (1991) classification of cultures are indicated. Hofstede administered questionnaires to 117,000 IBM employees. Answers to fourteen work goal items were factor-analyzed. The 40-country sample was subsequently expanded to a total of 50 national cultures and three regions. The classification describes nations on four dimensions: individualism, power distance, masculinity, and uncertainty avoidance.

All individual scores are z-scored individually and all regional scores regionally. For Iceland the scores of Denmark of the Hofstede classification are substituted. All partial EURO-D scales are coded as dummy-variables and adopted in the analysis in order to asses the effect of the partial scale on EURO-D.

Results

In the analysis in a forward procedure the program Mln (Rasbash & Woodhouse, 1995) was used. The analysis started with separate analysis for religious climate and cultural factors.

Firstly, Model 1 shows that the between-regional variance in depression is relatively high, being 9.2 percent (.098/(.959 +.098)). After introduction of gender and age as independent variables in Model 2, the results show that the hypotheses on gender- and age-relatedness of depression could be confirmed, and that there are significant regional differences in the size of the effects of gender and age on depression. Here, the evidence about the cross-regional differences is derived from the differences in the log-likelihoods.

The results can be summarized as follows (see Table 2).

a. On the average, gender and age do have the expected effects on depression. The depression-score is higher for women than in men (being .122) and increases with age (.073). The average effect of gender is higher than that of age. There is no interaction effect of gender and age.

b. There are significant differences between the regional areas in the effects of gender and age on depression as well in the (corrected) mean depression score. The evidence on the cross-regional differences in the regressions concerned has been derived from the differences in the likelihood values. Table 1 shows the region-specific values of the intercepts and slopes. In addition, Figures 2 and 3 depict those differences clearly.

Table 1. Values of intercepts and of gender-related and age-related slopes per region.

	Code	Intercept	Slope Gender	Slope Age
The Netherlands, NL	1	.097	.023	-.011
London, GB	2	.115	.102	.098
Liverpool, GB	3	.277	.020	.034
Berlin, G	4	-.173	4e-5	.012
Dublin, IRE	6	.021	7e-4	.007
Iceland, ICE	7	-.475	-.146	-.156
Munich, G	8	-.111	-.022	-.007
Verona, I	9	-.099	.088	.056
Zaragoza, E	10	.694	-.023	.009
France, F	11	-.237	.044	.014
Goteborg, S	12	-.037	-.048	-.038
Antwerp, B	13	-.069	-.058	-.018

c. Under Model 3 we investigated whether the religious climate variables can explain those between-regional areas effects, offering the following results:

Effect of gender - A nation's score on regular church attendance decreases the effects of gender (the coefficient is -.121), according to the mitigation effect hypothesis. The higher the score on national church attendance, the lower the depression differences between men and women. Moreover, the higher the percentage of protestants, the lower the effect of gender (-.069).

Effect of age - A nation's orthodoxy rate and rate of religious devotion influence the effect of age (.068 and .098, respectively): the higher the rates, the stronger the effect of age. This outcome is according to the provoking effect hypothesis.

Unknown effects - In addition to the effects mentioned, there are effects which originate from unknown factors and which are expressed in a nation's mean level of depression. The higher the percentage of Catholics in a nation, the lower the mean depression score (the coefficients are -.259). Moreover, the higher a nation's rate on orthodox beliefs and religious devotion, the lower the

Table 2. Outcome of the multilevel analysis

	Model 1		Model 2		Model 3	
	coeff	Std err	coeff	Std err	coeff	Std err
Fixed Part						
CONS	.079*	.091	.050*	.083	.433	.083
GEND			.122*	.023	.111*	.016
AGE			.073*	.022	.101*	.015
CPRS					-1.142*	.170
S-CARE					-2.218*	.407
CES-D					.468*	.102
Random Part						
Individual Level						
CONS/CONS	.959	.011	.935	.011	.934	.010
Regio Level						
CONS/CONS	.098	.041	.080	.033	.015	.007
GEND/CONS			.005	.007	-.005	.003
GEND/GEND			.005	.003	.002	.001
AGE/CONS			.007	.007	.000	.000
AGE/GEND			.004	.002	.000	.000
AGE/AGE			.004	.002	.000	.000
-2*log(lh)	46721.8		46323		46271	
Continuation model 3	INTERCEPT		SLOPE GENDER		SLOPE AGE	
	coeff	Std err	coeff	Std err	coeff	Std err
Religious Variables						
RC	-.259*	.069	-.015	-.024	.004	.017
PR	-.041	.090	-.069*	.034	.055	.041
AT	.434*	.128	-.121*	.042	-.063	.047
OR	-.809*	.125	.019	.038	.068*	.025
RD	-.369*	.122	.049	.034	.098*	.037

RC: Percentage RC, PR: Percentage PR, AT: percentage church attendance (>1x/week),
OR: mean score orthodoxy, RD: mean score religious devotion per country of the center.
*: significant fixed effect (Prob.= .05)

mean depression score (-.369 and -.809, respectively). The latter outcome is in line with the mitigating effect hypothesis. Moreover, the higher a nation's church attention rate, the higher the mean devotion score (.434), supporting the contrasting provoking effect hypothesis.

d. The separate analysis involving Hofstede's scores did not show any significant effect. The outcome is not presented here.

e. *Instrument effects* - There are significant effects of all instruments. CPRS and S-CARE underestimate a person's depression score in comparison with GMS (the coefficients are -1.142 and -2.218, respectively), and CES-D offers an overestimation (.468).

The outcome can be summarized in the Figure 4:

Figure 2. Regressions of EUROTOT on AGE (z-scored) per region.

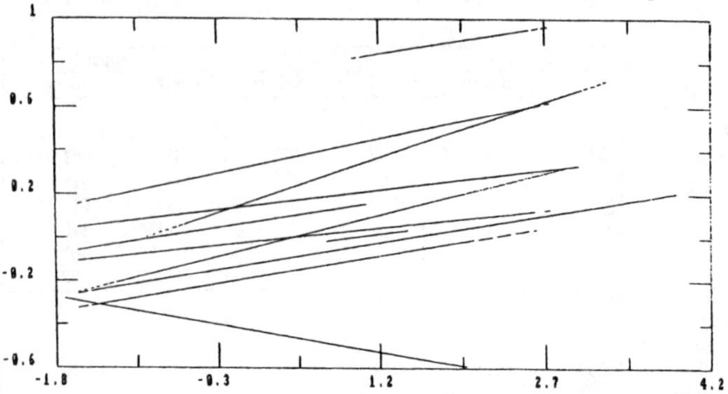

Figure 3. Regressions of EUROTOT on GENDER (z-scored) per region.

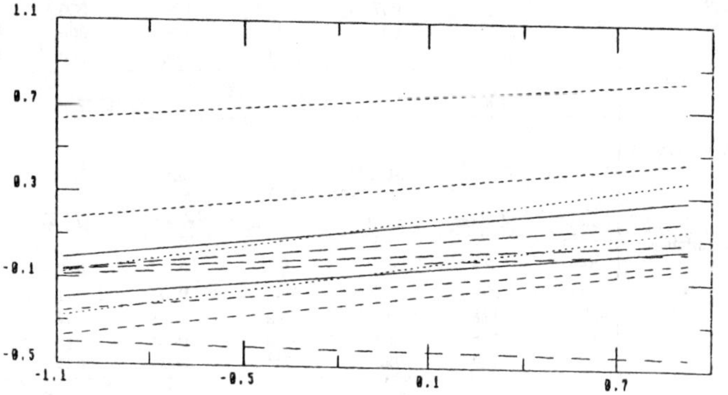

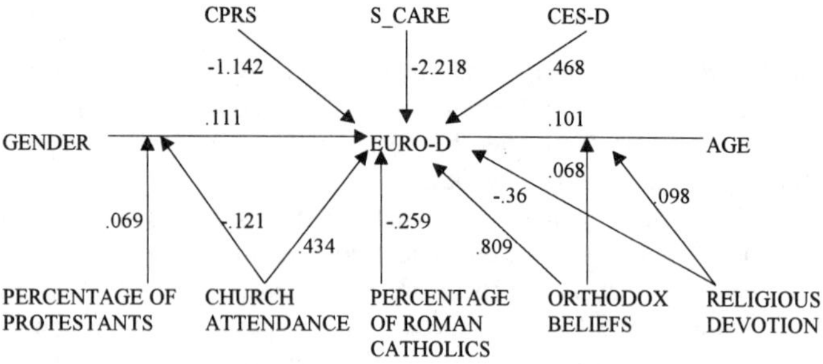

Figure 4. Outcome of the multilevel analysis

f. There are remaining differences in the individual depression scores, which is indicated in the table as individual CONS/CONS (the variance is .934). Moreover, after the analysis there are still differences in the means of depression between the regions (the variance is .015). The significance of between-region differences of the regression of age has disappeared in the analysis, but the significance of the between-region differences of the regression relating to gender is still present (the variance is .002).

Retrospective and Conclusion

It was hypothesized that a nation's religious climate will narrow the gaps in depression between men and women and according to age. The central contention was that religious climate is a mitigating condition for the individual processes which run from depressogenic personal circumstances (indicated by gender and age). As a contrast hypothesis, the depression-provoking effect of religious climate was used. The hypotheses were tested in three specific conditions: (a) elderly people, (b) in ten Western European countries, and (c) using both regional areas and countries. In the analysis several estimates for religious climate were used, in a comparative design, controlling for the instruments.

From the analysis in the above it turned out that the nature of the influence from religious climate that differs according to the background variables consists of gender or age. A nation's gender gap in depression is narrowed by national church attendance, supporting the mitigating effect hypothesis. However, a nation's age-related depression cleavage is broadened by national orthodoxy and religious devotion, supporting the provoking effect hypothesis. Moreover, it turned out that the effects that originate from unknown factors support both the mitigating effect hypothesis (regarding the percentage of Catholics, a nation's rate of orthodoxy and devotion) and the provoking effect hypothesis (regarding church attendance).

Our analysis indicates that it is impossible to decide that one single general hypothesis on the mitigating effect of religious climate on gender and age cleavages is valid. The gender-depression relation tends to be more susceptible for mitigating effects of the national religious climate, and the age-depression relation tends to be more susceptible for its provoking effects. That the mean depression score depends differently on different aspects of religious climate shows the validity of both hypotheses.

In the analysis a multilevel methodology has been used, which permits the unraveling of the effects of the different levels. Although there is no doubt about the model used, still some methodological questions remain unsolved. The relatively low the number of higher units (being twelve) makes the statistical testing not so powerful. Moreover, though the assessment of religious climate included various features, the resulting instrument may lack accuracy in how climate can be characterized. To avoid complexity, in the analysis we neglected the possibility that the religious climates of the countries of study are mutually dependent. As a result, the religious climate of a given country can exert influence on people of adjacent areas (this phenomenon is called spatial autocorrelation). From additional analyses it appeared that this influence is negligible.

It is concluded that a nation's religious culture represents a condition for the different effects between the various countries regarding gender and age as personal circumstances that are favorable to depression. This means that both the gender-depression hypothesis and the age-depression hypothesis can be considerably refined by extending them with religious climate as a national cultural factor. Gender and age differently depend on religious climate variables. This means that the mechanisms that operate with respect to gender and age and help to explain their relationships of depression are also different. Moreover, the outcome shows that religious climate as a whole is neither an enforcing nor a mitigating factor. How exactly the depressogenic mechanisms of physical and social difficulties work, which underlay the effects of gender and age on depression, depends on religious factors in particular and on cultural factors in general.

References

Asberg, M., Perris, C., Schalling, D. et al. (1978). CPRS: Development and applications of a psychiatric rating scale. *Acta Psychiatrica Scandinavica, Suppl. 271*, 1-69.

Beekman, A.T.F., Penninx, B.W.J.H., Deeg, D.J.H. et al. (1997). Depression and physical health in later life: Results from the Longitudinal Aging Study Amsterdam (LASA). *Journal of Affective Disorders 46*, 219-231.

Brown, G.W. & Harris, T.O. (1978). *Social origins of depression.* Tavistock, London.

Copeland, J.R.M., Dewey, M.E. & Griffith-Jones, H.M. (1986). A computerized psychiatric diagnostic system and case nomenclature for elderly subjects: GMS and AGECAT. *Psychological Medicine, 16*, 89-99.

Copeland, J.R.M., Beekman, A.T.F., Hooijer, C. et al. (1998). Depression in Europe: the geographical distribution among older people: the EURODEP collaboration. Submitted.

Durkheim, E. (1960 [1897]). *Le Suicide.* Presses Universitaires de France, Paris.

Ecksenberger, L.H., Lonner, W.J. & Poortinga, Y.H. (Eds.) (1979). *Cross-cultural contributions to psychology.* Lisse, Swets: and Zeitlinger.

Ellis, A. (1980). Psychotherapy and atheistic values: A response to A.E. Bergin's Psychotherapy and Religious Values. *Journal of Consulting and Clinical Psychology, 48*, 635-639.

Ellison, C.G. (1994). Religion, the life stress paradigm, and the study of depression. In J.S. Levin, J.S. (Ed.), *Religion in aging and health.* Thousand Oaks: Sage.

Ester P., Halman, L., & De Moor, R. (1994) *The individualizing society; Value change in Europe and North America.* Tilburg, the Netherlands: Tilburg University Press.

Gurland, B., Golden, R.R., Teresi, J.A., et al. (1984). The SHORT-CARE: An efficient instrument for the assessment of depression, dementia, and disability. *Journal of Gerontology, 39*, 166-169.

Harding, S., Phillips, D., & Fogarty, M. (1986). *Contrasting values in Western Europe: Unity, diversity and change.* Houndsmill, Basingstoke, England: Macmillan.

Hofstede, G. (1991). *Cultures and organizations: Software to the mind.* London: McGraw-Hill.

Idler, E.L., & Kasl, S.V. (1992). Religion, disability, depression, and the timing of death. *American Journal of Sociology, 92*, 1052-1079.

Koenig, H.G., Cohen, H.J., Blazer, D.G., Kudler, H.S. *et al.* (1995). Religious coping and cognitive symptoms of depression in elderly medical patients. *Psychosomatics, 36*, 369-375.

Pescosolido, B.A., & Georgianna, S. (1989). Durkheim, suicide, and religion: Toward a network theory of suicide. *American Sociological Review, 54*, 33-48.

Prince, M., Reischies, F., Beekman, A.T.F. *et al.* (1998). *The development of the EURO-D scale - A European Union initiative to compare symptoms of depression in 14 European centres.* Submitted.

Rasbash, J. & Woodhouse, G. (1995). *MLn: Command Reference.* London, Institute of Education, University of London.

Radloff, L.S. (1977). The CES-D scale: a self-report depression scale for research in the general population. *Applied Psychological Measurement 1*, 385-401.

Van de Vijver, F. & Leung,K. (1997). Methods and data analysis of comparative research. In: Berry, J.W., Poortinga, Y.H. & Pandey, J. (eds). *Handbook of Cross-Cultural Psychology, Vol 1. Theory and Method,* (pp. 257-300). Boston: Allyn and Bacon.

Weiss,M..G. & Kleinman, A. (1988). Depression in cross-cultural persepective: Developing a culturally informed model. In T.W. Berry, P. R. Dasen, & T. S. Sarawathi, (Eds). *Handbook of cross-cultural psychology, Vol II. Basic Processes and Human Development* (pp. 179-208). Boston, etc. Allyn and Bacon.

Wolk, S.I. & Weismann, M.M. (1995). Women and depression: An update. *Review of Psychiatry, 14*, 227-259..

Yap, P.M. (1971). Guilt and shame, depression and culture: A psychiatric cliché reexamined. *Community Contemporary Psychology, 1,* 35-53.

Psychological Recovery of Women with Cervical Cancer: The Role of Cultural Beliefs

Neena Kohli
Department of Psychology
University of Allahabad, India

Ajit K. Dalal
Department of Psychology
University of Allahabad, India

ABSTRACT

The main objective of this study was to examine cultural beliefs (both as causes of illness and as factors in recovery) to which women patients attribute their cervical cancer. The study also aimed to assess the link of causal and recovery beliefs to psychological recovery. The relationship was investigated in a cross-sectional study of three groups of 132 cervical cancer patients. The patients were randomly selected for three different stages of treatment at a local hospital. Based on responses in semi-structured interviews, we found that patients attributed fate, God and Karma as the cause of their cancer, but rated their doctor as a major factor in recovery. However, these beliefs had no link to psychological recovery of the patients. In general, recovery beliefs were more often associated with actual psychological recovery. The implications of these findings within Indian cultural context are discussed.

The most unique characteristic of the human psyche is its ability to withstand tragic life events successfully. One such tragic life event is the diagnosis of cancer. The diagnosis of cancer is the worst news a physician can bring. Many people believe that the diagnosis of cancer is synonymous with a painful, protracted death. People who suffer from cancer are confronted with many stressful situations. Apart from physical harm, cancer engenders a multitude of crises for the patients and their families, including stressed interpersonal relations, mounting medical expenses, anxieties and loss of control. Patients need enormous social and psychological resources to cope with the problems of treatment, adjustment to new realities, and rehabilitation. The way people cope with the tragic after-effects of cancer largely determines the course of their recovery. Lazarus and his colleagues (Lazarus, Averill, & Opton, 1974) have analyzed reactions to stressful events in terms of cognitive appraisal and coping. These psychological processes mediate encounters between the person and the environment that leads to adaptational outcomes.

In his theory, there are three types of appraisals, each of which serves in its own way to moderate the encounter. First, *primary* appraisal is a cognitive process of evaluating the significance of an encounter for one's well being.

Patients begin to seek answers to existential questions “Why me?”, and “Why now?” in their search for meaning in their illness. Second, *secondary* appraisal is the process of evaluating an encounter with respect to coping resources and options. Patients try to identify factors that will facilitate their recovery. The cognitive evaluation of the illness is done within the specific cultural context and influenced by native cultural models. Third, *reappraisal* occurs in response to internal psychological changes and environmental changes in the environment related to one’s coping efforts. It is at the reappraisal stage that cultural beliefs of the illness acquire greater salience.

The major objectives of the present study are (1) to examine the role of cultural beliefs (both as a cause of illness and as a factor in recovery) in the psychological recovery of women with cervical cancer at different stages of treatment; and (2) to establish links between lay explanations for causes of illness and lay explanations for recovery from illness with the actual psychological recovery of the patients.

The social psychology of attribution theory has not only suggested a classification system for explanations, but has elucidated the functions of various explanations (Heider, 1958; Kelly, 1971; Wortman, 1976). Empirical research has largely focused on the domain of interpersonal events yet similar processes are thought to affect people's interpretations of misfortunes such as unemployment (Furnham, 1982) and illness (Hewstone, 1988; Watts, 1982). The diagnosis of cervical cancer has a major disorienting influence on the patient. The world is no longer a predictable place and this uncertainty produces many existential crises. The transition from a healthy person to an ill person increases the individual’s vulnerability to further stressors. The first stressful period associated with cancer begins when the victim suspects that she might have the disease and then struggles with the decision as to how to respond to that suspicion. People vacillate between two positions saying alternately "I know it’s nothing" and " I know it’s cancer" (Holland, 1977). If a person's symptoms abate, usually the fear of cancer also abates. But if the symptoms continue, a second stressful phase usually ensures diagnostic testing to confirm or deny the presence of cancer. If the test results are positive, the third phase occurs: confrontation with the diagnosis of cancer. Attribution theory (Fiske & Taylor, 1984; Kelley, 1967) maintains that when one encounters a sudden threat or change in one's environment, one will initiate a causal search in an effort to understand the reasons for that threat or change (Pyszczynski & Greenberg, 1981; Wong & Winer, 1981). These attributions help patients understand, predict and control their environment. By understanding the cause of an event, one may also begin to understand the significance of the event and what it symbolizes in one's life. There is a growing body of literature examining the relationship between attributions and health-related functioning (Michela & Wood, 1985). In the case of cancer, no one knows the real cause. Yet causal thinking is prompted by the life-threatening illness. Taylor, Lichtman and Wood (1984) found that a majority of the cancer patients, their mates, relatives and close friends do identify the causes of cancer.

This causal search is not confined solely to specific medical explanations of the health problem. Patients also try to comprehend their illness experience within the larger social and cultural context (Radley, 1994). Each culture has its own belief system and the meaning of the illness is based on the socio-religious belief system prevalent in a particular culture. The way in which people react to a major life crisis, such as cancer, would depend on the theories and beliefs which people of a particular culture hold about the world and their illness. The connotation of disease is unique to the particular cultural context. Wortman (1983) posited that patients' beliefs about the world play an important role in shaping their reactions to sudden onset of illness or disability and hence the subsequent recovery process. Thus, a patient's explanation for illness etiology is often a social construction derived from the cultural models of illness. In the Indian setting, the research evidence suggests that tragic life events are more often attributed to metaphysical beliefs, that is belief in Karma, God's will and fate (Dalal, 1989; Mishra, 1997). Such metaphysical beliefs help people to accept their present suffering and keeps their hope alive for better future (Radhakrishnan, 1926).

The belief in Karma provides a convincing explanation for a host of undesirable life events. This belief is unique to the eastern world view. Karma is a net balance of good and bad deeds in previous lives (Paranjpe, 1998). The Hindu life spiral combines dharma, the law of the present life, with Karma. The basic ethical implications of the law of Karma follow from the assumptions that good actions lead to desirable consequences and vice-versa. According to Indian thought, the law of Karma became a basic and common assumption covering lawfulness within the material as well as the moral domains. In the Indian ethos, the doctrine of Karma, shapes the ideas, that an individual is responsible for his or her actions. This doctrine suggests a natural and inevitable causal connection between actions and their consequences.

Belief in God is a frequently cited metaphysical belief in times of crisis. God is seen as an external agent who controls rewards and punishments, not always according to what one deserves (Paranjpe, 1984). This is different from the doctrine of Karma. The belief in fate implies that all events in one's life are predestined and little can be done to alter them. The individual has no control over fate. Fate is also different from Karma because Karma does not imply any kind of resignation to one's destiny. Though conceptually different, these metaphysical beliefs have been used interchangeably in common parlance. Even in earlier research investigations, metaphysical beliefs have not been appropriately differentiated. It is important to our understanding of attributional patterns that these causal categories reflect their socio-cultural context.

This culturally derived worldview provides an understanding of not only the causes of illness but also the factors that are likely to contribute to recovery. Whereas causal beliefs are retrospective because of their emphasis on the past (antecedents), recovery beliefs have a prospective orientation because they emphasize the future (outcome). The relative salience of causal and recovery beliefs may vary depending upon the patient's phase of treatment. When patients initially report for treatment, they are still in a state of shock and disbelief. They are preoccupied with the existential question: "Why me?" Here the search for meaning is more salient. At a later stage, when the existential anxieties are over, the patient's concern may shift to physical recovery and here the recovery beliefs dominate. However, to date, this shift in beliefs has not been demonstrated empirically.

Most of the earlier investigations have focused exclusively on causal attributions for health problems (Weary, Stanley & Harvey, 1989), and have not distinguished between causal and recovery beliefs. Brickman and colleagues (1982) have proposed four models of helping and coping. They draw a distinction between attribution of responsibility for a problem (who is to blame for a past event) and attribution of responsibility for a solution (who is to control future events). In the first (called the moral model) actors are held responsible for both problems and solutions. In the compensatory model, people are seen as not responsible for problems, but responsible for solutions. In the medical model, individuals are seen as responsible for neither problems nor solutions. In the enlightenment model, actors are seen as responsible for problems but are unable or unwilling to provide solutions. Whether or not people are held responsible for causing their problems and whether or not they are held responsible for solving these problems, are the factors determining four fundamentally different orientations to the world. These different models of helping and coping exist in the minds of helpers, aggressors and recipients of help or aggression. They are also embodied in social institutions that mete out help or punishment. These models can be tested for causal and recovery beliefs. For example, one may consider oneself responsible for recovery (or non-recovery from illness) and not for the disease.

The present study explored the role of cultural beliefs (both as a cause of illness and as a factor in recovery) in the psychological recovery of women with cervical cancer. Diagnosis of cancer brings with it a series of common reactions to the stressful situation. Most cancer patients appear to go through several stages of emotional response to their diagnosis. No theoretical formulation contends that all individuals will respond identically to all aversive outcomes. Nonetheless, most theorists suggest that there will be some common pattern of reactions to undesirable life events at different stages. The key point is that stages of emotional response do exist and these may influence the choice of beliefs. The purpose was to link the stages of emotional response with the chosen sample. All patients were in the same stage of cancer but at different phases in their treatment. In the first phase of treatment, the women still has to come to terms with the situation. She begins to search meaning for her illness. The treatment-associated problems may or may not be a key focus. At this phase, causal beliefs may be more important to psychological health than recovery factors. In the third and final phase of treatment, the salience of beliefs may be different. Thus, the purpose of the present study was to see what patterns of causal and recovery beliefs emerge at the differing phases of treatment, and to examine the relationship of those beliefs with psychological recovery.

Method

Subjects

One hundred and thirty two Hindu female cervical cancer patients treated at a local hospital in Allahabad, India, constituted the sample for this study. All the patients were diagnosed as Stage III patients by the attending doctor. Stage refers to the spread of the cancer. Staging is important because the treatment plan depends not only on the type of tumor, but also on the extent of its spread. The treatment modalities for all the patients were radiotherapy. But the women were at different phases of treatment. Group 1 patients (n=50) were those patients who had just been inducted into the treatment program (first week of radiation). Group 2 patients (n=40) were towards the end of the treatment program (last week of radiation). These patients were given a supplementary dosage of radiation for a period of two weeks. Group 3 patients (n=42) were those who came for their first check-up after the completion of the course of treatment. These patients reported after about two months of treatment. We will refer to the patients interchangeable as group or phase: (e.g., Group 1/ Phase 1, Group 2 / Phase 2 and Group 3 / Phase 3 are terms used interchangeably). The duration of treatment in Phase 1 was four weeks and in Phase 2 it was two weeks. Between these phases there was a gap of two weeks.

The age of the patients ranged from 25 to 65 years, with a mean age of 46.5 years. Out of 132 patients, 110 patients were illiterate and 93 patients were from a rural background. These women had an average of 4 children, and 112 patients had a family income of less than Rs. 1000 per month. Three one-way analysis of variance were performed on three demographic background measures namely age, number of children and income. The F values show that the three groups of patients at three phases of treatment did not differ from each other in terms of age F (2, 129) = 1.07, $p > .05$ and number of children F (2, 129) = 1.32, $p > .05$. For income, there were significant differences among the three groups, F (2, 129) = 5.34, $p < .01$. Chi-squares were computed for two background variables, namely level of education (illiterate/ literate) and residential background (rural/ urban). None of the chi-square values were significant, implying that the groups were comparable on these background measures. Thus, the patients in all the three groups were comparable on all these background variables, except monthly income, where there was some difference.

Interview Schedule
We conducted semi-structured interviews were conducted. To facilitate communication, an interview schedule in Hindi language was prepared to tap information pertaining to (1) background of the patient, (2) history of illness and treatment, (3) lay explanations about the causes of illness, (4) lay explanations about the factors contributing to recovery from illness and (5) psychological recovery. The first few questions focused on the age of the patient, her background (educational and residential), family income and number of children. The next set of questions was related to the illness itself: history and nature of the illness, frequency and type of complaints, severity of the illness, remedial steps followed and expectation from treatment. Questions about causal attributions were the next set. The first item was an open-ended question asking patients to mention as to what could be the cause of one's illness. The patients were then asked to rate eight different causes to indicate the extent to which these were responsible for the illness. These causes (fate, God's will, Karmaphala, own carelessness, bodily weakness, mental stress, family circumstances and other's negligence) were rated on a five point rating scale, from "not at all" responsible (1) to "fully" responsible (5). Similarly, nine recovery factors, (fate, God's will, Karmaphala, self effort, worship, doctors, appropriate treatment, family and appropriate time), were rated by the patients concerning the possible contribution of these factors to their recovery.

The last set of questions was related to psychological recovery. To measure the psychological recovery of cancer patients, we employed a scale developed by Dalal et al. (1995). The scale has two sections. The first 8 item sub-scale assesses illness appraisal with statements related to patients' own evaluation of their illness/recovery primarily in comparison to illness/recovery of other patients in similar conditions. The patients were asked 'to what extent the statements were true in their case (very little to very much)?' Cronbach's alpha (α) was .74 for this sub-scale. The second 21 item subscale mapped emotional reactions or mood state of the patient. It included those thoughts and anxieties, experienced by the patient while convalescing in the hospital. These feelings included feelings of hopelessness, fear of doom and feeling hurt. The patient rated the frequency of these feelings from "never occurring" to "always occurring". Cronbach's alpha (α) for this subscale was .80. The overall psychological recovery scale as used in this study had a Cronbach's alpha (α) of .90.

Procedure

We obtained permission to conduct the interviews from the Head of the Oncology Department. The treatment status of the prospective participants was known to the researcher by way of the record file of the patient and from the attending doctor. The researcher, (first author), approached each patient personally either in the waiting room (for patients who came for radiation therapy) or in the office (for those who came for the first routine check-up). The patients were assured that their responses would in no way influence their treatment in the hospital. The patients were asked questions in a pre-assigned order, in a face-to-face interview. The responses were recorded verbatim. Because the majority of the patients were illiterate, care was taken to ensure understanding. The interview lasted about 40 minutes per patient. All interview data were collected by the same interviewer.

Results

Lay Explanations of the Causes of Illness

The patients were asked to appraise the probable causes of their illness. All the patients (N=132) gave at least one cause of their illness and 62 patients gave more than one cause. Content analysis of these causal descriptions revealed that illness related factors (symptoms) were mentioned by as much as 22% patients. Other frequently mentioned causes were: family circumstances (18.9%), God's will (16.7%), Fate (15.9%), negligence (12.9%), Karmaphala and Mental stress (10.6% each). Chi-square analysis was carried on for the three groups of patients at three distinct phases of treatment. The results of chi-square analysis revealed that there was no significant difference amongst the three groups in the identification of salient causes. For the open-ended question, phase of treatment had no effect on the choice of salient causes.

Along with the open-ended questions, the patient also rated eight given causes to indicate the extent to which each cause was responsible for their illness. To examine which causal beliefs was salient at which phase of treatment, eight one-way analyses of variance (ANOVAS) were computed. Of the eight causal beliefs, only fate, yielded a significant difference across phase of treatment, $F(2,129)=3.17, p<.05$.

To examine the pattern of causality within each group, the means computed for each belief were converted into specific causal categories (beliefs) means. The results presented in Table1 display the means for each causal belief and for each specific causal category for the three groups at three distinct phases of treatment. A look at the table shows that metaphysical beliefs have higher means as compared to causal attribution self and others, across all groups.

Table 1
Means of causal beliefs and causal categories for the three groups

Causal beliefs	Group 1/ Phase 1 (n=50)	Group 2/ Phase 2 (n=40)	Group 3/ Phase 3 (n=42)
Metaphysical	3.64	3.39	3.61
Fate	3.48	3.05	3.17
God's will	3.56	3.53	3.95
Karmaphala	3.88	3.60	3.71
Self	2.74	2.27	2.72
Own carelessness	2.66	2.09	2.45
Bodily weakness	2.56	2.23	2.50
Mental stress	3.00	2.48	3.21
Others	2.42	2.23	2.18
Family circumstances	2.62	2.33	2.33
Others negligence	2.22	2.13	2.02

Lay Explanations of the Factors Contributing to Recovery from Illness
The patients rated nine recovery beliefs indicating the extent to which each belief contributed to their recovery. To compare the groups on each recovery belief, nine one-way analyses of variance (ANOVA) were computed. None of the values were significant, indicating no differences in recovery beliefs across the three treatment.

To examine the pattern of recovery beliefs within each group, the means computed for each recovery belief were converted into specific recovery categories (beliefs) means. The results presented in Table 2, display the means for each recovery belief and for each specific recovery category for the three groups at distinct phases of treatment.

A look at the table shows that patients frequently attribute their recovery to others. Metaphysical factors are second in importance to recovery with patients rating themselves as least important to recovery. This is true for all the groups across the three phases of treatment.

Correlations Between Causal and Recovery Beliefs
Correlations were computed between causal and recovery beliefs to see the pattern of relationship amongst these beliefs. The results are presented in Table 3. Of the 72 correlations computed between causal and recovery beliefs, only 19 were significant. Thus, we have empirical support for separating causal and recovery beliefs.

Table 2. Means of recovery beliefs and recovery categories for the three groups

Recovery beliefs	Group 1/ Phase 1 (n=50)	Group 2/ Phase 2 (n=40)	Group 3/ Phase 3 (n=42)
Metaphysical	3.69	3.33	3.53
Fate	3.26	2.95	3.08
God's will	4.16	3.80	4.03
Karmaphala	3.66	3.23	3.47
Self	3.16	3.02	3.03
Self effort	3.46	3.13	3.33
Worship	2.86	2.90	2.73
Others	3.87	3.82	3.86
Doctors	4.42	4.33	4.41
Appropriate treatment	4.00	4.03	4.06
Family	3.10	3.00	3.10
Appropriate time	3.94	3.90	3.89

Psychological Recovery

The psychological recovery scores of the three patient groups are presented in Table 4.

Table 3. Correlations among causal and recovery beliefs (n=132)

Causal belief	Recovery beliefs						
	God	Fate	Karmaphala	Doctors	Appropriate treatment	Worship	Self effort
Fate	.30**	.21**	.14	.40**	.36**	.04	.00
God's will	.23**	.23**	.21*	.25**	.41**	.11	.10
Karmaphala	.11	.12	.16	.16*	.14	−.09	−.01
Own-carelessness	−.11	−.07	−.09	−.09	−.08	−.12	.11
Bodily weakness	−.05	−.09	−.08	−.08	.07	.04	.07
Mental stress	−.07	−.08	−.12	−.12	−.09	.02	.04
Family circumstances	−.12	−.14	−.15	−.15	−.09	−.09	−.11
Others negligence	−.15	−.20	.01	.01	−.31**	−.01	−.19*

* p < .05 **

The results show that Group 3 patients report higher means for illness appraisal than patients in Groups 1 and 2. There is a consistent progression across the three groups. The patients in Group 1 who have just begun treatment report the least positive view of their recovery. But as patients progress in treatment, their faith in recovery also increases (as is evident from the means of Group 2 patients). Similarly, patients of Group 3 who have completed the treatment report the greatest faith in their own recovery. This progressive trend is evident in the mood reactions sub-scale. This is not surprising because mood is more labile than cognitive appraisal. Patients can oscillate between hope and despair. Thus, a steady and consistent mood pattern was not expected.

Table 4. Means of the three groups on psychological recovery scale

Psychological Recovery Scale	Group 1/ Phase 1 (n=50)	Group 2/ Phase 2 (n=40)	Group 3/ Phase 3 (n=42)
Illness Appraisal (Subscale 1)	3.00	3.34	3.46
Mood reactions (Subscale 2)	3.17	3.38	3.31
Overall Psychological recovery (Subscale 1 and 2 combined)	3.09	3.36	3.39

Relationship Between Causal Beliefs and Psychological Recovery

To examine the relationship between causal reasoning and psychological recovery correlations were computed between this set of variables. These correlations are presented in Table 5. The results of Table 5 reveal that as far as psychological recovery is concerned, mental stress correlated in a negative way with psychological recovery at phases I and phase III of the treatment. There was no significant relationship between mental stress and psychological recovery as shown by the correlation obtained for group 2 (phase II) patients. There was a significant negative correlation between family circumstances and psychological recovery for patients who were at phase I of the treatment. No other causal beliefs shared any significant correlation with psychological recovery across the three phases of treatment.

Table 5. Correlations of causal beliefs with psychological recovery scale for the three groups

Causal beliefs	Psychological Recovery Scale (Two sub-scales combined)		
	Group 1/ Phase 1 (n=50)	Group 2/ Phase 2 (n=40)	Group 3/ Phase 3 (n=42)
Fate	– .04	.10	– .11
God	.24	.24	– .08
Karmaphala	– .15	– .20	.06
Own consciousness	– .08	– .17	– .02
Bodily weakness	– .25	– .27	– .17
Mental stress	– .36**	– .29	– .45**
Family circumstances	– .37**	.29	– .24
Other's negligence	– .21	– .03	– .14

** $p < .01$

Relationship Between Recovery Beliefs and Psychological Recovery

To examine the relationship between recovery beliefs and psychological recovery, correlations were computed between this set of variables. These correlations are presented in Table 6. The results of Table 6 reveal that Group 1 patients (Phase 1 of treatment) showed a significant position correlation between the psychological recovery and contribution of recovery factors, God and family. However, for Phase 2 patients, there was a significant positive correlation between appropriate treatment, and appropriate time with psychological recovery. For Group 3 patients, there was a significant positive correlation between recovery factors of self-effort, and appropriate treatment with psychological recovery. No other recovery belief correlated with psychological recovery for any group of patients.

Table 6. Correlations of recovery beliefs with psychological recovery scale for the three groups

Recovery beliefs	Psychological Recovery Scale (Two sub-scales combined)		
	Group 1/ Phase 1 (n=50)	Group 2/ Phase 2 (n=40)	Group 3/ Phase 3 (n=42)
Fate	.18	– .08	.30
God	.40**	– .02	– .09
Karmaphala	.14	.15	– .21
Self effort	.29	.17	.51**
Worship	.15	.13	.05
Doctors	– .02	.23	– .19
Appropriate treatment	.17	.50**	.38**
Family	.46**	.01	– .07
Appropriate time	.24	.39*	.13

* $p < .05$ ** $p < .01$

Discussion

The goal of the present study was to examine the explanatory models which poor rural Indian women use to understand their illness. We first assessed which cultural beliefs (causal and recovery) were most salient for each treatment group. Our second objective was to establish the link between causal and recovery beliefs with psychological recovery.

By examining the qualitative data from the open-ended question relating to causal explanations of the illness, we found that patients most frequently reported "symptoms" of the illness, such as excessive bleeding as the cause. There was an overlap between the meaning of an illness and assigning of causality. This may be due to patients' lack of knowledge about the illness and/or general lack of education. Family circumstances were rated as the second most frequent cause for illness symptoms. Most of the patients were from a very poor economic background (family income less than Rs.

1000 per month) and making ends meet is so predominant in their psyche that it reflects in their blaming their family conditions for the present crisis. Interestingly, it is not the family that is blamed. The assigning of causality is to family conditions which is outside one's control. Attribution to God's will and fate were also high as compared to Karmaphala

The Hindu patients did not spontaneously mention "Karma" when asked about the cause of the disease although belief in Karma is pervasive among the Hindu patients. In Ayurveda (the traditional Indian medicine system), cosmic beliefs are intertwined in the scientific context. "The *Carak Samhita* (one of the main texts for Ayurveda), talks of diseases resulting from the action of pervious lives and the futility of curative efforts till the effects of individual Karma have been exhausted after taking their own predetermined course" (Kakar, 1982, p. 225). In a post-hoc inquiry, many patients mentioned that they considered metaphysical beliefs to be too obvious and thought the researcher was not interested in knowing about such causes. Also, some patients felt inhibited about discussing their metaphysical beliefs with an educated researcher.

In a study by Dalal and Singh (1992) on tuberculosis patients, it was found that cosmic factors were not frequently mentioned in response to an open-ended item. Joshi (1995) in her study on Hindu insulin-dependent diabetic patients found that none of the patients spontaneously mentioned "Karma" when asked about the cause. However, in the structural rating responses patients assigned higher causality of Karmaphala. People take comfort in the concept of Karmaphala. This finding is similar to the ones obtained in earlier studies (Agarwal & Dalal, 1993; Dalal & Pande, 1988; Dalal & Singh, 1992, Joshi, 1995). Karma is deep-seated and enduring belief. But things that are deep-seated sometimes have to be brought to the fore. In the Indian worldview, causality extends beyond the natural world to the moral domain. A conscious effort on the part of the researcher is required to bring the discussion of Karma back to the everyday world.

In addition to Karmaphala, all the three groups of patients attributed their cancer to God's will and fate. This finding is consistent with those obtained in earlier studies (Agarwal & Dalal, 1993; Dalal & Pande, 1988; Dalal & Singh, 1992). Attributing the disease to metaphysical beliefs makes sense in a culture where religion pervades in all life domains. Metaphysical beliefs are embedded in mind and are not affected by specific distress or disease. Whenever people are in crisis, even the care-givers (e.g., family members) refer to these beliefs to explain suffering. Joshi (1988) and Weiss *et. al.,* (1986) found that the indigenous healing practices of the east emphasized supernatural causality including punishment, sorcery, spirit or God.

A clear cultural difference is found in attribution of illness in Western and Indian studies. Helman (1978) found that common cold was thought to be caused by environmental factors such as rain and cold winds. By contrast, fever was viewed as caused by "germs", "bugs" and "viruses". Blumhagen (1980) found that rural patients considered diet (such as eating red meat) as an important cause of hypertension. In Western societies, the emphasis upon life style choices and individuals responsibility for preserving their health and avoiding 'risk' has come to dominate explanations of illness. Self-indulgence and lack of self-discipline are viewed as the reasons why people become ill (Lupton, 1993). Thus, in the Western societies, the perceived causes of illness are mostly related to the material world, such as diet, health habits, viruses and self - whereas in India causal beliefs are embedded in the moral world. It seems that at the core of the explanatory model in the West are medical causes - whereas in India these are metaphysical beliefs.

While metaphysical beliefs were important causal explanations for the disease, these beliefs were not associated with recovery beliefs. For example, Karmaphala was considered as an important causal, but not a recovery factor by the patients. Such beliefs are consistent with the principle of Karma. This principle is supposed to explain what has already happened or is happening, but not what is going to happen (Gokhale, 1961). For all the three group of patients, the doctor was deemed important to recovery from cancer. Dalal and Singh (1992) also reported doctor as an important recovery factor. It is quite likely that hospital setting in which the patients were interviewed strengthened this belief. As noted by Krantz (1980) and Kornfeld (1972), hospitalization constitutes a stressful event for most people. It is quite possible that in a hospital setting, doctors are likely to be viewed by patients as the most powerful people on whom they are totally dependent for recovery from the disease.

In addition to the doctor, patients identified other recovery beliefs, e.g., appropriate treatment, family and appropriate time). Patients felt that their recovery was in the hands of others. These powerful others were seen as having control over the disease. The patients were confident these controlling agents would help them to recover. The patients consider themselves least responsible for recovering from illness. The groups however were not different on the choice of recovery beliefs although the salience of the recovery beliefs did differ across the groups.

With regard to psychological recovery, findings from correlational analysis point out, for the three groups of patients. God's will, fate and Karmaphala as causal factors did not correlate with psychological recovery. It appears that though metaphysical beliefs about the chronic illness are more frequently expressed in a particular cultural context, they do not necessarily (or directly) relate to psychological theory. This finding is consistent with an earlier finding on accident victims (temporarily disabled subjects) (Dalal & Pande, 1988) and (Dalal & Singh, 1992) on tuberculosis patients. Most empirical Western researches have shown that beliefs about the existence of God and his benevolent nature help individuals to cope with distress (Dimsdale, 1974; Folkman, Schaefer & Lazarus, 1979; Lipowski, 1970). But the findings of the present study showed no relationship. However, the causal belief of mental stress, likely due to the demands of others, did relate negatively with psychological recovery of Group 1 and Group 3 patients. Having a causal theory was predictive of bad adjustment. No other causal belief was predictive of either good or bad psychological recovery. Studies by Affleck et al., (1987a, b); Bulman and Wortman (1977) and Taylor et al., (1984) all point to the fact that attributing the cause of one's illness to others predicts poor physical and psychological adjustment.

As far as lay explanations about the factors responsible for recovery were concerned, the first group's recovery beliefs of God and family correlated positively with psychological recovery. In this sample, patients reported a strong faith in God and it may be that religious beliefs serve as a life stress buffer by enhancing faith in the specific coping strategies. People experiencing tragic outcomes are frequently told by a support group to have greater faith in God (Dalal, 1989). Family as a recovery factor is not surprising, because in India falling ill is a family event. The entire family mobilizes their resources to cope with the crisis. It is the family who brings the patient for treatment. It is not an unusual sight to find the corridors of hospitals thronged by family members.

For patients in Group 2, the recovery beliefs, appropriate treatment and appropriate time, correlated positively with psychological recovery. Tacit support for this finding is found in Taylor et al. (1984) work on breast cancer patients where they found that both the beliefs that one can control one's own cancer and the belief that the physician or treatment can control it are strongly associated with the disease, accelerates physical recovery and hence facilitates psychological recovery. The contribution of recovery belief: appropriate time in promoting psychological recovery endorses the patients beliefs in order and in a just world. Our culture reinforces acceptance, resignation to fate and quietude. By emphasizing appropriate time as being conducive to psychological recovery, the patients seek to make sense in a world that has been rendered meaningless.

For Group 3 patients, the recovery beliefs of self-effort and appropriate treatment showed a positive correlation with psychological recovery. The emphasis on self-effort as a factor in psychological recovery accelerates the process of self-enhancement. Traumatic events often reduce self-esteem (Briar, 1966; Pearlon & Schooler, 1978; Ryan, 1971) even when the individual had no responsibility for bringing the event about. Viewing the self as positive helps in rebuilding one's assumptive would, which has been shattered as a result of tragic events. Appropriate treatment as a recovery belief assumes importance because physical recovery is as important as psychological recovery. Only if the treatment is satisfying will the patient recover psychologically.

This study also tried to differentiate the differing stages of medical recovery of the patient and then examine the relationship between medical and psychological recovery. However, we found very differences among the three groups. It is very difficult to define medical recovery for these patients. What is recovery today may be recurrence tomorrow. The rate of recovery and the extent of recovery was synonymous for the doctor. It was one problematic issue, which can be seen as the limitation of this study.

However, the findings from present research provide a ray of hope. These findings can form the basis of designing effective health interventions for cervical cancer women. Issues like the cultural context, cultural beliefs of the patients, the hospital environment and setting can all form the basis of effective health interventions. A holistic approach to designing patient counseling would go a long way in reducing the distress and agony of these hapless patients.

References

Affleck, G., Tennen, H., Croog, S., & Levine, S. (1987a). Causal attribution, perceived benefits, and morbidity after a heart attack : An 8-year study. *Journal of Counseling and Clinical Psychology, 55*, 29-35.

Affleck, G., Tennen, H., Croog, S., & Levine, S. (1987b). Causal attribution, perceived control,and recovery from a heart attack. *Journal of Social and Clinical Psychology, 5*, 356-364.

Agarwal, M., & Dalal, A.K. (1993). Beliefs about the 'world' and recovery from myocardial infarction. *Journal of Social Psychology, 133(3)*, 385-394.

Blumhagen, D. (1980). Hypertension: A folk illness with a medical name. *Culture, Medicine and Psychiatry, 4*, 197-227.

Briar, S. (1966). Welfare from below: Recipient views of the public welfare system. *California Law Review, 54*, 370-385.

Brickman, P., Rabinowitz, V.C., Karuza, J., Coates, D., Cohn, E., & Kidder, L. (1982). Models of helping and coping. *American Psychologist, 37*, 368-384.

Bulman, R.J., & Wortman, C.B. (1977). Attribution of blame and coping in the "real world": Severe accident victims react to their lot. *Journal of Personality and Social Psychology, 35*, 351-363.

Dalal, A.K. (1989). *The effect of causal attribution for tragic events on communicating sentiments to the victims.* Unpublished manuscript, University of Allahabad, Allahabad, India.

Dalal, A.K., & Pande, N. (1988). Psychological recovery of the accident victims with temporary and permanent disability. *International Journal of Psychology, 23*, 25-40.

Dalal, A.K., & Singh, A.K. (1992). Role of causal recovery beliefs in the psychological adjustment to a chronic disease. *Psychology and Health, 6*, 193-203.

Dalal, A.K., Kohli, N., & Agarwal, M. (1995). *Development of a measure of psychological recovery of hospital patients.* Unpublished manuscript, University of Allahabad, Allahabad, India.

Dimsdale, J.E. (1974). The coping behavior of Nazi concentration camp survivors. *American Journal of Psychiatry, 131*, 792-797.

Fiske, S.T., & Taylor, S.E. (1984). *Social cognition.* New York: Random House.

Folkman, S., Schaefer, C., & Lazarus, R.S. (1979). Cognitive processes as mediators of stress and coping. In V. Hamilton & D.M. Wartburton (Eds.), *Human stress and cognition: An information processing approach* (pp.265-298). London : Wiley.

Furnham, A. (1982). Explanations for unemployment in Britain. *European Journal of Social Psychology, 12,* 335-352.

Gokhale, B.G. (1961). *Indian thought throughout the ages: A study of some dominant concept.* Bombay: Asia Publishing House.

Heider, F. (1958). *The psychology of interpersonal relations.* New York: Wiley.

Helman, C. (1978). "Feed a cold, starve a fever". Folk models of infection in an English suburban community and their relation to medical treatment. *Culture, Medicine and Psychiatry, 2,* 107-137.

Hewstone, M. (1988). *Causal attribution: From cognitive processes to collective beliefs.* Oxford: Basil Blackwell.

Holland, J.C. (1977). Psychological aspects of oncology. *Medical Clinics of North America, 61,* 737-748.

Joshi, M.S. (1995). Lay explanations of the causes of diabetes in India and the UK. In I. Markova & R.M. Farr (Eds.), *Representations of health, illness and handicap.* Switzerland: Harwood Academic Publishers.

Joshi, P.C. (1988). Traditional medical system in the central Himalayas. *The Eastern Anthropologist, 41,*(77-86.

Kakar, S. (1982). *Shamans, Mystics and Doctors: A psychological inquiry into India and its healing tradition.* London: Unwin Paperbacks.

Kelley, H.H. (1967). Attribution theory in social psychology. In D. Levine (Ed.), *Nebraska symposium on motivation* (Vol. 15). Lincoln: University of Nebraska Press.

Kelley, H.H. (1971). Attribution in social interaction. In E.E. Jones, D.E. Valins, & B. Weiner (Eds.), *Attribution: Perceiving the causes of behavior.* Morristown, NJ: General Learning Press.

Kornfeld, D.A. (1972). The hospital environment: Its impact on the patient. *Advances in Psychosomatic Medicine, 8,* 252-270.

Krantz, D.A. (1980). Cognitive processes and recovery from heart attack: A review and theoretical analysis. *Journal of Human Stress, 6(3),* 27-38.

Lazarus, R.S., Averill, J.R., & Opton, E.M. (1974). The psychology of coping: Issue of research and assessment. In G.V. Coelho, D.A. Mamkereg, St. J.E. Adams (Eds.), *Coping or alleviation.* New York: Basic Books.

Lipowski, Z.L. (1970). Physical illness, the individual and the coping process. *Psychiatry and Medicine, 1,* 91-102.

Lupton, D. (1993). Risk as a moral danger: The social and political functions of risk discourse in public health. *International Journal of Health Sciences, 23(3),* 425-35.

Michela, & Wood, J.V. (1985). Causal attributions in health and illness. In P.H. Kendall (Ed.), *Advances in cognitive-behavioral research and therapy* (Vol. 5). New York: Academic Press.

Mishra, R.C. (1997). Family support and health care in a culturally changing village community in northern India. *Social Science International, 13,* 10-18.

Paranjpe, A.C. (1984). *Theoretical psychology: The meeting of east and west.* New York: Plenum Press.

Paranjpe, A.C. (1998). *Self and identity in modern psychology and Indian thought.* New York: Plenum Press.

Pearlin, L.I., & Schooler, C. (1978). The structure of coping. *Journal of Health and Social Behavior, 19,* 2-21.

Pyszczynski, T.A., & Greenberg, J. (1981). Role of disconfirmed expectancies in the instigation of attributional processing. *Journal of Personality and Social psychology, 40,* 31-38.

Radhakrishnan, S. (1926). *The Hindu view of life.* Bombay: Blackie.

Radley, A. (1994). *Making sense of illness.* London: Sage Publications.

Ryan, W. (1971). *Blaming the victim.* New York: Pantheon Books.

Taylor, S.E., Lichtman, R.R., & Wood, J.U. (1984). *Adjustment to breast cancer: Physical, sociodemographic and psychological predictors.* Unpublished manuscript, University of California, Los Angeles.

Watts, F.N. (1982). Attributional aspects of medicine. In C. Antaki and C. Brewin (Eds.), *Attributions and psychological change: Applications of attributional theories to clinical and education practice*. London: Academic Press.

Weary, G., Stanley, M.A., & Harvey, J.H. (1989). *Attribution.* New York: Springer Verlag.

Weiss, M.G., Sharma, S.D., Gaur, R.K., Sharma, J.S., Desai, A., & Doongaji, D.R. (1986). Traditional concepts of mental disorder among Indian psychiatric patients. Preliminary report of work in progress. *Social Science and Medicine, 23(4),* 379-386.

Wong, P.T.P., & Winer, B. (1981). When people ask "Why" questions and the heuristics of attributional research. *Journal of Personality and Social Psychology, 40,* 650-663. world": Severe accident victims react to their lot. *Journal of Personality and Social Psychology, 35*, 351-363.

Wortman, C.B. (1976). Causal attributions and personal control. In J.H. Harvey, W.J. Ickes, & R.F. Kidd (Eds.), *New direction in attribution research* (Vol. 1, pp. 23-52). Hillsdale, NJ: Lawrence Erlbaum Associates.

Wortman, C.B. (1983). *Social support and the cancer patient.* Paper presented at the annual meeting of the American Cancer Society, St. Petersburg Beach, FL.

Cultural Manifestations of Self and Self-Concept

Self-Construal and Anger Action Tendencies in Hong Kong and the United Kingdom

Paul Redford
University of Sussex
School of Social Sciences

ABSTRACT

Action tendencies are a central component of an emotional experience, but they have rarely been studied, particularly across cultures. The present study examines the action tendencies associated with the emotional experience of anger in Hong Kong (n = 110) and the United Kingdom (n = 136). As predicted, individuals from the United Kingdom (UK) were more likely to report direct aggression action tendencies than individuals from Hong Kong. Furthermore, individuals from Hong Kong were more likely to report displaced aggression action tendencies than individuals from the UK. These cultural differences in action tendency cast doubt over the theory of display rules, suggesting that there may be differences across cultures in the action tendencies as well as the emotional display associated with anger. In an attempt to 'unpackage' this cultural influence the study also examines the hypothesis that individual differences in emotional experience across cultures can be accounted for by differences in self-construal. Partial support is found for this hypothesis.

In recent years emotion theorists have converged upon a componential model of emotion, which proposes that emotions are comprised of various components (Frijda, 1986; Scherer, 1984). There is also growing evidence that the experience of these components varies across cultures (Mesquita, Frijda, & Scherer, 1998). The present study aims to integrate emotion theory with Markus and Kitayama's (1991) proposition that self-construal may mediate the influence of culture on emotional experience. This is achieved through an examination of anger action tendencies and self-construal in the UK and Hong Kong.

Within Western cultures, anger is one of the most frequently experienced emotions (Oatley & Duncan, 1994; Scherer, Wallbott & Summerfield 1986; Tavris, 1982). It is an important emotion with many social and behavioural consequences. Furthermore, it plays an important role in regulating interpersonal behaviour such as social conflict (Averill, 1982; Deffenbacher, Oetting, Lynch, & Morris, 1996). Nevertheless, anger research is sparse and seldom addresses the influence of culture on the experience of anger. As Sharkin (1996) states:

> The experience of being angry is a common phenomenon of everyday living, yet empirical study of anger has been relatively limited. As a result, our understanding of anger has tended to be based more on assumptions than empirical data...[furthermore]... the cross-cultural analysis of anger has yet to receive much attention...It is my belief that we are neglecting to address a very important issue... (p. 166-167)

Frijda (1986) has suggested that an emotional experience can be separated into 7 components covering the subjective (feeling), cognitive (thinking) and behavioural (action) manifestations of emotion (See Table 1). This model of emotion allows for documentation and subsequent predictions concerning cultural similarities and differences, both within components and across components. Using this framework it is possible for some components to be universal at the same time that others exhibit cultural variation. For example, all cultures may display a similar facial expression when angry, but the events that evoke anger may vary across cultures. Conceptualising emotions as processes or syndromes (comprised of various components) provides a fruitful approach to the study of emotion (Averill, 1982; Frijda, 1986; Scherer 1984) that overcomes the universalist versus relativist dichotomy that has hampered cross-cultural emotion research (Mesquita & Frijda, 1992).

Table 1. Components involved in the elicitation and manifestation of an emotional experience. Adapted from Frijda (1986)

Component	**Brief Definition**
1. Antecedent Event	Events that elicit emotions.
2. Event Coding	Categorisation of an event into a certain type, or schemata.
3. Appraisal	How the event is understood in respect to an individuals well being, and ability to cope etc.
4. Physiological Reaction Patterns	Physiological body changes and representations of physiological changes.
5. Action Tendency	The impulse or inclination to behave or act in a certain way
6. Emotional Behaviour	Overt actual behaviour.
7. Regulation	Voluntary inhibitory control or enhancement. This can affect all emotion components above.

Research that has been conducted using the componential model of emotion has been dominated by the examination of emotion differentiation (i.e. what differentiates anger from fear, for example Scherer & Wallbott,

1994). This research seldom examines cultural differences in emotion. Furthermore, there is often a failure to identify cultural factors that may account for these differences (cf. Gudykunst, Ting-Toomey & Chau, 1988). Moreover, research utilising the component approach has primarily focused upon either the appraisal component or the expressive component (predominantly facial expression), and rarely addresses other components, if at all.

Culture and Self-Construal

Although cultural differences in emotional behaviour have been identified (Mesquita et al. 1998), cross-cultural psychologists have become increasingly aware of the need to 'unpackage' the concept of culture in order to identify the variables which may help explain differences in behaviour across cultures (Bond, 1994; Whiting, 1976). As Kagitcibasi asserts, it is necessary to understand "what it is about 'culture'" that accounts for differences across cultures (Kagitcibasi, 1994).

Until recently cultural differences in behaviour were frequently interpreted using a post-hoc explanation, often utilising Hofstede's (1980) culture-level value scores on his individualism/collectivism dimension. Unfortunately, most of these studies failed to test explicitly the endorsement of individual-level values within their sample. Current research has identified a number of individual level variables that may explain individual-level differences in behaviour across cultures. The self-concept has become one of the dominant focuses of this research (Markus and Kitayama, 1991; Triandis, 1989). As Singelis and Brown (1995) stated, "the construal of self (self-image) is an ideal candidate for the role of mediating culture's influence [on behaviour]" (p.358).

In their seminal review, Markus and Kitayama (1991) suggest that within Western societies the self is viewed as independent, motivated by internal desires, goals and wishes which are shaped by unique values, attitudes and opinions. Within non-western societies the self is viewed as embedded within the social context and defined by social relations (Markus & Kitayama, 1991; Shweder & Bourne, 1982; Triandis, 1989). Psychological measures such as the Twenty Statements Test have provided supporting evidence frequently finding that individuals from individualist cultures (Western, usually North American) make more references to personal, independent aspects of the self (e.g. traits, abilities, motives, and values), whereas individuals from collectivist (non-Western, usually Pacific Rim) cultures make more references to social and group aspects of the self (Bochner 1994; Bond & Cheung, 1983; Cousins, 1989; Ip & Bond 1995; Triandis, McCusker & Hui, 1990). Markus and Kitayama (1991) labelled these different conceptions of the self as *independent* and *interdependent*.

Although these constructs appear bipolar, scales constructed to measure independent/interdependent self-construals have found that the two scales are orthogonal (Gudykunst, Matsumoto, Ting-Toomey, Nishida, & Karimi, 1994; Singelis, 1994).

Individual variations in self conception have been linked to cultural-level variations in individualism and collectivism, with individuals from individualist cultures placing a higher emphasis on independent aspects of the self and individuals from collectivist cultures placing a higher emphasis on interdependent aspects of the self. Consequently, two cultures were chosen for the following study based on their scores on Hofstede's (1980) individualism / collectivism dimension. Hong Kong (China) ranked 37th on individualism, whereas the UK ranked 3rd. Therefore it was predicted that *individuals from the United Kingdom will place a higher emphasis on independent aspects of the self compared to individuals from Hong Kong* (Hypothesis 1) and that *individuals from Hong Kong will place a higher emphasis on interdependent aspects of the self compared to individuals from the United Kingdom* (Hypothesis 2).

The Self and Emotion

Markus and Kitayama (1991) and Triandis (1989) have proposed that individual differences in self-construal may account for individual differences in emotional experience across cultures. Markus and Kitayama argue that anger is a negative ego-focused (or self-focused) emotion which emphasises differences between individuals (independence). As such, it will be experienced and expressed more frequently within cultures that view the self as independent.

Action Tendencies

Action tendencies are central to an emotional experience. Action tendencies[1] are "...the individual's readiness or unreadiness to engage in interaction with the environment" (Frijda, Kuipers, & Schure, 1989, 213). Because different emotions can be expressed in similar ways (for example, crying when happy, sad, angry or in fear) it has been argued that the action tendency evoked by different emotions may be better at distinguishing between emotions than behaviour (Frijda, 1986). As Roseman, West and Swartz (1994) have suggested, "...it may be best to conceptualise the behavioural component of emotions as consisting of specific *action tendencies* rather than actions that must be performed when the emotion is felt" (p. 216, italics added). Emotions, therefore, have been conceived as *states of readiness to act*. Some theorists have even suggested that it is this state of activation that characterises an emotional experience and distinguishes emotions from states of pleasure or displeasure (Arnold, 1960). As Arnold (1960) puts it, emotions are "...the *felt tendency* toward anything intuitively appraised as good (beneficial), or away from anything intuitively appraised as bad (harmful)" (p. 182, italics added).

Frijda (1986) has argued that action tendencies are activated when events are appraised as emotionally relevant. General action impulses can be described as the impulse to "move toward", "move away", or "move against" (Frijda et al., 1989). These states may elicit actual behaviour or actions such as facial expressions, attack or retreat. However, changes in action tendencies do not always produce overt behaviour (Frijda, 1986). They are the *impulses* to act rather than the precursor to action. It has been argued that this state of activation is an adaptive behavioural response (Lazarus, 1991). For example, fear is characterised by situations involving (or perceived as involving) harmful stimuli. Consequently, the activation of flight (or escape) has obvious adaptive benefits.

The action tendency associated with anger is attack or retaliation (Lazarus, 1991). As Darwin suggested more than 125 years ago:

> Such gestures as the raising of the arms, with the fist clenched, as if to strike the offender, are common. Few men in great passion [anger]...can resist acting as if they intended to strike or punch the man violently away (1872/1998: 236).

Research has supported the notion that action tendencies such as to attack or aggress are associated with the experience of anger. In an early study of self-reported anger Gates (1926) found that the action tendencies during episodes of anger were aggressive (either direct physical aggression or verbal aggression), even though the actual instances of aggression were rare. This was supported by Davitz (1969) who found that a dominant response when angry is the *felt tendency* to engage in physical aggression. However, attack is only one action tendency associated with anger. Gates reported other action tendencies associated with anger such as 'to injure inanimate objects' or 'to run away, leave the room'. Averill (1982) identified four types of impulses that are felt during an angry episode; 1) Direct aggression (verbal, physical or removal of some benefit); 2) Indirect aggression (telling a third party, harming someone close to the object of your anger); 3) Displaced aggression (aggression towards a non-human object); Non-aggressive responses (calming activities, talking it over peacefully). These have been supported in subsequent single culture studies (e.g., Tangney, Wagner, Marschall, & Gramzow, 1991). Averill found that although the direct aggression impulse was common, the most frequent behavioural responses was to engage in calming activities, with actual aggression relatively rare. Averill also found that other impulses were frequently felt during an angry episode. However, neither Averill nor Tangney et al. examined the influence of culture on action tendencies.

Measurement of Action Tendencies

Action tendencies are difficult to measure. Research has been dominated by overt action and has rarely studied states of activation except through the measurement of physiological arousal. A number of researchers have measured action tendencies, although they have not always described the measures explicitly as measures of action tendency.

Frijda (1986) proposed a list of action tendencies involved in different emotional experiences, for example “I wanted to approach, make contact” (approach), “I wanted to stay away”(avoidance), “I wanted to hurt or insult” (antagonistic). These have been tested empirically (Frijda, 1986; Frijda et al. 1989). Frijda et al. asked participants to recall an emotional experience (from a list of set emotions) and mark the extent to which they felt like engaging in a number of actions and action tendencies (drawn from Frijda, 1986). They found that distinct appraisal patterns and distinct action tendencies were associated with different emotional experiences. Anger was associated with “moving against” (boiling inwardly, antagonistic feelings), hyperactivation (excitation) and what Frijda et al. Called “don’t want”, which reflects the tendency to want the situation to be different. However, some of the items on this measure appear to assess constructs distinct from action tendencies. Examples: “I interrupted what I was doing”, “I held the ropes”, “I laughed”, “I cried” all refer to actual actions rather than action tendencies. Additionally, “I wanted something not to be so” (don’t want) reflects a desired goal or future state and “I boiled inside” appears to measure an internal feeling state.

Roseman et al. (1994) aimed to differentiate between action tendencies, action and goals in emotional experiences. Again, like Frijda et al. (1989) Roseman et al. asked participants to recall an instance in which they experienced a specified emotion and asked the participants to recall what they felt like doing. They found that the action tendencies for anger were “feeling like yelling” and “feeling like hitting someone”. Even though the actual instances of aggression were rare the action tendencies reported during experiences of anger were to attack and hurt. However, both Frijda et al. and Roseman et al. focused on the differentiation between emotions and did not study cultural differences.

Most of the studies cited above have used structured self-reported experiences of emotion. Although other methods are available, structured self-report is potentially the most useful (Averill, 1982; Scherer & Tannenbaum, 1986). This allows researchers to study what individuals “felt like” doing as well as what actions they may have actually engaged in (Averill, 1982).

Culture and Action Tendencies

Given the central importance of action tendencies in the experience of emotion there is a surprising paucity of cross-cultural research on this topic. As Mesquita and Frijda (1992) report in their extensive review "no systematic comparisons [across cultures] have been made of forms of action readiness" (p. 190). Mesquita et al. (1998) cite Scherer and Wallbott's (1994) results as evidence of research examining action tendencies across cultures, yet Scherer and Wallbott did not have any measure of action tendency. The results that Mesquita et al. cite are drawn from a self-report measure of "expressive reactions", a measure of expression rather than action tendency. However, recent research has provided some insight into variations in action tendencies across cultures.

In a study conducted in India using Averill's (1982) questionnaire, Singh and Mishra (1997) found that the dominant action tendencies amongst both males and females were verbal, symbolic and actual aggression aimed at the offender. However, the prevalence of other action tendencies were not reported, and a comparison with a similar non-Indian sample was not conducted.

Kassinove, Sukhodolsky, Tsytsarev, and Solovyova (1997) used a variation of Averill's (1982) anger questionnaire which included a measure of what participants "felt like doing" as well as what they "actually did" in Russia and the United States. Significant differences were found between action tendency responses obtained in the two countries. In comparison to the Russian participants the American participants were significantly more likely to want to "fight or hit a person", "hit or destroy something", "yell and argue", "make sarcastic remarks" , and "make a complaint". These responses all represent direct aggression action tendencies.

In studies of conflict it has been found that respondents from collectivist cultures demonstrate more conflict avoidance than those from individualist cultures (Ohbuchi & Takahashi, 1994). Moreover, individuals from Western (typically individualist) cultures prefer direct, confrontational and assertive means of handling conflicts, whereas individuals from Eastern (typically collectivist) cultures show a preference for indirect, avoidance or denial strategies in conflict situations (Itoi, Ohbuchi, & Fukuno, 1996; Markus, Kitayama, & Heiman, 1996; Trubisky, Tong-Toomey, & Lin, 1991). Leung (1987) suggested that within collectivist cultures there is a strong emphasis on group harmony and face saving behaviour, as a consequence indirect methods for resolving conflict are used to maintain group harmony and face. Additionally, it has been suggested that these variations in conflict resolution strategies may be mediated by differing conceptions of the self across cultures (Triandis, 1995). In individualist cultures, where the dominant view of the self is independent, individuals perceive conflict as a natural and inevitable aspect of social life as "everyone is different". Conflicts reflect differences and as a consequence emphasise the independent nature of the self. In collectivist cultures, where the dominant view of the self is interdependent, harmony is emphasised and therefore tactics to avoid conflicts are paramount.

Anger is an emotion evoked in conflict situations. Consequently, behaviours used to resolve conflict may be similar to behaviours exhibited and felt when angry. It has been suggested above that individuals from individualist cultures prefer direct confrontational behaviours when faced with conflict. It was therefore predicted that *individuals from the United Kingdom are more likely to feel like expressing their anger through direct aggression than individuals from Hong Kong* (Hypothesis 3). Conversely, it was argued above that individuals from collectivist cultures prefer indirect, avoidance tactics when faced with conflict, therefore it was predicted that *individuals from Hong Kong are more likely to feel like expressing their anger through displaced aggression*[2] *than individuals from the United Kingdom* (Hypothesis 4).

Implications for Display Rules

The theory of display rules proposed by Ekman (1972), and now widely accepted, implicitly assumes similarity of action tendencies across emotions and across cultures. The main study cited by Ekman (1972) as providing supporting evidence examined the influence of the presence/absence of an experimenter on the emotional reactions of individuals from the USA and Japan. The results (according to Ekman, 1972; although see Fridlund & Duchaine, 1996) supported the theory that individuals from the USA show the same display of emotion both in the presence and absence of an experimenter, whilst participants from Japan show different expressions of emotions whilst in the presence and absence of an experimenter, respectively. The theory postulates that the same emotions were evoked in both situations and the Japanese felt the same impulses as the Americans, yet they did not display them because of the influence of Japanese display rules. This theory relies on the premise that the evoked emotion (in this case disgust, which was not explicitly measured) has a fixed action tendency (the inclination to act in a certain way) which may (or may not) lead to specific behaviour depending on the context and the appropriateness of display. It may be, however, that emotions vary across cultures in their action tendencies.

Psychologists and anthropologists have found that expressions of anger vary across cultures. Anthropologists have even suggested that some cultures such as the Uktu Eskimos express anger rarely, if at all (Briggs, 1970). Ekman's (1972) theory explains these differences as variations in the social rules of emotional display. This implies that the action tendencies associated with anger are the same across cultures.

According to the "display rules" theory action tendencies should be less subject to cultural rules than overt behaviour. It may be socially inappropriate to express direct aggression when angry. These rules, however, may not influence action tendencies. Moreover, if cultural differences in action tendencies did emerge it would cast some doubt on the theory that culture only influenced emotional display, suggesting that both the expression and the experience of emotion were influenced by culture. For example individuals from different cultures may not only act in different ways when angry but actually "feel like" acting in different ways.

Culture, Self and Action Tendencies

As suggested earlier, a number of theorists have proposed how differing conceptions of the self may help explain individual differences in emotional behaviour across cultures (Markus & Kitayama, 1991; Triandis, 1989). One of the main features of an independent self is an emphasis on direct communication. Consequently, it has been proposed that individual differences in independent self-construal may account for differences across cultures in communication styles. This hypothesis was supported in a study by Kim, Sharkey and Singelis (1994), who found that individuals with higher independent self-construals preferred direct explicit communication, whereas individuals with higher interdependent self-construals preferred interactions that take others feelings into account. This preference for direct styles of communication exhibited by individuals with a higher independent self-construal, may also be exhibited in their action tendencies. It was therefore predicted that *individual- level independence will account for cultural differences in direct aggression action tendencies* (hypothesis 5). As the literature concerning interdependent self-construals was unclear, no prediction was made concerning the influence of interdependent self-construal on action tendency.

Method

Participants

United Kingdom Sample. A total of 136 students (undergraduate and post-graduate) from the University of Sussex (90 women, 46 men) participated. Demographic information was obtained from all participants. Their mean age was 25.8 (SD = 7.43).

Hong Kong Sample. A total of 110 students from the Chinese University of Hong Kong (55 women, 55 men) participated. Demographic information was obtained from all participants. Their mean age was 20.1 (SD = 1.21).

A significant age difference was found between the two samples ($p<0.01$). The UK sample was significantly older than the Hong Kong sample. Therefore, age was entered as a covariate in subsequent analyses.

Instruments and Procedure

Self-Construal

Participants completed the 29-item Independent Interdependent Self-Construal Scale (IISC, Gudykunst et al., 1994). An official Chinese version was used with the Hong Kong sample. The results of the IISC were subject to a within country fixed factor analysis. Items that did not obtain at least a 0.3 factor loading in each country were dropped from subsequent analyses (Van de Vijver & Leung, 1997). This resulted in a 9-item independent self-construal scale (United Kingdom, α = .72; Hong Kong, α = .66), and a 11-item interdependent self-construal scale (United Kingdom, α = .79; Hong Kong, α = .78).

Emotional Experience

Participants were asked to recall an event in which they had experienced anger (based on Scherer, Wallbott, & Summerfield, 1986). Participants then completed questions concerning the event that addressed different components of the emotional experience[3]. These were drawn from Averill's (1982) work on anger, Scherer et al.'s cross-cultural study of emotion, and questions drawn from the literature. The relevance of these questions had been checked in a pilot study conducted in both the UK and Hong Kong (n=50).

Action Tendency

The participants completed a 16-item scale adapted from Averill (1982). This scale asks participants to report the extent that they "felt like" engaging in certain actions whilst angry. Each item was measured on a 5-point scale (1 = not at all, 3 = somewhat, 5 = very much). Participants also reported whether they actually did engage in certain actions whilst angry (yes/no). This scale was translated into Chinese by a native Chinese bilingual and was then back-translated by a second bilingual using the method described by Brislin (1970). Discrepant item translations were then altered through discussion with the first translator. The anger action tendency scale was subject to factor analysis. This revealed four interpretable factors that supported previous findings in the literature. These were: 1) Direct Aggression, e.g., *"felt like becoming physically aggressive towards the object of my anger"*, *"felt like making an obscene gesture"towards them"*; 2) Indirect Aggression, e.g. *"felt like telling a third party to gain revenge"*, *"felt like damaging property of those involved"*" 3) Displaced Aggression, e.g. *"felt like expressing my anger through non-physical aggression (e.g. slamming doors, stamping feet"*', *"felt like becoming angry at something else (non-human)"*; 4) Calm (non-aggressive behaviour), e.g. *"felt like doing something away to calm myself down"*, *"felt like talking it over calmly"*.

Results[4]

Culture and Self-construal

It was hypothesised that participants from the UK would place a higher emphasis on independent aspects of the self than participants from Hong Kong (H1). It was also hypothesised that participants from Hong Kong would place a higher emphasis on interdependent aspects of the self compared to participants from the United Kingdom (H2). These hypotheses were tested using the independent and interdependent self-construal scales (see Figure 1). A 2 (country: Hong Kong, United Kingdom) by 2 (self-construal: Independent, Interdependent) ANOVA was performed with a repeated measure on the latter variable. A significant main effect for self-construal was found [$F(1, 237) = 46.52$, $p <. 001$], such that irrespective of culture participants reported significantly higher endorsement of independent aspects of the self. A significant self-construal by country interaction effect was found [$F(1,237)=39.20$, $p < .001$]. Pairwise comparisons indicated that the UK sample endorsed significantly higher independent aspects of the self than the Hong Kong sample ($p < .001$). Conversely, participants from Hong Kong endorsed more interdependent aspects of the self than participants from the UK ($p < .01$). As there was a significant age difference between the two samples a second analysis was conducted with age entered as a covariate and was found to have no effect.

These analyses support Hypothesis 1 and Hypothesis 2. The results show that individuals from the UK place a higher emphasis on independent aspects of the self compared to individuals from Hong Kong. The results also show that individuals from Hong Kong place a higher emphasis on interdependent aspects of the self compared to individuals from the UK.

Culture and Action Tendency

It was predicted that participants from the UK would be more likely to feel like expressing their anger through direct aggression than participants from Hong Kong (direct aggression action tendency). It was also predicted that participants from Hong Kong are more likely to feel like expressing their anger through displaced aggression than participants from the UK. A MANOVA was conducted to test for differences across cultures in anger expression action tendencies. The main effect for culture was significant (Wilks' $\lambda = .91$, F, $[4, 227] = 5.72$, $p < .001$). Pairwise comparisons revealed that the UK respondents felt like using direct aggression significantly more than the Hong Kong respondents ($p < .001$), and that Hong Kong respondents felt like expressing

Figure 1. Independent Self Construal Scales

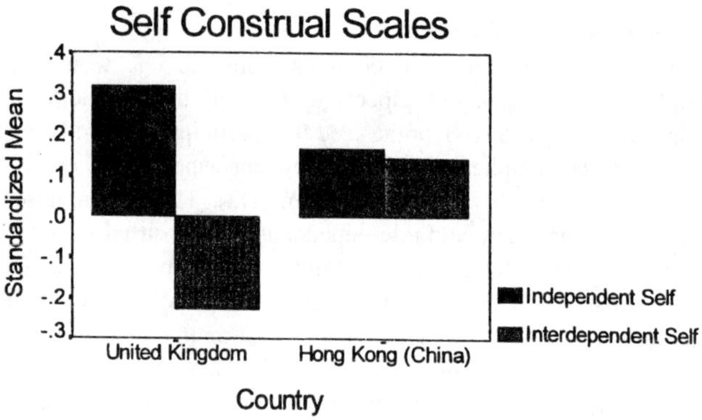

their anger through displaced aggression more than the UK respondents ($p < .001$). These findings supported Hypotheses 3 and 4 (see Figure 2).

Figure 2. Action Tendencies in the Expression of Anger

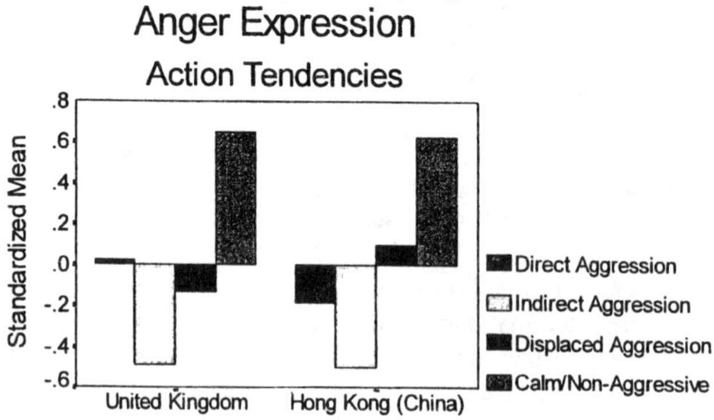

Self-Construal and Action Tendency

The final hypothesis predicted that individual level independent self-construal would account for differences in direct aggression action tendency. A between-country hierarchical multiple regression was conducted. As the aim of the analysis was to test differences in action tendency and not differences in behaviour, the first variable entered into the regression equation was actual direct aggression (whether or not they had actually expressed their anger through direct aggression). This controls for differences in actual behaviour, and allows for the possibility of identifying the relationship between self-construal and action tendency. Independent self-construal was then entered as it was predicted that this would have the strongest relationship with direct aggression. Interdependence, culture, and the interactions of culture with independence and interdependence were entered sequentially into the regression equation. As predicted, after controlling for actual behaviour, independence was positively associated with direct aggression action tendency (t [1, 223] = 2.77, $p < .005$, ß = .16). Neither interdependence (t [1, 222] = -0.03, ns, ß = -.00), nor culture (t [1, 221] = -1.97, ns, ß = -.12) reached significance after entering independence. The present analysis "unpackaged" culture, suggesting that independent self-construals can account for cultures effect on action tendency. This supports Hypothesis 5.

However, the interaction between culture and independent self-construal was also significant (t [1, 220] = 2.24, $p < .05$, ß = .13). This finding was unexpected. This interaction indicates that the relationship between independence and direct aggression action tendency is not consistent across each of the cultures. To explore this relationship a within country analysis was conducted to eliminate the effect of culture. Again the first variable entered into the regression equation was action (whether or not they had actually expressed their anger through direct aggression).

The hypothesis was supported within the Hong Kong sample. It was found that after accounting for actual behaviour independent self-construal accounted for a significant amount of the variance (t [1, 107] = 3.43, $p < .001$, ß = .27) . This provides stronger support for the hypothesis, suggesting that individuals within Hong Kong with a higher independent self-construal are more likely to feel like directly expressing their anger. The interdependent self-construal did not prove to be significant (t [1, 106] = -0.06, ns, ß = -.01) (Table 4).

Within the UK the independent self-construal was not significant after accounting for actual emotional behaviour (t [1, 116] = 0.15, ns, ß = .01) (Table 5) .

The within-country analysis explained the interaction effect found in the first regression. The interaction effect found that individuals with higher independent self-construals within Hong Kong are more likely to feel like being directly aggressive. However, within the UK no relationship was found between an individuals self-construal and their action tendency. Therefore hypothesis 5 was only partially supported.

Discussion

The aim of this study was to explore the relationship between culture and individual self-construal, the relationship between culture and action tendency, and to examine whether the relationship between culture and action tendency could be accounted for by individual level self-construal. Overall, support was found for the predictions.

Culture and Self-Construal

It was found that individuals from the UK (an individualist culture) were more likely to endorse independent aspects of the self compared to individuals from Hong Kong (a collectivist culture). Conversely, individuals from Hong Kong are more likely to endorse interdependent aspects of the self compared to Individuals from the UK. This finding is becoming increasingly common within the cross-cultural literature (Gudykunst et al, 1994; Gudykunst, Matsumoto, Ting-Toomey, Nishida, Kim, & Heyman, 1996; Singelis, 1994; Singelis & Brown, 1995) . As Hong Kong has been identified as a collectivist culture and the UK an individualist culture it is tempting to suggest that individual level self-construals are related to cultural level collectivism. However, this finding needs to be corroborated in many more countries than is currently available to provide stronger support for this hypothesis. Nevertheless, this finding does help researchers identify individual-level processes that are influenced by culture. It also may provide an individual-level variable that can be used to explore individual differences across cultures.

It is interesting to note that within both cultures independent aspects of the self were endorsed more highly than interdependent aspects of the self.

Culture and Action Tendency

Anger is of central importance in everyday social life (Deffenbacher, 1998). However, attempts to research anger empirically have only just begun (Sharkin, 1996). The current research identified that the structure of anger action tendencies was similar in both cultures. The most frequently felt tendency in both Hong Kong and the UK was calm/non aggressive responses. This supports Averill (1982) who found that in an American sample calm/non-aggressive responses were the most common. The least-endorsed action tendency in both cultures was indirect aggression. This supports the finding that indirect aggression is rarely used as a response whilst angry (Tangney et al., 1991). This similarity in structure supports a universalist orientation suggesting that there are specific action tendencies associated with the emotional experience of anger. However, although the structure may be universal, cultural differences in action tendencies were identified.

Individuals from Hong Kong were more likely to feel like expressing their anger through displaced aggression compared to individuals from the UK. Furthermore, individuals from the UK were more likely to feel like expressing their anger through direct aggression compared to individuals from Hong Kong. These findings supported the hypothesis that although there may be common action tendencies across cultures, cultures vary in the extent that they feel (or endorse feeling at least) different action tendencies. This is the first time that the influence of culture on action tendency has been tested explicitly. The results support the findings that individuals from an individualist culture are more likely to engage in direct methods of communication and emotional expression (Markus et al., 1996). The results also elaborate on previous findings in that individuals from an individualist culture are more likely to have the impulse to engage in direct aggression compared to individuals from a collectivist culture (Hong Kong). Furthermore, these findings support previous research that has identified a preference for indirect methods of communication amongst individuals from collectivist cultures (Leung, 1987). Again, the findings of the present study build upon this by suggesting that individuals from a collectivist culture are more likely to have the impulse or action tendency towards displaced aggression (the most indirect form of action tendency).

These results cast further doubt over the theory of display rules. The theory of display rules suggests that culture influences emotional expression not action tendency, assuming implicitly that the action tendencies associated with emotion are the same regardless of culture, even though the actual display varies. However, the findings of the present research suggest that culture also influences the action tendencies during an emotional experience. This finding is striking considering that reporting feelings should be less subject to reporting bias than reporting actions.

Additionally, this research provides ecologically valid results. Asking people to describe situations in which they have felt and acted emotionally (anger in the current research) may be more appropriate across cultures than research in which hypothetical situations are constructed (usually within one country) and individuals are asked to report how they *would* feel/act in such a situation, or the likelihood that they would engage in certain behaviours or express certain facial patterns. Although, obviously these areas of research have their benefits.

Culture, Self and Action Tendency

To explain the differences in action tendency a measure of independent-interdependent self-construal was used. This tested explicitly the theory proposed by Markus and Kitayama (1991) and Triandis (1989). Within the Hong Kong sample it was found that independent self-construal was associated with direct aggression action tendency. This illustrates that individuals who conceive of the self as independent are more likely to feel like expressing their anger through direct aggression. Again, this finding challenges the display rules theory showing that within-culture variation, as well as cross-cultural variation can be accounted for by individual differences in self-construal. The display rules explanation is based on the premise that individuals feel like expressing their emotions but do not. However, the findings of this study indicate that self-construal influences what the individual feels like expressing.

The present study found that self-construal was not associated with direct aggression action tendency in the UK sample. This finding is more difficult to explain. A number of possible explanations can be suggested. It may that it is a statistical artefact. This could be due to the UK sample scoring highly on both the measure of independent self-construal, and the measure of direct aggression action tendency. If this were the case there may be low variance in the two scales reducing the correlation between them. Alternatively, it may be that the theory is wrong. However, previous research and support for the theory within the Hong Kong sample suggests that this explanation should not be accepted at present. Another possibility is that the measures do not measure the constructs adequately. Self-construal research has been dominated by North American versus Pacific Rim comparisons. It may be that the constructs of independent / interdependent self-construals have properties that are unique to these cultures. It may be that the relationships between self-construal and emotions may not hold within a UK or even European sample. Other variables that help "unpackage" culture may be needed to account for individual level differences in emotional behaviour. A more comprehensive measure that may be more sensitive to individual differences across cultures could possibly identify a more complex relationship between culture and individual emotional behaviour. It may be that the relationship between culture and individual action tendency is mediated by a different variable within a UK sample. For example, Schwartz (1992) has proposed that individual level values may be one possible mediator between culture and individual behaviour

Conclusions

The present research attempted to explore the complex relationship between culture and emotion, through an integration of both emotion and cross-cultural theories. The study provides a number of pertinent results. Firstly, evidence was provided showing that culture influences anger action tendencies. This builds upon research that has identified cultural differences in emotion display, but that has rarely has examined action tendencies. Additionally, similarities across cultures in the structure of action tendencies associated with the experience of anger were identified. In both cultures calm/non aggressive action tendencies were the most common and indirect aggression action tendencies the least common. This supports a universalist orientation in the structure of anger action tendencies. Finally, the present study found that the cultural differences in action tendencies could be explained by individual differences in self-construal, a proposition that has seldom been tested. These results suggest that self-construal may be effectively used to "unpackage" culture's influence on emotional experience. Although work still needs to be conducted, the results presented here provides further understanding concerning the complex relationship between culture and emotion.

References

Arnold, M. B. (1960). *Emotion and personality* (2 Vols.) New York: Columbia University Press.

Averill, J. R. (1982). *Anger and aggression:An essay on emotion.* New York: Springer.

Bochner, S. (1994). Cross-cultural differences in the self concept: A test of Hofstede's individualism/collectivism distinction. *Journal of Cross-Cultural Psychology, 25*, 273-83.

Bond, M. H. & Cheung T. S. (1983). The spontaneous self-concept of college students in Hong Kong, Japan, and the United States. *Journal of Cross-Cultural Psychology, 14*, 153-71.

Bond, M. H. (1994). Emotions and their expression in Chinese culture. *Journal of Non-verbal Behavior, 17*, 245-262.

Briggs, J. (1970). *Never in anger.* Cambridge, MA: Harvard University Press.

Brislin, R. W. (1970). Back-translation for cross-cultural research. *Journal of Cross-Cultural Psychology, 1*, 185-216.

Cousins, S. (1989). Culture and selfhood in Japan and the US. *Journal of Personality and Social Psychology, 56*, 124-31.

Darwin, C. (1872/1998). *The expression of emotion in man and animals (Third Edition).* London: Harper Collins Publishers.

Davitz, J. L. (1969). *The Language of emotion.* New York: Academic Press.

Deffenbacher, J. L., Oetting, E. R., Lynch, R. S. & Morris, C. D. (1996). The expression of anger and its consequences. *Behaviour, Research, and Therapy, 34*, 575-590.

Ekman, P. (1972) Universals and cultural differences in the facial expression of emotion. In J. Berman (Ed.). *Nebraska Symposium on Motivation* (Vol. 19, pp. 207-284). Lincoln: University of Nebraska.

Fridlund, A. J., & Duchaine, B. (1996). Facial expressions of emotion and the delusion of the hermetic self. In R. Harré and W. G. Parrot, *The emotions: Social, cultural and biological dimensions* (pp. 259-284). Thousand Oaks, CA: Sage.

Frijda, N. H. (1986). *The emotions*. Cambridge: Cambridge University Press.

Frijda, N. H., Kuipers, P., & ter Schure, E. (1989). Relations among emotion, appraisal, and emotional action readiness. *Journal of Personality and Social Psychology, 57*, 212-228.

Gates, G. S. (1926). An observational study of anger. *Journal of Experimental Psychology, 9*, 325-331.

Gudykunst, W. B., Matsumoto, Y., Ting-Toomey, S., Nishida, T., & Karimi, H. (1994). *Measuring self-construals across cultures: A derived-etic analysis*. Paper presented at the International Communication Association, Sydney.

Gudykunst, W. B., Matsumoto, Y., Ting-Toomey, S., Nishida, T., Kim, K., & Heyman, S. (1996). The influence of individualism-collectivism, self-construals, and individual values on communication styles across cultures. *Human Communication Research, 22*, 510-543

Gudykunst, W. B., Ting-Toomey, S., & Chau, E. (1988). *Culture and interpersonal communication*, Newbury Park, CA: Sage.

Hofstede, G. (1980). *Culture's consequences: International differences in work-related values*. Beverly Hills CA: Sage

Hui, C. H., & Triandis, H. C. (1989). Effects of culture and response format on extreme response style. *Journal of Cross-Cultural Psychology, 20*, 296-309.

Ip, G. W. M. & Bond, M. H. (1995). Culture, values, and the spontaneous self-concept. *Asian Journal of Psychology, 1*, 30-36.

Itoi, R., Ohbuchi, K., & Fukuno, M. (1996). A cross-cultural study of preference of accounts: Relationship closeness, harm severity, and motives of account making. *Journal of Applied SocialPsychology, 26*, 913-934.

Kagitcibasi, C. (1994). A critical appraisal of individualism-collectivism: Toward a new formulation. In U. Kim, H. C. Triandis, C. Kagitcibasi, & G. Yoon (Eds.), *Individualism and collectivism: Theoretical and methodological issues* (pp. 52-65). Thousand Oaks, CA: Sage.

Kassinove, H., Sukhodolsky, D. G., Tsytsarev, S. V., & Solovyova, S. (1997). Self-reported anger episodes in Russia and America. *Journal of Social Behaviour and Personality, 12*, 301-324.

Kim, M. S., Sharkey, W. F., & Singelis, T. M. (1994). The relationship between individuals' self-construal and perceived importance of interactive constraints. *International Journal of Intercultural Relations, 18*, 117-140.

Lazarus, R. S. (1991). *Emotion and adaptation*. New York:Oxford University Press.

Leung, K. (1987). Some determinants of reactions to procedural models for conflict resolution: A cross-national study. *Journal of Personality and Social Psychology, 53*, 898-908.

Leung, K., & Bond, M. H. (1989). On the empirical identification of dimensions for cross-cultural comparison. *Journal of Cross-Cultural Psychology, 20*, 133-51.

Markus H. R. & Kitayama S. (1991). Culture and the self: Implications for cognition, emotion and motivation. *Psychological Review*, *98*, 224-53.

Markus, H. R., Kitayama, S. & Heiman, R. (1996). Culture and 'basic' psychological principles. In E. T. Higgins & A. W. Kruglanski (Eds.) *Social psychology: Handbook of basic principles*. (pp. 857-913) New York: Guildford Press.

Mesquita, B. & Frijda, N. H. (1992). Cultural variations in emotion: A review. *Psychological Bulletin*, *112*, 179-204.

Mesquita, B., Frijda, N. H., & Scherer, K. R. (1998). Culture and emotion. In J. W. Berry, P. R. Dasen, & T. S. Saraswathi (Eds.). *Handbook of cross-cultural psychology* (Second Edition, Volume 2, pp. 255-297.) Boston: Allen and Bacon.

Oatley, K. and Duncan, E. (1992). Strutured diaries for emotions in daily life. In K. T. Strongman (Ed.), *International Review of Studies on Emotion*, (Vol. 2, pp. 249-294). Chichester: Wiley.

Ohbuchi, K.-I, & Takahashi, Y. (1994). Cultural styles of conflict management in Japanese and Americans: Passivity, covertness and effectiveness of strategies. *Journal of Applied Social Psychology*, *24*, 1345-1366.

Richardson, K. F. (1918). The psychology and pedagogy of anger. *Educational Psychology Monographs*, *19*.

Roseman, I. J., West, C., & Swartz, T. S. (1994). Phenomenology, behaviors, and goals differentiate discrete emotions. *Journal of Personality and Social Psychology*, *67*, 206-221.

Scherer, K. R. (1984). Emotion as a mulitcomponent process: A model and some cross-cultural data. In P. Shaver (Ed.)., *Review of personality and social psychology* (Vol. 5, pp.37-63). Beverly Hills, CA: Sage.

Scherer, K. R. & Tannenbaum, P. H. (1986). Emotional experiences in everyday life: A survey approach. *Motivation and Emotion*, *10*, 295-314.

Scherer, K. R., Wallbott, H. G. & Summerfield, A. (Eds.). (1986) *Experiencing emotion: A cross-cultural study*. Cambridge: Cambridge University Press.

Scherer, K. R., Wallbott, H. G. (1994). Evidence for universality and cultural variation of differential emotion response patterning. *Journal of Personality and Social Psychology*, *66*, 310-328.

Schwartz, S. H. (1992). The universal content and structure of values: Theoretical advances and empirical tests in 20 countries. In M. P. Zanna (ed.) *Advances in experimental social psychology*, *25*, (pp.1-65) , New York: Academic

Sharkin, B. S. (1996). Understanding anger: Comment. *Journal of Counseling Psychology*, *43*, 166-169.

Shweder R. A. & Bourne, E. J. (1982). Does the concept of the person vary cross-culturally? In A. J. Marsella, & G. M. White (Eds.) *Cultural conceptions of mental health and therapy*, (pp. 97-137). Dordrecht, Holland: Reidel

Singelis, T. M. & Brown, W. J. (1995). Culture, self-construal, and collectivist communication. Linking culture to individual behavior. *Human Communication Research*, *21*, 354-389.

Singelis, T. M. (1994). The measurement of independent and interdependent self-construals. *Personality and Social Psychology Bulletin*, *20*, 580-591.

Singh, J. K. & Mishra, G. (1997). The experience of anger and aggression in Indian youth: Some preliminary observations. *Trends in Social Science Research, 4*, 231-242.

Tangney, J. P., Wagner, P. E., Marschall, D., & Gramzow, R. (1991). *The Anger Response Inventory* (ARI). Fairfax, VA: George Mason University

Tavris, C. (1982), *Anger: The misunderstood emotion.* New York: Simon and Schuster.

Triandis, H. C. (1989). The self and social behavior in differing social contexts. *Psychological Review, 96*, 506-520.

Triandis, H. C., McCusker, C. & Hui, C. H. (1990). Multimethod probes of individualism and collectivism. *Journal of Personality and Social Psychology, 59,* 1006-1020.

Trubisky, P., Ting-Toomey, S., & Lin, S-L. (1991). The influence of individualism-collectivism and self-monitoring on conflict styles. *International Journal of Intercultural Relations, 15*, 65-84.

van de Vijver, F. & Leung, K. (1997). *Methods and data analysis for cross-cultural psychology*. Thousand Oaks, CA: Sage.

Whiting, B. B. (1976). The problem of the packaged variable. In K. F. Reigel and J. A. Meacham (eds.), *The developing individual in a changing world*, The Hague: Mouton.

Acknowledgements

Many thanks to Michael Bond and Lai Ming for their invaluable help with the Hong Kong data collection. Thanks to Peter B. Smith for his guidance throughout this project. Thanks also to Kate Cavanagh for her helpful comments on earlier drafts of this paper, and to both Andrew Ward-Minter and Jess Pimenta for their help with the final editing.

Notes

[1] In the literature 'action tendencies', 'action readiness', and 'action impulses' are all used interchangeably. For clarity only the term 'action tendencies' will be used in this paper.

[2] Although individuals from collectivist cultures have been shown to prefer 'indirect' communication and 'indirect' methods to resolve conflict, 'indirect aggression' as defined above is more 'direct' than displaced aggression in that indirect aggression is aimed at actual people or at property involved in the anger provoking situation whereas displaced aggression is aimed at inanimate objects that are not involved in the anger provoking situation.

[3] The results presented in this paper are part of a larger research project examining the influence of culture on each component of the emotional experience of anger.

[4] It has been reported that some cultures vary on their use of rating scales (Hui & Triandis, 1989). These systematic variations may produce spurious results. One method to reduce the influence of response bias is to standardise scores within individuals and across items as described by Leung and Bond (1989). All the data were standardised using this method.

Culture and Gender Influences on Self-Concept and the Bases of Self-Esteem: Four Turkish Studies

Diane Sunar
Boğazici University
Psychology Department

ABSTRACT

Interrelations among self-concept, bases of self-esteem, gender, age, and individualism-collectivism were investigated in four studies with Turkish respondents, using the Twenty Statements Test (TST) to assess self-concept, the ASSEI to assess bases of self-esteem, and the IndCol (I-C) scale to measure individualism-collectivism. Gender and age differences were found in two categories of TST responses. Compared to males and students, females and adults gave more allocentric and small group responses. Collectivistic respondents and females gave greater importance to interpersonal/relational bases of self-esteem than Individualistic respondents and males. There were no age, gender, or I-C differences in the importance of personal characteristics as bases of self-esteem. The pattern of results over the four studies suggests that contextual variables may be important, and that the conceptualization of individualism-collectivism as a single dimension makes it difficult to state clear predictions concerning the separate and joint effects of gender and culture on self-concept and self-esteem.

The aim of this paper is to explore the impact of gender and individualism-collectivism on self-concept and self-esteem in the Turkish cultural context. To this purpose, findings from four different studies which bear on these relationships are presented, and some implications for individualism-collectivism research are discussed.

Aspects of Self-Concept and Self-Esteem

Ever since the pioneering work of William James, most self researchers have assumed that the self includes various components or aspects, and that self-esteem is based on particular characteristics and performances which may be valued differently from person to person. Nevertheless, until recently, self-esteem has generally been measured in a global fashion, taking little or no account of specific bases of self-esteem or their weights. However, recent research has shown that it is profitable, on both conceptual and empirical grounds, to distinguish bases of self-esteem and the weight attributed to them by individuals. Similarly, work on self-concept (defined here as the terms in which a person conceptualizes the self) has shown the usefulness of a multifaceted and phenomenological approach.

This more complex approach to the study of self also requires instruments which reflect the complexity. The Adult Sources of Self-Esteem Inventory (ASSEI) provides a convenient method for measuring the importance of a wide range of possible bases or domains of self-esteem, along with the respondent's satisfaction with the self in each of the domains. Likewise, the Twenty Statements Test--TST (also known as the Who Are You test--WAY) provides an extremely useful means of eliciting the different aspects of a respondent's self-concept. All of the studies to be reported here used one or both of these two measures.

Gender, Culture and the Self

While consistent overall differences in global self-esteem between males and females are not usually found (Hattie, 1992), considerable evidence has begun to accumulate that there is gender variation in the terms used to describe self-concept and in bases of self-esteem (see, e.g., Hattie, 1992; Josephs, Markus, & Tafarodi, 1992). However, since this variation is thought to be due in large part to the person's identification with culturally mandated roles and evaluation of his/her performance in these roles according to culturally defined standards, the issue of cultural variation is immediately implicated. In fact, studies in some non-Western cultures have not found the expected gender variation (e.g., Luk & Bond, 1992; Watkins, Adair, Akande, Gerong, McInerney, Sunar, Watson, Wen, & Wondimu, 1998), which suggests that gender differences in self-concept may arise only in particular cultural contexts.

It has been argued that the operative cultural dimension is individualism-collectivism. In this perspective, there is considerable overlap between collectivistic self-conceptions, which stress interrelatedness with others, and the self-conceptions of women which, at least in individualistic cultures, also tend to stress relations with others. Thus it is expected that there should be less gender variation in self-concept in collectivistic cultures, since in those cultures both men and women will conceptualize themselves in relational terms (see also Luk & Bond, 1992; Watkins et al., 1998).

However, recent studies have suggested that the connection between culture and gender in the production of self-concept and self-esteem may not be so straightforward. Kashima, Yamaguchi, Kim, Choi, Gelfand, and Yuki (1995), studying five cultures, concluded that cultural differences and gender differences stemmed from different sources; specifically, cultural differences were found to reflect degree of agency in action, while gender differences were found to reflect degree of emotional relatedness. Watkins, et al. (1998), in a study covering nine cultures, found that males and females differed in the predicted way in some individualistic cultures but not others, and that there were unpredicted but significant gender differences in some collectivistic cultures. Also, Watkins, Adair, Akande, Cheng, Fleming, Gerong, Ismail, McInerney, Mpofu, Regmi, Singh-Sengupta, Watson, Wondimu, and Yu

(1996), examining sixteen cultures, found that only the individualist cultures followed the predicted pattern of gender differences in self-concept, while respondents from collectivist cultures emphasized social relationships (other than family) less than predicted.

In short, studies which cast a wide net in terms of number of cultures sampled have not found simple patterns in the relationships among culture, gender, self-concept, and self-esteem. At this point it appears that research needs to go in two directions: first, more rigorous and ever more broadly based studies comparing large numbers of cultures; and second, more intensive studies of particular cultures. The set of studies presented in this paper, focusing on the Turkish cultural context, serve as an example of the second approach.

Turkish Background

Surveying the literature based on Turkish respondents, it appears that theories of the self have not been heavily researched in Turkey. One of the first attempts to focus directly on gender and self-esteem among Turkish respondents is Study 2 below (Inelmen, 1996).

In contrast, there is a growing interest in the individualism-collectivism dimension in Turkish culture. Turkey was classified in Hofstede's (1980) study as collectivistic, with a score of 37, and Kağitcibasi (1996) has asserted that Turkish culture is a "culture of relatedness". Using qualitative methods, Seckin (1996) has found highly interdependent self-concepts in young Turkish women. On the other hand, Göregenli's (1995) research using the IndCol measure suggests that Turkish culture is neither strongly collectivistic nor strongly individualistic. Thus it may be advisable to measure respondents' personal level of individualism-collectivism (as in Study 4 below: Anamur, 1998).

Four studies were carried out, each with different aims and combinations of measurements, and used completely different samples. The aspects of each study which bear on the relations of gender, individualism-collectivism, self-concept and self-esteem are presented. Students included in the samples were attending a university, except in Study 3 which sampled high school seniors. The age range for nearly all students was from 17 to 23 years of age, and their home communities were urban. Most of the university respondents were enrolled in introductory psychology courses that were available to students from various departments.

All of the adults in the studies were from Istanbul and ranged in age from their 20s to 60s. Their occupations varied and included professional athletes , physicians, and professors. All had at least a high school education, and many were university educated.

Methods

All four studies used the ASSEI, and two of them also used the TST. The ASSEI consists of 20 items (for example, "looks and physical attractiveness" and "having a close relationship with someone") which are rated first for their importance to the respondent's self-esteem, and second for the respondent's satisfaction with the self with regard to each aspect. The 20 items may be regarded as comprising two subscales, constituted by classifying each item according to whether it refers, like the first example, to "personal characteristics" (PCs), or, like the second example, to "interpersonal characteristics" (IPCs). In each of the four studies, both importance of and satisfaction with PCs and IPCs were scored.

The measure of self-concept, the TST, consists simply of 20 answers to the question "Who are you?", with the order and format of the answers determined by the respondent. In the two studies which used the TST, responses were classified into the following categories: idiocentric, allocentric, small group, and large group (see Watkins, et al., 1998, for a description of these categories).

In Table 1, for each study, the aim of the study, the composition of the sample, and the instruments used are presented.

Results

For all the results presented below, analyses are either ANOVA or MANOVA, unless otherwise noted. The main results of all four studies are summarized in Table 2.

Study 1

On the TST, females gave more allocentric responses than males (8.2 vs. 5.3, $p < .01$). On the ASSEI, (a) no overall differences were found either between males and females or between adults and students on either PCs or IPCs; (b) some item differences were found both between males and females and between adults and students.

Study 2

Females scored higher than males on IPC importance (87.26 vs. 80.59, $F = 15.60$, $p = .0001$) and on IPC satisfaction (82.66 vs. 77.29, $F = 9.12$, $p = .003$). There were no overall gender differences on PC importance or PC satisfaction.

Table 1. Aims, Respondents, and Instruments in the Four Studies

Table 1. Aims, Respondents, and Instruments in the Four Studies

AIMS	RESPONDENTS	INSTRUMENTS
STUDY 1: To measure self concept and self esteem in a Turkish sample	164 students (62 M, 102 F) 50 adults (20 M, 30 F)	TST ASSEI
STUDY 2: To examine relationships among gender, sex role identification and self esteem	139 students (59 M, 80 F)	ASSEI Coopersmith Self Esteem Inventory Bem Sex Role Inventory
STUDY 3: To investigate relationships between personality characteristics and bases of self esteem	84 students (35 M, 49 F) 255 adults (137 M, 118 F)	ASSEI NEO-FFI
STUDY 4: To examine relationships among I-C, gender, and bases of self esteem	300 students (150 M, 150 F)	TST ASSEI IndCol

Study 3

Females scored higher than males on IPC importance ($\underline{F} = 3.86$, $\underline{p} = .05$), and they showed a trend towards scoring higher on IPC satisfaction ($\underline{F} = 3.35$, $\underline{p} = .07$). No overall gender differences were found on PC importance or PC satisfaction.

Study 4

On the TST, females gave more allocentric responses than males, $\underline{F}(1,296) = 13.54$, $\underline{p} = .0001$, and more small group responses, $\underline{F}(1,296) = 10.48$, $\underline{p} = .001$.

There were no differences between Individualist and Collectivist respondents on any of the categories of self-description on the TST. However, there was a significant interaction between gender and Ind-Col on idiocentric self-descriptions: Individualist males gave more idiocentric responses than Individualist females, but Collectivist females gave more idiocentric responses than Collectivist males, $\underline{F}(1,296) = 6.91$, $\underline{p} = .009$.

There was also a significant interaction between gender and IndCol scores on large-group self descriptions: Individualist males gave only slightly more large-group responses than Individualist females, but Collectivist males gave significantly more large-group responses than Collectivist females, $\underline{F}(1,296) = 8.22$, $\underline{p} = .004$.

15.59, p = .0001. Also, Collectivist respondents scored higher than Individualist respondents on IPC importance, $F(1,296) = 11.49$, $p = .001$ (but scores for Collectivist males were not different from scores for Individualist females). Collectivist respondents also scored higher than Individualist respondents on IPC satisfaction, $F(1,296) = 7.38$, $p = .007$.

Conclusions

Self-Concept (TST) Responses

Among Turkish respondents, social roles and status related to factors such as gender , age or employment, appear to be more important determinants of allocentric and small-group responses than scores on the I-C scales. More specifically, females and adults gave more allocentric and small-group responses than males and students across the I-C categories. These individual-level findings replicated the Turkish findings of Watkins et al. (1998), but they differ -- as they did in that study -- from the overall culture-level pattern in which gender was not associated with variability in allocentric responses except in interaction with culture.

One implication may be that, as noted above, Turkish culture does not clearly fit into either the individualist or the collectivist categories, with the result that individual variables and/or local or social class norms may be more determinative than broad cultural variables in forming allocentric self-conceptions. The fact that all respondents were urban dwellers, and all had at least a high school education, probably contributed to a more individualistic tendency than would be found in a more representative sample . Alternatively, or at the same time, the suggestion by Watkins et al. (1998) that individualism-collectivism does not provide a straightforward explanation for cultural variation in self-concept should be considered.

ASSEI Scores: Importance of PCs and IPCs

Findings regarding PCs were essentially uniform across the four studies, with no significant differences in PC importance or PC satisfaction according to gender, age, or I-C scores. For all groups, IPCs were more important than PCs.

The finding of greater attribution of importance to IPCs by females, and their greater satisfaction with themselves in regard to IPCs, supports the arguments of Josephs et al. (1992) regarding culturally defined gender roles, especially in light of the lack of overall difference between adults and students on these variables. Nevertheless, the failure to find overall gender differences in IPC importance in Study 1 raises the caution that particular contextual variables may be important, and that, again as suggested by Watkins et al. (1996), it may not be possible to predict the separate and joint effects of gender and culture in a straightforward manner on the basis of current theory.

especially in light of the lack of overall difference between adults and students on these variables. Nevertheless, the failure to find overall gender differences in IPC importance in Study 1 raises the caution that particular contextual variables may be important, and that, again as suggested by Watkins et al. (1996), it may not be possible to predict the separate and joint effects of gender and culture in a straightforward manner on the basis of current theory.

Table 2. Summary of the Main Results of the Four Studies

Measure	Study 1	Study 2	Study 3	Study 4
TST				
Idiocentric				Sex X I-C interaction
Allocentric	$F>M^2$			$F>M^4$
Small Group				$F>M^3$
Large Group				Sex X I-C interaction
ASSEI				
PC importance	F=M	F=M	F=M	F=M
PC satisfaction		F=M	F=M	
IPC importance	F=M	$F>M^4$	$F>M^1$	$F>M^3$ $C>I^3$
IPC satisfaction		$F>M^3$	F>M	$C>I^2$

^{1} $p < .05$
^{2} $p < .01$
^{3} $p < .001$
^{4} $p < .0001$

M = male
F = female
I = Individualistic
C = Collectivistic

Further work with individualism-collectivism will very likely show that it is not a single dimension, but rather two relatively independent dimensions. Triandis (1994) suggested that collectivism itself has at least two aspects or types, which he called "horizontal" and "vertical" collectivism. Likewise, Schwartz (1994) pointed out that, from the point of view of values, there are at least two different types of individualism. In other words, both ends of the dimension can be differentiated into two or more types. Just as masculinity-femininity has been reconceptualized as two dimensions rather than a single dimension, individualism-collectivism may prove amenable to a similar reconceptualization.

Many writers have posited two basic needs in human beings: for separateness, independence or "agency", on the one hand, and for closeness, interdependence, or "communion" on the other. The social arrangements, values, and psychological orientations which support the first need constitute individualism. Those which support the second constitute collectivism. If different perspective, Sampson has criticized the individualistic bias of American psychology with at least an implicit recognition that collectivism in not the only alternative (see for example, Sampson, 1985). New interpretations of the impact of both gender and culture on self-concept and self-esteem will depend at least partly on further advances in our understanding of the cultural construct of individualism-collectivism.

References

Anamur, Z. (1998). *Individualism-collectivism, self-concept and sources of self-esteem*. Unpublished master's thesis, Boğazici University, Istanbul, Türkiye.

Bond, M. H. (1994). Into the heart of collectivism: A personal and scientific journey. In U. Kim, H. C. Triandis, Kağitcibasi, S.-C. Choi & G. Yoon (Eds.), *Individualism and collectivism* (pp. 66-76). Newbury Park, CA: Sage.

Göregenli, M. (1995). Individualism-collectivism orientations in the Turkish culture: A preliminary study. (In Turkish.) *Turk Psikoloji Dergisi, 10*, 1-14.

Hattie, (1992). *Self-concept*. Hillsdale, NJ: Erlbaum.

Hofstede, G. (1980). *Culture's consequences: International differences in work related values*. Beverly Hills, CA: Sage.

Inelmen, K. V. Ö. (1996). *Relationship of sex-role orientation to two measures of self-esteem*. Unpublished master's thesis, Boğazici University, Istanbul, Türkiye.

Josephs, R. A., Markus, H. R. & Tafarodi, R. W. (1992). Gender and self-esteem. *Journal of Personality and Social Psychology, 63*, 391-402.

Kağitcibasi, C. (1994). A critical appraisal of individualism and collectivism: Toward a new formulation. In U. Kim, H. C. Triandis, Kağitcibasi , S.-C. Choi & G.Yoon (Eds.), *Individualism and collectivism* (pp. 52-65). Newbury Park, CA: Sage.

Kağitcibasi, C. (1996). *Family and human development across cultures: A view from the other side*. NJ: Erlbaum.

Kashima, Y., Yamaguchi, S., Kim, U., Choi, S.-C., Gelfand, M.J. & Yuki, M. 1995). Culture, and gender, and self: A perspective from individualism-collectivism research. *Journal of Personality and Social Psychology, 69*, 925-937.

Luk, C.L. & Bond, M.H. (1992). Explaining Chinese self-esteem in terms of the self-concept. *Psychologia, 35*, 147-154.

Schwartz, S.H. (1994). Beyond individualism/collectivism: New cultural dimensions of values. In U. Kim, H.C. Triandis, C. Kağitcibasi, S-C. Choi, & G. Yoon, (eds.), *Individualism and collectivism: Theory, method, and applications* (pp. 85-119). Newbury Park, CA: Sage.

Seckin, B. (1996). *A narrative analysis of the construction of self in a group of Turkish university undergraduates: A self amidst tradition and change.* Unpublished master's thesis, Boğazici University, Istanbul, Türkiye.

Sunar, D.G. (1994). *Changes in child rearing practices and their effect on self-esteem in three generations of Turkish families.* Paper presented at the American Psychological Association Annual Convention, Los Angeles, CA.

Triandis, H.C. (1990). Cross-cultural studies of individualism and collectivism. *Nebraska Symposium of Motivation* (pp. 41-133). Lincoln, NE: University of Nebraska Press.

Triandis, H.C. (1994). *Culture and social behavior.* New York: McGraw-Hill.

Watkins, D., Adair, J., Akande, A., Gerong, A., McInerney, D., Sunar, D., Watson, S., Wen, Q., & Wondimu, H. (1998). Individualism-collectivism, gender, and the self-concept: A nine culture investigation. *Psychologia, 41*(4), 259-271.

Watkins, D., Adair, J., Akande, A., Cheng, C., Gerong, A., Ismail, M., McInerney, D., Mpofu, E., Regmi, M., Singh-Sengupta, S., Watson, S., Wondimu, H., & Yu, J. (1996). Cultural dimensions, gender, and the nature of self-concept: A fourteen country study. Paper presented at the XIIIth Congress of the International Association for Cross-Cultural Psychology, Montreal.

Acknowledgements

The research for Study 1 was partially supported by Boğaziçi University Research Fund Project #94B0753, and that for Study 3 was partially supported by Boğaziçi University Research Fund Project #96B0945. Kıvanc Inelmen and Zeynep Anamur graciously provided data from their MA thesis studies (Study 2 and Study 4); many thanks to both of them. Thanks are also due to the following for their help in data collection and analysis in Study 3: Didem Akın, Ilgın Başar, Etel Behmuaras, Yeşim Burul, Hüma Çelen, Tanya Dursun, Beril Eraydın, Hande Eslen, Elzi Halmen, Galma Jahic, and Gül Kaya.

Nomological Network of Relationship Harmony for Chinese

Chun Li
Chinese University of Hong Kong

Virginia S. Y. Kwan
University of California, Berkeley

Michael Harris Bond
Chinese University of Hong Kong

ABSTRACT

Relationship harmony focuses on the degree of harmony achieved in interpersonal relationships. This study is part of a program to establish the nomological network surrounding the construct of relationship harmony for the Chinese in preparation of further cross-cultural studies. Relationship harmony has been found to correlate with self-reported Openness, Emotional Stability, Helpfulness, Restraint, and Extroversion. Collective self-esteem was also positively correlated with relationship harmony, a result which suggests that it is related to the importance of participants' ethnic identity and how they perceive others to rate their ethnic group. However, relationship harmony as initially assessed was correlated with only one dimension of personality as perceived by peers. This gap suggests that relationship harmony must also be measured in terms of specific relationships within one's social circle and not merely by self-assessments. An alternate way to tap relationship harmony is thus proposed, and the possible linkages of this new measure are discussed.

Relationship harmony is the degree of harmony achieved in the dyadic relationships within a person's social network. Social harmony is a concept referring to the balance and absence of ill feelings achieved in one's interpersonal relationships. Relationship harmony differs from other constructs concerning interpersonal relationships (cf. Diener & Diener, 1995; Leung & Leung, 1992; Michalos, 1991) in that it is a relationship-oriented rather than an individual-oriented construct. It is an evaluation of the degree of harmony achieved in relationships, as opposed to the pleasure or satisfaction one can derive from those relationships. Since measuring only one relationship will be insufficient to tap one's general relationship harmony with others, relationship harmony has been measured by averaging the self-reported relationship harmony with the five most important people in the participant's life (Kwan, Bond & Singelis, 1997).

Relationship harmony provides insight about the importance of relationship for people across cultures. The importance of harmonious relationships has been advanced by psychologists working in a collectivist

Chinese society (Kwan et al., 1997), where "the degree of interdependence a society maintains among individuals" is emphasized (Hofstede, 1983, p.83). For a collectivist cultural group like the Chinese, the predictive power of relationship harmony for life satisfaction over and above self-esteem is foreseeable. However, added predictive power of relationship harmony in predicting life satisfaction over and above self-esteem also exists for Americans and a number of other cultural groups (et al., Stewart, Rao, Bond, McBride-Chang, Fielding & Kennard, 1998). While self-esteem is a predictor derived from the logic of individualistic Western culture, relationship harmony is a complement derived from collectivist Asian culture. Such findings suggest that, no matter in individualistic or collectivist cultures, people can be satisfied both because they are proud of themselves and because they have achieved harmonious relationships with others. The only difference is that individualistic Americans may view self-esteem as relatively more important; while collectivist Chinese will regard both relationship harmony and self-esteem as vital to their well being (Kwan et al., 1997).

Nomological Network

For further cross-cultural comparisons, it will be necessary to look into the nomological network of relationship harmony within one culture. Only with an established network within a culture can the functional or relational differences be easily revealed when the construct is introduced to another culture. Also, after examining how relationship harmony can be located among the existing constructs, we may find more alternate ways to operationalize relationship harmony, which in turn will increase our understanding of the concept. Thus, the present study is part of a program to establish the nomological network surrounding the construct of relationship harmony.

Past Findings and Current Objectives

Relationship harmony, measured by self-ratings, has been studied with self-rated constructs in both Chinese and American cultures. As a predictor of life satisfaction, relationship harmony, not surprisingly, correlates with subjective well being (Kwan et al., 1997; Stewart et al., 1998). Also, as a mediator between personality dimensions and life satisfaction, relationship harmony was positively related to extroversion and conscientiousness and negatively related to neuroticism as measured by the NEO-FFI (Kwan et al., 1997). Finally, both independent and interdependent construals were also shown to be positively correlated with one's relationship harmony (Kwan et al., 1997).

Within the nomological network established thus far, relationship harmony has a close relationship with life satisfaction and personality dimensions that are rated by the self and at the same time associated with the self only. However, since relationship harmony is a relationship-oriented construct, it should also involve others, not just the self. Moreover, relationship harmony stresses the importance of rating the relationship rather than individual feelings and forces the participants to concentrate on the social network surrounding the self. Such an orientation towards one's social connections rather than individual fulfillment should be reflected in the evaluation of not only the self but also in one's evaluations by others. Hence, the second intent for this study is to establish linkage between relationship harmony and other social constructs.

Other-Rated Personality

Measuring oneself from others' perspectives is pertinent to the study of personalities. Hogan (1995) stated that, "Socioanalytic theory distinguishes between personality from the perspective of the observer and from the perspective of the actor" (p.166) and conceptualized the other-rated personalities as one's reputation. Hogan (1995) also showed that the reputation of an individual can be assessed with acceptable reliability (cf. Funder & Sneed, 1993) and used to forecast future behavior. Thus, other-rated constructs will provide measurable, predictive power that may help us to expand the nomological network surrounding relationship harmony.

Since relationship harmony measures the relationship established between the actor and others, the assumptions held by both the actor and the surrounding others should contribute to the degree of harmony achieved. For example, it has been demonstrated that self-rated extroverts tend to report more harmonious relationships (Kwan et al., 1997). If Extroversion, as a tendency to reach out to others, to be warm and sociable, is reckoned as facilitating harmonious relationships, a person generally perceived by others as an extrovert should also have higher degree of relationship harmony. In other words, no matter whether perceived by the self or by the others, the presence of 'Extroversion' as a favorable factor possessed by any party to a relationship should help to promote a harmonious relationship.

Similar logic can also be applied to other personality dimensions such as Helpfulness or Neuroticism. For Helpfulness, at least one other person must be present for an actor to manifest caring, consideration and attention. Such a manifestation is in fact a chain of actions or attitudes exchanged during the interaction between two persons. As perceived Helpfulness of the other has a positive effect on friendship (Lee & Bond, 1988), the perception of being helpful should help to avoid ill feelings and promote relationship harmony. Self-rated Neuroticism has been found to correlate with relationship harmony negatively (Kwan et al., 1997). If one who considers the self as neurotic is prone to less harmonious relationship, a person considered by others as neurotic may also have the reputation of being fickle and temperamental. Such an oscillating manner will be considered as difficult to manage and will undoubtedly hinder the cultivation of a balanced relationship. On the other hand, people with stable emotion will allow the others to act in a predictable way that will help to promote relationship harmony.

Therefore, one way to expand the nomological network of relationship harmony will be to include personality ratings given by observers surrounding an individual. In this study, we are going to collect personality ratings from the actor and from the observers by using the Sino-American Person Perception Scale (Yik & Bond, 1993). Firstly, we will replicate the link between relationship harmony and self-rated personality. Secondly, other-perceived personality will also be assessed to see how other-rated personality is related to relationship harmony. It is hypothesized that these results involving relationship harmony will validate Kwan et al.'s (1997) findings and parallel those from self-rated personality dimensions such as those for Extroversion, Intellect, and Emotional Stability.

Other-Rated Liking and Contribution

Since relationship harmony focuses on the quality of the social network achieved by a person, it may not only affect others' perception of a person in terms of personality dimensions, but also elicit positive social evaluations from others. A common form of interpersonal evaluations is liking (Berg, 1984). It is speculated that the ability to cultivate a less conflicting relationship will provide a better chance for others to like oneself. In the present survey, the participants were in a working environment; therefore, the assessment of each person's contribution rated by group members has also been included. This will provide us with the grades given to each individual by their group-mates. Since a positive evaluation will reflect a competent, helpful image for the actor, it is speculated that such a reputation generalizes to other situations. This reputation will in turn suggest that the actor will rate his/her relationship with others as more harmonious in general.

Self-Rated Social Constructs

The importance of social group memberships to individual's self-concept and social behavior is acknowledged in social identity theory (e.g., Tajfel & Turner, 1979). Tajfel and Turner proposed that there are two distinct aspects of the self-concept: personal identity and social identity. Based on social identity theory, Luhtanen and Crocker (1992) measured the social identity aspect. They developed an instrument to measure collective self-esteem, an aspect of one's social identity. Since collective self-esteem focuses on the social identity of an individual, people endorsing higher collective self-esteem should be those who put more energy and effort in maintaining their connectedness with others in their social group. Undoubtedly, such directed effort in the relationship will help to improve one's relationship with others. People who put more effort to maintaining relationship with others will also achieve relationships with better quality. Thus, collective self-esteem should be closely related to the relationship harmony, which emphases the quality of relationship set up in an individual's social environment.

Recently, Bettencourt and Dorr (1997) have found that collective self-esteem is a mediator of the relationship between allocentrism and subjective well-being. Also, Kwan et al. (1997) found that relationship harmony is a stronger mediator of interdependent self-construal compared to independent self-construal in its effect on life satisfaction. Acting as mediators in similar contexts, collective self-esteem and relationship harmony should be closely related. Thus, the present study will ask the participants to rate the social construct of collective self-esteem, which will enable us to explore the relationship between collective self-esteem and relationship harmony.

Method

Participants

Participants were 128 students in the Chinese University of Hong Kong, they were asked to take part in the study in partial fulfillment of their social psychology course requirements. There were 98 females and 30 males, and their ages ranged from 19 to 22 years old. All of the participants were Hong Kong Chinese.

The participants were asked to form groups composed of 4 or 5 persons. Of the 24 groups formed, there were 10, 5-female groups, 8, 4-female-1-male groups, 3, 3-female-2-male groups, 2, 2-female-2male groups, 1, 2-female-3male, 1, 1-female-4-male, and 1, 5-male group. Each group was required to meet at least once a week and to complete three group assignments in addition to attending regular class meetings. A large portion of their individual grade was based on the group projects and other group members rated their individual contributions to their group. This realistic work group setting allowed the participants to have adequate opportunities to observe one another.

Instruments

Interpersonal Relationship Harmony Inventory. The Interpersonal Relationship Harmony Inventory (Kwan et al., 1997) was used to evaluate the degree of an individual's achieved interpersonal relationship harmony. The participants were asked to specify the target's name, gender and relationship for the five, most important, dyadic relationships in their lives. In addition, participants indicated the degree of harmony characterizing each relationship ranging from 1 "very low" to 7, "very high". A relationship harmony index was calculated by taking the mean of the 5 harmony ratings.

Collective Self-Esteem. The Collective Self-Esteem Scale (CSES; Luhtanen & Crocker, 1992) consisted of 4 sub-scales, each containing 4 items. The race-specific form of the CSES (Crocker, Luhtanen, Blaine & Broadnax, 1994) was used. The membership esteem subscale evaluated how participants perceived their worthiness as members of the Hong Kong

Chinese group; the private esteem subscale evaluated participants' perception of how good Hong Kong Chinese are; public esteem subscale evaluated participants' perception of how others view Hong Kong Chinese; and the importance to identity subscale evaluated the importance of being Hong Kong Chinese to participants' self-concept. All responses were made on 7-point scales with anchors of 1, "strongly disagree', and 7, "strongly agree".

The alpha coefficients of the four subscales showed an acceptable level of internal consistency from .53 for identity .to .73 for private. The alpha for the composite scale was also acceptable (.75). An averaged score for all 4 subscales of collective self-esteem was computed for further analyses.[1]

Other-rated liking scores. The other-rated liking scores were collected to investigate to what extent the participants were liked by their group members in general. All participants were asked to rate each group member on a 7-point scale with anchors 1, "really dislike" and 7, "really like". A liking score for each participant was thus computed by averaging the ratings that were given by all their group members.

Other-rated contribution. All participants had learned some important information about other members' skills and shortcomings in the course of completing their group assignments. Thus, each group designed its own evaluation form to evaluate each of its member's contributions to the group assignments. Each group independently chose the components and weights of criteria to be included in the evaluation form. The most frequently selected criteria were variants of participation, responsibility, creativity, attentiveness, and communication skills. All participants rated themselves and each member in their groups based on those criteria. An individual averaged score from all members was used as each individual's group grade, which constituted 20% of the total course grade. To control for group effect, we have centered the groups' means so that every group will have the same mean for further analysis.

Sino-American Person Perception Scale (SAPPS). The SAPPS (Yik & Bond, 1993) was composed of both indigenous and imported personality trait items. It consisted of 32, bipolar adjective scales comprehensively measuring the perceived dimensions of personality in the Chinese culture. The items are mixed randomly with half of the positive poles on the right side and the remaining half on left side of the scale. There are eight dimensions in the SAPPS, namely Openness to Experience, Emotional stability, Extroversion, Application, Intellect, Helpfulness, Restraint, and Assertiveness.

All the 128 participants were asked to rate themselves and each group member in their group on 7-point scales. The alpha coefficients for self-ratings of SAPPS showed an acceptable level of internal consistency for four-item scales ranging from .56 for Helpfulness to .85 for Openness to

---

[1] The seventh item in the public subscale has been deleted due to its negative part-whole correlates with the scale. The correlation between the subscales with and without this item is .9 (p <.05).

Experience, which was comparable to previous study in the same population (Yik, 1993).

Results

Self-Rated Individual SAPPS

Each participant's personality was measured by a comprehensive personality inventory: Sino-American Personality Perception Scale (SAPPS, Yik & Bond, 1993). The results were similar to those formed by using the NEO-FFI (Kwan et al., 1997). Relationship harmony correlated with self-reported Emotional Stability, r (128) = .24, and Extroversion, r (128) = .21, (p's <.05). Also, additional dimensions were found to correlate with relationship harmony: Helpfulness, r (128) = .32, Restraint, r (128) = .29, and Openness, r (128) = .21, (all p's <.05).

Self-Rated Collective Self-esteem

Collective self-esteem was also correlated with relationship harmony at r (128) =.19, (p <.05). Among the four components of collective self-esteem, the identity and public components correlated with relationship harmony, r (128)=.29 and r (128) =.28, respectively, (p's <.05).

Others-Rated SAPPS, Liking and Grade

Respondent's relationship harmony was only correlated with Extroversion as rated by other group members, r (128)=.19, (p <.05). Contrary to our predictions, it was not correlated with the remaining other-rated personality dimensions, achieved liking, or one's group contribution score.

Discussion

Expanded Nomological Network

Self-rated personality. The connection between relationship harmony and self-rated dimensions of personality is further confirmed in the present study by using the SAPPS rather than the NEO-FFI used in the Kwan et al. (1997) study. Relationship harmony has been found to correlate with self-reported Openness, Helpfulness, Restraint, Emotional Stability, and Extroversion of the SAPPS—a lexical measure of personality. Besides confirming the linkage between relationship harmony and the latter two dimensions found by Kwan et al. (1997), the results also demonstrate the possible linkage with other self-rated personality dimensions.

Self-rated collective self-esteem. Collective self-esteem also has a positive correlation with relationship harmony. This is consistent with our hypothesis that people with positive racial collective self-esteem will have more harmonious relationships with others who are from the same ethnic group in the present study. However, the relatively low correlation may also be the results of the sample size and power. This problem will be addressed later. By examining the significantly correlated subscales, it is suggested that if a person considers racial identity important to the self-concept, that person's relationship harmony will be higher. A similar increase in relationship harmony also will occur if a participant thinks people outside Hong Kong will rate Hong Kong Chinese positively.

Missing Links

Within the group level, each group member has been asked to give ratings on one another's personality, to indicate whether they like each other, and to evaluate the contribution of each group member; however, relationship harmony was correlated with only one dimension of personality as perceived by peers. This set of outcomes indicates that self-reported relationship harmony with one's most important five others did not correlate with other constructs of one's reputation or social personality as achieved in a medium-term group setting. Furthermore, whether one is liked or rated as performing well in an academic work team is also not related to one's relationship harmony.

The findings give rise to a problem that needs to be explained. As relationship harmony focuses on the interpersonal balance maintained by a person, the perception that one possesses several favorable traits should reflect one's achievement of stable harmonious relationships. This assumption is confirmed when favorable self-rated traits like Helpfulness and Intellect are shown to be linked to relationship harmony (Lee & Bond, 1998). However, if others are asked to rate similar traits, the linkages with relationship harmony are drastically reduced.

Such results may be due to the inconsistency between the people included in the relationship harmony inventory and the group members giving the ratings. People's personalities manifested to their most important five persons may be very different from their reputation as achieved in such group settings. When one is asked to rate the relationship harmony with the five most important others, one may focus on the interpersonal, intimate nature of the relationship. However, in the present study, the relationship harmony with group members will tend to be task-oriented. Also, the relationship harmony with the five most important others is obtained by asking participants to evaluate five, one-to-one relationships; while the relationship harmony in the group settings is closer to a many-to-one relationship. Thus, the ratings collected from the group members tend to be bounded by the group setting and are apparently not related to relationship harmony as achieved with non-group members.

Another possible explanation may be that the personalities manifested by an individual are in fact very similar across different social settings. The fact that relationship harmony correlates with self- but not other-rated personalities may be due to the difference between self and other perception.

It may be that, although one acts in the same way across situations, the difference we have found is due to the low correlation of one's personality as measured by the self and the others (Kolar, Funder, & Colvin, 1996).

Limitations

Since we tried to minimize the control over such realistic work group setting, we did not assign people into groups. This results in a biased male to female ratio of about 1 to 3.3 and only 1 group consisted of only males, making it impossible to test for the gender effect.

For the present findings, the correlations found were not very impressive. The highest correlations confirmed has been .35 (between relationship harmony and collective self-esteem) which accounts for only 12.25% of the variability. Whether these findings have been due to the sample size and power or they do reflect some connections around relationship harmony can still be investigated.

Future Studies

Since relationship harmony seems as presently measured to be linked with self-reported measures only, it is suggested that relationship harmony can be measured in terms of specific relationships within the group. We propose to assess such achieved relationship harmony, linking it to both self- and other-perceived measures derived from group members in future studies. By following the procedures mentioned, people included in the relationship harmony measures and those providing the other-perceived constructs will be the same people, thereby providing a stringent test to compare the relationship between other-rated constructs and the self- and other-reported relationship harmony.

The present study has expanded the nomological network of self-rated relationship harmony with self-rated personality ratings and collective self-esteem. However, one's other-rated personality, liking and contribution evaluation did not correlate with relationship harmony at all. Thus, a new method to measure other-rated constructs as well as relationship harmony is proposed. This newly proposed domain-specific measure of relationship harmony would allow us to further explore the nomological network from both individual and other perspectives.

References

Berg J. H. (1984). Development of friendship between roommates. *Journal of Personality and Social Psychology, 46,* 346-356.

Bettencourt, B. A., & Dorr, N. (1997). Collective self-esteem as a mediator of the relationship between allocentrism and subject well-being. *Personality and Social Psychology Bulletin, 23*, 955-964.

Crocker, J., Luhtanen, R., Blaine, B., & Broadnax, S. (1994). Collective self-esteem and psychology well-being among white, black, and Asian college students. *Personality and Social Psychological Bulletin, 20*, 503-513.

Diener, E. & Diener, M. (1995). Cross-cultural correlates of life satisfaction and self-esteem. *Journal of Personality and Social Psychology, 69*, 851-864.

Funder, D. C. & Sneed, C. D. (1993). Behavioral manifestations of personality: An ecological approach to judgmental accuracy. *Journal of Personality and Social Psychology, 64*, 479-490.

Hofstede, G. (1983). *Culture's consequences: International differences in work-related values.* Beverly Hills, CA: Sage Publications.

Hogan, R. (1995). A socioanalytic perspective on the five-factor model. In J. S. Wiggins (Ed.), *The five factor model of personality: Theoretical perspectives* (pp.163-179). New York: Guilford Press.

Kolar, D. W., Funder, D. C., & Colvin, C. R. (1996). Comparing the accuracy of personality judgments by the self and knowledgeable others. *Journal of Personality, 64*, 311-337.

Kwan, V. S. Y., Bond, M. H., & Singelis, T. M. (1997). Pancultural explanation for life satisfaction: Adding relationship harmony to self-esteem. *Journal of Personality and Social Psychology. 73*, 1083-1051.

Lee, R. Y. P. & Bond, M. H. (1998). Personality and roommate friendship in Chinese culture. *Asian Journal of Social Psychology, 1,* 179-190.

Leung, J. P. & Leung, K. (1992). Life satisfaction, self-concept, and relationship with parents in adolescence. *Journal of Youth and Adolescence, 21*, 653-665.

Luhtanen, R. & Crocker, J. (1991). Self-esteem and intergroup comparisons: Toward a theory of collective self-esteem. In J. Suls & T. A. Wills (Eds.), *Social comparison: Contemporary theory and research* (pp.211-234). Hillsdale, NJ: Lawrence Erlbaum.

Luhtanen, R. & Crocker, J. (1992). A collective self-esteem scale: Self-evaluation of one's social identity. *Personality and Social Psychology Bulletin, 18*, 302-318.

Michalos, A. C. (1991). *Global report on student well-being (Vols. 1-4).* New York: Springer-Verlag.

Rosenberg, M. (1965). *Society and the adolescent self-image.* Princeton, NJ: Princeton University Press.

Stewart, S. M., Rao, N., Bond, M. H., McBride-Chang, C., Fielding, R., & Kennard, B. D. (1998) Chinese dimensions of parenting: Broadening Western predictors and outcomes. *International Journal of Psychology, 33*, 345-358.

Tajfel, H., & Turner, J. C. (1979). An integrative theory of intergroup conflict. In W. Austin & S. Worchel (Eds.), *The social psychology of intergroup relations* (pp. 33-48). Pacific Grove, CA: Brooks/ Cole.

Yik, M. S. M. (1993). *Self- and peer ratings of personality traits: Evidence of convergent and discriminant validity among Hong Kong university students.* Unpublished master thesis: Chinese University of Hong Kong.

Yik, M., & Bond, M. H. (1993). Exploring the dimensions of Chinese person perception with indigenous and imported constructs: Creating a culturally balanced scale. *International Journal of Psychology, 28*, 75-95.

Cultural Identity Development and Global Self-Esteem in Indigenous and Migrant Background Australian Adolescents

Elsa R. Germain
James Cook University of North Queensland
School of Psychology & Sociology

ABSTRACT

This study explores the effects that cultural adjustment to a dominant culture context may have on the development of cultural identity and ultimately on global self-esteem in early and late adolescent youth of ethnic minority background. The study sought to assess the inter-relationship between perceived cognitive, social, and physical self and cultural membership that ultimately contribute to the development of self-identity and global self-esteem. In addition, attitudes toward acculturation and achieved cultural identity were expected to be a function of maturation. Experiences of racism, parental characteristics and geographical status were also considered as critical features shaping cultural identity. Convenience samples of 400 junior and senior high school students residing in regional North Queensland Australia were surveyed. Of these, 106 were identified as being of culturally and linguistically diverse background (CLDB). Results indicated that cultural identification appears to be significantly influenced by the combined effects of experiences of racism, segregation views on adjustment, and cultural exploration. In turn, global self-esteem was influenced significantly by the combined effects of marginalisation attitudes to acculturation, age, and cultural identity search.

Verkuyten (1992) has suggested that psychological adjustment problems experienced by youngsters from a cultural minority background are unique and quite distinct to those of youth of a mainstream cultural background, and older immigrants who tend to subscribe more clearly to one culture More specifically, the development and retention of migrant ethnic identity among adolescents have been addressed by several researchers (Hurtado, Guring & Peng,1994; Laperriere, Compere, Dkhissy, Dolce & Fleurent,1994; Liebkind 1993; Phinney, DuPont, Espinosa, Revill, & Sanders,1994; Rumbaut,1994, Saenz, Hwang, Aguirre & Anderson,1995; Nesdale & Rooney,1997). In particular, the relationship between ethnic identity and self-esteem has been explored by Phinney (1990) and others (Rotheram-Borus & Phinney,1990). Phinney and Chavira (1992) also examined the effects of age on cultural identity development. They found that identity developed over time, with older youth evidencing greater cultural identification and higher self-esteem. However, only a few studies have focused on the combined effects that attitudes to acculturation (Berry et al., 1992), and acculturating behaviours have on cultural identification (Liebkind,1993;1996). This was one of the main aims of the present study. Of additional interest was the link between cultural identity and self-esteem, as well as the effects that phenotypical characteristics, and critical experiences such as racism have on cultural exploration and identification in minority culture adolescents.

Cultural Identification

A so called *achieved identity* is the result of a period of exploration and experimentation that takes place typically during adolescence (Erickson,1968). Four major realms of development including biological, psychological, social-cognitive and emotional, have been highlighted as contributing to the formation of an individual identity. Of these, Hattie (1992) who described the self as being primarily a cognitive appraiser has underscored the cognitive component. He stated that identity is entwined with knowledge about the self. Moreover, Duval and Wicklund (1972) have argued that self-evaluation can be elucidated by the standards or traits and attitudes of *correctness* that each individual possesses. Social identity is achieved when an individual is aware of belonging to certain social groups together with some affective and value significance to him/her of the group membership (Tajfel, 1981). Moreover, ethnic self-awareness may be heightened or blurred depending on the degree of perceived *dissonance* or *consonance* with the larger social context (Rumbaut,1994). It is also possible that ethnicity or ethnic identity per se may become optional for some (Rumbaut,1994) as it has become for many well established migrants arriving in Australia after World War II. However, how optional cultural identity may be largely depends not only on the extent of assimilation but also on phenotypical characteristics (visible ethnicity). Phenotypic characteristics consistent with a given cultural background may influence how individuals construe a cultural reality and indeed the choice to belong to one's own group or the mainstream's group. Portes and Zhou (1993, cited in Rumbat, 1994) have posed a critical question, namely to what sector of a given society does a particular minority culture group assimilate? The present study extended this query to, to what social group within the multicultural context does adolescents of CLDB identify with and how does the process of adjustment to a dominant culture shape the experience?

Cultural Identity as a Process

Various models propose a number of cultural identification stages. For instance, Marcia (1980) proposes at least four stages: *pre-encounter, encounter, immersion*, and *internalization* that can be the function of maturation. In addition, cultural or ethnic self-identification has been thought to be triggered by a critical experience such as prejudice or racism. In an attempt to resolve negative feelings resulting from stereotyping and value discrepancy, adolescents may engage in cultural identity search. Cultural identification is then developed through the exploration of features such as language, participation in cultural activities, attitudes to self and others in reference to cultural membership, and social networks (friendships, and interpersonal relationships) (Phinney, 1990). Similarly, Phinney, Lochner, and Murphy (1990) propose three distinct stages of ethnic identity: (1) ethnicity is not an issue and therefore is unexplored; (2) increasing awareness about ethnicity; and (3) coming to terms with ethnic issues (acceptance). Moreover, Phinney and Devic-Navarro (1995) have proposed the use of the Multigroup Ethnic Identity Measure to ascertain the degree of bicultural identification in cultural minority adolescents. The measure assesses three aspects of ethnic identity, (a) a sense of belonging and attitudes towards one's ethnic group; (b) ethnic identity achievement, based on exploration and commitment; and (c) traditional behaviours and customs.

The impact of cultural elements in the formation of identity is complex and uncertain according to Rosenthal (cited in Phinney et al., 1990). To facilitate unravelling the contribution that culture makes in adolescent development, it may be useful to explore not only self appraisal but also its connection with group experiences such as parental characteristics, cultural participation, and geographical status. The latter has been analysed by McClenahan, Cairns, Dunn, and Morgan (1991). The authors investigated preference for geographical location as a measure of ethnic/national identity in children from Northern Ireland. They found that the technique of geographical preference based on religious orientation provided a suitable way of measuring ethnic/national identity preference in children.

Cross-cultural Adjustment Theories

A distinction has been made between two related processes, *acculturation* and *ethnic identity* development. Cultural adjustment or acculturation refers to the changes in cultural attitudes, values and behaviours that result from contact between two distinct cultures (Berry, Trimble & Olmedo 1986). Ethnic identity on the other hand refers to the ethnic component of social identity (that part of an individual's self concept which derives from knowledge of membership of a social group or groups) together with the value and emotional significance attached to that membership" (Tajfel, 1981, p. 255). Thus, ethnic identity may be thought of as an aspect of acculturation, in which the focus is on how individuals of ethnic minority background relate to their own group as a subgroup of the larger society (Phinney, 1990). The ways in which an acculturating individual wishes to relate to the dominant society have been termed *acculturating strategies* (Berry et al., 1992). When the central ideas of *participation* within a given larger cultural context and *contact maintenance* with one's own cultural group are conceptualised, a framework yielding a set of distinct outcomes or attitudes to acculturation can be identified (Berry et al., 1992). Attitudes to acculturation are embodied in the following concepts, (1) *Integration*, where there is an interest in maintaining both original culture values and contact with the larger context; (2) *Assimilation*, when the original culture is not maintained and the adoption of the larger culture values takes place; (3) *Marginalisation*, in which there is little interest in original culture maintenance and little opportunity by choice or exclusion to participate in the larger culture context; and (4) *Separation*, when value is placed on maintaining the original culture and continuous contact with minority in-groups. Berry (1990) has designed a 72-item scale to measure these attitudes to acculturation. Moreover, the author has pointed out that the scale tap onto group-level factors and individual-level factors which shape adaptation. These factors can be said to be universal but also specific to the cultures in contact.

Research Focus

This study attempted to explore the relationship that attitudes to acculturation to a dominant cultural context may have on cultural identity and ultimately global self-esteem in early and late adolescence minority culture youth. The research focused on the major concepts underlying cultural identity formation as described by Phinney (1989, 1990), and more specifically by the Phinney and Devich-Navarro's (1996) Bicultural Identification model. Also of main interest were the theoretical concepts underlying cultural adjustment as measured by Berry's Attitudes to Acculturation Strategies Scale (Berry, 1996). Empirical analysis involved the evaluation of these variables and their inter-relationships using attitudes to acculturation and age as independent measures for cultural identity and ultimately self-esteem. Additional factors considered in this study were experiences of racism, respondents' phenotypical characteristics, parental characteristics, and geographical status. The following questions were posed: Do attitudes to acculturation influence cultural identity search and ultimately cultural identification? Are individuals who experience racism more likely than those who do not, to engage in cultural exploration leading to a cultural identification? Do youngsters who have achieved a cultural identity have higher self-esteem than those who have not? Are the processes of cultural identification and cultural identity exploration influenced by age? Do factors such as visible ethnicity, participation in in-group activities and geographical status influence the process of cultural identity development? Following the assumptions made by the theories briefly explored, attitudes to acculturation were expected to influence cultural identification and consequently self-esteem. Moreover, cultural identification was expected to be linked to cultural identity search and experiences of racism. Phenotypical characteristics (whether youngsters were visibly identifiable as of ethnic minority background), parental cultural background, cultural participation and geographical status were also expected to influence cultural identity search and ultimately cultural identification.

Method

Participants

Stratified samples of convenience were selected consisting of a total of 400 children from four different high schools each (junior and senior grades). Target schools included two state, non-denominational, co-educational schools, and two private, Catholic schools, (all boys and all girls). The State schools were located in rural areas of North Queensland, Australia, namely at the townships of Ingham and Ayr. The Catholic schools were situated in Townsville, a relatively large regional centre with a population of approximately 110,000.

A total sample of 106 culturally and linguistically diverse background (CLDB) adolescents was identified. The criteria for selection was respondents identifying themselves as being born in a non-English-speaking (NES) country, or having at least one parent born in Australia of Indigenous descent (Aboriginal, Torres Strait Islander or South Sea Islander), or being of second generation NES migrant background or having at least one parent born in a non-English-speaking country. Youngsters in the sample were categorised into two age groups, namely early adolescence (12-15 year olds) and late adolescence (16-19 year olds). Younger males were over-represented in the sample (58%). Chi square analysis showed a significant difference with respect to age; there were more males within the 12-15 year old category, with the female respondents being more or less equally distributed across the two age groups. A large proportion of the 12-15 year olds (82%) attended a private-Catholic school, while the majority of 16-19 year olds (62%) attended a public-state school. Socio-economic family status was comparable across the age groups, with the majority of respondents in both age groups (46%, and 52%, respectively) reporting unskilled parental occupation. There was no difference across the two age categories with respect to geographical status, with the majority of respondents reporting living in an urban area (64%, 67%). The overwhelming majority of CLDB respondents reported being born in Australia 77%(n=81), with 19% (n=20) being born overseas in a non-English speaking country, and approximately 4% (n=4) being born overseas in an English-speaking country but of NES background parents. Languages spoken at home included traditional Aboriginal dialects such as Wyk Mungkan, Kuuk Taayorre, and Wik Ngan Cherra, and TSI languages. Other languages reported included Basque, Bislama, Chinese, Croatian, French, Hindi, Italian, Maori, Spanish, Swedish, Tagalog, Thai, Tokelau, and Vietnamese. The most frequently reported language spoken at home was Italian (29%). A total number of 39 (38%) youngsters reported being from a two-culture household (mother or father born in an overseas country), 36 (35%) reported both parents being born overseas, and 27 (26%) reported both parents were born in Australia. Of these 20 were identified as Indigenous Australians, and the other 7 were considered to fit into the category of CLDB after close analysis of the data revealed that they were second generation migrants living in a NESB household (e.g., other than English language reported being spoken at home). The term Indigenous was used liberally in that it was applied not only to Aboriginal and Torres Straits Island background youngsters but also to those of South Sea Island background. Four cases were missing. The overwhelming majority of respondents (n=93, 91%) said they lived in a nuclear family, with no significant difference between early and late adolescence youngsters.

Measures

Cultural Adjustment was measured by an abbreviated version of Berry's (1992) *Attitudes to Acculturation Strategies Scale*. The scale measures attitudes to acculturation or acculturating strategies that pertained, as stated in the literature review, to the way acculturating individuals wish to relate to the dominant culture. The original scale consists of 72 items containing statements designed to tap on to the four attitudes to acculturation. These are organised in a sematic differential response format, ranging in responses from 1 ("strongly disagree") to 5 ("strongly agree"). The scale can be said to have high face validity, and is currently one of the most widely used instruments in recent cross-cultural studies (see for example Kwak & Berry, 1998; Neto, 1998; Sam, 1998; Nguyen et al., 1998). Items selected for the present study consisted of 12 randomly selected statements of which three were selected for each of the four categories. This yielded a composite score for each of the four attitude categories, namely *integration, assimilation, segregation* and *marginalisation*. The higher the score in a given category, the stronger the attitude in a given acculturation strategy. The response format for the original scale was altered for this study in that an additional value was added to the range of responses from 5 to 6. So the actual range was from 1 ("strongly disagree") to 6 ("strongly agree"). The rationale behind this addition was that an even number range of responses may yield a clearer picture with respect to attitudes, as respondents would not have the option of ticking a middle score. Examples of items pertaining to each of the four categories are as follows: (1) *Assimilationist* attitudes, "Because we live in Australia we do not need to know migrant and Indigenous Australian languages. We should focus our attention on speaking English fluently;" (2) *Marginalisation* attitude, "Events such as the Multicultural Fest, The Laura Festival (Aboriginal-Australian Festival) and so on are just events supported by government to keep minorities quiet;" (3) *Separation* attitudes, "If I had a choice I would marry someone who was brought up in my own culture;" and (4) *Integration* attitudes, "I would encourage high school children to learn not only about the history of mainstream Australians, but also that of Indigenous Australians and other ethnic groups because it is important to know where we all come from."

Age of respondents was categorised as early adolescence (between 12-15 years) and late adolescence (between 16-19 years).

Cultural Identity Search referred to the exploration process by which adolescents learn about their cultural background and eventually make a commitment to a given cultural identity. Cultural identity search was measured by Phinney's (1992)14-item Multigroup Ethnic Identity Measure. The measure has a reliability α = .81 with high school students. It has three sub-scales that assess three facets of ethnic identity: (1) sense of belonging to and attitudes towards one's ethnic group (i.e.,"Have you ever tried to find out more about your culture of origin?"). These five items had a response format of *yes* or *no*; (2) ethnic identity achievement based on exploration and commitment (i.e.,"How important is it to find out about your culture of origin?") The response format for these seven items was *1="very important" to 6="not at all important;"* (3) participation or "ethnic behaviours and customs" (Phinney & Devic-Navarro, 1995, p. 7) pertaining to one open-ended question (i.e., "How did you go about learning about your original culture?" "What kinds of activities help you learn about your culture?") and yielding the number and nature of activities consistent with actively learning and participating in one's original culture. The total range of the number of responses given was 1-6, which was considered as the number of cultural participation activities.

Cultural identification was measured by one of five possible answers to the question "In terms of culture or ethnic group, what do you consider yourself to be?" Responses included "Australian," "original culture," "both," "unsure," and "none".

Global Self-esteem was measured using the Personal Attribute Inventory for Children (Parish, 1978) a self-report instrument consisting of a 48-item adjective checklist. The scale was designed to measure children's self-concept, and has a test-retest reliability of .73 for a sample of school children over a four-week period.

Second language spoken at home. This was considered to be an essential element of active participation in traditional cultural activities. Second language spoken at home was simply measured by asking the question "Do you speak a language other than English at home?" The response format was either *yes* or *no.* Respondents were also asked to identify languages spoken (other than English).

Phenotypical characteristics were measured with the single request to "tick the face that most closely resembles your physical features".

Respondents were presented with 12 illustrations, six of boys and six of girls, depicting phenotypical characteristics consistent with Caucasian, Asian and Black human features. The illustrations were modelled on photographs of people identified as of the backgrounds specified from a social anthropology text (Nanda, 1994). Responses were grouped into two categories, visibly ethnic (Asian and Black) or visibly Caucasian (Caucasian). The illustrations were pilot tested with a group of 16 ethnic minority adolescents (5 Indigenous Australians, 5 Filipinos, 4 Chinese and 2 Vietnamese) between the ages of 13 and 17, who were participating at the time in a community project entitled the Youth Transit Project as an initiative from the Migrant Resource Centre in Townsville to assist Indigenous and refugee background youth (mostly Asian) access community services. All sixteen respondents in the pilot study were able to "recognise" their phenotypical features in the illustrations successfully.

Experiences of racism was simply measured by a “yes” or “no” response to the question, "Have you ever experienced racism?"

Parental characteristics. This included family composition, socio-economic status (employment status and type), other than English languages spoken by parents, and English-language ability (if English was identified as their second language). Three categories of family composition were derived, both parents born in Australian, both parents born overseas, and of mixed marriage.

Geographical status. Two geographical locations were identified for this measure, regional and rural and simply pertained to the place of residence of respondents, either Townsville or Ingham and Ayr respectively.

Demographics. Including school year attended by respondents, country of birth, cultural background (whether of Indigenous, migrant or Anglo-Australian background), length of stay in Australia if born overseas, and languages other than English spoken by participants.

Procedure

All students enrolled in junior (six year 8 classes) and senior (four year 12 classes) high school grades in two public (at Ingham and Ayr) and two private high schools (at Townsville) were asked to respond to a questionnaire containing demographic items including geographical status; Berry’s Attitude to Acculturation Strategies Scale (1990); the Multi-ethnic Identity Measure (Phinney & Devic-Navarro, 1995); a cultural identity measure; the Personal Attribute Inventory for Children (Parish, 1978); a stimuli of six illustrations eliciting self-perceived visible ethnicity or phenotypical characteristics; a measure eliciting experiences of racism; and information on parental characteristics. The questionnaire was organised to minimise reactivity and socially desirable responses by reminding participants that there were no “right” or “wrong” answers but “opinions” which were the focus of interest in the study. A total of four hundred and fifteen students across the four participating high schools completed a questionnaire during school time under the supervision of the class teacher. Teachers were previously informed of the study, and were also given the opportunity to review the questionnaire and ask questions if any aspect of the instrument was not clear prior to distributing it among the participants. Each of the classes participating contained within 35 to 55 students of which approximately 25% were of Non-Anglo Australian background. A total of 400 questionnaires were deemed useable. Questionnaires took approximately 45 minutes to complete. The instrument was in English as all respondents were fluent English speakers. Written parental consent for children to participate in the study was obtained prior to data collection. Confidentiality was assured and respondents were asked not to provide personal details that may identify them in the questionnaires. Parents and participants were also assured that if participants became upset in the process of responding to the questionnaire they would be referred to the school counsellor. Respondents were informed that participation was voluntary and that their responses to the questionnaire would not be shown to teachers, parents or school administrators. Participants were instructed to respond to the questionnaire without talking to their fellow students since the purpose of the study was to obtain personal views and beliefs on a number of issues related to cultural identity. Youngsters were directed to ask questions to the class teacher if any aspect of the questionnaire was unclear.

One hundred six of the participants identified themselves as being of ethnic minority background or of culturally and linguistically diverse background (CLDB), with 20 of these being Indigenous Australians. Data pertaining to the remaining 294 Anglo-Australian participants (AA) were used in inter-group comparison analysis which is the topic of another paper and will not be discussed here. Cultural identity was considered to be a process of cognitive appraisal achieved through either the *individual* (personal level) or *collective* (group level) experience. In addition, *attitudes to acculturation* and *achieved cultural identity* were expected to be functions of maturation.

Results

Preliminary analysis involved two steps. Firstly, univariate and bivariate inspections of the data revealed no serious violation of assumptions underlying statistical tests used in the analysis of results. In addition, responses to the 12 items pertaining to Attitudes to Acculturation were subjected to a validity check by means of a Chi square analysis for each of the four dimensions assessed by the scale and reported cultural participation as measured by the third section of Phinney and Devic-Navarro's (1995) Multi-ethnic Identity Measure as described previously. Results did not confirm fully theoretical assumptions made by the scale's author (Berry, 1990). Results indicated a significant relationship between attitudes to *assimilation* and cultural activities participation, $\chi^2(1,65)= 6.232$, $p<.05$. However, analysis results for the remaining three measures, *integration, marginalisation,* and *segregation* were not statistically significant. Thus, results including Attitudes to Acculturation measures were interpreted with caution.

Some assumptions made by the theoretical constructs with respect to cultural identity were supported by the results. The expected relationship between Attitudes to Acculturation scores and an achieved cultural identity, mediated by cultural identity search and experiences of racism was evaluated using a step-wise regression analysis. Results indicated a significant combined contribution effect of *segregation* attitudes to acculturation with a correlation coefficient of .436 (R^2 =.19) on cultural identity, an R value of .497 (R^2 = .24) for cultural identity search, and an R value of .547 (R^2 = .3) for experiences of racism. It appears that the greatest contribution is that of racism (accounting for 30% of the variance) closely followed by *segregation* attitudes (24% of the variance), and cultural exploration (19% of the variance). Thus, cultural identification appears to be significantly influenced by the combined effects of experiences of racism, *segregation* attitudes, and cultural exploration. The remaining attitudes to acculturation measures had no significant effect on cultural identification. Age had no effect on cultural identification, either as an individual factor or combined with other factors.

The third step in the analysis involved examining the relationship between cultural identity and global self-esteem. One-tail Pearson correlation tests results indicated a significant relationship between global self-esteem and cultural identity search (R = .286 R^2 = .08, $p< .05$), however, there was no relationship between self-esteem and achieved cultural identity. A final step in the analysis process examined the relationship that group and individual experiences such as cultural participation activities, parental characteristics, geographical status, visible ethnicity and experiences of racism may have on ethnic identity and identity search.

Group Experiences

Cultural activities participation and ethnic identity search. Chi-square analysis of a second language spoken at home and cultural identification search yielded significant results $\chi^2(1, 90) = 12.34$, $p = .0004$. Of the total number 33 youngsters who reported speaking a second language at home (37%), twenty-seven (82%) tended to report engaging in cultural identity search. Those who did not speak a second language at home (n = 57, 63%) tended to report not engaging in cultural identity search either (n = 32, 56%). With respect to cultural activities participation and cultural identity search, results of a One way ANOVA indicated a significant difference across the groups, $F(1,64) = 13.74$, $p = .0004$. Youngsters tending to report cultural activities participation also tended to report having engaged in cultural identity search more than those who did not participate in cultural activities (34%). Post-hoc analysis revealed the difference to be significant (Scheffe $F = 13.74$, $p = .05$).

Cultural activities participation and cultural identity., A second language spoken at home, and the number of cultural activities engaged in were significantly related with cultural identity. Chi square analysis of cultural identity and second language showed a significant relationship between the variables $\chi^2(3,103)=28.56$, $p=.0001$, Cramer's $V = .527$. Youngsters tending to report an "Australian" identity tended to report not speaking a second language at home (94%). In contrast, youngsters who did not identify with or were unsure of a cultural identity (70%) tended to report speaking a second language at home more than respondents in the other two categories (64% "Original culture" identity, and 53% "Bi-cultural" identity). Post-hoc analysis confirmed these observations partly. By far the largest differences between expected and observed cell values were found in the "Australian" identity category (post-hoc cell contribution= 5.18) and "Unsure/none" identity category (post-hoc cell contribution= 2.85).

In turn, oneway ANOVA results of cultural activities participation and cultural identity showed a significant relationship $F(3,66)=3.728$, $p=.015$, with those reporting an achieved original culture identity tending to report the highest number of activities ($M = 3.87$, $SD= 1.80$). In contrast, those reporting an "Australian" identity said they engaged in a lower number of in-group activities ($M = 2.17$, $SD = 1.13$). A post hoc comparison analysis yielded a Scheffe $F = 2.985$, $p = .05$. Those who reported being "unsure" of or not identifying with any culture reported participating in a higher number of cultural activities than those identified as "Australian" ($M = 2.83$, $SD = 1.47$). However, a post hoc comparison revealed that the difference was not significant.

Family composition, geographical status and cultural identity exploration. Chi-square results indicated no significant relationship between these variables, with children from all family groups tending to report comparable results for both family composition and geographical status.

Family composition, geographical status and cultural identification. Chi square results revealed a significant association between the variables $\chi^2(6,102)= 31.89$, $p = .0001$. The majority of respondents from mixed-marriage families tended to identify with being "Australian", whilst respondents with parents born overseas tended to report more an "original" culture identity. Minority youngsters of Australian born parents (second generation migrants or Indigenous Australians) tended to report being unsure of or not identifying with a particular culture. Chi square results showed no significant differences across the cultural identity groups with respect to geographical status.

Individual Experiences

Phenotypical characteristics (visible ethnicity) and cultural identity exploration. Chi-square results indicated a significant relationship between respondents phenotype and cultural identity search, v^2 (1,84)= 4.21, p=.04. As expected, visibly ethnic youngsters tended to report engaging in cultural identity search more so than the Caucasian looking children.

Visible ethnicity and cultural identity. Chi-square results indicated a significant relationship between the variables $\chi^2(3,96)= 9.54$, $p = .02$. Caucasian looking children tended to report an "Australian" identity more so than the visibly ethnic respondents who, interestingly, tended also to report a bicultural identity rather than an achieved original culture identification as expected.

Experiences of racism and cultural identity search. Chi-square results of racism and cultural identity search revealed a significant relationship between the χ^2 (1,89) = 5.52, p = .01, with those respondents indicating having experienced racism also tending to report engaging in cultural identity search (68%). In contrast the majority of those who did not experience racism reported not engaging in cultural identity exploration (58%).

Experiences of racism and cultural identity. Chi-square analysis of racism and cultural identity yielded a significant result , χ^2 (3,91) = 8.52, p = .03. The majority of respondents who identified as "Australian" tended to report never having experienced racism (55%), while in sharp contrast, the overwhelming majority of those identified as of original culture reported having experienced racism (90%). The majority of youngsters identified as either “bicultural” (68%) and “unsure/no identification” (67%) reported having experienced racism. It is important to note also that a large proportion (63%) of youngsters in the sample overall, whether visibly ethnic or Caucasian, reported having experienced racism.

Further analysis based on the results already presented was carried out addressing interaction effects of visual ethnicity, and racism on cultural identity search. Two-way ANOVA results indicated no interaction effects.

Discussion

Berry's (1992) assumptions of cultural adjustment as measured by his Attitudes to Acculturation strategies scale were not fully validated by the results, as the scale achieved significance in only one of the four attitudes to acculturation strategies *(marginalisation)* . A failure to fully validate the scale may be related to the abbreviation procedure to which the original scale was subjected rather than with its actual validity. The scale was reduced from 72 to only 12 items, thus, in all likelihood reducing its internal consistency. An additional reason for the failure to validate the scale might have been that the CLDB sample was composed of a number of distinct cultural background individuals. The scale was designed primarily to be used with homogeneous groups after adjusting the scale for contextual features of the cultures in contact. According to Berry, group-level factors and individual-level factors shape adaptation. Moreover, these factors can be said to be universal but also specific to the cultures in contact. It is possible that the concepts measured by the scale may not be interpreted consistently across different cultural background participants.

The impact of the low validity of the modified version of Berry's scale on the conclusions reached in the present study is considerable and analyses involving attitudes to acculturation measures have been interpreted with caution. Naturally, some of the results of the study cannot be conclusive for this reason, nonetheless, indication of degree of agreement or disagreement with the various attitudes to acculturation statements as measured by the scale were deemed to be useful when making certain observations about results. A replication of this study using the scale in its original form would certainly increase the chances of validating the instrument as required before more reliable findings can be established. Future studies considering the use of this scale should take the above comments into consideration as well as the recommendations made by Nguyen et al (1998). They suggested that although the psychometric properties of various acculturation scales, including Berry's, report factors that appear generalisable across groups (e.g., language usage, social affiliation, and ethnic identity), these factors and their corresponding question items do not necessarily equate across studies. Thus, it is not known if similarly named factors are indeed equivalent.

Overall, results supported most of the assumptions made by the theories on cultural identity examined in the literature review. Individual experiences that may influence the development of a cultural identity include experiences of racism and greater agreement with *segregation* attitudes to acculturation. It appears that youngsters who tend to hold stronger segregation views and have experienced racism identify more clearly with their original culture. It is possible that youngsters react to negative experiences such as prejudice and discrimination by re-affirming a commitment to the original culture. Segregation views may emanate from the reality of having scant opportunities outside their own cultural realm and so it may reflect a view based on an imposed reality rather than merely an attitude.

Global Self-esteem

Contrary to what the literature indicates, an achieved cultural identity was not found to be associated with high self-esteem (Hattie,1992). According to

Phinney and others, bi-cultural adolescents who have not examined and resolved issues pertaining to their cultural identity will exhibit lower self-esteem and will be at a greater risk of experiencing adjustment problems. This was not supported by the evidence in this study in that there were no differences in self-esteem scores between those who reported an achieved identity and those who did not. Thus, self-esteem may have little to do with being aware of a clear original identity within a minority group. It may be that during adolescence individuals do not consider cultural values particularly poignant or relevant to their reality living as they do in a dominant context, and where it is more functional or of greater "value" -if regrettable- to try and adhere to majority values. In other words, self-esteem may have more to do with how closely young people adhere to the reference group (dominant culture) values rather than the values of the membership group (ethnic minority). Following from this, it may be feasible to suggest that a redefinition of the manner in which the membership group values are perceived may promote youngsters to consider their membership group also as their reference group.

Language, Cultural Participation and Identity

The term "Australian" appears to have been interpreted by participants to mean Anglo-Celtic background rather than as a term capturing the nature of what the Australian national identity is supposed to be: a multicultural, but cohesive group of people deriving strength from their diversity. For example, youngsters perceiving themselves as "Australian" tended not to report a second language spoken at home. On the other hand, those reporting a second language at home in turn tended to report not identifying with any culture or being "unsure" of an identity. Thus, it is possible that those who reported a second language may be experiencing a social reality in more than one way (Vygotsky, 1978) and are therefore unsure of their identity. Cultural participation by means of partaking in traditional activities followed a slightly different pattern to that of language. Youngsters who identified as being of an original culture also tended to report higher number and a greater variety of original cultural activities. As expected, those identified as "Australian" reported the least participation. It appears that sharing common practices with a social group tends to reinforce the reality of belonging to that group. Thus, it follows that active participation, which may also involve speaking a second language, may be far more impactive in shaping a cultural identity than speaking a second language alone.

Parental Characteristics and Identification

Parental characteristics were found to be significant in shaping cultural identity. Again, the term "Australian" appears to have been interpreted by participants to mean Anglo-Celtic background, as results indicated that having a parent born in Australia of Anglo-Celtic background appears to be more significant in shaping an "Australian" identity than it is having both parents born in Australia of either Indigenous descent or first or second generation non-English speaking migrants. It is also possible that the acquisition and maintenance of an "Australian" identity depend on mainstream acceptance and support which is facilitated if at least one parent is of "Australian" background. Following from the previous paragraph, if indeed youngsters have consistently understood the term to mean white-Anglo-Celtic, then it can be concluded that having a parent with these characteristics and background may facilitate the perception of membership into the dominant culture. In contrast, a clear original cultural identity was reported by children of both parents born overseas in which case there would be an assumed consistency of values and parental styles. Parental consistency of values, it would seem, may be powerful enough to help maintain an original culture experience within a dominant context. A puzzling finding, however, was the unexpected weak association between cultural identity search and family composition involving both parents born overseas. It may be reasonable to assume that youngsters living with two parents or significant others who were born overseas would tend to report a greater number and range of these activities. However, children with this background tended to report as many cultural activities participated in as those from other family composition categories. This may be due to the fact that the original cultural reality within the family is a given that might not need exploring because it is constantly experienced nonetheless.

Geographical Status

Results did not support the assumption that the more isolated the youngsters (i.e., living in remote areas), the lesser the opportunity to engage in meaningful culture-promoting activities. This could be in fact reflecting the Australian government's policy of settling newcomers in poorly populated areas to avoid the so-called "ghetto" effects experienced in larger urban communities such as Sydney, Brisbane, and Melbourne. Indeed communities such as those surveyed for this study contain relatively large numbers of immigrants (19%-25%), newly arrived and well established, and these social structures may be facilitating contact and participation. Indigenous Australians (8%) may present a different picture, however, in that many of them have been displaced from their "country" of birth (judging by the variety of languages identified in the sample) and have therefore probably lost contact with elders and other in-group members that may facilitate identity retention. The number of indigenous Australians participating in this study was too small to allow for meaningful conclusions. Nonetheless, issues such as Aboriginality, displacement and cultural dislocation as experienced by Indigenous Australians merit more attention in future research.

Cultural Identity and Visible Ethnicity

As expected visible ethnicity was a major factor in shaping cultural identification. Those children who reported being visibly Caucasian tended to describe themselves as "Australian." However, children who identified themselves as being visibly "Indigenous" or "Asian" (e.g., Chinese, Vietnamese, Islanders, Indigenous Australians) tended to report biculturality rather than original culture identification. Alternatively, it may be more adaptive and functional not to identify with any given culture even though the youngster may be visibly of an ethnic minority background. This is consistent with what other researchers have found, namely that cultural identity may be related to but not dependent on perceived group membership (Phinney & Alipuria, 1995). Factors such as the impact of phenotypical features, parental characteristics and the adherence to more than one cultural reality may contribute to the process of adjustment but may not necessarily be associated with an achieved cultural identity.

Experiences of Racism

Racism was found to be a critical experience in terms of triggering off the process of cultural identity exploration as described by Phinney (1991). Racism was also strongly related to visible ethnicity as expected. However, a surprisingly large majority of CLDB participants reported experiencing racism, regardless of whether they were visibly ethnic or not (63%). Moreover, those who perceived themselves to be "Australian" tended to report a lower incidence of racism. This may indicate that there may be pressure to conform to social norms and if youngsters do not subscribe to the cultural identity of the majority they may suffer discrimination and prejudice as a consequence. Thus, experiences of racism for many of minority culture youngsters may be strongly related to language, participation and ultimately perceived cultural identity. The more an individual identifies/embraces an original minority culture reality the greater the chances that he or she will be discriminated against by the majority. Unfortunately, multiculturalism and its accompanying philosophy of tolerance do not appear to be evident in the experiences described by respondents in this study.

Contrary to what is suggested in the literature, results indicated that racism is not the only catalyst for cultural identity search and achieved identification in minority culture adolescents. Positive, in-group, identity-shaping experiences such as speaking a second language at home and partaking in social and cultural activities appear to be strongly associated with cultural identity search. So, it can be said that the onset of perceived cultural membership is not necessarily and exclusively associated with negative experiences involving one's minority group but rather a process that may be triggered by positive, self-enhancing group experiences. This conclusion has implications for ethnic identity development, retention and maintenance as it is prescriptive in enhancing the value of traditional practices and participation. The latter can be said to facilitate the understanding and acceptance of one's cultural identity and membership, and to strengthen the personal commitment to that identity. Thus, it could be said that practice and participation in traditional or culture-specific activities may not only assist ethnic minority youth to develop an identity but they may also protect young people against the negative effects of racism.

Language and physical features were also confirmed to be salient factors in the process of identification in the visibly ethnic adolescents. This can be understood within the context of the self-concept, involving a number of realms such as physical and social features. This was also the case for Caucasian-looking youngsters who tended to identify more with the mainstream culture.

To recapitulate, results indicated that the process of identity development involving cultural identity search resulting in achieved cultural identity is not necessarily likely to be the result of a crisis such as experiences of racism (Phinney,1992). In cases where racism is experienced, in an attempt to resolve negative feelings resulting from stereotyping and value discrepancy adolescents may be engaging in cultural identity search. In cases were positive experiences have been associated with cultural membership (e.g., visiting the country, attending special festivities etc.), cultural identity search was also found to be linked to cultural participation such as speaking an original language and in-group activities. Thus, it may be the case that cultural exploration may not necessarily be a preceding step in participation and consequently identification but rather a co-occurring feature of identification itself.

Although the present study helps to clarify aspects of cultural identity theory, a number of limitations must be identified. The use of an abbreviated form of Berry's Attitudes to Acculturation Strategies Scale appears to have lowered the internal consistency and therefore limited the study's power to reach meaningful conclusions. Similarly, the use of samples of convenience consisting of mixed background participants may have clouded the results with respect to attitudes to acculturation strategies. Moreover, it was difficult to establish meaningful findings underlying Indigenous Australian youth issues because of the small number of participants with that background. Future research should ideally focus exclusively on Indigenous youth who may experience cultural identity in a vastly different way to that of immigrant background youth. Largely related to the previous statement, most of the models and instruments used have been designed by North American researchers and tested on North American samples including African Americans and Hispanic youth. What is required is perhaps a comprehensive qualitative study that can provide the foundations of a model reflecting the subjective experience of identity as construed by Indigenous youth.

In spite of its limitations, the present study clarifies a number of issues outlined by cultural identity theory and models of biculturalism. For instance, there is no discussion in the literature of how phenotyoical characteristics may impact on the experience of identity (Phinney & Devic-Navarro, 1995). The present study found that so-called visual ethnicity is a major contributing factor in perceived cultural identity and cultural identity search. The study also contributes to the argument that challenges the connection between self-esteem and cultural identity. Another strength of the study is that minority groups residing in rural and remote areas in North Queensland Australia have very limited opportunities to participate in research of the nature of this study. This is not to say that any research is better than no research, but rather that a start has to be made in empirically addressing the major issues underlying the experiences of ethnic minorities living in rural and remote areas in Northern Australia. The study has also brought to the forefront the plight of many Indigenous Australian youngsters who are experiencing cultural dislocation, and confusion with regards to who they are and where they fit in society.

References

Berry, J.W. (1996). *Attitudes to Acculturation Strategies Scales.* Unpublished Scales, personal communication.

Berry, J.W. (1990). A functional approach to the relationship between stereotypes and familiarity. *Australian Journal of Psychology, 22,* 29-33.

Berry, J. W., Dasden, P.R., Poortinga, Y., & Segall, M.H. (1992). *Cross-cultural psychology:research and applications.* New York: Cambridge University Press.

Berry, J.W., Trimble, J., & Olmeda, E. (1986). The assessment of acculturation. In W.J. Lonner, & J.W. Berry (Eds) *Field methods in cross-cultural research* (pp. 291-324) London: Sage

Duval, S., & Wicklund, R.A. (1972). *A theory of objective self awareness.* New York: Academic.

Erikson, E. (1968). *Identity: Youth and crisis.* New York: Norton.

Hattie, J. (1992). *Self-concept.* London: Lawrence Erlbaum.

Hurtado, A., Guring, P., & Peng, T. (1994). Social identities: A framework for studying the adaptation of immigrants and ethnics. The adaptation of Mexicans into the United States. *Social Problems, 41*(1),129-151.

Kwak, K., & Berry, J.W. (1998). *Generational differences on acculturation attitudes and values among Vietnamese and Korean families.* Paper presented at the14th International Congress of Cross-cultural Psychology, Bellingham, WA, USA.

Laperriere, A., Compere, L., Dkhissy, M., Dolce, R., & Fleurent, N. (1994). Mutual perceptions and inter-ethnic strategies among French, Italian and Haitian adolescents of a multi ethnic school in Montreal. *Journal of Adolescent Research, 9,*193-217.

Liebkind, K. (1993). Self-reported ethnic identity, depression and anxiety among youth Vietnamese refugees and their parents. *Journal of Refugee Studies, 6,*25-39.

Liebkind, K. (1996). Acculturation and stress: Vietnamese refugees in Finland. *Journal of Cross-cultural Psychology, 27*, 161-180.

Marcia, J. (1980). Identity in adolescence. In J. Adelson (Ed). *Handbook of Adolescent Psychology* (pp. 159-187). New York: Wiley.

Marcia, J., Waterman, A., Matteson, D., Archer, S., & Orlofsky, J. (1994). *Ego identity: A handbook for psychosocial research.* New York: Springer-Verlag.

McLenahan, C., Cairns, E., Dunn, S., & Morgan, V. (1991). Preference of geographical location as a measure of ethnic/national identity in children in Northern Ireland. *Irish Journal of Psychology, 12*(3),346-354.

Nanda, S. (1994). *Cultural anthropology* (5th ed.). Belmount, CA: Wadsworth.

Nesdale, D., Rooney, R., & Smith, L. (1997). Migrant Ethnic identity and psychological distress. *Journal of Cross-cultural Psychology, 28*, 569-588.

Neto, F. (1998). *Young immigrants acculturation attitudes in Portugal and Portuguese adolescents' attitudes toward immigrants.* Paper presented at the14th International Congress of Cross-cultural Psychology, Bellingham, WA, USA.

Parish, T.S. (1978). Personal Attribute Inventory for Children. In K.Corcoran & J. Ficher (1987). *Measures for clinical practice: A source book* (pp. 405-407). New York: The Free Press.

Phinney, J.S. (1992). The multigroup ethnic identity measure: A new scale for use with diverse groups. *Journal of Adolescent Research, 7*(2), 156-176.

Phinney, J.S. (1990). Ethnic identity in adolescents and adults: review of the research. *Psychological Bulletin, 108*, 499-514.

Phinney, J.S. (1989). Stages of ethnic identity development in minority group adolescents. *Journal of Early Adolescence, 9*(1-2), 34-49.

Phinney, J.S., & Alipuria, L.L. (1995). At the interface of cultures: Multiethnic/multiracial high school and college students. *Journal of Social Psychology.*

Phinney, J.S., & Devic-Navarro (1995). Variations in bicultural identification among African American and Mexican American adolescents *(in press)*

Phinney, J.S., Du Pont, S., Espinosa, C., Revill, J., & Sanders, K. (1994) Ethnic identity and American identification among ethnic minority groups. In A. Bouvy, F. van de Vijver, P.Boski, P. Schmitz (Eds.), *Journeys into cross-cultural psychology* (pp. 167-183). Amsterdam: Swets & Zeitlinger.

Phinney, J.S., & Chavira, V. (1992). Ethnic identity and self-esteem: An exploratory longitudinal study. *Journal of Adolescence, 15*(3), 271-281.

Phinney, J. S., Chavira, V., & Tate, J.D. (1993). The effect of ethnic threat on ethnic self-concept and own-group ratings. Journal of Social Psychology, *133*(4), 469-478.

Phinney, J.S., Lochner, B., & Murphy, R. (1990). Ethnic identity development and psychological adjustment in adolescence. In A. Stiffman & L. Davis (Eds.) *Ethnic issues in adolescent mental health.* Newbury Park, CA: Sage.

Rosenthal, D. A., & Feldman, S.S. (1992). The nature and stability of ethnic identity in Chinese youth: Effects of length of residence in two cultural contexts. *Journal of Cross-cultural Psychology, 23*(2), 214-227.

Rotheram-Borus, M.J. (1990). Adolescents reference-group choices, self-esteem, and adjustment. *Journal of Personality and Social Psychology, 59,* 1075-1081.

Rotheram-Borus, M.J., & Phinney, J.S. (1990). Patterns of social expectations among Black and Mexican-American children. *Child Development, 61,* 542-556.

Rumbaut, R.G. (1994). The crucible within: Ethnic identity, self-esteem and segmented assimilation among children of immigrants. *International Migration Review, 28,* 748-94.

Saenz, R., Hwang, S.S., Aguirre, B.E., & Anderson, R.N. (1995). Persistance and change in Asian identity among children of intermarried couples. *Sociological Perspectives, 38,* 175-194.

Sam, D. (1998, August). *Ethnic identity and acculturation preferences among four ethnic groups in Norway: Relationships and their predictors.* Paper presented at the 14th International Congress of Cross-cultural Psychology, Bellingham, WA, USA.

Tajfel, H. (Ed) (1981). *Human groups and social categories.* London: Cambridge University Press.

Verkuyten, M. (1992). Ethnic group differences and the evaluation of ethnic identity among adolescents in the Netherlands. *Journal of Social Psychology, 132,* 741-750.

Vygotky, L.S. (1978). *Mind in society: The development of higher psychological processes.* Cambridge, MA: Harvard University Press.Nguyen, D.D., Ilani, S., Chang, R. (1998, August). An empirical categorisation of general factors in acculturation scales. Paper presented at the 14th International Congress of Cross-cultural Psychology, Bellingham, WA, USA.

Contributions of Special Relevance to Children and Youth

Early Child-Rearing and Social Motives After Nine Years: A Cross-Cultural Longitudinal Study[1]

Hans-Joachim Kornadt
University of the Saarland, Germany
Department of Education

in cooperation with
Yoshiharu Tachibana
Gifu University, Japan
Department of Education

ABSTRACT

Striking differences in criminality between countries are known. Those differences can be explained from the perspective of a motivation theory, especially if they are seen in their cultural context. The study covers an interval of nine years and compares data from subjects living in European, East-Asian and South-East-Asian cultures. Quantitative and qualitative differences in the aggression motive and in altruism were found. There were also differences in early child-rearing between the cultures. The results showed a longterm relationship between early child-rearing and the aggressiveness and altruism of the children nine years later. The most important variable was whether the mother was able to establish a relationship of secure attachment with her child. This was more the case for Japanese than German mothers and is embedded in a general cultural pattern. However, new data reveal different attitudes of Japanese mothers, possibly indicating a process of social change.

Statistical data about criminality report striking differences between countries (Landau, 1984), especially between Western and East-Asian cultures. For instance, the overall crime rate in the USA is roughly four times higher than in Japan. The number of homicides in London is four times and in New York twelve times higher than in Tokyo. The number of robberies in Tokyo in a year is less than the number reported in New York in two days (Kornadt, 1994).

Those facts stimulated the first author to carry out this cross-cultural study about aggressiveness and about conditions of child development which might contribute substantially to the differences.

---

[1] Parts of the study have been supported by several grants from the German Science Foundation (DFG) and Volkswagen-Foundation to the first author, and the Japanese Society for the Promotion of Science (JSPS) to both authors. The first author wants to thank Professors Hayashi, Kyoto; Professors Mar'at, Bandung; Professors Foppa, Bern; and Professor Trommsdorff and their teams for their cooperation.

The study was based on two main hypotheses derived from the motivation theory (Heckhausen, 1991) and its elaboration regarding aggression (Kornadt, 1982). The aggression motive, seen as the core of aggressive behavior, is postulated as being a complex functional system comprising several elements. Some of them are biologically rooted reaction tendencies to frustration. Others are acquired through socialization experiences during the course of development. The formation of individual motivational differences is mainly influenced by early experiences in mother-child interactions. In particular, the variables assumed to be most relevant influence the development of secure or insecure attachment (Cummings et al., 1986). This impacts the amount and kind of anger-activating frustration the child experiences and her/his tolerance for frustration. Furthermore, the child will develop cognitive schemata such as:

- the world is considered as hostile, so that one has to pursue one's own interests against others;
- or, the world is considered to be friendly, leading to pro-social behaviors.

Other variables in mother-child interactions are those that contribute to the attribution of benevolent or malevolent intentions in others and which convey values of aggression or compassion.

Accordingly, in the present study, data were collected about the aggression motive and early childhood rearing techniques of mothers. Hypotheses concerning relevant variables of mothers' child-rearing behavior were developed after the pilot study was conducted. Included in the study were samples from the countries of Switzerland, Germany, Japan, and representatives of Balinese and Batak cultures. The study was carried out in cooperation with Japanese, Swiss and Indonesian collegues (Kornadt et al., 1992). The pilot study was conducted between 1979-1983 to develop and test the instruments and the methodology. From 1985-1989 the first phase of data collection was begun. Between 1994-1998 the second phase was completed with all samples except the Swiss.

Method

Design

The design of the combined cross-sectional and longitudinal study is depicted in Figure 1.

Figure 1. Design of the Cross-Cultural-Study:

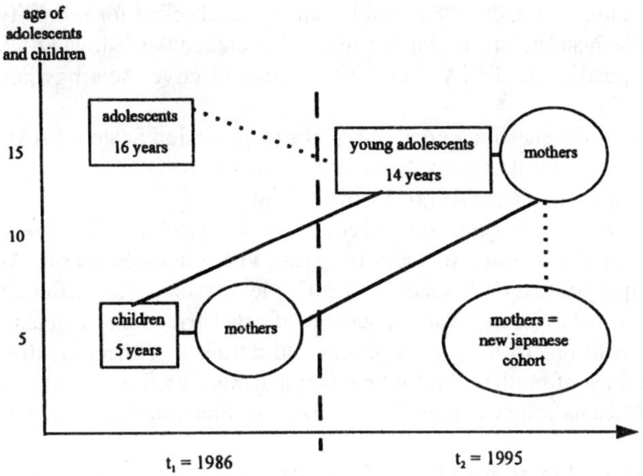

Subjects

Included in the study were samples from the five groups mentioned above. Subjects in the first sample were male and female adolescents of about sixteen years of age, and mothers with children from four to six years old. The mothers and children were studied again after a nine year period (see Table 1).

Table 1. Subjects

First Measurement: 1986					
n =	Germany	Switzerland	Japan	Bali	Batak
adolescents (16 years)	137	111	226	235	225
mother-child-pairs	98	30	67	66	63
Second Measurement: 1995					
n =	Germany	Switzerland	Japan	Bali	Batak
young adolescents (14 years)	45	-	59	43	25
mothers	45	-	53	43	25
mothers, new cohort	-	-	20	-	-

Instruments

The measurements were constructed mainly according to the motivation theory of aggression (Kornadt, 1982, 1989), and were checked for reliablity and validity. The instruments used in the research included the following.

1. Aggression-specific TAT (A-TAT) with an objective scoring key (Kornadt, 1982).
2. Aggression-specific questionnaire (Saabr□cken Aggression Scale = SAS), Retrospective adolescent socialization questionnaire (RASQ), Actual parent questionnaire (APQ) (Kornadt, 1989).
3. A set of scenario-techniques were specifically designed for the cross-cultural comparisons. Some of them (Aggression-Situation-Scenario, A-Sit and Helping-Situation-Scenario, H-Sit) yield scores for different components of behavior motivation, such as affect, attribution, or goals, particularly with regard to aggressiveness and altruism . Others identify relevant variables of mother-child interaction and were used with mothers or with adolescents retrospectively (Socialization-Situation-Scenario, So-Sit).

All data was collected by teams of investigators from the respective cultures who were specifically trained by the first author. Mothers and children were studied at their home. The adolescents (16 and 14 years old) were studied in their schools.

Results

The first measurement t_1 (1986) resulted in various quantitative and qualitative data about the aggression motive of adolescents, their retrospectively reported child-rearing experiences, the child-rearing practices of mothers with four to six years old children from the same cultures as the adolescents (but not their mothers) and about the aggressiveness of their children. The second measurement (follow-up study) taken when the children were about 14 years old resulted in data about their aggressiveness and altruism. The child-rearing practices of their mothers was also measured again.

Aggressiveness - First Measurement

The first measurement showed differences in aggressiveness of adolescents from the cultures studied (Kornadt, 1991). Since A-TAT differentiates between aggression and aggression inhibition it was clear that low aggression scores were not simply due to inhibition. They indicated low motivation for aggression (see Figure 2).

Figure2. Aggression and aggression inhibition (A-TAT) of subjects from different cultures

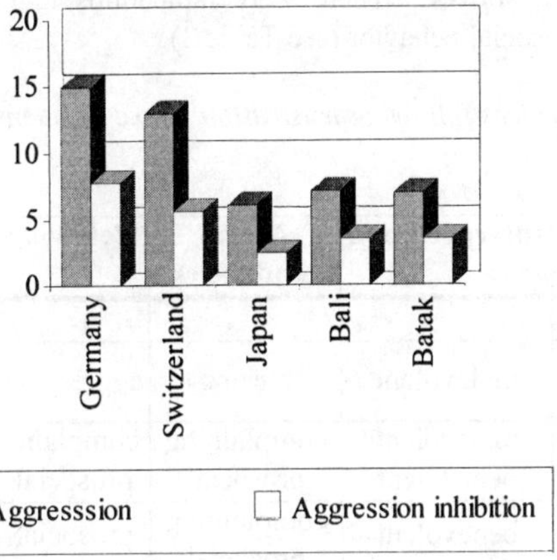

Even more interesting are qualitative differences in components and sequence of aggressive motivation. The internal processes of reacting to being frustrated were analyzed. Normally, after experiencing frustration there is an affective reaction (e.g. anger), the intention of the frustrator is interpreted (e.g. malevolent) which results in motivation to reach a certain goal related to behavioral reactions (e.g. retaliation). The scores revealed cultural specificities. For the differences between German and Japanese samples see Table 2.

Table 2. Culture specific motive components. Reactions following frustration, adolescents 1986 (A-Sit):

	Germany	Japan
shame / guilt	0 %[1]	30%
attribution: due to frustrators personality, unpersonal, unintended	1 %	42%
prosocial goals & action tendencies	1%	15%
prosocial behavior or giving in	7%	49%

Note[1]. Percentage of subjects

Using a configural frequency analysis technique (KFA, Lienert & Oeveste, 1985) on the A-Sit results, it was found that frustrations among European participants were most frequently followed by anger, whereas the Asian participants experienced sorrow. There were indications that for Asians, frustration results in prosocial behavior (see Table 3).

Table 3. Reaction sequences following frustration - most frequent configurations (KFA)

Culture	Affect	Interpretation	Action tendencies	Behavior
Switzerland Germany	anger	malevolent	hurting	aggression
Japan	anger / sorrow	malevolent benevolent	complaining prosocial	complaint prosocial
Bali / Batak	anger / sorrow	benevolent	complaining prosocial	prosocial

Note. All configurations are highly significant $p < .001$

Child-rearing

The results of the first measurement on child-rearing showed cultural differences in the variables postulated. For instance, mothers interpreted the disobedience of their children differently (in case the child does not obey).

- They may believe their children want to be oppositional ("burdensome"), mothers get angry, punish the children, and hurt their self-esteem.
- Mothers excuse their children as being too immature ("excusable"), they can help their children, e.g. to do what should be done and to avoid conflicts (see Figure 3).

Mothers differed in the way they dealt with children's needs. Some mothers were able to harmonize their own needs with those of the children, thereby avoiding conflicts and frustration. Other mothers tended to stress their own rights and interests in contrast to those of their children, thus creating a conflict instead of avoiding it. By criticizing their children and insisting on their rights, mothers may escalate the conflict. Differences in responses of Japanese and German participants are shown in Figure 4.

On the aggregate level, these cultural differences in child-rearing techniques correspond to the cultural differences in aggressiveness as predicted. In cultures where child-rearing variables indicated secure mother-child attachments, aggression scores were lower and vice versa. The significant correlations ranged between $r = -.81$ to $r = .58$ ($n = 8$ subcultures).

Figure 3. Attribution: Mother's interpretation of her child's misbehavior (APQ t_1=1986)

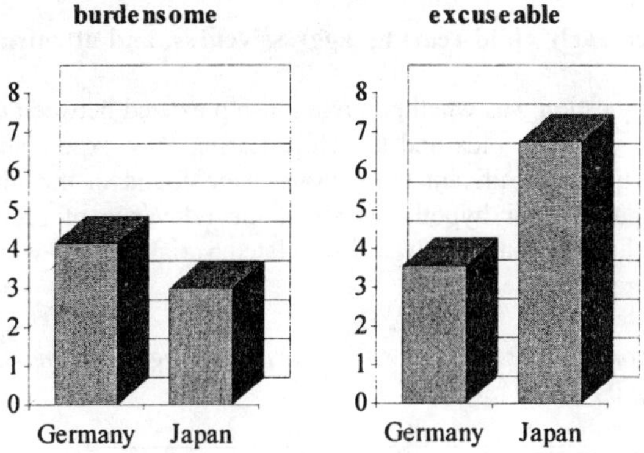

Figure 4. Cultural differences in child-rearing techniques (SO-SIT 1986), positive and negative handling of needs

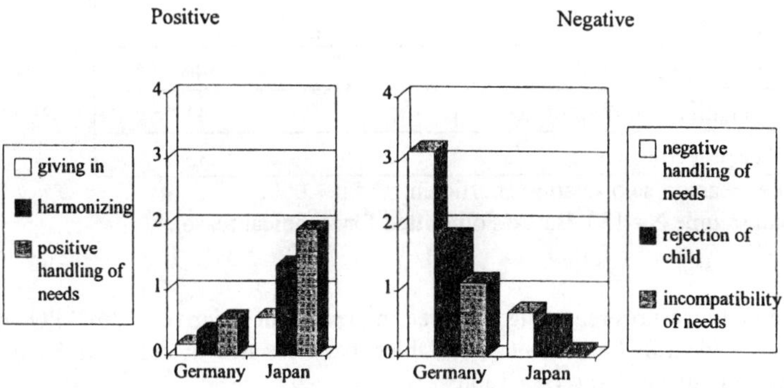

Nine year follow-up study

Of course, correlations on the aggregate level do not really prove of a longterm effect of child-rearing on the social motives at the individual level. Therefore, the same mothers and their children were studied nine years after the first measurement to obtain data on single mother-child pairs.

At the time of the follow-up study, the children were about 14 years old. Comparing the data that measured their aggressiveness with that obtained from the study of adolescents nine years before, the same differences existed between Japanese and German adolescents at t_2 as in t_1. This can be interpreted as an indication that our samples might be typical of the respective cultures. It could be said that the t_2 data replicated and validated the first measurements on aggressive behavior.

Relationship between early child-rearing, aggressiveness, and altruism: nine years later

The most interesting question was whether a relationship existed between the aggressiveness of the 14 years olds and the child-rearing they experienced nine years earlier. Highly significant correlations were found in the total sample, thereby supporting our hypotheses about the relevance of secure attachment. Due to limited space, only a few related variables that were mentioned earlier are reported here.

Table 4. Long-term correlations between child-rearing and aggressiveness. Correlations covering a 9-years intervall

Mother - child rearing t_1	**Child´s aggression t_2** (r =)
harmonizing of needs	- .38 ***
excuseable interpretation of childs behavior	- . 41 ***
conveying empathy	- .46 ***
negative handling of needs	.41 ***
lasting conflicts	.33 ***

Note. Pearson´s correlation coefficient *** p< .000.
Total sample N= 133, Batak´s ommitted for technical reasons

The first measures regarding child-rearing techniques (derived from APQ and So-Sit) identified a number of variables that were significantly correlated to the aggressiveness at t_2 (see Table 5).

As for altruism measured at t_2 with the H-Sit, results were generally the same. Selecting from the various types of altruistic behavior, the study concentrated on altruism based on empathy, “true altruism” according to Batson (1991). Similar relationships between early child-rearing techniques and children’s behavior indicated a complex condition that can be described as the difference between secure and insecure attachment. A regression analysis for the combined group of Japanese and German subjects revealed that three predictors of child-rearing variables

Table 5. Early child-rearing and the aggressiveness of their children 9 years later Construct-scores (APQ & So-Sit (1986)and A-TAT (1995))

child-rearing conditions positively correlated ("encouraging" aggressiveness):

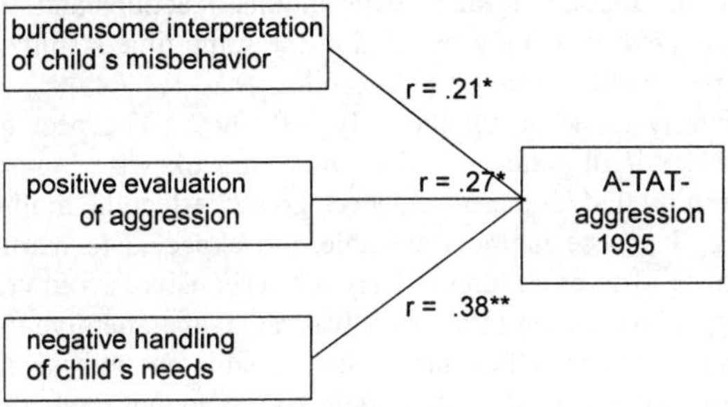

child-rearing conditions negatively correlated ("discouraging" aggressiveness):

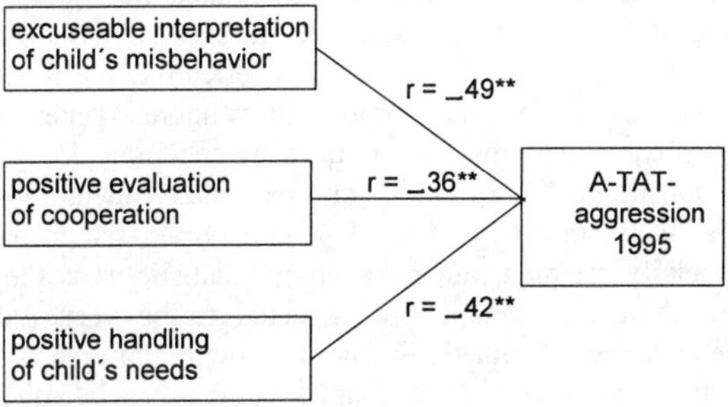

Note. Pearson´s correlation coefficient ** p< .00, * p< .01
Sample: Japanese and German subjects N = 83

explained 24% of the variance in empathy-based altruism over the nine year time span: mothers' interpretations of children's behavior (Beta 4.86); children's resistance (1.45); children's negative affect (-1.83).

These and other data demonstrate that there is indeed a longterm relationship between early child-rearing and the development of social motives. The correlations and the regression analysis confirm the central hypotheses about the influence of early mother-child relationships.

Conclusion

Cultural context

Of course, we do not simply postulate a kind of imprinting which remains stable over a decade. Rather, we assume that an *interaction cycle* is established, comprising mutual attitudes, expectations, reactions and affects, which becomes stabilized over the years, and at the same time stabilizes the motives and other personality variables in the child.

Certainly the family alone is not the only influence. The peer group, social norms and behavioral patterns in the culture are likewise important. One has to keep in mind that all these influences greatly affect the mothers as well. For instance, Japanese mothers are able and expected to harmonize their needs with those of their children. They are responsive, avoid conflict by gradually giving in, are patient rather than frustrated, and attentive to their chi ldren's fundamental needs. All of this is only possible on the basis of one prerequisite. For several years, when their children are young, mothers must be willing to devote their lives completely to the children's wellbeing. Maternal dedication requires much social support, including high regard for the role of mothers in the respective culture. At the same time cultures also provide corresponding developmental themes and related traditional child rearing techniques, customs and values (Super & Harkness, 1998). Such a social "climate" not only rewards mothers for effective child rearing behavior, in many ways the climate also reinforces low aggressiveness in the children. It is also probable that prosocial motives are encouraged.

Japanese traditions present an example for particular reflection (e.g. Fogel, 1991; Lebra & Lebra, 1974). The Japanese culture is primarily collectivistic and socially oriented rather than individualistic as is the case with most Western cultures. People are expected to be very polite, thoughtful, and considerate of others, including young children. Such practices maintain and convey clear norms, and support prosocial roles like being a good mother (Kornadt & Trommsdorff, 1990). These social values have a high priority in the culture. They are rooted in religious beliefs, especially in Buddhism and Confucianism.

With reference to comparisons between German and Japanese maternal child-rearing practices, the second measurement revealed that in nearly all important variables there were few changes from the first to the second assessment. Mothers' basic attitudes toward their children seem to reflect little change over time in both cultures.

Social change?

However, there were a few and maybe important exceptions to note. One exception was findings regarding the variable "harmonizing of needs". The Japanese mothers were much higher than the Germans at the first measurement. But the difference between the two disappeared completely after nine years.

Two explanations are possible. On the one hand, it could be that the mothers reacted to the children's higher developmental age in the second study. To harmonize a mother's needs and wishes with those of fourteen year old boys or girls is certainly more difficult than to harmonize with the more basic needs of four to six years old children. On the other hand, the findings may also point to changes in the attitudes of Japanese women regarding their willingness to give up their interests in favor of their children's. More generally, it is possible to question if contemporary women are changing their views regarding the traditional role of mothers. It seems likely that a lower acceptance of and devotion to the traditional role of mothers has occured in Japan.

Another important result of the study was found in reference to the encouragement of aggressiveness among children. The great differences that had been found between Japanese and German mothers at t_1 disappeared. Japanese mothers reached the German mothers' level at the t_2 measure (see Figure 5). The opposite was true for encouraging cooperation.

Here, the changes of mothers' attitudes seem unlikely to be related to their children's ages. It is not plausible that mothers consider aggression as more acceptable just when the children are

Figure 5. Changing in values of mothers: cultural comparisons concerning the encouragement of being aggressive (Japan:Germany t1: p<.05; t2: p=n.s.) and cooperative (Japan:Germany t1, t2: p=.05)

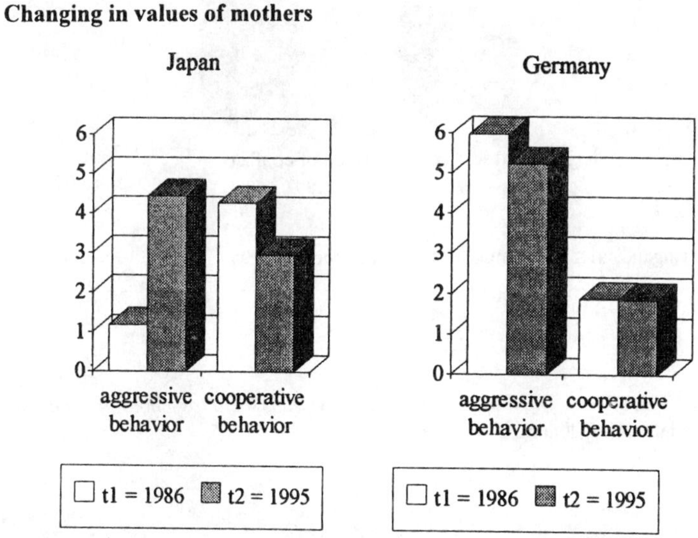

reaching puberty, especially since aggression can become a problem at this developmental age, particularly for males. It seems, therefore, more likely to interpret this result as an indicator of social change in Japan.

This interpretation is supported by data we have collected from a new sample of Japanese mothers ($n = 20$) with four to five year old children, data that is comparable to the study of mothers completed nine years ago. The two samples can be seen as comparable cohorts measured nine years apart. "Modern mothers" (1995 sample) interacted more angrily with their children, and conflicts escalated more often than had been the case in the original group nine years earlier (see Figure 6).

There are many influences that may be contributing to changes in Japanese society. These include political policies and practices that encourage more individualistic and hedonistic behaviors, economic developments, and influences from abroad. It seems likely that the beginning of social change is indicated by the data. The measured changes in basic child-rearing variables might have widespread and longterm effects far beyond the realm of social motives.

Figure 6. Two cohorts of Japanese mothers, reaction in conflict (APQ)

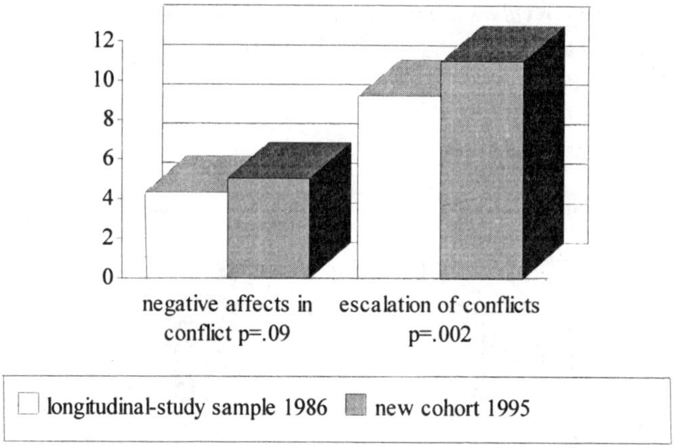

References

Batson, C. D. (1991). *The altruism question: Toward a social psychological answer.* Hillsdale, NJ: Erlbaum.

Cummings, E.M., Hollenbeck, B., Iannotti, R., Radke-Yarrow, M., & Zahn-Waxler, C. (1986). Early organization of altruism and aggressiveness: Developmental patterns and individual differences, (pp. 165-188). In C. Zahn-Waxler, E.M. Cummings, R. Iannotti, *Altruism and aggression*. Cambridge: Cambridge University Press.

Fogel, E. F. (1991). *Japan's new middle. class.* Berkeley, CA: University of California Press.

Heckhausen, H. (1991). *Motivation and action.* New York: Springer.

Kornadt, H.-J. (1982). *Aggressionsmotiv und Aggressionshemmung* (Band 1). Bern: Huber.

Kornadt, H.-J. (1989). *Aggressivität und Erziehung im Kulturvergleich.* Unpublished research report. Saarbrηcken: Universität des Saarlandes.

Kornadt, H.-J. (1994). Social sciences at the German Institute for Japanese Studies. In J. Kreiner (Ed.), *Japan in global context (pp. 55-61).* München: Iudicium Verlag.

Kornadt, H.-J., Hayashi, T., Tachibana, Y., Trommsdorff, G., & Yamauchi, H. (1992). Aggressiveness and its developmental conditions in five cultures. In S. Iwawaki, Y. Kashima, & K. Leung (Eds.), *Innovations in cross-cultural psychology* (pp. 250-268). Amsterdam: Swets & Zeitlinger.

Kornadt, H.-J., & Trommsdorff, G. (1990). Naive Erziehungstheorien japanischer Motter - deutsch-japanischer Kulturvergleich. *Zeitschrift for Sozialisations forschung und Erziehungssoziologie, 10,* 357-376.

Landau, S.F. (1984). Trends in violence and aggression: A cross-cultural analysis. *International Journal of Comparative Sociology, 24,* 133-158.

Lebra, T. S., & Lebra, W. P. (1974). *Japanese culture and behavior.* Honolulu, HA: The University Press of Hawaii.

Lienert, G.A., & Oeveste, H. (1985). Configural frequency analysis as a statistical tool for developmental research. *Educational Psychological Measurement, 45,* 301-307.

Super, C. M., & Harkness, S. (1997). The cultural structuring of child development. In J. W. Berry (Ed.), *Handbook of cross-cultural psychology: Basic processes and human development (Vol. 2)* (pp. 1-39). Boston: Allyn & Bacon.

North African and French Children Placed in Care: A Comparative Study of Psychosocial and Educational Outcomes

Marie Anaut
Université Lumière-Lyon 2
Institut de Psychologie

Bernard Chouvier
Université Lumière-Lyon 2
Institut de Psychologie

Jeanne Tyrrell
Université Lumière-Lyon 2
Institut de Psychologie

ABSTRACT

In France, when there is unsatisfactory parenting, children and adolescents are separated from their biological families by social services and placed in the care of in foster families whose duty is to raise and educate them. Some placed children are from ethnic minorities and different cultures. Research indicates that children of North African origin are more likely to be placed in institutional care rather than in foster families, although there is no evidence to explain why this occurs. Based on a representative French sample, the current investigation presents a profile of placed children in terms of demographic factors, family background, educational progress and psychosocial development. Although the biological parents came from either North Africa (26%) or France, all of the children were born in France and have lived there since early childhood. These children were placed in either residential care, or with French cultural families. We compare the children of North African origin with the French children in terms of psychosocial and intellectual development.

Every year in France, there are about 120,000 children and adolescents who are separated from their birth families because of educational deficiencies or maltreatment. Some of them are sexual abuse victims. When the children are considered to be so vulnerable as to require placement away from home, the children are entrusted to the care of foster families or in Children's Homes. Many studies have examined the characteristics of placed children, in the United Kingdom (Rushton & Minnis, 1997; Quinton, Rushton Dance, & Mayes, 1998; Ward, 1998) in France (Anaut, 1997; Assally, Corbillon & Duyme, 1989; Lebovici, 1995), in Canada (Flynn & Biro, 1998) or in the

U.S.A. (Weiss & Jacob, 1988 ; Whittaker & Pfeiffer, 1994). Some of these studies have examined the social, emotional and intellectual aspects of development, and have produced some disturbing findings concerning the educational and psychosocial outcomes for children looked after away from home.

The experience of cross-cultural placement has received relatively little attention. Comparative studies between placement in foster families and in residential care show that usually, in France, North African children are more often placed in residential care than in foster families (Mignacca, Guers, Pithon & Demailly, 1989). The birth families maintain contact with the separated children. The North African youngsters are, therefore, confronted with two very different cultural values (birth family culture and French culture). It is not known why North African children are more likely to be placed in homes, and there is little published information concerning the characteristics of these children or the outcomes of placement.

The current findings are part of a larger study that was supported and funded by French Social Services (Chouvier et al., 1997). The original survey concerned 1100 deprived families whose children had been placed in foster families (52.5%) or in residential units (47.5%) for neglected care. Twenty-six percent of the sample were children whose parents moved to France from North Africa.

Aim of Study

The purpose of the study was to compare certain psychosocial and educational characteristics of North African children (whether placed in family or institutional care) with those of French children. Specifically, we compared children on the basis of their ages, intellectual level, educational progress, use of psychotherapy, and the presence of a family history of placement.

Method

Participants

A representative sample of 80 children and adolescents placed in foster families or in residential care was studied. A profile of the sample appears in Table 1, which includes basic demographic data, as well as information about the children, their parents and the reason for placement ; 21 of the children were of North African origin, and 59 were French children. A preliminary analysis of the proportions of children placed in each type of home (family or residential) revealed that there was no significant association between nationality and type of placement (χ^2 (1, $\underline{N}$=80) =.60, $\underline{p}$=.44)).

Materials and Procedure

The study included a questionnaire and individual psychological assessment for every child. For cross-culturally placed children whose parents came from North Africa, we specifically studied the child's IQ, school history, use of psychological services, and parental foster care placement. The results are compared with similar data from the French children.

Results

Children were compared on the basis of age, intellectual quotient (IQ) scores, and progress in school. We also looked at whether they were receiving psychotherapy, and if either biological parent had been placed as a child. First, we compared "North African" children and French children on each of these factors. Where possible, we conducted a more detailed analysis, to compare children, not only on the basis of nationality, but by type of placement. Tables 2 and 3 display comparative data about North African and French children placed in family care and in residential care.

Table 1. Characteristics of the sample of 80 children and adolescents placed in foster homes or residential care

Gender	55% boys and 45% girls
Range of ages	Between 1 year 2 months and 17 years 11 months
Average age	10 years 6 months
Type of placement	52,5% foster family 47,5% residential home
Status of placement	11% provisional placement 89% legal recommendation
Principal reasons for placement of child	Educational or moral reasons 34% Inadequate care of child 17% Psychological factors 14% Mental illness of mother 10% Disagreement between parents 8% Physical abuse or suspected abuse of child 7% Maternal alcoholism 6% Mental handicap of mother 3%
Children's education	57% repeating at least one year of school 33% in special education 2% in secondary education
Intellectual quotients (mean IQ scores)	Boys : IQ = 93.1 Girls : IQ = 88.2 1st generation (Mother "not placed") : IQ = 90.4 2nd generation (Mother " placed ") : IQ = 93.6
Profile of intellectual levels of children in sample	56.5% with IQ within normal range 13 % with an IQ indicative of mental deficiency (=>IQ of 69 or less) 9.5 % of children with exceptional intelligence (=> IQ of 130 or more)
Mental health of children	32% receiving psychotherapy 46% judged to be in need of psychotherapy
Mental health of biological parents	42% of mothers with mental health problems 26% of fathers with mental health problems
Parental employment (biological parents)	23% of mothers were working 32% of fathers were working
Average length of placement at time of study	5.8 years

Ages
The French children were slightly older with a mean age of 11.25 years (SD=4.5 years) compared with North African children ($\underline{M}$ =9.25 years; SD=4.6 years). However, this difference was not of statistical significance ($\underline{F}(1,78) = 3.08$, $\underline{p} \leq .08$). Similarly, there was no significant difference between children in terms of their age at placement $\underline{F}(1,78) = .02$, $\underline{p} \leq .90$.

IQ
The children did not differ significantly in terms of IQ ($\underline{F}$(3,65 =2.09, $\underline{p}$=.11). However, post-hoc testing (Fisher's test) revealed that North African children ($\underline{M}$ =102.9) who were placed in families had significantly higher IQ scores than French children placed in families ($\underline{M}$ =85.5; $\underline{p} \leq .03$) .

Progress in school
We compared children on the basis of whether or not they were repeating a year of school. Due to small numbers in one of the four categories, it was not possible to do a two factor chi-squared test. The difference between French and North African children was not statistically significant, (χ^2 (1, $\underline{N}$=75) =2.45, $\underline{p} \leq .12$., However, Table 2 shows that *none* of the nine North African children placed in family care have repeated a year of school. This is a marked contrast to the percentages of children repeating a year in the other categories (67% of North African children in residential care, and 59% of French children in family care).

Psychotherapy
There was no difference in terms of the proportions of North African and French children who were receiving psychotherapy (χ^2 (1, $\underline{N}$=79) = 1.38, $\underline{p}$=.24). Once again, due to small numbers in one category, it was not possible to do a more detailed chi-squared test. However, North African children placed in families have the lowest rates of psychotherapy (11%) compared with children in the other categories (28% of North African children in residential care, and 31% of French children in family care).

Maternal history of placement
Data were missing for 11 biological mothers. Sixty-two percent of mothers of French children had previously been placed, compared with only 26% of mothers of North African children. A chi-squared test indicated that this association was of statistical significance (χ^2 (1, $\underline{N}$=69) = 5.77, $\underline{p}$<.05).

Paternal history of placement:
Data were missing for 38 biological fathers. Thirty-three percent of biological father of French children had been placed as children, compared with 22% of

North African fathers. A chi squared test indicated that this difference was not statistically significant (χ^2 (1, 42) = .05, p=.82).

Results and Discussion

There are some interesting findings from this study of placed children. First, there was no overall difference in IQ scores according to cultural background. However, the children of North African origin placed in foster families have higher IQ scores than children in the three other groups. In contrast, the North African children placed in residential care have the lowest IQ scores. The statistical analysis showed that North African children placed with families had significantly higher IQs than the French children placed in families. In France, there is no routine testing of IQ before being placed, so it is unlikely that IQ influenced the type of placement offered to children

Table 2. Children placed in Foster Families : A comparison of educational and psychosocial characteristics

Children of North African origin (n=9)	**French children (n=33)**
Ages: from 2 years 11m to 14 years 10 m.	Ages: from 2 years 6 m to 17 years 3 m.
IQ (Intellectual Quotient) Average scores on Wechsler Scale: IQ Verbal = 101 IQ Performance = 104 IQ General = 102	IQ Average scores on Wechsler IQ Verbal = 85.8 IQ Performance = 88.6 IQ General = 85.5
Schooling : 0% repeating a year	Schooling : 59% repeating a year
11% of children in psychotherapy	31% of children in psychotherapy
25% of biological mothers placed in care as children	52% of biological mothers placed in care as children
0% of biological fathers placed in care as children	35% of fathers placed in care as children

several years beforehand. In terms of intellectual development, it appears that North African children benefit from being placed in families rather than institutional care.

There was no overall difference in educational problems according to cultural background. However, Table 2 shows that none of the nine North African children placed in families has repeated a year of school. This is a marked contrast to the North African children in residential care (59%), and the French children in either type of placement (59% in family care, and 70% in residential care)). The children in this sample had already been placed for an average of 5.8 years. Thus, it appears that in terms of educational outcomes, North African children benefit most from being placed with families.

Table 3. Children Placed in Residential Homes : A comparison of educational and psychosocial characteristics

Children of North African origin (n=12)	French children (n=26)
Ages : from 1 year 2 m to 17 years 11 m.	Ages: From 1 year 9 m to 17 years 9 m.
IQ (Intellectual quotient) Average scores on Wechsler scale IQ Verbal = 88.9 IQ Performance = 90.3 IQ General = 88.6	IQ Average scores on Wechsler scale IQ Verbal = 92.5 IQ Performance = 96.5 **IQ General = 94.3**
Schooling : 67% repeating a year	Schooling : 70% repeating a year
28% of children in psychotherapy	42% of children in psychotherapy
27% of mothers placed in care as children	74% of mothers placed in care as children
33% of fathers placed in care as children	31% of fathers placed in care as children

The use of psychotherapy is an indicator of adjustment and wellbeing, and there was no overall cultural difference in the use of psychotherapy. Nevertheless, visual inspection of Tables 2 and 3 reveals that North African children placed in families have the lowest rates of psychotherapy (11%) compared with children in the other categories (28% of North African children in residential care, and 31% of French children in family care). The small numbers of children in the North African group meant it was impossible to do a more detailed statistical analysis, but there appears to be a tendency towards lower consultation rates when North African children are placed with families.

We also examined the personal history of the biological parents to establish if they had been placed as children. The majority of French children had mothers who had been placed as children (62%). Only 26% of mothers of North African children had a history of being placed as children. This difference was of statistical significance, although the difference in previous placement rates is complicated to interpret. Variations in placement rates may reflect different approaches in North Africa and France to the management of family problems (for the previous generation of children). Another explanation is that the mothers of North African children are at a higher risk of experiencing problems adjusting to living in France, irrespective of whether they had problems as children (hence the need for placing their children in care). There was no difference in the percentages of biological fathers who had been placed as children. However, data were missing for nearly half of the fathers, so this result should be interpreted with some caution.

The data for this study were collected when most children had been placed for several years, and the measures are limited but useful indicators of developmental outcomes. There is an overall tendency for children who were placed in families to have better outcomes than children placed in residential care. This trend is even more marked for North African children. However, as explained in the introduction, children of North African origin are more likely than French children to be placed in residential care (Mignacca, Guers, Pithon & Demailly, 1989). There are no published studies of why this is so, although our experience suggests that some families prefer to foster French children, rather than children from other ethnic groups. Given the positive outcomes in terms of the psychosocial and education progress of North African children placed in families, further research is required to understand the process of determining the type of placements offered, and to study how children adjust to placements.

Finally, this study was limited to a sample of 80 children. It was not possible to obtain similar data from the beginning of the child's placement and thus we are unable to assess the development of the children during the years prior to our study. It is possible that pre-existing developmental problems determined the type of placement provided for each child. We did not explore the influence of the foster family environments on children's development. Also, the availability of families willing to foster North African children may be limited. However, it would be interesting to compare the characteristics of families who welcome children of different ethnic origin, with those who chose French children.

Conclusion

The current findings suggest that placed children have better psychological and social development when they have been living in French foster families than in residential care (irrespective of their cultural origins). North African children seem to benefit most from being placed in foster families rather than residential care. They have superior IQ scores, fewer educational problems and are less likely to be receiving psychotherapy. These results are important because usually, in France, social workers choose to place North African youngsters most often in residential care than in foster families. We encourage more research in order to understand the dynamics of North African child placement, and to understand the factors that influence the psychosocial development and educational progress of all placed children.

References

Anaut, M. (1997) *Entre détresse et abandon: la répétition transgénérationnelle chez les enfants placés.* Paris: CTNERHI/ P.U.F.

Assally, J-P., Corbillon, M., & Duyme, M. (1989) Transmission intergénérationnelle et comportement parental, *Revue de Neuropsychiatrie de l'Enfance et de l'Adolescence, 37*, 7.

Chouvier B., Anaut M. & et al., (1997), *Etude des enfants placés dans le département de la Loire, (Rapport CRPPC).* Université Lumière-Lyon 2, Institut de Psychologie, Lyon, France.

Flynn, R. & Biro, C.(1998), *Evaluation des résultats de l'aide sociale à l'enfance (ERAE*), Ecole de Psychologie, Univerité d'Ottawa, Canada.

Lebovici S. (1995), *Maltraitance : maintien du lien ?*, Paris, Fleurus.

Mignacca, Guers, Pithon, Demailly, (1989), Etude des processus de décision en matière de placement. In *L'enfant placé actualité de la recherche française et internationale,* Actes du Colloque MIRE-GERIS, Paris, CTNERHI.

Quinton D., Rushton A., Dance C. & Mayes D. (1998), *Joining new families : A study of adoption and fostering in middle childhood,* Chichester, Wiley.

Rushton, A. & Minnis, H. (1997), Annotation : Transracial placements, *Journal of Child Psychology and Psychiatry*, *38*, 147-159.

Ward, H. (1998), Assessing Outcomes in Child Care : An International Perspective, [Special Issue], *Children and Society,* XII (3).

Weiss, H.B. & Jacob, F.H. (1988) *Evaluating Family Programs,* New York, Aldine de Gruyter.

Whittaker, J.K. & Pfeiffer S.I. (1994) Research priorities for residential group child care. *Child Welfare, LXXIII*, 583-601.

Educational Beliefs of Mothers and Day Care Teachers in Former East- and West-Germany

Tatjana Meischner
Free University of Berlin
Institute for Early Childhood Education

Wolfgang Tietze
Free University of Berlin
Institute for Early Childhood Education

Holger Wessels
Free University of Berlin
Institute for Early Childhood Education

ABSTRACT

The educational beliefs of familial and institutional educators of preschool children from the former East and West Germany were compared in this study. In addition to common German patterns, we looked for divergent beliefs as a result of political, ideological and educational separation over the past fifty years. In the former East Germany, there was a strong political and ideological influence on the educational field based on the political goal of the state to develop a socialistic personality in children. Although we are reluctant to identifythe East/West educational belief differences as culturally specific, we try to compare them through a combination of exploratory and confirmatory factor analysis procedures. Results show that only a part of the investigated educational beliefs can be meaningfully compared in the the areas of cognitive skills as educational goals and controlling educational practices. Eastern and western pre-school educators share the view that these educational goals are rather unimportant for their work with children. No definite statements could be made with regard to other educational goals and practices investigated because of uncomparable (items relationships and) factor structures within the samples.The low degree of overlap of scale items demonstrates the need for indepth investigation of indigenous East- and West-German ideas with regard to the child as an autonomous individual and his/her functioning as a part of social group. The results are important with regard to both methodological aspects of East-West comparisons within the same "culture" as well as for curricula and training programs within the field of preschool education.

In this paper, we compare the educational beliefs of mothers and day care teachers of preschool children from the former East and West Germany. The importance of investigating educational beliefs among teachers, parents and other educators arises predominantly from their connection with pedagogical practice and the developmental outcomes on the part of the children. We understand educational beliefs as attitudes, ideas and opinions about the nature of the child, about the educational goals and practices for different ages and about the role of the educators in the process of a child's development.

Educational beliefs are the product of a co-constructive process between the society and its members. This implies that beliefs are influenced by historical, cultural, socio-economical and political conditions as well as by individual views and ideas. Additionally, with the development of pedagogy as a profession requiring professional training and education, the differentiation between educational beliefs of familial (parents and other relatives) and institutional (teachers) educators is worthy of investigation.

The topic of this paper is a comparative investigation of the educational beliefs of familial as well as institutional educators of preschool aged children from the former East and West Germany. This assessment of mothers' and teachers' educational beliefs is part of a larger research project on the quality of preschool education in Germany (Tietze et al., 1998). In this study, the pedagogical quality in general and the quality of institutional day care in particular is understood as a multidimensional construct, with the educational beliefs as one of the important dimensions.

Although the political and organizational structures of the preschool education system in the former East Germany have been integrated with those of West Germany soon after the reunification in 1989, it is not yet clear whether daycare pedagogical quality is now comparable in both parts of the country. Results of our research show similarities as well as differences with regard to numerous aspects of day care quality in the former eastern and western parts of the country.

This comparison is somewhat unique in that we are comparing the beliefs of two groups of educators and parents who share the same language and, historically, the same cultural background. At the same time, we have to take into consideration the breakdown of this cultural continuity for more than forty years. In the former East Germany, there was a strong political goal for education to mirror the socialist political goal of the state.

Boehnke and Merkens (1994) reflect on different strategies for quantitative comparisons of samples from East and West Germany in their investigation of value orientations of adolescents from East and West Berlin. Using the same data set, they find large differences between value orientations of adolescents from East and West Berlin can be shown when an *emic* approach is employed, but minimal differences when an *etic* approach is used. With regard to the use of factor analytic procedures, they conclude that subjecting the combined data set (East and West subsamples together) to an exploratory factor analysis emphasizes the similarities between the data set, while factorizing every (sub-)sample separately emphasizes the differences between the samples.

Following the conceptual and operational framework proposed by Berry

(1989), we are searching for empirically derived commonalities within the investigated beliefs of the educators from former East and West Germany. Toward this goal, we first employ explorative factor analysis for each subsample separately, to look at the uniqueness. Second, we apply confirmatory factor analysis to investigate whether the factor structures in the East and the West are the comparable enough for meaningful group comparisons.

An empirical foundation for possible overlap of educational beliefs in eastern and western educators is evident in the publications describing the aims and ideas of preschool education in both German states. Liegle (1990) identifies two basic *similarities*: the orientation to education for *all children* and comprehensive *fostering* of their development. The *specific* background for the development of educational beliefs of educators in the *former GDR* was characterised by the *unified picture of the individual and society* as well as by the *close link-up between the tasks of day care for preschool children and of the school system.* The special background for day care teachers in the former *West Germany* was characterised by the view of the *children's perspective* and the *independent educational task of day care* without special links to the tasks of the school system.

Accordingly, a unified educational programm for preschool children in the GDR existed with relatively high emphasis on school-relevant aspects of children's development as well as high emphasis on the *leading role of the teacher* in the educational process. By contrast, in West Germany there is no unified and obligating curriculum for all day care centres. The child is seen as having *more responsibility* for his/her development in the "risk society" of the West Germany, rather than placing special emphasis on cognitive skills' training in day care centers (Laewen, 1998).

In our investigation of the educational aims for preschool children (4 to 6 years), and pedagogical beliefs about child behavior, we have to ask: Are there areas or *aspects* within the investigated beliefs we *can meaingfully compare* in the East and in the West, or are the beliefs too divergent to be compared? What is the *relation* between eastern and western educators with regard to *comparable dimensions* of their educational beliefs? Do day care teachers show the same East-West-relation as mothers or are there specifics within the investigated beliefs of familial and institutional educators of preschool children in Germany?

Finally, we discuss whether differences found in the educational beliefs of mothers and teachers five years after the formal unification can be related to their affiliation to the former eastern vs. western part of the country. The discussion of results obtained adresses not only the content of the educational beliefs investigated but also the question of the comparability of the data in general.

Method

Participants

The sample was recruited from 103 day care groups from the former East and West Germany. The day care centres come from four regions of Germany chosen to represent the range of sociocultural conditions (north vs. south, city vs. small town or rural area from eastern and western part, respectively) as well as different day care traditions (full vs. half day care centres) in unified Germany. A comparison with official data (in Germany called "Mikrozensus") shows the similarity of our sample with the overall German data with regard to such features as proportion of different kinds of sponsorship and operating times (full vs. half day centre) as well as socio-economical status of families investigated (income, professional and civil status of parents).

From each of the 103 day care groups, one day care teacher and parents of four randomly selected children (two boys and two girls) were interviewed by trained interviewers. Because all participating day care teachers were female, we limited our investigation of parental beliefs to mothers to avoid a possible gender related artifact. Tables 1 and 2 show the selected characteristics of our parental (Table 1) and teacher (Table 2) samples.

Two aspects have to be pointed out with regard to these characteristics. First, the East German mothers of four year old children are younger than the West German mothers of children of the same age. This is not an artifact of the sample but a social reality, well known from other assessments. Women in Eastern Europe bear children at an earlier age than women in West Europe. Another remarkable detail of these data is a very low variance in the years of schooling by eastern day care teachers. It refers to the fact that there was a unified way of professional education to become a day care teacher in the former GDR, whereas in West Germany different educational ways could lead to this profession. Table 2 shows also that a proportion of teachers were mothers at the same time. We interviewed them in their role as day care teacher rather than splitting the group of teachers into those with and without children.

Measures

The questionnaire used for interviewing mothers and teachers consisted of 35 items. Twenty-four items concern features related to personality traits, social and creative abilities, cognitive and school related skills. Of these 24 items 13 concern educational purposes relevant for preschool children of about 4 - 6 years of age and 11 items concern educational purposes for children of about 6 years ready to start school. The other 11 items concern educational practices including

Table 1. Sample of mothers from the former East and West Germany

	former East	former West
Number	172	243
Age		
x	29.45	31.89
s	4.81	4.7
Number of own children		
x	1.8	1.9
s	0.77	0.76
Years of schooling	11.9	11.3
x	2.99	2.8
s		

Table 2. Sample of teachers from the former East and West Germany

	former East	Former West
Number	41	62
Age		
x	43.98	40.06
s	7.35	9.1
Number of own children		
x	1.6	0.5
s	0.9	0.82
Years of schooling		
x	9.9	10.2
s	0.57	1.00

controlling and supportive practices as well as practices that encourage child independence. In the interview, participants were asked to rate the importance of different educational goals and principles. For all three parts (educational principles and methods, educational goals for preschool children and educational goals for children starting school) an 8-point scale was used, ranging from 1 (least important) to 8 (most important). The interview questions are derived from a scale used in a previous study on 800 mothers and 800 educators (Oliva & Palacios, 1992) itself based on a previous instrument by Hess, Kashiwagi, Azuma, Price and Dichson (1980).

Data Analysis

Confirmatory Factor Analysis (CFA) offers an approach to data analysis when the factor structure is known or can be hypothesized. Here the hypothesized factor structure can be imposed on the sub-samples in a multi-group analysis. Model fit and additional statistics can be obtained to evaluate whether the factor structure holds in both sub-samples or not and what misspecifications the model demonstrates when the model fit is poor. When a factor structure cannot be derived from theory or previous research, this approach becomes more complicated. One way to obtain a factor structure would be to determine the factors based on one sample using an exploratory factor analysis and then test this factor structure using CFA in the second sample. A problem using this strategy occurs when not all items of the questionnaire are assigned to factors in the exploratory factor analysis. Then, the analysis does not provide any information on the question whether the items excluded due to e.g. double-loadings or small loadings on all factors are the ones containing the (sub-sample) culture-specific information.

To answer the questions mentioned above, we chose to employ a two step procedure combining exploratory and confirmatory factor analysis.The first step, an exploratory factor analysis, was carried out for both groups separately and the factor structures were then compared. In the second step, these factor structures were used in CFA as the hypothesized factor model against which the other sample was compared. For the western sample we used the factor structure obtained in the exploratory factor analysis of the eastern sub-sample to evaluate whether the eastern factor structure holds in the western sub-sample. Similarly, for the eastern sub-group, the western structure was used.

This strategy can provide a wealth of information about the samples.For example, exploratory factor analysis may identify different factor-structures in both sub-samples. In this case, we would expect the CFA to indicate that the factor model obtained for the one sub-sample does not hold in the other sample. Thus, we could not compare responses across the two samples. Another possibility is that, based on the exploratory factor analysis, we find identical or quite similar factor structures for both samples. In this case, we would expect the CFA to show that the factor model obtained for the one sub-sample also holds in the other sub-sample. A third possibility is that a factor structure partially (e.g. some factors) holds in both samples but that other factors are not the same in both samples. To we compared the factor values of "comparable" factors through MANOVA (multivariate variance analysis) procedures.

Results

Factor Analytic Procedures - Mothers

In the first step, exploratory factor analysis was performed for groups of *mothers* from East and West separately. A four factor solution was found for each group. The scree-test indicated that a four factor solution was appropriate for each group. A comparison of the factors in both different groups shows that the first three factors are quite similar. One of the three similar factors was identical for both samples. The fourth factor in both groups was entirely different.

In the second step, Confirmatory Factor Analysis (CFA) was employed to validate the derived factor structures. These analyses were carried out separately for each group using the Analysis of Moment Structures (AMOS) Program (Arbuckle, 1997). Because factors in CFA need at least three markers/items for a factor to be identifyable, a three factor model was fit for the *Eastern* sample and the fourth factor, consisting of two items, had to be dropped. Evaluation of this model indicates an unsatisfactory fit between the model and the data. Examination of the "modification indices" reported by AMOS suggested that the first factor might in fact be better represented by two factors instead of one: the first of these factors was marked by the items "to learn to read and write", "to know how to count", and "to get good marks" while all other items loaded on the second factor. After splitting the first factor into two, a (new) four factor model showed a substantially improved model fit.

The same procedure was employed for the *Western* sample. Again, the first analysis modeling the four factors indicated an unsatisfactory fit. Similar to the Eastern sample, the evaluation of the modification indices supported dividing the first factor, resulting in a five factor solution. In addition, the squared multiple correlations (SMS) and modification indices suggested that the item "structured school learning" did not fit well on the last factor and, along with the item "work in class according to rules", cross-loaded on factors 1 and 4. Hence, this factor was eliminated from the analysis.

Summarizing our results thus far, we can conclude that a four factor model holds in both the Eastern and the Western sample with quite similar or somewhat similar factors in in both groups. The derived fifth factor was composed of cross-loaded items and was dropped for both samples. Thus, at least for 13 items of the applied item pools resulted in a comparable factor structure for both samples.

We next conducted Confirmatory Analytic procedures to determine whether the factors found in one sample could be applied to the other sample (eastern and western mothers‘ samples). We found that the factor structure obtained through exploratory factor analysis of the western sample could be fit adequately to our eastern sample (and vice versa). Based upon these results we concluded that *three factors* in the two samples (Table 3) were sufficiently similar to warrant comparison of the factors. Another (fourth) factor adressed social competence in both samples. However, of six items loading on this factor in either subsample, only two items overlapped for both samples (*to have good friends* and *to let act freely*).

Table 3. Factors shared by eastern and western mothers' samples including items' loadings

Names of Factors/Scales	Items: How important is it ...	Items Loadings	
		East	West
controlling educational practices	1. to obey parents/teachers	-.617	-.687
	2. to listen to adults	*	-.640
	3. to punish for something bad	.552	.579
	4. to keep from bad company	.649	.631
	5. to smack for bad behavior	*	.647
	6. to stop before making mistake	.550	.625
schoolrelated cognitive skills for preschool children	1. to know how to count	.536	.558
	2. to get good marks	.701	.514
	3. to learn to read and write	.647	.574
schoolrelated cognitve skills for children starting school	1. to write some words	.768	.780
	2. to solve arithmetic problems	.690	.766
	3. to know most of letters	.717	.789
	4. to count up to 50	.646	.746

*These items have a factor loadings less than 0.5 in the eastern sample.

Data Comparison with Teachers

Because small samples size precluded separate analyses for Eastern and Western teachers, we treated the teachers as one group. This means that we tested whether the factor structure derived from the eastern mother sample holds for the teachers as well and then did the same with the factor structure derived from the western mother sample.Results of these analyses indicated that the factor structure derived from the western mother sample could be adequately fit to the teachers' data. However, the factor structure derived from the eastern mother sample did not provide a good fit for the eastern teachers' data. This problem is not uncommon in CFA and is most likely due to the small number of teachers in our sample. Unfortunately, this problem limited us to further evaluate only the factor structure derived from the western mother sample.

We interprete these results as justifying using the factors obtained on the western mothers sample to analyse educational beliefs in all four investigated groups: mothers from the former eastern and western part of the country and day care teachers from the former East and West. Unfortunately, due to cross-loadings and items not loading on a factor, the factors to compare include only a part of the original items. As much as possible given the limitations of the data, we compared the educational beliefs in east and west. (Table 3). The common items belonging to these factors were fit together in three indexes or scales which could be named "controlling educational practices" (6 items), "school related cognitive skills for preschool children" (3 items) and "school related cognitive skills for children starting school" (4 items). For the items from our questionnaire related to social behaviours of children and supportive/encouraging educational practices, no secure comparison base within the framework of factor analyses could be found.

Factor Mean Comparison

For the three factors shared by all participants groups, Table 4 presents factor means of the educational beliefs of mothers and teachers in the former East and West. We summarize these results as following: First, these means, (which are between 1.6 and 3.7 on a scale from 1 to 8), indicate that mothers and teachers consider all three educational goals and practices to be of little relevance to education. Similarly, schoolrelated cognitive skills for preschool and starting school children were rated as unimportant educational goals for educators (means between 1.6 and 3.5). Further, controlling educational practices do not appear to be very important for mothers and day care teachers (means between 3.2 and 3.7 on the 8-point scale).

Table 4. Factor means by mothers and teachers from the former East and West

	Mothers		Teachers	
	East	West	East	West
Controlling education practice	3.5	3.7	3.3	3.2
School related cognitive skills for preschools	3.5*	3.3*	2.3	2.4
School related cognitiv skills for starting school	2.7	2.8	2.1	1.6

*Significant East-West difference (<5%)

With regard to single scales, only one significant East-West-difference could be found: eastern mothers valued school related cognitive skills for preschool children higher than western mothers did ($F(3,5) = 4.28$, $p < .039$). The day care teachers from the former East and West showed no significant differences in their rating of the three separated scales.

Systematic differences were found between the views of familial and institutional educators rather than between east and west. Mothers valued school related cognitive skills for preschool and starting school children higher than day care teachers did, indicating by differences of means of about 0,6 till to 1,2 points of the scale. The same is true for controlling educational practices with 0,2 to 0,5 scale point differences. All differences are highly significant (F from 12.51 to 55.59;$p < 00$).

Summary and Discussion

In this paper we investigated similarities and differences within the educational beliefs of mothers and day care teachers from the former East and West Germany.For this purpose, we took the conceptual and methodological considerations discussed by Berry (1989) and Boehnke and Merkens (1994) into account. Extending these approaches, we utilized the relatively new approach of Confirmatory Factor Analysis to obtain additional information about the factor structures and to evaluate, to what extent these structures were comparable.

As a result, we could identify specific factor structures within the samples of western and eastern mothers and day care teachers that were comparable and that differed. Unfortunately, we had to collapse the eastern and western teachers' groups for factor analysis procedures because of small sample size. Through CFA procedures, we could identify the factor structure of the western mothers' sample as applicable for all three samples: western mothers, eastern mothers and teachers. On the basis of these factors, three scales were built: cognitive skills for preschool children, cognitive skills for children starting school and controlling educational practices.

With regard to the content of the educational beliefs, as described by these factors, there were no significant differences in factor ratings among the investigated groups with the exception of higher values for school related cognitive skills for preschool children for eastern mothers than for western mothers. Therefore, we find an almost homogeneous view with regard to such dimensions as controlling educational practices, cognitive skills for preschool children and cognitive skills for starting school children across the groups of educators. All three groups (eastern mothers, western mothers and teachers) see the educational purposes and practices associated with these factors as rather unimportant for education. This is an interesting finding given the very strong directives to teachers in the former GDR. Further, it is interesting that the most consistent difference is between day care teachers and mothers with mothers valuing the above described dimensions more than day care teachers.

Due to the lack of statistical comparability for the majority of the items (21 of 35 items), no definite conclusion with regard to beliefs about social behaviors of children, personality traits, social learning in groups, or encouraging childrens` independence and autonomous thinking could be drawn. However, based on these preliminary results, we have support for separate analyses by East and West sample as well as by role – teacher versus parent. Further research should follow these area of educational beliefs more precisely with a larger sample. Our relatively small sample size of eastern mothers ($\underline{n}$=175) and a small sample of teachers ($\underline{n}$=103) prevented us from carrying out an independent factor analysis for eastern and western day care teachers' data. We see the need for indepth investigation of indigenous East- and West-German ideas with regard to the child as an autonomous individual and his/her functioning as a part of a social group

We see the results of our study as further evidence of the challenge in dealing with German-German data in a meaningful way, neither exaggerating the similarities within "German culture", or overemphasizing the differences between the "eastern and western world". The results show that developing the concepts for preschool education in the "new" German state, not only shared as well as divergent beliefs in both parts of the country can be referred to, but also some systematic differences between the educational beliefs of familial compared to institutional educators have to be taken into consideration.

References

Arbuckle, J. (1997). *Analysis of Moment Structures* 3.61. Chicago, IL: Smallwater

Berry, J.W. (1989). Imposed etics-emics-derived etics: The operationalization of a compelling idea. *International Journal of Psychology, 24*, 721 - 735

Boehnke, K. & Merkens, H. (1994). Methodologische Probleme des Ost-West-Vergleichs am Beispiel der Wertforschung zu Kollektivismus und Individualismus. *Zeitschrift für Sozialisationsforschung und Erziehungssoziologie, 14, 3*, 212 - 226

Hess, R.D., Kashiwagi, K., Azuma, H., Price, G.G. & Dichson, W.P. (1980). Maternal expectations for mastery of developmental tasks in Japan and the United States. *International Journal of Psychology, 15*, 259 - 271

Liegle, L. (1990). Struktur und inhaltliche Probleme des Bildungswesen. Vorschulerziehung. In *Materialien zur Lage der Nation herausgegeben vom Bundesministerium für innerdeutsche Beziehungen.* Vergleich von Bildung und Erziehung in der Bundesrepublik Deutschland und in der Deutschen Demokratischen Republik (pp. 157 - 170). Köln: Wissenschaft und Politik

Oliva, A. & Palacios, J. (1992). *Teachers ideas about children and their education (Questionnaire).* Department of Developmental and Educational Psychologist, University of Seville

Tietze, W. (Hrsg.), Meischner, T., Gänsfuß, R., Grenner, K., Schuster, K.-M., Völkel, P. & Rossbach, H.G., (1998). *Wie gut sind unsere Kindergärten?* Berlin: Luchterhand Verlag

Mother-Child Conflict Resolution Styles Among Chinese College Students in Taiwan

Annie Y. Tsai
University of California, Los Angeles
Department of Psychology

Hsiu-ting Yu
National Taiwan University
Department of Psychology

Ashley Maynard
University of California, Los Angeles
Department of Psychology

ABSTRACT

The purpose of this study was to examine mother-child conflict resolution styles among Taiwanese° college students in Taiwan using an indigenous approach. Specifically, Hwang's (1998) Chinese Model of Conflict Resolution was tested. Chinese college students chose mainly Compromise and Confrontation as conflict resolution styles instead of Endurance/Forbearance and Obey Publicly, Defy Privately, as Hwang's model would have predicted. In addition, to explore an alternative model of Chinese mother-child conflict resolution, other culturally-relevant factors such as face-saving, mother-child relationships, and the indigenous emotion Choicelessness (*wunai*) were also studied. Participants responded to questions following each of four conflict scenarios. Data were analyzed by structural equation modeling (SEM) to produce a new, indigenous model of the variables affecting the resolution of conflicts in Chinese mother-child interactions. This model shows that saving mother's face is causally related to conflict resolution styles Compromise and Confrontation. Face-saving also serves as a mediaing variable through which other variables could indirectly affect conflict resolution.

In the United States, where children are socialized to become independent individuals, children tend to be more rebellious as they grow older and gain more control over their own lives (Robin & Foster, 1989; Gehring, Wentzel, & Munson, 1990). On the other hand, in more collectivistic Chinese cultures

° Because culturally, Taiwan and China share the same Confucian heritage that this study is based on, results from a Taiwanese sample are generalized onto the entire Chinese population. The terms "Taiwanese" and "Chinese" are also used interchangeably in this context for the same reason. Although most students in Taiwan identify themselves as Taiwanese politically, they all identify themselves as Chinese culturally.

where children are socialized to develop interdependent and hierarchical relationships within the family (Ho, 1981, 1986; Bond & Hwang, 1986), as children grow older they may adhere more to Chinese cultural values of conflict avoidance through deferential and respectful behavior. Thus, it is hypothesized that in dealing with intergenerational conflicts, Chinese children seek to use harmony-seeking resolution styles.

Confucian Teachings of Harmony Maintenance

Confucianism is the moral doctrine and guiding principle in all forms of social interaction in Chinese culture (Tu, Hejtmanek, & Wachman, 1992). It is based on the fundamental assumption that a person is defined and exists through his/her relationship to others. These relationships are structured hierarchically, thus ensuring the social order through each person playing his/her proper role and fulfilling the requirements of that role (Bond & Hwang, 1986)

In a study of Chinese students, Yang (1981) found that decisions for students' behaviors were predominantly based on the anticipated reactions of other people to that action. He also found that students tended to use non-offensive strategies that seek to maintain harmony and prevent embarrassment. Numerous other studies also have found that the Chinese are socially oriented, or relationship-centered, and that they have a tendency to act in accordance with expectations and norms for the purpose of maintaining harmony in a relationship (Chinese Culture Connection, 1987; Chen, 1994).

Mother-Child Relationships

Confucian values mandate specific requirements for how children are to treat their parents. Parents always occupy a superior position to children, no matter how old the child is. Yau and Smetana (1993) found that Chinese-American adolescents give greater priority to parental expectations than to their own personal desires in conflict situations. It was hypothesized that the degree to which Chinese children are willing to sacrifice their personal desires during conflict should be dependent on the status of their relationship with their parents.

We chose to focus only on mother-child relationships because Chinese fathers usually do not communicate directly with their children regarding issues of conflict (Kim, 1996; Chu, 1989). Conversations with fathers tend to be more about day-to-day issues and do not involve intense emotions. For more serious matters, fathers' wishes are usually expressed through mothers. Similarly, the child's concerns and needs are generally addressed only to mothers (Ho, 1986).

We asked students how close they are with their mothers, and how much authority their mothers have over them (c.f. Chu, 1989). It was hypothesized that increased closeness with the mother and increased authority of mother would be associated with increased harmony-seeking conflict resolution styles.

Face-Saving

The cultural doctrine and norm of "face-saving" to maintain harmony directly influence parent-child interactions (Chu, 1983, 1989; Huang, 1996). The term *mianzi*, or face, can be understood as a superficial front which denotes an individual's social position, prestige, or authority (Hu, 1994). When people "lose face", or don't have any *mianzi*, they may experience shame or embarrassment (Hwang, 1998), anger, anxiety, or self-blame (Chu, 1983). A loss of face could also hurt an individual's self-esteem, thereby increasing feelings of uneasiness and tension (Hwang, 1987).

As a result, in most Chinese social interactions, a primary objective for every person is to pay attention to the preservation of another's face. This is especially true for saving the face of someone who is superior in position in the social hierarchy (Bond & Hwang, 1986). Thus, *mianzi*, or face saving, should serve as a major mediating variable and an important consideration for mother-child conflict resolution.

Emotionality

Consistent with cultural values of avoiding the loss of face and maintaining harmonious relationships, the restraint of emotional expressions is heavily stressed and taught to Chinese students. Graham (1983) found that Chinese students tend to control and suppress emotional difficulties and look upon any loud, explosive behavior as offensive. As a result, this study specifically asked participants to report levels of emotions they **felt** rather than emotions they **displayed**. For example, high intensities of more passive emotions such as shame or regret should lead to greater consideration for mother's face in order to restore the feeling of harmony in the relationship.

Wunai. The emotion *wunai* requires further explanation because it is an indigenous Chinese emotion. *Wunai*, which could be translated as "choicelessness," is the feeling of powerlessness in having no choice resulting from being in a particular position or relationship. These positions or relationships demand that specified behaviors, roles, obligations, and duties be carried out. Choicelessness is the feeling of having no choice or power due to obligations called for by existing cultural values, rather than really not having any choice. *Wunai*, like shame or regret, would also be categorized as a passive emotion.

Importance

Because not all issues of conflict are weighed equally in students' minds, we also assessed how important each conflict scenario was to participants. It was hypothesized that a more important issue would elicit more intense affective responses.

This study, testing indigenous Chinese methods of conflict resolution, sought to determine culturally normative methods of conflict resolution for Taiwanese college students. To do this, we examined how variables already discussed (Face saving, closeness to mother, authority of mother, intensity of emotions felt, and importance of specific conflict) were related to different conflict resolution styles. We addressed these issues using a culturally-sensitive approach (Greenfield, 1996; Kim, 1994) where concepts, methodologies and procedures are based on the Chinese way of life and modes of communication.

For this reason, this study used and tested an indigenous model of conflict resolution based on traditional Chinese cultural values (Hall, 1969; Hwang, 1998). Hwang's model has two dimensions "pursuing vs. discarding personal goal" and "maintaining vs. disrupting interpersonal harmony" (see Figure 1).

Based on these two dimensions, Hwang defined five possible conflict resolution styles, with "Compromise" as the midpoint in both harmony and goal. The other four extremes were, "Confrontation" (low on harmony, high on personal goal), "Obey Publicly, Defy Privately" (high on harmony and personal goal), "Severance" (low on harmony and personal goal), and "Forbearance/Endurance" (high on harmony, low on personal goal). In accord with Confucian values, Hwang (1998) predicted that students' conflict resolution styles would most frequently tend toward maintaining harmony in parent-child relationships, i.e., Obey Publicly, Defy Privately or Forbearance/Endurance.

Figure 1. Chinese Conflict Resolution Model (Hwang, 1998)

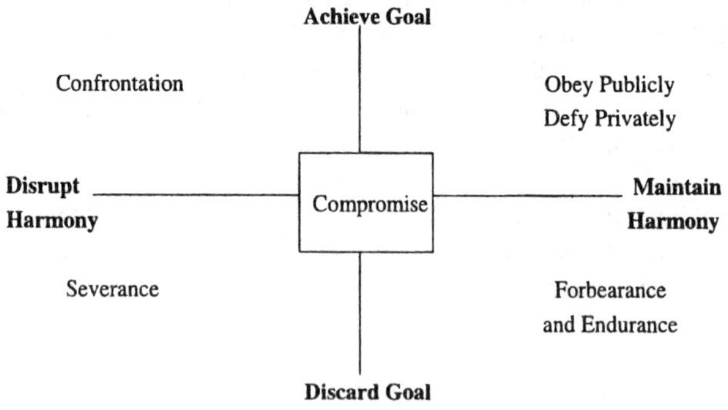

Method

Participants

A total of 129 students from Taiwan (63 women and 66 men, mean age = 20.51 years, SD = 1.37) volunteered to participate in the study as part of their requirement for an introductory psychology class. These students are from National Taiwan University which is comparable to a top university in the United States. At the time of data collection, half of the participants (64) lived with their parents.

Materials

For the purpose of refining our questionnaire, a pilot study and two focus groups were conducted. Each focus group had eight participants (four males, four females), comparable to our sample, who were college students at National Taiwan University. They were asked questions about the relevance of the conflict issues and the different emotions felt. They were also asked whether any questions from our questionnaire seemed inappropriate, ambiguous, or difficult to understand. These responses were used to refine and develop the questionnaire further.

The entire questionnaire consisted of three sections. In the first section, four different conflict scenarios, each with follow-up questions were presented. The order of scenarios were counter-balanced and randomly distributed such that each scenario had an equal chance to appear first, second, third, or fourth. The second section included two questions that assessed participants' relationships with their mothers. The final section involved demographic and personal information.

Conflict scenarios were chosen because they had the most relevance to issues of family conflict according to both Taiwanese literature (Chen, 1994; Huang, 1996) and focus groups that were conducted about which issues should be used. The four scenarios selected were all verbal debates about different situations: (1) the student coming home late from a social activity, (2) re-taking the college-entrance exam to qualify for a higher ranked major, (3) the student's need to buy a scooter, and (4) the mother eavesdropping on a personal phone conversation.

The conflict resolution style employed in dealing with each scenario was assessed with participants picking one out of six multiple choice options offered. The first five options were from Hwang's (1998) five conflict-resolution styles. The last option was "other:_____" which allowed participants to write in their own resolution tactic if they felt that none of the previous five options matched their own resolution style.

This last open-ended response was later coded as one of the five resolution styles (see Fig. 1). Two people independently coded all the open-ended responses with an inter-rater reliability of 90.1% (with a 20% chance rate of agreement).

For each conflict scenario, participants rated the intensity of six emotions (anger, shame, regret, *wunai*, fear, sadness) and importance of the conflict. They also rated closeness with mother and authority of mother. All were measured on a 10-point scale ranging from 0 to 9.

Design and Procedures

The four conflict scenarios were counterbalanced and randomly distributed so that each scenario had an equal chance to be the first, second, third, or fourth scenario in the questionnaire. All participants were allowed as much time as necessary to finish the questionnaire. Everyone finished in less than forty minutes, and was thanked for their participation.

Results

Table 1 contains the means and standard deviations for variables used in testing the theoretical model. Based on all four scenarios, the most frequently-used conflict resolution styles were Compromise (45.5%) and Confrontation (23.8%). Because they account for 69.3% of the responses, these were the conflict resolution styles used in our theoretical model.

We used a structural equation modeling (SEM) program, EQS (Bentler, 1995), to test a formal model of direct and indirect effects of these variables on the outcomes of the mother-child conflicts. SEM permits estimation of models that include multiple mediators and latent variables (Hoyle & Smith, 1994).

The maximum likelihood estimation of the conceptual model for conflict outcomes is shown in Figure 2. The Comparative Fit Index (CFI) was .96 (where CFI can range from 0 to 1, and values over .90 are typically considered indicative of good-fitting models; Ullman, 1996). The X^2 test also indicated that this model is a good description of these data ($X^2 = 47.12$, $\underline{p} = .08$, where the X^2 test should be non-significant, meaning that there is probably not a better model to be found). Each of the parameter coefficients, or links, in the model is statistically significant at the $\underline{p} < .05$ level. Overall, this model shows that saving mother's face functions as a mediating variable between importance of conflict, inwardly experienced emotions, closeness to mother, and the conflict resolution strategy.

Table 1. Predictive Variables

Variables	Mean	SD
Importance	5.72	1.27
Emotions		
Anger	6.00	1.49
Wunai	5.17	2.01
Sadness	4.40	2.21
Fear	1.68	1.50
Shame	1.58	1.36
Regret	1.30	1.28
Relationship with mom		
Authority	4.05	2.42
Closeness	6.49	1.88
	4.58	1.72
Face giving	4.58	1.72

Note. Judgments were made on a 10-pont scale
(0=none or not at all, 9=extremely or very)

Figure 2. Theoretical Model of Chinese Mother-Child Conflict Resolution Style

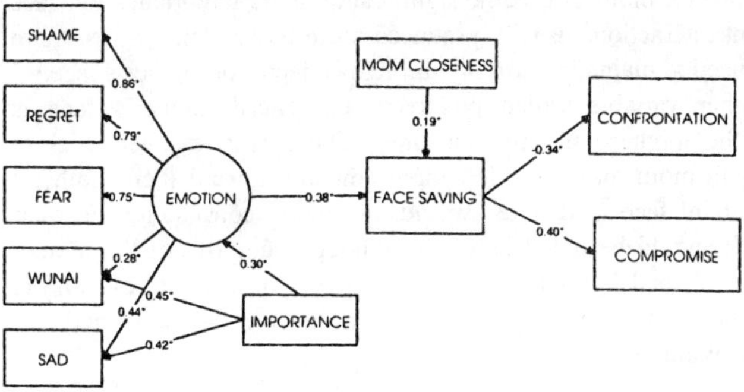

Variables Influencing Concern for Mother's Face

Importance of conflict, emotion, and closeness with mother all influence concern for mother's face. Importance of the conflict affects the degree of emotion felt. The model shows that as conflict scenarios increased in importance to students, the emotions felt became more intense. The originally hypothesized model did not include the specific links from importance to sadness and *wunai*; however, the Lagrange Multiplier test indicated that the overall fit of the model could be improved by adding these parameters. Sadness and *wunai*, culturally acceptable emotions to the Taiwanese students, increased even more than the other emotions as the importance of the conflict increased. These five emotions, unlike anger, are all passive, inward emotions. Students who reported experiencing these emotions intensely felt worse about having had a conflict with their mothers than those who had reported lower intensities. Thus, they should have felt a stronger need to re-establish harmony to feel connected with their mothers (Lung, 1996). One way to do this was by maintaining their mother's face. Consistently, those who felt more shame, regret, fear, *wunai*, or sadness gave significantly more consideration to saving mother's face.

Degree of anger felt was measured in the study and was a variable in our original model, weighing on the factor of emotion. However, anger did not relate to face-saving in the same way as other emotions. In fact, anger did not weigh on the factor of emotions (beta weight = .05, ns) and it was ultimately rejected as a parameter by statistical analyses. One possible explanation for anger being dropped by the model is that compared to the other emotions that are more passive and inward in nature, anger is more of an active and outward emotion. It would make sense that it did not function in the same manner as more passive emotions.

As the importance of the conflict and emotions increased, the issue of face maintenance for mothers became significantly more important. Because more important interactions usually produced more threatening results, there was a greater need to maintain harmony through concern for mother's face.

The other variable which positively influenced mother's face is closeness of the mother-child relationship. Those who enjoyed a close relationship with mom may have felt more empathy toward their mothers' need to maintain face and thus would be more considerate in their interactions. It should be noted here that although authority of the mother was a variable we had hypothesized to play a role in a model of conflict resolution, authority did not have any significant links in the model and was dropped by the Wald test.

Concern for Mother's Face and Conflict Resolution

Taken together, importance of the conflict, degree of emotion felt, and closeness with mother all affected concern for mother's face, which in turn affected the conflict resolution style. Our theoretical model includes the two most used conflict resolution strategies: Confrontation and Compromise.

Confrontation was defined as seeking personal goals at the price of harmony in the relationship. This model suggests that as students' concern for mother's face decreases, their likelihood of using confrontation as a resolution style increases. Therefore, when students were not considering their mother's face, they would sacrifice harmony in their relationship in order to obtain their own goals. On the other hand, students who considered their mother's face more would be more harmony seeking and more self-sacrificing, using more Compromise, which was defined as seeking some harmony by yielding some personal goals. As such, the model shows that a high degree of concern for mother's face has a positive association with Compromise, meaning that more consideration for mother's face translated into seeking harmony by yielding a few steps.

Discussion

In this study we sought to test Hwang's (1998) predictions based on his Chinese model of conflict resolution derived from traditional Confucian values of hierarchical relationship and harmony maintenance. In addition, other variables that affect conflict resolution processes that had not been addressed were also examined for an alternative, more complete model. These variables included relationship with mother (closeness and authority), importance of the conflict, and intensity of emotions experienced (anger, shame, regret, choicelessness, sadness, and fear).

In our structural equation model of Chinese mother-child conflict resolution styles, face-saving for mother was the key variable that influenced the two most frequently chosen conflict resolution styles, Confrontation and Compromise. Face-saving had a mediating effect between variables such as inward emotions (e.g., shame), closeness to mother, and importance of conflict and the chosen conflict resolution styles.

The differences between our original hypothesized model and the final model are worthy of some discussion here. First, that anger was dropped from the model may surprise Euro-American readers who may have witnessed adolescents in fits of anger and rebellion with their parents. Anger is the variable typically studied in American mother-child conflicts (Prinz et al., 1979; Robin & Weiss, 1980). Anger, however, is an outward emotion often suppressed in Chinese mother-child conflicts. Our model confirms this fact by showing that concern for mother's face is the central, mediating variable between the adolescent's own emotional experience and the outcome of the conflict. Anger may have been felt intensely but that emotion does not seem to play a role in consideration for mother's face or choice of conflict resolution style.

The second major difference between our original model and the final outcome is the deletion of the authority of the mother as a parameter. Though we had originally thought that authority of the mother would influence both importance of conflict and emotions felt, authority of the mother had to be removed as a parameter to make the model work. This result confirms Chao's (1994) finding that Chinese children's respect for and obedience toward their parents is based on the closeness of the relationship rather than the authority of the parents. Hence, it is not surprising to find closeness with the mother to weigh importantly in the model, with authority not carrying any weight at all.

Generally speaking, results showed that, contrary to Hwang's (1998) predictions, Chinese college students did not readily conform to prescribed resolution styles as preached by Confucian doctrines (e.g., Endurance and Forbearance). They opted for Compromise the most rather than Endurance/Forbearance or Obey Publicly, Defy Privately.

According to Yang (1986), one explanation to account for these findings would be that under the impact of societal modernization the Chinese population is changing, becoming more individual-oriented rather than social-oriented. Compromise defined as seeking to maintain harmony while trying to satisfy personal goals seems more compatible as a resolution for today's Chinese college students. However, they are still different from Euro-Americans, who tend to use Confrontation the most (Robin & Foster, 1989).

In modern Chinese society, it seems then that pragmatism (satisfying cultural expectations and personal goals) is the best way to resolve conflicts with parents rather than unconditional self-sacrifice as mandated in doctrines of filial piety (Yeh, 1995). In conclusion, it is important to realize that Chinese society and personality are changing. The Chinese college population of today may understand traditional teachings passed on through Confucian heritage, but how they utilize this knowledge is a more complex matter that merits further investigation.

References

Bentler, P. M. (1995). *EQS Structural equations program manual.* Encino, CA: Multivariate Software, Inc.

Bond, M. H. & Hwang, K. K. (1986). The Social Psychology of Chinese People. In M. H. Bond (Ed.), *The psychology of the Chinese people*. (Pp. 213-231). Oxford: Oxford University Press.

Chao, R. K. (1994) Beyond parental control and authoritarian parenting style: Understanding Chinese parenting through the cultural notion of training. *Child Development, 65*, 1111-1119.

Chen S. W. (1994). Social relationships and the choices of conflict resolution procedures: In a perspective of patterns of the properties of relationships. Unpublished Master thesis, National Taiwan University. (In Chinese.).

Chinese Culture Connection (1987). Chinese values and the search for culture-free dimensions of culture. *Journal of Cross-Cultural Psychology, 18*, 143-164.

Chu, R. L. (1983). Empirical research on the psychology of face. Unpublished doctoral thesis, National Taiwan University. (In Chinese.).

Chu, R. L. (1989). Parent-child interaction and its consequences for children. *Bulletin of the Institute of Ethnology Academia Sinica, 25*, 181-246. (In Chinese.).

Gehring, T. M., Wentzel, K. R., & Munson, J. (1990). Conflict in families of adolescents: The impact of cohesion and power structures. *Journal of Family Psychology, 3*(3), 290-309.

Graham, M. A. (1983) Acculturative stress among Polynesian, Asian, and American students on the Brigham Young University - Hawaii campus. *International Journal of Intercultural Relations, 7*(1), 79-103.

Greenfield, P. M. (1996) Culture as a process: Empirical methodology for cultural psychology. In Y.H. Poortinga & J. Pandey (Eds.), *Theory and method: Vol. 1. Handbook of cross-cultural psychology* (2nd ed.) (pp. 301-346). Boston: Allyn & Bacon.

Hall, J. (1969). Conflict Management Survey. Rochester, New York: Technometrics.

Ho, D. Y. F. (1981). Traditional patterns of socialization in Chinese society. *Acta Psychologica Taiwanica, 23*(2), 81-95.

Ho, D. Y. F. (1986). Chinese patterns of socialization: A critical review. In M. H. Bond (Ed.), *The psychology of the Chinese people* (pp. 1-37). Oxford: Oxford University Press.

Hoyle, R. H. & Smith, G. T. (1994). Formulating clinical research hypotheses as structural equation models: A conceptual overview. *Journal of Consulting and Clinical Psychology, 62*, 429-440.

Hu, H. C. (1994). The Chinese concept of 'face'. *American Anthropologist, 46*, 45-64.

Huang, L. L. (1996). *Harmony and conflict in Chinese social relationships: Theory and empirical analysis*. (in Chinese). Unpublished doctoral dissertation, National Taiwan University.

Hwang, K. K. (1987). Face and favor: The Chinese power game. *American Journal of Sociology, 92*(4), 944-974.

Hwang, K. K. (1998). Guanxi and Mientze: Conflict resolution in Chinese society. *Intercultural Communication Studies, 7*(1), 17-42.

Kim, U. (1994). Introduction to individualism and collectivism: Conceptual clarification and elaboration. In U. Kim, H. C. Triandis, & C. Kagitcibasi (Eds.), *Individualism and collectivism: Theory, method, and applications (pp. 19-40)*. Newbury Park, CA: Sage.

Lung, A. (1996). Family conflict and resolution in Chinese American and Caucasian families. Unpublished doctoral dissertation prospectus, University of California Los Angeles.

Prinz, R. J., Foster, S. L., Kent, R. N. & O'Leary, K. D. (1979). Multivariate assessment of conflict in distressed and nondistressed mother-adolescent dyads. *Journal of Applied Behavior Analysis, 12*, 691-700.

Robin, A. L., & Foster, S. L. (1989). *Negotiating adolescence: A behavioral family systems approach to parent-adolescent conflict.* New York: Guilford Press.

Robin, A. L., & Weiss, J. G. (1980). Criterion-related validity of behavioral and self-report measures of problem-solving communication skills in distressed ad non-distressed parent-adolescent dyads. *Behavioral Assessment, 2*, 339-352.

Tu W., Hejtmanek, M., & Wachman, A. (Eds.) (1992). *The Confucian world observed: A contemporary discussion on Confucian humanism in East Asia.* Honolulu, Hawaii: Institute of Culture and Communication, The East-West Center.

Ullman, J. B. (1996). Structural equation modeling. In B. G. Tabachnick & L. S. Fidell (Eds.), *Using multivariate statistics* (3rd ed.) (pp. 709-812). New York: Harper Collins.

Yang, K. S. (1981) Social orientation and individual modernity among Chinese students in Taiwan. *Journal of Social Psychology, 113*, 159-170.

Yang, K. S. (1986). Chinese personality and its change. In M. H. Bond (Ed.), *The psychology of the Chinese people* (pp. 106-160). Oxford: Oxford University Press.

Yau & Smetana (1993) Chinese-American adolescents' reasoning about cultural conflicts. *Journal of Adolescence Research, 8*(4), 419-438.

Yeh, G. H. (1995). Solution types in filial dilemmas and their various correlates. *Bulletin of the Institute of Ethnology Academia Sinica, 79*, 87-118.

Author Note

The authors would like to express appreciation to Patricia Greenfield, Cathy R. Chu, and Yi-Yue Yeh; Ting-ho Huang, Lan-fang Shih, and Pauline Hsieh

Exploring the World of Meaning of ESL Students

Lilian C. J. Wong &
F. Ishu Ishiyama
Department of Counseling Psychology
The University of British Columbia

Paul T. P. Wong
Graduate Program in Counseling Psychology
Trinity Western University

ABSTRACT

This chapter argues that there is a need to consider cultural context and acculturation in counseling and assessing children from different ethnic backgrounds. It describes two assessment tools used to explore the world of personal meaning of English as a second language (ESL) students: Ishiyama's Validationgram and Wong's Personal Meaning Profile. Three cases of Chinese immigrants' children were chosen to illustrate how these instruments enabled us to look beneath the surface meanings of behavioral problems and uncover the deeper meanings of ESL children's frustrated needs and acculturative stress. More importantly, all three cases revealed an indomitable human spirit in spite of the many school and family difficulties faced by ESL students. The present meaning-centered approach to counseling and assessment has several advantages: (1) it focuses on the strengths, resilience and spirituality of clients; (2) it relies on narrative and story telling; and (3) it addresses racial identity development, family relationships, and cultural context from the child's perspective.

The recent influx of immigrants has placed considerable demands on the school systems for English as a second language (ESL) classes and created a demand for culturally appropriate counseling and assessment. Since culture shapes children's psychosocial development, it is important that counselors and school psychologists understand the unique challenges faced by ethnic minority students (Lee, 1995; Herring, 1997).

Moving to a new country involves acculturative stress (Berry & Annis, 1974). Migration may result in disorientation, stress, anxiety, and grief over the loss of cultural heritage. Cultural dislocation entails a complex experience of uprootedness, cultural conflicts, and loss of personal meaning (Ishiyama, 1995a, 1956b, Westwood & Lawrance, 1990). Therefore, when counseling immigrants there is a need to focus on validation and restoration of a sense of self. Ishiyama (1995a) recommends that "the counselor needs to explore the personal meaning of a transition experience with the client and to recognize its impact on the client's life" (p. 134).

Studying in a foreign country can create additional adjustment problems (Ishiyama, 1989; Pedersen, 1991). According to Schram and Lauver (1988), international students often experience (a) *alienation* (feelings of powerlessness to achieve desired outcomes), (b) *meaninglessness* (inability to make sense of what is happening to them), and (c) *social estrangement* (feelings of loneliness). Students who study ESL in the public schools may be particularly vulnerable to acculturative stress because of their young age and racial/ cultural identity crisis (Ibrahim, Ohnishi & Wilson, 1994); this at-risk group would need special attention from school counselors.

Although considerable attention has been given to counseling international college students (Leong & Chou, 1996), the same attention has not been given to ESL students in the public school systems. This chapter focuses on recent immigrants' children. It first briefly reviews the literature on the difficulties of cross-cultural counseling and assessment of children. Then it describes two instruments employed to explore the subjective meanings of ethnic minority students. Finally, it presents a case study of three immigrant students to illustrate how these instruments can enhance our understanding of the values, emotional needs and lived experiences of ESL students.

Cross-Cultural Issues in Counseling and Assessment of Children

Cross-cultural counseling and assessment are fraught with difficulties (Lonner & Berry, 1986; Lonner & Ibrahim, 1996). The task is made even more difficult in working with ESL students, not only because of their deficiencies in English, but also because of their reluctance to share family secrets with strangers. This challenge calls for new ways of assessing their needs and life situations.

Recently, Sue (1996) has documented various ethnic biases in counseling and assessment. Some of the sources of these biases include therapists' biased diagnoses of the psychological functioning of minorities, the lack of cross-culturally valid assessment instruments, and minorities' culturally different response sets. Sue emphasizes the need to understand the cultural background of the client in assessment: "Because of the growing multiethnic nature of our society and the increasing importance of assessment in all phases of life, there is an urgent need to direct our attention to the issues facing ethnic minority populations. A relatively small amount of research effort has been devoted to the valid assessment of these populations. The time is ripe for us to expend substantial efforts to address cross-cultural assessment issues" (p. 33).

Samuda (1998) highlights the disadvantages of minority students with regard to standardized testing: "Too often, the main use of testing has been to serve a sorting and labeling function. Concomitantly, minority children have been placed into programs of minimal curriculum content on the basis of spurious results. . . . Minority children, as a group, have always scored lower on standardized tests. That statement holds good regardless of the ethnicity of the group" (p. 3).

Similarly problems exist in counseling. Minority students are likely to be viewed in a negative light when counselors and therapists assume that their own worldviews and cultural assumptions provide the only appropriate framework for assessment and counseling. Ibrahim (Ibrahim, 1993; Ibrahim et al. 1994) emphasizes the need to understand culturally different clients' beliefs, values and worldviews that affect their decisions. She and her colleagues recommend that worldviews be one aspect of informal and qualitative assessment of the client's cultural identity, which refers to how individuals define themselves from a cultural perspective (Ibrahim et al., 1994).

According to Lonner and Ibrahim (1996), cultural identity also includes considerations regarding the client's generational status, age, stage of life, etc. "An appraisal of these dimensions adds to the counselor's understanding of the client's worldview by providing a phenomenological experiential context for the assumptions held by the client" (p. 296).

Ethnocentric bias is also evident in therapeutic goals, which are typically based on Western models of psychotherapy. In counseling minority students, such bias is also shown in the attempts of assimilation. For example, Leong and Chou (1996) point out that "Ethnocentrism is a significant problem because many American counselors may assume that the goal of counseling is to make international students adapt and adjust to the American way of life" (p. 228).

Prior Attempts to Overcome Cultural Biases in Assessment

In order to meet the educational and mental health needs of minority students, attempts have been made to overcome cultural biases. For example, Mercer and Lewis (1978) developed the System of Multicultural Pluralistic Assessment (SOMPA). It incorporates three assessment models: medical, social, and pluralistic. "The social system model is concerned with the child's ability to adapt and function in social situations. It attempts to measure how well a child meets social expectations at home, at school and in the community" (Lewis, 1998, p. 227). The pluralistic model uses information gathered through parental interview to determine the estimated learning potential of the testee. This represents the first attempt to reduce cultural biases and stigmatization in assessing culturally and linguistically diverse children.

Armour-Thomas and Gopaul-McNicol (1998) recognize that values and beliefs within a culture influence cognitions and decide what constitutes an appropriate goal. "Culture defines not only what its members should think or learn but also what they should ignore or treat as irrelevant" (p. 56). They argue "that observed behaviors at any point in a child's development are more precisely defined as culturally dependent cognitions. As members of the species *Homo sapiens*, we are born into this world with certain dynamic characteristics, including cognitive potentials that create a biological predisposition for human development. How these characteristics develop, along what pathways, and toward what end states, however, are determined by the reciprocal interplay of these characteristics with equally dynamic experiences within particular zones of the culture wherein the child develops and functions" (p. 77).

From this biocultural perspective, intelligent behavior reflects the extent culture has differentially shaped biologically constrained cognitive potentials. The biological system is assumed to interact with four major cultural niches — namely, home, peer group, school, and community within the context of the larger society. This four-tiered biocultural assessment system consists of (1) Psychometric assessment, (2) Psychometric potential assessment, (3) Ecological assessment, and (4) Other intelligences, such as musical intelligence, and interpersonal intelligence.

What is of special interest to the school counselor is ecological assessment. This approach consists of assessing several domains of the child's life: family/community support, performance in the school, home, and community, stage of acculturation, and teacher questionnaire. The child is observed in his/her cultural niches — home, community and school. The examiner discusses all the tasks that the child was able to perform in these settings with his/her parents and teachers. The above authors cited numerous studies demonstrating that intellectual functions and school success were related to familial support, parental attitudes, and values (the worth of schooling).

In addition to assessing other intelligences, minority children are also assessed in their stage of acculturation. This nonpsychometric assessment focuses on adjustment difficulties minority children may be experiencing — how they cope with living in a new place and cultural changes (linguistic, social networks) and how these experiences result in psychological changes (alteration in their mental status due to culture shock and psychological transition from their own cultural values to host-cultural values). The stress and impact of acculturation are particularly important in assessing and counseling ESL children, most of whom have immigrated to the host country only recently.

Paniagua (1994) argues that assessment and treatment of culturally different clients need to include assessment of acculturation effects. Dana's (1993) assessment model emphasizes the need to assess the client's level of acculturation and to select assessment devices or models that are culturally appropriate. Lonner and Ibrahim (1996) have also emphasized the need "to consider qualitative factors such as the client's worldview, cultural identity, and level of acculturation as assessment factors" (p.293). Lee (1996) proposes that assessment and counseling of students should be from culture-specific viewpoints and school psychologists need to learn about salient characteristics of other cultures.

More recently, Ivey and Ivey (1999) recommend the use of the community genogram to learn about the culture and social context of clients. Clients are asked to draw their communities and then tell positive stories about their community genogram. For example, Mary Ivey asked Tamara, one her elementary students, to draw a circle to represent her community. This circle indicated that Tamara's family and church were her primary support systems and revealed the central role of spirituality in her life. The community genogram can be used therapeutically to draw out from clients their sources of support and strength.

In short, a consensus is emerging that in counseling and assessing culturally different children, we need to understand their home environments, social contexts, and the meanings they attach to their life situations. This chapter reports a case study employing two instruments (Validationgram and Personal Meaning Profile) to explore the private world of meanings of three ESL students. These instruments are designed to draw out stories and narratives from students about their values and subjective perceptions of their life situations. Since culture is primarily based on shared meanings, values and beliefs, these two meaning-centered instruments can be helpful in integrating ESL students' cultural context with psychological assessment and school counseling.

Method

Subjects

Three children (2 boys and 1 girl) from recent Chinese immigrants were selected to illustrate the usefulness of meaning-centered assessment. They were all designated by the school districts as ESL students. All three of them experienced some difficulties in school and at home.

T. J., a slim eleven-year-old boy, was small for his age. He was the only child of university-educated, wealthy Chinese parents, who immigrated to Canada from Taiwan about one and a half years ago. Mother was very concerned about his disobedience at home and his mediocre school performance. At home, he spent excessive time on "Nintendo" games and Chinese storybooks. At school, he did not follow instructions well and had very few friends.

Bill, a lanky twelve-year-old, immigrated to Canada with his family from Hong Kong about three years ago. His father was very unhappy about the educational system and child rearing practices in Canada, and wanted to enforce strict discipline over his children. His father had used "smacking" to discipline Bill, but was warned by the authorities for possible charges of child abuse. The father was very frustrated with his low achievement motivation, disobedience and lying. Bill was hostile towards his father and openly defiant towards his teacher.

Jane, a twelve-year-old girl, was timid and cooperative. Her family immigrated to Canada from Hong Kong about two years ago. Her father returned to Hong Kong to do business and visited his family from time to time. Jane lived with her mother and a younger sister. Her mother did not speak much English. Her teacher was concerned about her high degree of anxiety and her tendency to over-react to feedback on her academic performance. The teacher also reported incidents of plagiarism on assignments.

Instruments and Procedure

The participants were first asked do the Validationgram (Ishiyama, 1995a) and then completed the Children's Personal Meaning Profile adapted from Wong (1998). The senior author conducted all assessments in the context of counseling.

Ishiyama's Validationgram

This instrument is based on Ishiyama's (1989) self-validation model, which serves as a conceptual framework for understanding cross-cultural issues. The model emphasizes themes and the sources of validation as well as various dimensions of the self. The four major domains comprise the validation network, which is expected to enhance one's sense of self and personal meaning. "Validationgram is a semi-structured activity designed to help clients articulate the world of meanings and values and explore associated feelings" (Ishiyama, 1995a, p. 138). The validationgram worksheet has a large circle divided into four quadrants representing the four domains of validation: Relationship, Place, Things and Activity. The inner circle represents Self. Respondents are asked to use a few adjectives to describe themselves, and then write down items of importance to them in each of the four quadrants in such a way that the closer an item to the center, the more personal significance it has. The completed validationgram represents the client's network of validation sources.

In the present study, the assessor worked with the children in completing the validationgram. While working on the validationgram, the assessor encouraged the children to elaborate on the answers they provided.

The main objectives were (1) to understand what was important (i.e., valuable and validating) to the children from their perspective, and (2) to facilitate the children's spontaneous sharing of their feelings and perceptions without any influence from the assessor.

Children's Personal Meaning Profile (PMP-C)

The present study employed a children's version of the Personal Meaning Profile (PMP; Wong, 1998), which measures seven sources of personal meaning: Achievement, Intimacy, Relationships, Religion, Self-transcendence, Self-acceptance, and Fair Treatment. The present children's version (PMP-C) was adapted for elementary school children. In addition to rating the seven main sources of meaning, probing questions were asked to explore specific issues. For example, regarding intimacy, respondents were asked: "How important is it to you to have a very close relationship with someone? That is, to have someone who really cares about you, and with whom you can share everything? Do you have someone like that? How about your parents or brothers and sisters? Did you have someone very close to you back in your own country?" (A copy of the PMP-C may be obtained from the authors).

While the Validationgram focuses on concrete events and things important to the children, the PMP-C focuses on less tangible matters. More importantly, the PMP-C not only identifies what children value, but also reveals whether they are able to experience what they value. In other words, the PMP-C indicates the gaps between children's values and their actual experiences.

Results and Discussion

T. J., A Frustrated, Lonely Boy

Working on the validationgram, T. J. described himself as "smart" but "mean", because "people told me that I am selfish, bad, annoying, get mad easily." Regarding Relationship, he named his parents and two boys from the neighborhood. He did not feel attached to any place, as the family had lived in several cities. The things that he valued most were money and video games. He had very limited sources of validation.

The PMP-C revealed large discrepancies between what he valued and what he actually received. For example, he valued relations and friends, but he had to play by himself most of the time. He valued fair treatment, but claimed that classmates had treated him unfairly. He said that it was very important to believe in God, but he found going to church very boring. He de-emphasized the importance of achievement (rating it 3 on a scale of 1 to 5), but he really wanted to do well in everything. He also rated self-acceptance a

"3" and he wished to be the son of a trillionaire. When he did something wrong, he felt bad ("feeling funny inside") and wished to be somebody else.

Judging from the thoughtful and analytical way in which he answered questions, and his ability to articulate his ideas in spite of his limited vocabulary, he appeared to be an intelligent boy. His parents also suggested that he is a smart boy, because of his quick, inquiring mind and his past school achievement in his home country. His mediocre school performance is likely due to language difficulties and low motivation. His inability to meet high parental expectations has led to a self-defeating strategy: if he does not do well in school because of laziness, then he can maintain the image of being smart.

He feels frustrated in several areas of his life because of unfulfilled high expectations. His acting-out behavior and temper tantrums likely stem from his high frustration. Behind the facade of defiance is a lonely boy crying out for acceptance, validation, and emotional support. His dream of great wealth reflects his attempt to gain approval and respect through financial success, which is emphasized by his father.

His network of social support is very limited. At home, he plays by himself most of thc time. At school, he often gets into trouble with his classmates. He is not involved in any extra-curricular activities. Occasionally, he plays with a couple of Chinese children in the neighborhood.

In terms of acculturation, his family chooses the strategy of separation (Berry, 1990). All their contacts and friends are Chinese. Given the large Chinese community in Vancouver, BC, many Chinese immigrants can live in a parallel world, with little or no interaction with the majority society. T. J. has adopted a similar attitude and shows no interest to interact with Caucasian students at school. His devotion to Chinese storybooks is his way of escaping into a world familiar to him — a world he has to leave behind not by his choice. His feelings of alienation and isolation in school, compounded by unfair treatment by classmates, are bound to have some negative effects on his academic motivation. In sum, his behavioral and academic problems at home and school are at least partially due to his negative acculturation experiences.

Bill, A Rebel Against His Own Culture

In completing validationgram, Bill described himself as annoying, independent, and risk-taking. His close relationships consist of his mom and all other friends from school. His home meant little to him. He listed his friends' homes and the park as important places. The things he valued most were money, TV, and a computer. His important activities were playing with friends, watching TV, getting on-line on the computer, and playing basketball and hockey. His major source of validation comes from his friends.

The PMP-C indicated that friends are most important: "If you don't have anyone close to you, feeling like killing yourself." He felt good about himself because he was good at basketball, hockey and had lots of friends, but disliked being "short" and Chinese. "I don't want to be Chinese". He wished to be like his Caucasian friends. It was very important to him to be treated fairly, but he felt that he was not treated fairly by his teacher, father, and his paternal grandfather. Bill believed God as a creator who loves people: "With God, you have somebody to talk to".

Bill was caught in the clash between two cultures. He rebelled against his father's strict discipline and disliked being Chinese. He felt oppressed and frustrated for not having the same freedom as his Caucasian friends: "Why should I have to come home right away after school? This is very unfair!"

Bill chose the acculturation strategy of assimilation (Berry, 1990), while his family preferred segregation. This created a great deal of conflict at home. The more he wanted to identify with his Caucasian friends, the more he resented his Chinese heritage. He did poorly at school in order to get back at his father. His behavioral and academic problems stem primarily from his rebellion against the traditional Chinese culture as epitomized by his father.

A Talented Girl Who Hates Being Herself

The Validationgram showed that Jane was aware of her talent in music, but she described herself as being stupid and lazy. The piano was the most important thing to her. Her favorite activities were playing the piano and sports. Her family ranked first in her relationship, followed by an unnamed boy in her class and other friends. Her home and school were the most important places to her.

The PMP-C revealed that Jane highly valued relationship, but had difficulty naming a person whom she felt close to. She nominated her diary as her "closest confidant", where she could pour out her feelings. She did not have any close friends, "because I'm Chinese." She was secretly infatuated with a Caucasian boy. She complained about being teased by her classmates, who often treated her unfairly, but she had learned to ignore them.

Achievement was very important to her and she worked very hard to succeed but gets "mad when others are better than I." She felt very proud to accompany the school choir on the piano. She intensely disliked her looks. "I like nothing about myself — my face, my whole body. I don't like my skin, color too dark, mouth too big, eyes too small." She really wanted to be like a girl in her class: "She is so pretty, and I want to be like her from neck to feet." She lamented that she was too slow in learning English. She did not like being so lonely. Even though she excelled at piano, she still said: "Don't like being so stupid and lazy, need to practice over and over again on piano."

She believed that religion might play a more important role when she grew older.

Jane excelled in music and school, but she had a very negative self-concept and suffered from anxiety, because of high expectations and fierce competitiveness. The one reported instance of plagiarism was prompted by her worry about getting a low grade in her written English assignment.

She tried to please her parents and her Caucasian classmates, but succeeded in neither. She tried to stay close to one or two Chinese girl friends, but mother insisted that she should make friends with "Canadians" so that she could improve her English. Her deep sense of alienation was evident in that her best friend was her diary. She hated her "Chinese" looks, because she had bought into the Western values of being glamorous and sexy. She wanted very much to be like those popular Caucasian girls who flirted with boys, but she could not even express her affection to the only boy she loved. She did not feel good about herself, in spite of all her accomplishments in music and mathematics. She was confused about her identity and felt very anxious about failure and rejection. Race and culture became Jane's constant handicaps in her striving to achieve success and acceptance in a foreign country.

Conclusions

All three ESL children displayed some behavioral problems. The two boys were defiant and did poorly at school. The girl did well in school, but suffered from high anxiety and resorted to plagiarism. But there was a common thread in their difficulties — acculturative stress. Many of their problems can be traced to their recent immigration status and the crises within their racial identity development.

Their parents' adherence to the traditional Chinese culture created an intense inner conflict in them at school. Bill was able to become assimilated with his Caucasian classmates, but by adopting their values of freedom and independence, he had to rebel against his own father. T. J. clung to the traditional Chinese culture and was completely isolated at school. Jane wanted to be like her Caucasian classmates, but she could not free herself from her traditional Chinese values. Their experiences of racism (such as teasing) only exacerbated their feelings of isolation and alienation.

Their difficulty with English, coupled with high parental expectations, further contributed to their stress, frustration, and anxiety. The two boys coped with their acculturative stress by acting out and becoming openly rebellious. The girl coped with her stress by trying desperately to please her parents.

For all three participants, almost all of their problems at school may be attributed in some way to their difficulties in adjusting to the host culture.

In order to achieve multicultural competencies in assessment and counseling there is an urgent need to understand the effects of acculturation and racial identity development (Dana, 1993; Lee, 1996; Lonner & Ibrahim, 1996; Paniagua, 1994).

A number of psychologists have proposed ways to assess acculturation (e.g., Armour-Thomas & Gopaul-McNicol, 1998), but they tend to rely on interviewing parents and teachers. The present study has demonstrated the Validationgram and PMP-C can be effectively used to reveal the inner struggles of ESL children and the deeper meanings of their behavior problems.

On a more positive note, in spite of their difficulties at home and in school, there was within each child an indomitable spirit of resilience. For T. J. and Bill, their acting out was their way of defining and defending their emerging selfhood in the throes of clashing cultures. For Jane, her quiet determination to excel despite her language handicap was her way of proving her self-worth.

These three children are in essence telling us: "We value love, relationship, achievement, fairness; we want to help others and we value belief in God. We accept our failings, but we will never give up trying to improve ourselves. These are our positive inner resources. Right now, we are unhappy, because we are torn between two cultures. We are unhappy, because we look different from our classmates, and we don't know who we are. Please understand our struggles and help us!"

We have demonstrated that a meaning-centered approach to assessment and counseling can increase our understanding of how ESL children adjust to the challenges of growing up in a host culture. We also hope that this chapter will stimulate more research on children's acculturative stress and the multicultural issues in counseling and assessment. "The world is increasingly becoming one global village. More and more, the industrial nations of the world will face the need to absorb immigrants into the economic, social, and industrial fabric. If we are to optimize the potential of all individuals, we must find the ways and means of identifying and cultivating the capabilities of all individuals, regardless of their origin or background" (Samuda, 1998, p. 19).

References

Armour-Thomas, E. & Gopaul-McNicol, S. (1998). *Assessing intelligence: Applying a bio-cultural model*. Thousand Oaks, CA: Sage Publications.

Berry, J. W. (1990). Psychology of acculturation. *Nebraska Symposium on Motivation, 37*, 201-234.

Berry, J. W., & Annis, R. C. (1974). Acculturative stress: The role of ecology, culture, and differentiation. *Journal of Cross-Cultural Psychology, 5*, 382-405.

Dana, R. H. (1993). *Multicultural assessment perspectives for professional psychology*. Boston: Allyn & Bacon.

Herring, R. D. (1997). *Multicultural counseling in schools: A synergetic approach.* Alexandria, VA: American Counseling Association.

Ibrahim, F. A. (1993). Existential worldview theory: Transcultural applications. In J. McFadden (Ed.), *Transcultural counseling: Bilateral and international perspectives* (pp. 23-58). Alexandria, VA: American Counseling Association Press.

Ibrahim, F. A., Ohnishi, H., & Wilson, R. P. (1994). Career assessment in a culturally diverse society. *Journal of Career Assessment, 2*, 276-288.

Ishiyama, F. I. (1989). Understanding foreign adolescents: Difficulties in cross-cultural adjustment: A Self-Validation model. *Canadian Journal of School Psychology, 5*, 41-56.

Ishiyama, F. I. (1995a). Use of validationgram in counseling: Exploring sources of self-validation and impact of personal transition. *Canadian Journal of Counseling, 29*, 134-146.

Ishiyama, F. I. (1995b). Culturally dislocated clients: Self-validation and cultural conflict issues and counseling implications. *Canadian Journal of Counseling, 29*, 263-275.

Ivey, A. E., & Ivey, M. B. (1999, February). Integrating cultural and contextual issues into the interview: The community genogram. *Counseling Today*, pp. 38, 40.

Lee, C. C. (1995). *Counseling for diversity: A guide for school counselors and related professionals*. Boston: Allyn & Bacon.

Leong, F. T. L., & Chou, E. L. (1996). Counseling international students. In P. B. Pedersen, J. G. Draguns, W. J. Lonner, & J. E. Trimble (Eds.). *Counseling across cultures* (4th ed.) pp. 210-242. Thousand Oaks, CA: Sage.

Lewis, J. E. (1998). In R. J. Samuda, R. Feuerstein, A. S. Kaufman, J. E. Lewis, R. J. Sternberg, & Associates. (1998). *Advances in cross-cultural assessment (*pp. 218-241). Thousand Oaks, CA: Sage.

Lonner, W. J., & Berry, J. W. (Eds.) (1986*) Field Methods in Cross-Cultural Research, Vol. 8.* Beverly Hills, CA: Sage.

Lonner, W. J., & Ibrahim, F. A. (1996). Appraisal and assessment in cross-cultural counseling. In P. B. Pedersen, J. G. Draguns, W. J. Lonner, & J. E. Trimble (Eds.). *Counseling across cultures* (4th ed.) pp. 293-322. Thousand Oaks, CA: Sage.

Mercer, J. R., & Lewis, J. F. (1978). *System of Multicultural Pluralistic Assessment.* San Antonio, TX: The Psychological Corporation.

Paniagua, F. A. (1994). *Assessing and treating culturally diverse groups: A practical guide*. Newbury Park, CA: Sage.

Pedersen, P. B. (1991). Counseling international students. *The Counseling Psychologist, 19*, 10-58.

Samuda, R. J. (1998). Cross-cultural assessment: Issues and alternatives. In R. J. Samuda, R. Feuerstein, S. Kaufman, J. E. Lewis, R. J. Sternberg, & Associates. *Advances in cross-cultural assessment* (pp. 1-19). Thousand Oaks, CA: Sage.

Schram, J. L., & Lauver, P. J. (1988). Alienation in international students. *Journal of College Student Development, 29*, 146-150.

Sue, S. (1996). Measurement, testing, and ethnic bias: Can solutions be found? In G. R. Sodowsky & J. Impara (Eds.). *Multicultural assessment in counseling and clinical psychology (pp. 7-36)*. Lincoln, NE: Buros Institute of Mental Measurement, University of Nebraska-Lincoln.

Weswood, M. J., & Lawrence, S. (1990). Uprooted: Towards a counselor understanding of the refugee experience. *International Journal for the Advancement of Counseling, 13*, 145-153.

Wong, P. T. P. (1998). Implicit Theories of Meaning and the Personal Meaning Profile. In P. T. P. Wong & P. Fry (Eds.), *The human quest for meaning: Handbook of psychological research and clinical applications*. New Jersey, NY: Lawrence Erlbaum.

Perspectives on Work and Organizational Factors

Culture and Organizational Differences

Pieter J.D. Drenth
Vrije Universiteit
Amsterdam, The Netherlands.

Deanne N. Den Hartog
Vrije Universiteit
Amsterdam, The Netherlands.

ABSTRACT

Cross-cultural organizational psychology is concerned with two basic questions: First, do organizations located in different countries differ with respect to organizational characteristics, behavior of members or the interrelationship between these two, and, second, can these differences be explained in terms of culture? Increasing globalization and internationalization characterize today and tomorrow in the industrial world. An intriguing question in cross-cultural organizational psychology is whether this internationalization leads to a more common organizational culture world wide, in other words, to increased convergence? The position argued here is that although organizational structures and strategies may converge, organizational practices and the way these are worked out, perceived, and appreciated across countries, are still quite dissimilar. Research from the GLOBE study on leadership is described as an example. This research shows that although attributes associated with charismatic leadership are universally valued, this does not imply similar enactment of such characteristics across cultures. In general terms, internationalization does induce convergence of certain organizational characteristics. However, looking more specifically at behavior and processes reveals many cultural specific qualities and ways of enactment of such characteristics.

Internationalization is a keyword in present-day marketing, business strategy and corporate planning. Competition and cooperation have become international and this is not restricted to multinationals or only specific sectors of the economy. Recent political developments, such as the opening of the countries in Central and Eastern Europe, the growing unification of Europe and the increasing rate of migration of workers from countries with poor living conditions or repressive political regimes, will further reinforce this tendency towards globalization and internationalization of the industrial world of today.

Reactions of organization members seem to be somewhat paradoxical. On the one hand we see a strong corporate identification (I am an IBMer, I am a Shell man), and on the other hand it is striking that, according to a study of Laurent (1983), British, French and German managers working for an American multinational firm were--in terms of their expressed values and their behavior--more British, French and German than their respective compatriots working for domestic firms. Moreover, in the hype of internationalization we should not forget the failures of international merges, in all likelihood because extremely strong cultural differences could not be resolved or overcome. The Dutch-German mergers Fokker and Daimler, and Hoogovens and Hoechst, and the Anglo-French merger Metal Box Company and Carnaud are cases in point.

An intriguing question is, therefore, whether this internationalization also leads to a more common organizational culture worldwide. We see McDonalds, Coca Cola, and Holiday Inns everywhere around the globe. There is worldwide use of Microsoft, Euro-Mastercards, Philishaves and Volkswagens, and the scientific/technological innovations developed in Japan or Korea need little time to travel to the rest of the world. But does that also mean that organizations in different cultures will more and more look alike, and that the cultural factors are indeed negligible or of dwindling importance in the light of the dominant economic and technological factors that seem to force organizations to converge? Or do we have to recognize that organizational structures and strategies may converge but that organizational practices, and the way these are worked out and also perceived and appreciated, are still quite dissimilar across countries?

Companies in different cultures increasingly appreciate the importance of valid selection procedures. However, as a survey by Shackleton and Newell (1991) shows, in the UK more emphasis is put on objective testing, references and group-interview, whereas in France more attention is given to personality assessment and one-to-one interviews. Obviously, in the UK, more importance is attached to an objective estimate of the person-task fit, and in France to the ability to function successfully in hierarchical networks and webs of relations. In Japan, the objective of performance appraisal is to encourage teamwork, whereas in most Western companies its objective is to stimulate better performance and achievement (Hoecklin, 1994). Most companies nowadays employ some form of a career development plan, but the way this plan is realized differs extensively across countries, depending on what individuals in different cultures expect and want from their career (Laurent & Derr, 1989). Erez (1994) has repeatedly shown that the same measure in the area of Human Resource Management is interpreted differently and has different effects in different cultural contexts.

The same objects, concepts or measures may have a different meaning in different cultures. A mobile phone in Jakarta may be a symbol of importance, in London an instrument to inform a client that one is delayed for a meeting due to traffic problems. Dining in McDonalds in Beijing may indicate status, in Washington that one only has time for a fast bite. Organizational concepts, such as participation, control, cooperation and trust may not mean the same in different cultures. In the West participation usually refers to having influence on the outcome of a decision by taking part in it in one form or another (Heller et al., 1988). On Java, the concept refers to a cooperative form of decision-making; in Japan to the consensus oriented approach through the bottom-up procedures and lobby-consultations of the ringi-system (Heller & Misumi, 1987). It may very well be that behind the same word a world of different connotations, perceptions, and attitudes lies hidden.

The discussion indicated in the previous paragraph can be seen as an alternative reading of the well-known "convergence hypothesis". This hypothesis was initiated by Kerr and his collaborators at the Harvard University in the early 60"s (Kerr, et al. 1960), and has been described extensively in the literature (e.g., Child & Kieser, 1979; Cole, 1973; Dore, 1972; Form, 1979; Kerr et al., 1964; Kerr, 1983; Lammers, 1983; Maurice, 1979; Neghandi, 1979; Pascale, 1978; Pugh, Clark & Mallory, 1996; Ronen, 1986). This hypothesis surmises that organizations in many different countries increasingly resemble one another, as factors such as increasing industrialization, technological developments, communication and information means, education and general standards of living all seem to converge, whereas the importance of factors that would have a diverging effect, such as differences in natural resources, development level, demographic constitution and specific cultural factors is decreasing. National cultural factors are seen as having an important conservative influence, but their impact on organizations is supposed to diminish in the light of the technological and economic dominance.

A few critical remarks can made with respect to the convergence hypothesis (see also Drenth & Groenendijk, 1998). First, it is not always clear which characteristics are concerned in the discussion on convergence. Kerr (1983) distinguishes between, on the one hand, highly abstract and aggregated categories of production and consumption, involving pragmatic, adaptive solutions (knowledge, mobilization of production factors, organization of production, work, lifestyle and pay), showing broad convergence in East and West European countries, and on the other, continuing heterogeneity with respect to concrete variables such as attitudes, feelings and emotions, linked to pre-industrial beliefs and behaviors. Between these extremes, we find mixed results with respect to economic and political structures in organizations, as they are influenced by elites. Therefore, it depends on the nature and the level of abstraction of the variables under consideration whether or not convergence can be observed.

Secondly, strictly speaking, the empirical substantiation of the convergence hypothesis in its full breadth is hard. The conception is based on the following premises: divergent cultural factors are weaker than convergent technological and economic factors, the latter have more influence on organizations than the former, this gradually leads to organizations coming to resemble one another. The second of these three premises comes close to the idea of the technological imperative or technological determinism. This, however, has been repeatedly criticized in the literature (Hickson et. al, 1969; Mohr, 1971; IDE, 1981; Lammers, 1983). Moreover, cross-sectional comparisons revealing similarities or dissimilarities in themselves do not show the quality of the convergence hypothesis. The needed systematic longitudinal studies are rare, and those that have been carried out (Fliegel et al., 1979; IDE, 1992) have not provided much support for the convergence hypothesis. Let us see to what extent the convergence hypothesis as a result of internationalization holds.

Cross Cultural Organizational Psychology

The previous discussion has brought us to the core theme of this paper: culture and organizational differences. It is also one of the central topics of cross cultural organizational psychology. Cross cultural organizational psychology is concerned with two basic questions: First, do organizations located in different countries differ with respect to organizational characteristics, behavior of members or the interrelationship between these two? Second, can these differences be explained in terms of culture?

In order to answer both questions it is not enough to investigate whether organizations differ cross-nationally. The problem is that not all national differences can be considered cultural differences, in spite of the fact that these two words often are used synonymously. Nations may differ in language, legislation, education, religion, geography, climate as well as on economical, technological, and many other variables. These may be related to culture but cannot be equated with it (Drenth, 1996). Even worse is the approach to define culture as everything that cannot be explained through other identified factors: culture as residual, as rest factor in the black box. Culture should be defined on basis of a reasoned choice. We will follow Kroeber and Parson (1958), who reformulate Kluckhohn"s classical definition a bit more sharply as "patterns of roles and norms embedded in certain paramount values."

A practical and methodological difficulty presents itself in attempts to measure culture. Of course, this could be done in terms of rules of behavior, traditions and institutionalized roles. However, both culture and the dependent variable "organizational behavior and attitudes" are often measured using questionnaires, attitude and value scales. The bulk of cross-cultural studies in organizational psychology is concerned with attitudes, values, needs and expectations of organization members (see Haire et al., 1966; Hofstede, 1980; MOW, 1981; Ronen & Shenkar, 1985). The question whether the differences found really reflect cultural differences runs the risk of becoming tautological, since both are measured with comparable, or even identical questions.

There are two ways to avoid this problem (Drenth & Groenendijk, 1998). First, culture can be defined, as was indicated above, in macro-level terms, such as religious preferences, political traditions, customs and conventions, educational level, and can thus be distinguished from individual attitudes, opinions and values at the micro-level (Ajiferuke & Boddewijn, 1970). Second, culture could be measured at the individual level, but then a clear choice should be made which type of attitudes, norms or opinions are to be considered as "culture," and which are not. For the former, one could accept the rule that they (a) are relatively stable over time, and (b) will provide a more comprehensive description and explanation of behavior and attitudes in different situations.

The relevant literature reveals that a number of cultural dimensions have shown their usefulness and relevance in understanding national and cultural differences in behavior and attitudes in organizations. Without claiming completeness and indisputableness, an analysis in terms of explanatory power or organizational effects suggests the following cultural dimensions to be relevant for understanding cross-cultural differences in organizations (Hofstede, 1984, 1991; House et al., 1999; Inglehart, 1997; Schwartz & Sagiv, 1995; Triandis, 1994; Trompenaars, 1993; Van Leest, 1997):

1. Collectivism versus individualism (is primary concern in life in oneself and immediate family or in wider groups to which one belongs);
2. Egalitarianism versus power distance (should power be distributed equally or unequally in society and organizations);
3. Uncertainty avoidance (do people feel threatened by ambiguous situations and are they trying to avoid uncertainty through beliefs and rules or not);
4. Masculine control versus harmony (rational and power control of people and environment versus harmonious and affective relations with other people and nature);
5. Universalism versus particularism (can what is good and true be defined and applied everywhere, or do unique conditions and relationships always have to be taken into consideration in order to determine what is good and true);
6. Discipline versus individual autonomy (soberness and adherence to moral values versus an emphasis on intellectual and moral independence);
7. Neutral versus affective relationships (the extent to which culture allows people to express their emotions or forces them to keep their emotions and affections under strict control);
8. Achievement versus ascription (are people evaluated by their functional performance or by their roles, status or formal characteristics);
9. Materialism versus post-materialism (emphasis on economic goals and financial rewards versus aiming at a much broader defined well-being objective and non-material values).

10. Future orientation (the extent to which the (not immediate) future is an important orientation in the choice of behavior and decision making).

An interesting question is how these cultural dimensions exert influence on organizational behavior; via formal characteristics or via the individual attitudes, values and behavior of the organization members? Drenth (1996) describes that there is not much evidence for a direct influence of culture on formal organizational characteristics. He suggests focusing on an organizational concept closer to the level of behavior of the people in organizations, which is also, through the (culturally determined) attitudes and values of the latter, more closely linked to culturally connected variables. This is what may be called "organizational processes" (see Aiken & Bacharach, 1979; Smith & Tayeb, 1988). Organizational processes should be distinguished from employee attitudes, the former being objectively observable processes, and the latter referring to what goes on in people"s heads. Organizational processes are also distinct from formal organizational characteristics, the latter describe a "formal prescribed set of roles and rules," the former what actually takes place.

The Case of Leadership

One of the most obvious and clear examples of cultural contextualization of general principles can be found in the area of leadership. On the one hand, leadership is an instrument of management, a system of control and influence, and the aforementioned equalization or convergence of organizations may also apply to this aspect of the organization"s control system. On the other hand, a leader-subordinate or leader-group relationship is a thoroughly interpersonal and social phenomenon, and therefore, deeply embedded in the social and cultural environment. It is difficult to envision how attempts to influence or stimulate (groups of) workers could be abstracted from this cultural context. Anecdotal evidence on leader behavior in different countries, as well as cross-cultural studies, into the phenomenon of "organizational leadership" show its cultural boundedness.

Yukl (1998) points out that most research on leadership during the past half century was conducted in the United States, Canada and Western Europe. Peterson and Hunt (1997) note that the frequent use of the labels "leader" and "leadership" and their many connotations are distinctly American. However, they also hold that, when taken more broadly, the interest in how powerful parties conduct themselves is not narrowly American. Hofstede (1993) states that US management theories contain several idiosyncrasies not necessarily shared by management elsewhere, for example, a stress on market processes, a stress on the individual, and a focus on managers rather than workers. Similarly, House (1995) notes that almost all prevailing theories of leadership and most empirical evidence is rather North American in character, that is, "individualistic rather than collectivistic; emphasizing assumptions of rationality rather than ascetics, religion, or superstition; stated in terms of individual rather than group incentives, stressing follower responsibilities rather than rights; assuming hedonistic rather than altruistic motivation and assuming centrality of work and democratic value orientation" (p. 443). Many cultures do not share these assumptions. "As a result there is a growing awareness of the need for a better understanding of the way in which leadership is enacted in various cultures and a need for an empirically grounded theory to explain differential leader behavior and effectiveness across cultures" (House, 1995, pp. 443-444). However, developing such an "empirically grounded theory" faces a multitude of problems.

One such problem relates to possible cross-cultural differences in the meaning of concepts mentioned earlier. Even the term "leadership" itself is interpreted differently across cultures. "Leader" and "leadership" have a positive connotation in Anglo-Saxon countries, conjuring up heroic images of outstanding individuals. Meindl's work on the "romance of leadership" shows the American "romantic" attachment to and overestimated importance of the leadership role (e.g. Meindl, Ehrlich & Dukerich, 1985; Meindl, 1990). However, the direct translation of leader to German is "Führer". Obviously, the historically laden connotation of this term is far more negative. In some other countries the word leader brings to bear images of recent dictatorship. In such countries, the term "manager" rather than "leader" often takes on the positive connotation "leader" has in English. Such examples show that obtaining a similar meaning of words, even through careful translation, can not be taken for granted. This poses obvious measurement problems - how can we be sure we are even measuring the same construct and if we are not, to what should found differences be attributed - and remains an area of concern in cross-cultural (leadership) research.

Culture dimensions (e.g. power distance, individualism-collectivism) yield many hypotheses regarding cross-cultural differences in leadership. For example, high uncertainty avoidance, with the resulting emphasis on rules, procedures and traditions may place other demands on leaders than low uncertainty avoidance, with the resulting attitude of tolerance of ambiguity and innovative behavior. More "masculine" cultures are probably more tolerant of strong, directive leaders than harmony oriented or "feminine" cultures, where a preference for more consultative, considerate leaders seems more likely (Den Hartog et al., 1999).

An interesting example of studying such cross-cultural aspects of leadership is the on-going work on event management, which presents an analysis of role relationships putting the role of leaders in the context of other sources of meaning (e.g., Smith & Peterson, 1988; Smith, Peterson & Misumi, 1994). In handling events, managers can use different sources of information and meaning (e.g., rules, national norms, superiors, peers, subordinates). Among other things, Smith et al. (1994) show that managers in high power distance countries report more use of rules and procedures than do managers from low power distance countries.

Charismatic Leadership: Universally Valued or Locally Applicable?

Much leadership research over the last decade has focused on charismatic, transformational, inspirational or visionary leadership (e.g., Yukl, 1998). The charismatic/transformational leader "articulates a realistic vision of the future that can be shared, stimulates subordinates intellectually, and pays attention to the differences among the subordinates" (Yammarino & Bass, 1990, p. 151). Such leaders broaden and elevate the interests of followers, generate awareness and acceptance among the followers of the purposes and mission of the group, and motivate followers to go beyond their self-interests for the good of the group (e.g., Bass, 1985; Bass & Avolio, 1989; Den Hartog, Van Muijen & Koopman, 1997; Yukl, 1998).

Recent research focuses on whether charisma is universally endorsed and valued or whether charismatic/transformational leadership is only likely to emerge and be effective in certain societies (Bass, 1997; Den Hartog et al., 1999). Following from the observation that managerial practices and motivational techniques that are legitimate and acceptable in one culture (or time period) may not be in another (Erez, 1994), one proposition is that differences in national culture influence the emergence and effectiveness of charismatic leaders. That is, charismatics will "appear in societies with traditions of support for them and expectations about their emergence" (Bass, 1990a, p. 196).

A contrasting and perhaps more controversial proposition is that (a preference for) such leadership may - to a certain extent - be universal (Bass, 1997). Transformational/charismatic leadership has been shown to meaningfully exist and correlate positively with different outcomes in countries as diverse as The United States, Canada, Japan, Taiwan, India, The Netherlands and Austria (Bass, 1997). Also, Bass and Avolio (1989) show that attributes respondents associate with their "ideal" leader are highly correlated with transformational leadership. This was also found in New Zealand and Taiwan (Singer & Singer, 1990). A large-scale study into cultural differences and similarities in implicit theories of (effective) leadership (the GLOBE study, House et al., 1999) offered an excellent opportunity to test these opposing propositions. In the next section we will briefly describe this cross-national study.

The GLOBE Study

Although different cross-cultural research projects take leadership into account, Global Leadership and Organizational Behavior Effectiveness (GLOBE) Research Program is the largest project of its kind to date. Robert House conceived the idea for a global research program concerned with leadership and organizational practices in the summer of 1991. Since then,

GLOBE has evolved into a multi-phase, multi-method study in which some 170 investigators from over 60 cultures representing all major regions in the world collaborate to examine the inter-relationships between societal culture, organizational culture and practices, and organizational leadership. For a detailed overview of GLOBE, including its objectives, hypotheses and methods (House et al., 1999).

The initial aim of the GLOBE project was to develop societal and organizational measures of culture and leadership attributes that are appropriate to use across cultures. This was accomplished in the first phase of the project (Hanges et al., under review). The second phase entails gathering data on and testing of hypotheses concerning relationships between societal culture dimensions, organizational culture dimensions and culturally-endorsed implicit leadership theories as well as relationships specified by structural contingency theory of organizations (e.g., Donaldson, 1995). Data collection in this second phase is now completed and the analyses to test the hypotheses are currently being conducted.

Den Hartog et al. (1999) use findings from the GLOBE research on culturally endorsed implicit theories of leadership to test the hypothesis that charismatic/transformational leadership attributes will be universally endorsed as contributing to outstanding leadership. Results show that this is indeed the case. Such attributes include foresight, encouraging, communicative, trustworthy, dynamic, positive, confidence builder, and motivational. Several other charismatic attributes, including enthusiastic, risk taking, ambitious, self-effacing, unique, sincere, sensitive, and compassionate, are culturally contingent. None of the items universally perceived as impediments to outstanding leadership describe transformational/charismatic leadership.

Such evidence regarding "universality" is by no means meant to imply that there are no marked differences across cultures in the expression of such transformational/charismatic attributes. Bass (1997) holds that in the case of transformational leadership "universal" means a universally applicable conceptualization, which does not preclude the cultural boundedness of the specific behaviors indicative of this style. For example, Bass (1997) states that "Indonesian inspirational leaders need to persuade their followers about the leaders' own competence, a behavior that would appear unseemly in Japan" (p. 132). However, according to Bass, not withstanding the fact that it can be expressed in different ways, the concept of inspiration appears "to be as universal as the concept of leadership itself" (p. 132).

Similar examples of enacting positively valued attributes in a different manner in different countries ensue from the GLOBE research. Martinez and Dorfman (1998) gathered GLOBE data in Mexico. An example of behavior that was highly valued by the Mexicans, but might not be appropriate in other contexts was a high degree of involvement of a leader in the private lives of his employees. An example from their interviews is a leader calling the doctor when the husband of an employee was in hospital to make sure an operation was legitimate. However, such a behavior would be felt to be an invasion of privacy in other countries. Such examples clearly show that the behaviors indicative of consideration or compassion will differ strongly in different cultures even if the positive evaluation of the construct "consideration" in itself is found across different cultures (see Den Hartog et al., 1999). In terms of the convergence hypotheses this seems to imply that although demands on managers in different countries may increasingly converge, the appropriate and effective behaviors and ways of interacting needed in order to meet such demands remain markedly different.

Conclusions

As was stated earlier, cross cultural psychology is concerned with two basic questions: 1. Do organizations in different countries differ with respect to organizational characteristics, the behavior of their members or the interrelationships between the two? and, 2. If so, can these differences be explained in terms of culture?

Regarding organizational leadership, the tentative answer to both questions is affirmative. Although the GLOBE study reports both culturally contingent characteristics (e.g., ambitious, risk taking) and universally valued leadership characteristics (e.g., foresight, communicative), neither the universal nor the culturally contingent positive evaluation of characteristics implies similar enactment of such characteristics across cultures. Behaviors that indicate consideration in one country may be taken as an invasion of subordinates" privacy elsewhere. Visions can be communicated in an aggressive, flamboyant tone or in a rather more soft-spoken manner. Not only is "risk taking" valued is some but not in other cultures, behavior that is (perceived as) risk taking in one culture may not be in another (Den Hartog et al., 1999).

More research is obviously needed in this area. Especially in determining to which extent found differences are indeed due to culture rather than to other (related) national differences. However, there are many indications that cultural differences strongly influence the demands placed on leaders and the meaning specific behaviors take on. A good example is leadership in egalitarian societies versus societies with high power distance. The GLOBE study and other studies show that in some countries, a high value is placed on egalitarianism. This is reflected in the demands placed on leaders within the society. Although Bass (1996) insists that transformational leadership can take more as well as less participative forms, the latter may not be as acceptable in egalitarian societies. The Dutch, for instance, emphasize consensus and acceptance of visions by lower level employees (Thierry, Den Hartog, Koopan & Wilderom, 1999). Research on transformational leader behavior shows that, in the Netherlands, consultation or participative leadership can be seen as a component of transformational leadership (Den Hartog, 1997). Similarly, Ashkenasy and Falkus (1998), state that studies on transformational leadership in Australia suggest it is somewhat distinct from its American counterpart, based on the ubiquitous value placed on egalitarianism by Australians (Feather, 1994). Although transformational leadership is found to be effective and valued in both countries, the pervasive sense of egalitarianism places demands on the enactment of such leadership.

A general conclusion may be that internationalization does induce a convergence of certain organizational characteristics. But if one looks more specifically at the behaviors and organizational processes one discerns many cultural specific qualities and ways of enactment.

References

Aiken, M. & Bachara, S.B. (1979). Culture and organizational structure and process: a comparative study of local government administrative bureaucracies in the Walloon and Flemish regionsof Belgium. In C.J. Lammers & D.J. Hickson (Eds.), *Organizations alike and unlike*. London: Routledge & Kegan Paul.

Ajiferuke, M. & Boddewijn, J. (1970). Socio-economic indicators in comparative management.*Administrative Science Quarterly, 15*, 453-458.

Ashkenasy, N.M. & Falkus, S. (1999) The Australian Enigma. In R.J. House & J. Chhokar (Eds.). *Cultures of the world, A GLOBE anthology of in-depth descriptions of the cultures of 14 countries* (Vol. 1).

Bass, B.M. & Avolio, B.J. (1989). Potential biases in leadership measures: How prototypes, leniency and general satisfaction relate to ratings and rankings of transformational and transactional leadership constructs. *Educational and Psychological Measurement, 49*, 509-527.

Bass, B.M. (1985). *Leadership and performance beyond expectations*. New York: Free Press.

Bass, B.M. (1990a). *Handbook of leadership: Theory, research and managerial applications*, (3rd ed.). New York: Free Press.

Bass, B.M. (1990b). Editorial: Toward a meeting of minds. *Leadership Quarterly*, 1.

Bass, B.M. (1996). A new paradigm of leadership: An inquiry into transformational leadership. Alexandria, VA: U.S. Army Research Institute for the Behavioral and Social Sciences.

Bass, B.M. (1997). Does the transactional - transformational paradigm transcend organizational and national boundaries? *American Psychologist, 52*(2), 130-139.

Child, J. & Kieser, A. (1979). Organization and managerial roles in British and West Germancompanies: an examination of the culture-free thesis. In C.J. Lammers & D.J. Hickson, (Eds.), *Organizations alike and unlike*. London: Routledge & Kegan Paul.

Cole, R.E. (1973). Functional alternatives and economic development: An empirical example of permanent employment in Japan. *American Sociological Review, 38*, 424-438.

Den Hartog, D.N. (1997). *Inspirational leadership*. Vrije Universiteit Amsterdam. KLI doctoral dissertations series, 1997 - nr 2. Enschede: Ipskamp.

Den Hartog, D.N., House, R.J., Hanges, P.J., Dorfman, P.W., Ruiz-Quintanilla, S.A., & 170 co-authors (1999). Emics and etics of culturally-endorsed implicit leadership theories: are attributes of charismatic/transformational leadership universally endorsed. *Leadership Quarterly*, in press.

Den Hartog, D.N., Van Muijen, J.J. & Koopman, P.L. (1997). Transactional versus transformational leadership: An analysis of the MLQ. *Journal of Occupational and Organizational Psychology, 70*(1), 19-34.

Donaldson, L. (1995). *American anti-management theories of organization.* Cambridge: Cambridge University Press.

Dore, R. (1973). British factory - Japanese factory. London: Allen & Unwin.

Drenth, P.J.D. & Groenendijk, B. (1998). Organizational psychology in cross-cultural perspective.In P.J.D. Drenth, Hk. Thierry, & Ch.J.de Wolff (Eds.*), Handbook of work and organizational psychology* (Vol. III.). Hove: Psychology Press.

Drenth, P.J.D. (1996). "Cultures consequences" in organizations. In P.J.D. Drenth, P.L. Koopman, & B. Wilpert (Eds.*), Organizational decision-making under different economic and political conditions.* Amsterdam: North-Holland.

Erez, M. (1994). Toward a model of cross-cultural industrial and organizational psychology. In H.C. Triandis, M.D. Dunette & L.M. Hough (eds*). Handbook of industrial and organizational psychology* (2nd ed., Vol. 4), 559-607. Palo Alto, CA: Consulting Psychologists Press.

Feather, N.T. (1994). Attitudes towards high achievers and reactions to their fall: Theory and research concerning tall poppies. In M.P. Zanna (Ed.) *Advances in social psychology* (Vol. 26, pp. 1-73). New York: Academic Press.

Fliegel, F., Sofranko, A.J., Williams, J.D., & Navin, C.S. (1979). Technology and cultural convergence: A limited empirical test. *Journal of Cross-Cultural Psychology, 10*, 3-22.

Form, W. (1979). Comparative industrial sociology and the convergence hypothesis. Annual Review of Sociology, 5, 1-25.

Haire, M., Ghiselli, E.E. & Porter, L.W. (1996). *Managerial thinking: An international study.* New York: Wiley.

Heller, F.A. & Misumi, J. (1987). Decision making. In B.M. Bass & P.J., D. Drenth (Eds). *Advances in organizational psychology*. Newbury Park, CA: Sage.

Heller, F.A., Drenth, P.J.D., Koopman, P.L. & Rus, V. (1988*). Decisions in organizations: A three country comparative study*. London: Sage.

Hickson, D.J., Pugh, D.D., & Pheysey, C. (1969). Operations technology and organizational structure: An empirical reappraisal. *Adm. Science Quartely, 14*, 378-379.

Hoecklin, L. (1994). *Managing cultural differences.* Wokingham: Addison-Wesley.

Hofstede G. (1993). Cultural constraints in management theories. *Academy of Management Executive, 7*(1), 81-94.

Hofstede, G. (1980). *Culture's consequences: International differences in work-related values.* Beverly Hills, CA: Sage.

Hofstede, G. (1991). *Cultures and organizating: Software of the mind.* London: McGraw-Hill House, R.J. (1995). Leadership in the 21st century: A speculative enquiry. In A. Howard (Ed.) *The changing nature of work.* San Francisco: Jossey Bass.

House, R.J., Hanges, P.J., Ruiz-Quintanilla, S.A., Dorfman, P.W., Javidan, M., Dickson, M., Gupta, V. & 170 co-authors (1999). Cultural influences on leadership and organizations: Project GLOBE. In W.Mobley (Ed.) *Advances in global leadership* (Vol.1). JAI Press, in press.

House, R.J., Wright, N.S. & Aditya, R.N. (1997). Cross-cultural research on organizational leadership: A critical analysis and a proposed theory. In P.C. Early & M. Erez (Eds.) *New perspectives on international industrial/organizational psychology.* San Francisco: The New Lexington Press.

IDE-International Research Group (1981a). *Industrial democracy in Europe.* Oxford: Oxford University Press.

IDE-International Research Group (1981b). *Industrial relations in Europe.* Oxford: Oxford University Press.

IDE-International Research Group (1992). *Industrial democracy in Europe revisited.* Oxford: Oxford University Press.

Inglehart, R. (1997). *Modernization and post-modernization. Princeton.* Princeton UniversityPress.

Kerr, C. (1983). *The future of industrial societies: Convergence or continuing diversity.* Cambridge, MA: Harvard University Press.

Kerr, C., Dunlop, J.T., Harbison, F. & Myers, C.A. (1964). *Industrialism and industrial man.* New York: Oxford University Press.

Koopman, P.L. & B. Wilpert (Eds.), *Organizational decision-making under different economic and political conditions.* Amsterdam: North-Holland.

Kroeber, A.L. & Parsons, T. (1958). The concepts of culture and of a social systems. *American Sociological Review, 23*, 582-583.

Lammers, C.J. (1983). *Organisaties vergelijkenderwijs.* Utrecht: Spectrum. Laurent, & Derr, C.B. (1989). The internal and external career: a theoretical and cross-cultural perspective. In M. Arthus, D. Hall, & B. Lawrence (Eds). *Handbook of career theory.* Cambridge: Cambridge University Press.

Laurent, A. (1983). The cultural diversity of Western conceptions of management. International Studies of Management and Organizations, 13, 75-96.

Leest, P.F. van (1996). *Persoonlijkheidsmeting bij allochtonen.* Lisse: Swets & Zeitlinger.

Martinez, S. & Dorfman (1998, summer) The Mexican Entrepreneur: An ethnographic study of the Mexican empressario. *International Studies of Management and Organizations, 28*, 97-123.

Maurice, M. (1979). For a study of "the societal effect": Universality and specificity in Organization research. In C.J. Lammers & D.J. Hickson (Eds.), *Organizations alike and unlike.* London: Routledge & Kegan Paul.

Meindl, J.R. (1990). On leadership : An alternative to the conventional wisdom. *Research in Organizational Behavior, 12*, 159-203.

Meindl, J.R., Ehrlich, S.B. & Dukerich, J.M. (1985). The romance of leadership. *Administrative Science Quarterly, 30,* 78-102.

Mohr, L.B. (1971). Organizational technology and organizational structure. *Administrative Science Quartely, 16*, 444-459.

MOW International Reserach Team (1987). *The meaning of working*. London: Academic Press.

Negandhi, A.R. (1979). Convergence in organizational practices: An empirical study of industrial enterprise in developing countries. In C.J. Lammers & D.J. Hickson (Eds.), *Organizations alike and unlike.* London: Routledge & Kegan Paul.

Pascal, R.T. (1978). Communication and decision-making across cultures: Japanese and American comparison. *Administrative Science Quartely, 23*, 91-110.

Peterson, M.F. & Hunt, J.G. (1997). International perspectives on international leadership. *Leadership Quarterly, 8*(3), 203-231.

Pugh, D., Clark, T. & Mallory, G. (1996). Organization structure and structural change in European manufacturing organizations. In P.J.D. Drenth, P.L.

Ronen, S. & Shenkar, O. (1985). Clustering countries on attitudinal dimensions: A review and synthesis. *Academy of Management Review, 10*, 435-454.

Ronen, S. (1986). *Comparative and multinational management*. New York: Wiley.

Schwartz, S.H. & Sagiv, L. (1995). Identifying culture-specifics in the content and structure of values. *Journal of Cross-Cultural Psychology, 26*, 92-116.

Shackleton, V.U. & Newell, S. (1991). Management selection: a comparative survey of methods used in top British and French companies. *Journal of Occupational Psychology, 64*, 23-36.

Singer, M.S. & Singer, A.E. (1990). Situational constraints on transformational versus transactional leadership behavior, subordinates" leadership preference, and satisfaction. *Journal of Social Psychology, 130*(3), 385-396.

Smith, P.B. & Peterson, M.F. (1988). *Leadership, organizations and culture*. London: Sage.

Smith, P.B. & Tayeb, M. (1988). Organizational structure and processes. In M.H. Bond (Ed.). *The cross-cultural challenge to social psychology.* Newbury Park, CA: Sage.

Smith, P.B., Peterson M.F. & Misumi, J. (1994). Event management and work team effectiveness in Japan, Britain and the USA. *Journal of Occupational and Organizational Psychology, 67*, 33-43.

Thierry, H., Den Hartog, D.N., Koopman, P.L. & Wilderom, C.P.M. (1997) Culture and leadership in a flat country: The case of the Netherlands. In R.J. House & J. Chhokar (Eds.). Cultures of the world: A GLOBE anthology of in-depth descriptions of the cultures of 14 *countries*, (Vol. 1).

Triandis, H. (1994). *Culture and social behavior*. New York: McGraw Hill.

Trompenaars, F. (1993). *Riding the waves of culture*. London: The Economist Books.

Yammarino, F.J. & Bass, B.M. (1990). Long-term forecasting of transformational leadership and its effects among naval officers: some preliminary findings. In K.E. Clark & M.B. Clark (Eds.), *Measures of leadership* (pp.151-170). West Orange, NJ: Leadership Library of America.

Yukl, G. (1998). *Leadership in organizations*. (4th ed.). Englewood Cliffs, NJ: Prentice-Hall.

A Cross-Cultural Investigation into Three Measures of Work Orientation

Adriaan M. Viviers
University of South Africa
Department of Industrial Psychology

ABSTRACT

The construct Work Orientation comprises three different concepts - organizational commitment, job satisfaction and job involvement. The aim of this research is to investigate the potential relationship between the three concepts and establish whether an optimal orientation pertains to different cultural groups in South Africa. The hypothesis states that the concepts correlated, representing a Work Orientation construct which manifested itself differently within the two sub-samples, namely the White and the Black group. A set of measures, comprising the Organizational Commitment Questionnaire, Job Involvement Questionnaire and Job Descriptive Index, was distributed to 1,983 students. Of the larger sample, 934 students returned the questionnaire. Factor and reliability analyses were performed and invalid items rejected. All questionnaires were found suitable for further analyses. Spearman correlations were determined, followed by a structural analysis of latent variables. The results of the study show that the variables significantly correlated for both the White and the Black groups and manifested meaningfully within Work Orientation. The findings reflect an optimal Work Orientation among two cultural groups in South Africa.

The construct Work Orientation is not a formal theoretical concept generally found in Industrial/Organizational Psychology literature. It is rather a composite term referring to a variety of concepts. Work Orientation is described as an employee's optimal orientation towards work, based on positive feelings, perceptions and experiences gained through work related aspects of a particular job (Viviers, 1996). Work Orientation includes those aspects which allow for individual optimization through the expression of employee potential within the working environment and the personal growth as well as fulfilment an employee could experience through his/her work. Work Orientation reflects the positive perception of work and the desire of an employee to identify psychologically with a particular job.

An optimal orientation regarding work reflects the broader social and psychological meaning and value an employee attaches to a particular job. It is not only embedded in the employee's motivation to work per se, but how competently, according to his/her perception. Work provides the employee with an opportunity to utilize his/her potential/abilities/talents. It also allows the employee to experience a productive and optimal work existence, which in turn contributes to a sense of meaningful existence in a challenging and demanding world.

The construct refers to a salutogenic orientation (Antonovsky, 1979,1984,1993). Salutogenesis implies the omnipresence of stressors and the ability of man to survive and remain relatively healthy despite the bombardment of stressors. Optimization plays a vital role in this orientation. The construct Work Orientation can furthermore be linked to the construct *Fortigenesis* (Strümpfer, 1995), as both project an orientation towards optimization in the world of work. Fortigenesis can be seen as an extension of salutogenesis and is the dedicated attempt by an employee to utilize generalized resistance resources in order to handle work related stress. Strümpfer (1990:270) sees the employee, striving towards optimization, as:

- making cognitive sense of the workplace, perceiving its stimulation as clear, ordered, structured, consistent and as predictable information;
- perceiving his/her work as consisting of experiences that are bearable, with which (s)he can cope, and as challenges that (s)he can meet by availing him-/herself of personal resources or resources under the control of legitimate others; and
- making emotional and motivational sense of work demands, as welcome challenges, worthy of engagement and investment of his/her energies.

Work orientation concepts

Work Orientation, within the confines of this study, represents three concepts with theoretical underpinnings as in work done by Mowday, Steers and Porter (1979) - *Organizational Commitment*; Lodahl and Kejner (1965) - *Job Involvement*; and Smith, Kendall and Hulin (1969) - *Job Satisfaction.*

Strong organizational commitment is seen as the strength of an employee's identification with the organization. This manifests itself in terms of the employee's strong belief in and acceptance of the goals set and values upheld by the organization, a willingness to walk the extra mile in the interest of the organization and a definite desire to remain a member of the organization.

Job involvement is viewed as the extent to which an employee identifies with the job, the importance of the job in terms of self-image and the degree to which his/her achievements influence self-esteem.

Job satisfaction is viewed as the degree of satisfaction an employee experiences regarding a number of work related areas. These include satisfaction with colleagues, the work itself, supervision, remuneration and promotion opportunities.

A strong organizational commitment, active job involvement and high job satisfaction normally reflect an optimal orientation towards work and by implication life. Work is viewed in this regard as positive and meaningful with the possibility of self-actualization.

Objective

The objective of this investigation is to establish whether Work Orientation, as defined above, pertains to different cultural groups within South Africa. Due to the perception that various cultural groups perceive and view the world of work from a different paradigm namely, a modern Western commercial orientation versus a more traditional African approach, empirical evidence is required to verify this perception.

Method

Participants

Questionnaires were distributed to a total of 1, 983 Organizational Psychology students at the University of South Africa. Of the larger sample, 934 students returned the questionnaire. The sample was then divided into two working samples for the purpose of this research, namely a "Whites" group (*N*=731) and a "Black" group (*N*=203). The difference in sample sizes approximately reflects the proportional enrollments among white and black students (68.77% white students and 31.23% black students) for the course.

The age of the subjects ranged mostly between twenty and forty years (Whites = 82.3% and Blacks = 86.2%). Gender was more or less equally represented by males and females (Men = 53.68% and Women = 46.32%). All participants hold matriculation certificates (Grade12) and have passed the entry level course in Industrial/Organizational Psychology. As students enrolled at a distance teaching university (studying evenings and weekends), all respondents were simultaneously full-time employees within the various business enterprises/sectors of the South African labor market. All students were proficient in the languages used in the questionnaires, namely English and Afrikaans.

Measures

A set of measures comprising Mowday, Steers and Porter's (1979) *Organizational Commitment Questionnaire*, Lodahl and Kejner's (1965) *Job Involvement Questionnaire* and Smith, Kendall and Hulin's (1969) *Job Satisfaction Questionnaire*, was compiled.

Due to the heterogeneous cross-cultural nature of the sample (Whites and Blacks), factor and reliability analyses were performed on the measures and invalid items rejected. All questionnaires were found to be suitable for further analyses.

Hypothesis

The hypothesis is stated that organizational commitment, job involvement and job satisfaction are significantly correlated in representing a Work Orientation construct. The observed variables manifest themselves significantly differently within the two sub-samples. The assumption was that the factor loadings (parameter estimates) would be similar for both groups, but that the error variances would differ within the respective sub-samples. The expected difference between the error variances was ascribed to cross-cultural differences between the groups.

Statistical analyses

Spearman correlations (SAS program) between the Work Orientation concepts were determined. This was followed by confirmatory factor analysis (LISREL-analysis, Jöreskog & Sörbom, 1993) of Work Orientation as a latent variable. According to Kaplan (1999), differences between unequal sub-samples may well be ascribed to inequality among the sample sizes, rather than true differences. Group comparison by means of structural equation modeling with LISREL-analysis, however provides for unequal sample sizes to be specified in the program.

Results

The results reflected in the following tables (product moment correlation coefficients for the White and the Black group) indicate that organizational commitment, job involvement, as well as job satisfaction, are significantly correlated. Satisfaction with remuneration did not, however, correlate with these variables. These findings applied to both the White and the Black group, although one might assume that a difference in socio-ecomonic status exists.
The correlation matrixes for both samples were used as input data for the LISREL-analysis. In view of insignificant correlations regarding remuneration as a determinant of job satisfaction within the sub-samples, this scale was rejected after confirmatory structural analysis. It is reasoned that salary structures within the South African context, which at the time of the research was rather non-negotiable, could not be an accurate reflection of job satisfaction. The low average score obtained in testing satisfaction with remuneration scales for the two respective groups, confirmed the above finding and reflected an indication of dissatisfaction with salaries. An analysis prior to elimination of remuneration satisfaction, indicated a poor fit between the theoretical model and the data.

Parameter estimates and *t*-values indicated a fairly good fit between the theoretical (Work Orientation) model and the data characteristics (RMSEA = 0.085; GFI = 0.97). The hypothesis of no differences between the manifestation of Work Orientation within the sub-samples could therefore not be rejected. LISREL-analysis indicated that organizational commitment, job involvement and job satisfaction are all significantly correlated for both groups and that the

Table 1. Product Moment Correlation Coefficients for Work Orientation Questionnaires for Whites

Questionnaire	OCQ	JIQ	JDI Work	JDI Remuneration	JDI Promotion	JDI Supervision	JDI Colleagues
OCQ	1.00	0.58	0.57	0.21	0.35	0.38	0.32
JIQ		1.00	0.59	0.08	0.30	0.29	0.22
JDI Work			1.00	0.07	0.36	0.44	0.44
JDI Remuneration				1.00	0.10	0.04	0.04
JDI Promotion					1.00	0.41	0.31
JDI Supervision						1.00	0.44
JDI Colleagues							1.00

Table 2. Product Moment Correlation Coefficients for Work Orientation Questionnaires for Blacks

Questionnaire	OCQ	JIQ	JDI Work	JDI Remuneration	JDI Promotion	JDI Supervision	JDI Colleagues
OCQ	1.00	0.47	0.47	0.21	0.33	0.38	0.31
JIQ		1.00	0.43	0.17	0.32	0.37	0.32
JDI Work			1.00	0.20	0.39	0.55	0.49
JDI Remuneration				1.00	0.16	0.19	0.15
JDI Promotion					1.00	0.45	0.38
JDI Supervision						1.00	0.51
JDI Colleagues							1.00

Figure 1. Parameter estimates and t-values of work orientation concepts for the White group

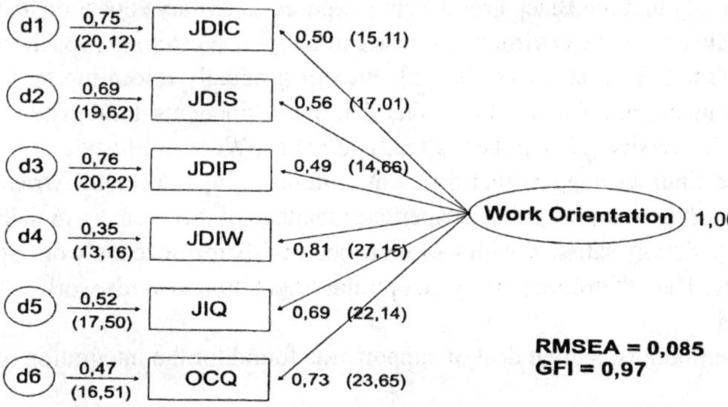

Figure 2. Parameter estimates and t-values of work orientation concepts for the Black group

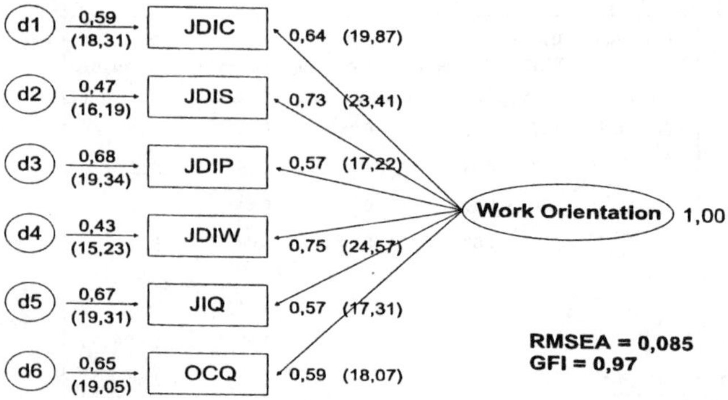

above variables manifested themselves meaningfully within Work Orientation.

Discussion

The findings reflect the significance of these concepts within the study of Organizational Psychology and more specifically, an optimal orientation towards work within the White and Black sub-samples. Optimal Work Orientation implies that employees regard the experience of work as a positive experience. This in turn, implies that the job and the organization, as potent sources of creative energy, are able to create a fulfilling or "optimal" lifestyle, irrespective of cultural differences.

The results indicate that both the White and the Black group, in other words, two diverse cultural groups in South Africa, maintain and comply to the Western paradigm regarding Work Orientation. This was expected of the White group, being brought up in the Western tradition as instilled through links with an European past and the influence of immigrants. This was, however, not expected from the Black cultural group, having grown up in more traditional and often rural settings with strict traditions and values based on African customs. The results imply that the Black group, being exposed to tertiary education and a modern industrial work environment, tends to adopt a Western approach to Work Orientation. This could be the influence of gradually relocating to an urban environment, but also due to the fact that the respondents are registered students at a university. This in itself already reflects a Western lifestyle.

These findings suggest that different cultural groups in South Africa, commit themselves to organizations, experience feelings of involvement in their jobs and are generally satisfied with various aspects of their respective working environments. They therefore portray an optimal orientation towards work and life in general.

In the findings, a great deal of support was found for the integration of these three theoretical concepts within Industrial/Organizational psychology. The specific concepts investigated, namely organizational commitment, job involvement and job satisfaction, represent an underlying view of work as an opportunity towards optimal functioning. Empirical evidence suggests that the three concepts are inter-correlated and together represent the construct of Work Orientation.

Work Orientation implies that employees need to confront the experience of work in a positive light. Employees need to become psychologically orientated in regarding the job and the organization as an opportunity to enjoy the challenge of work optimally. This in turn, may emerge as a potent source of creative energy and may lead to a gratifying, "optimal" lifestyle.

There are however, indications that all the questionnaires were not equally effective in measuring Work Orientation. More comprehensive measures of the various concepts may exist. More research is required in investigating these measures of Work Orientation among a broader spectrum of the population, possibly not only in the South African context, but also internationally. A more balanced sample of randomly selected subjects would also strengthen research findings.

References

Antonovsky, A. (1979). *Health, stress and coping.* London: Jossey-Bass Publishers.

Antonovsky, A. (1984). A call for a new question - salutogenesis - and a proposed answer - the sense of coherence. *Journal of Preventive Psychiatry, 2* (1) 1-11.

Antonovsky, A. (1993). Complexity, conflict, chaos, coherence, coercion and civility. *Social Science and Medicine Journal, 37* (8), 969-981.

Jöreskog, K. & Sörbom, D. (1993). LISREL version 8.12a for WINDOWS.

Kaplan, D. (1999). Statistical power in structural equation models.[Lecture notes]. Retrieved March 10, 1999 from the World Wide Web: http//www.gsu.edu/~mkteer/power.html.

Lodahl, T.M. & Kejner, M. (1965). The definition and measurement of job involvement. *Journal of Applied Psychology, 49* (1), 24-33.

Mowday, R.T., Steers, R.M. & Porter, L.W. (1979). The measurement of organizational commitment. *Journal of Vocational Behaviour, 14* (2), 224-247.

SAS (1990). Version 6, 4th edition. North Carolina: SAS Institute Inc.

Smith, P.C., Kendall, L.M. & Hulin, C.L. (1969). *The measurement of satisfaction in work and retirement: A strategy for the study of attitudes.* Chicago: Rand McNally & Company.

Strümpfer, D.J.W. (1990). Salutogenesis: A new paradigm. *South African Journal of Psychology, 20* (4), 265-276.

Strümpfer, D.J.W. (1995). The origins of health and strength: From 'salutogenesis' to 'fortigenesis'. *South African Journal of Psychology, 25* (2), 81-88.

Viviers, A.M. (1996). *Salutogenesis in organizational context.* Unpublished DCom dissertation. University.

Assessing Multicultural Supervision Competencies

Paul T. P. Wong
Trinity Western University
Graduate Program in Counselling Psychology

Lilian C. J. Wong
The University of British Columbia
Department of Counselling Psychology

ABSTRACT

The need for cross-cultural supervision competencies in training culturally-skilled counselors is explained. The development of the Multicultural Supervision Competencies Questionnaire (MSCQ) outlined and initial evidence of its reliability is presented. The MSCQ is a 60-item questionnaire covering four multicultural supervision competencies: Attitude, Knowledge, Skills and Relationship. Twenty questionnaires were completed by graduate students in Counseling Psychology regarding their practicum or internship supervisors who were from a different ethnic cultural background. The results show that this sample of supervisors had rather low levels of cross-cultural competencies. The internal reliability of the MSCQ was high, with Alpha values in the .90s for all four subscales and the total MSCQ scores. The usefulness of the MSCQ in cross-cultural counselor education and supervision research was discussed.

Since supervision is the only way to prepare students for clinical practice, it is a vital part of counselor education. There is a burgeoning literature on supervision (Bernard & Goodyear, 1998; Heppner & Roehlke, 1984; Holloway, 1995; Ronnestad & Skovholt, 1993; Worthington, 1987), but there has been very little research on cross-cultural issues in supervision. The scanty literature on cross-cultural supervision reveals low levels of satisfaction in minority supervisees (Cook & Helms, 1988), and varying degrees of discrimination (McNeill, Hom & Perez, 1995).

Multicultural supervision competencies (MSC) deserve recognition for two reasons. Firstly, there is an urgent need for cross-culturally competent supervisors, because more and more graduate students come from diverse ethnic groups (Bernard & Goodyear, 1998; Leong & Chou, 1996). Culturally-insensitive supervisors can unintentionally harm minority students (Corey, Corey, & Callanan, 1998; Kaiser, 1997). According to McNeill, Hom and Perez (1995), there was a dearth of information on the training needs of racial and ethnic minority trainees. They also pointed out that "culturally diverse trainees are then faced with a struggle to assert their unique needs and make others aware of the multicultural implications of course material, counseling theories, and interventions. Most often, however, students are forced to attend to and accept this insensitivity for fear of repercussion because of the power differential between professor and student" (p.253).

Secondly, it is difficult for majority students to acquire multicultural counseling skills when their clinical supervisors do not meet the minimal standards of cross-cultural competencies. Based on informal surveys of departmental and field supervisors, the majority of supervisors have not had any cross-cultural training, especially in the area of multicultural supervision.

There has been some discussion on cross-cultural training (Lonner, 1997; Pedersen, 1997; Sue, 1997). Generally, training approaches can be classified as either didactic or experiential. Pedersen's (1997) triad training model is an example of the didactic approach, whereas learning from face-to-face contact with other individuals from other cultures is a case of experiential learning. Lonner (1997) outlines three pathways to multicultural competencies: Experiential, Academic, and Formal Culture Training. What has been missing in the discussion is the role of clinical supervision. A cross-culturally competent supervisor provides both didactic and experiential learning. In addition, a mentoring-minded supervisor also provides modeling, guidance, encouragement, and friendship to promote trainees' professional and personal development.

The main purpose of this chapter is to describe the development of the Multicultural Supervision Competencies Questionnaire and to provide some empirical evidence on supervisors' levels of cross-cultural competencies.

It is interesting to note that while the literature on multicultural counseling continues to grow (e.g. Pedersen, , 1997; Pedersen, Draguns, Lonner, & Trimble, 1996; Sue, Ivey, & Pedersen, 1996), multicultural supervision has not received the same level of attention. Only in the last few years did psychologists begin to recognize ethnic and cultural issues in supervision (e.g., Leong & Wagner, 1994; McNeill, Hom & Perez, 1995; Priest, 1994). For example, Fukuyama (1994) explored critical incidents in multicultural supervision of interns and identified two major themes: 1) culture and cultural differences, and 2) racism and racial identity issues. Bernard (1994) concludes: "the development of the profession and the relevance of counselor education programs will be severely compromised if we do not advance the knowledge and practice of multicultural supervision" (p. 170).

Multicultural supervision needs to be researched in its own right, because it is more complex than multicultural counseling, as shown in Table 1.

The dynamics of interactions are much more complex in a multicultural supervision situation. This is because any one or two of the triad

— supervisor, supervisee and client — may come from a different ethnic or cultural background. For example, a White professor may be supervising an Asian counselor who has a Black client. In such situations, more knowledge and skills are needed.

It is also important to recognize that counseling differs from supervision in several ways. (1) The goal of counseling is to facilitate change in the client, whereas the goal of supervision is to protect the welfare of the client and facilitate the professional development of the supervisee. (2) The major role of a counselor is counseling; teaching only plays a minor part. In contrast, supervision involves multiple roles: counselor, teacher, consultant, and mentor; teaching plays a prominent role. (3) Counseling is concerned with assessing the client's condition, whereas supervision is concerned with both the evaluation of supervisee's competence as well as assessment of the client's condition. (4) Counseling requires clinical competence, whereas supervision requires both clinical competence and supervision competence.

Given the above differences in tasks and skill requirements, an experienced clinician is not necessarily a competent supervisor. Similarly, a multiculturally competent counselor does not automatically become a multiculturally competent supervisor without additional training.

Table 1. Contrast Between Multicultural Counseling and Multicultural Supervision.

Multicultural Counseling	Multicultural Supervision
Needs to be aware of client's worldview.	Needs to be aware of client's and supervisee's worldviews.
Needs culturally appropriate counseling skills.	Needs culturally appropriate counseling and supervision skills.
Racial/cultural differences affect the relationship between counselor and client.	Racial/cultural differences affect both counselor-client and supervisor-counselor relationships.
Cultural biases may harm client.	Cultural biases may harm client and supervisee.
Involves conflicts of cultural assumptions and values.	Involves conflicts of cultural assumptions and values plus conflicts of theoretical orientations and counseling approaches.

In sum, multicultural supervision deserves a great deal of attention from the standpoints of counselor education and supervision research. We believe the development of a valid and reliable instrument to measure MSC will contribute to both cross-cultural training and research.

Currently, there are several instruments for assessing multicultural counseling competencies (please see Pope-Davis & Dings, 1995 for a review), but none of these is explicitly designed to measure multicultural supervision competencies. Among the reasons why it is important to develop the MSCQ are: (1) it allows the supervisee an opportunity to provide feedback to the supervisor, (2) it facilitates multicultural training of supervisor and counselor, (3) it determines the suitability of supervisor to work with culturally different supervisees, and (4) it facilitates quantitative research on multicultural competencies in supervision.

Method

Subjects

The subjects were 15 graduate students from counseling psychology programs in Vancouver and the Lower Mainland, British Columbia, Canada. Most of them had completed their practicum. A few had also completed their internship. They were allowed to evaluate more than one supervisor, if they had received cross-cultural supervision from two or three individuals during their clinical training. A total of 21 MSCQs were completed, but one was discarded because of missing data. Participants included Chinese, Japanese, and Indo-Canadians.

The Development of the Multicultural Supervision Competence Questionnaire

The MCSQ was primarily based on the three cross-cultural competencies described by Sue, Arrendondo and McDavis (1992), namely, Attitudes, Knowledge and Skills. Relationship was added to the MSCQ because the supervisory relationship is essential to effective supervision (Bradley, 1989; Holloway, 1995). The Multicultural Counseling Inventory (Sodowsky et al., 1994) also identified Relationship as a key factor in cross-cultural competence in addition to Awareness, Skills and Knowledge.

Differences in values, worldviews, and communication styles often lead to cultural conflicts and interpersonal difficulties. According to Pedersen's (1997) Interpersonal Grid, individuals from different cultures may have the same or different behaviors, and the same or different expectations, forming four quadrants. Congruence occurs only in the first quadrant where both individuals have the same expectations and same behaviors. Conflicts occur in all other three quadrants. Different expectations and misperceptions can contribute to a multicultural conflict (Rubin, Kim, & Peretz, 1990). That is why the ability to develop a good relationship is essential in reducing and preventing cultural conflicts in supervision.

The four subscales of the MSCQ (Attitude, Knowledge, Skills and Relationship) represent four multicultural competencies. A total of 67 items were initially used to develop the four subscales. The items, generated by the authors, were based on the literature of multicultural counseling and supervision as well as the authors' experiences in this area. These items were then arranged randomly. Table 2 shows exemplary items for the four constructs.

Table 2. Exemplary Items for the Subscales of the MSCQ

I. Attitudes and beliefs
- Demonstrates openness and respect for culturally different supervisees.
- Does not seem to be aware of own implicit cultural biases in counseling and supervision.

II. Knowledge and understanding
- Shows some knowledge about the cultural traditions of various ethnic groups.
- Understands the worldviews of supervisees and clients from other cultures.

III. Skills and practices
- Takes into account cultural biases in assessments and clinical judgments.
- Is very rigid and dogmatic regarding what constitutes the proper approach of counseling.

IV. Relationship
- Is able to overcome cultural and linguistic barriers in working with minority students and clients.
- Is willing to advocate for minorities who experience institutional discrimination.

Procedure

Respondents were contacted individually by telephone or in person. They were asked to identify a recent supervisor who was from a different ethnic or racial background as the object of evaluation. A 5-point Likert scale was used, where 1=Strongly Disagree, 5=Strongly Agree, and 3=Undecided. Statements were worded both in the positive and negative directions; however, scoring was in the positive direction such that scores larger than 3 indicated the presence of cross-cultural supervision competence.

Results and Discussion

On the basis of Cronbach's Alphas and feedback from the participants, 7 items were eliminated: 3 from the Attitude subscale, 2 from Skills, and 2 from Relationship. Results were based on the final version of 60 items. The Alpha values and the means and SD of the MSCQ are shown in Table 3.

Table 3. Reliability Coefficients and Means of the Subscales of the MSCQ

Level	Alpha	No. of Items	Mean	SD
Attitude	.9655	12	3.4917	1.08
Knowledge	.9266	9	3.3306	0.90
Skills	.9802	22	3.3636	1.04
Relationship	.9771	17	3.4471	1.16
Total	.9924	60	3.4075	1.05

The results showed that the MSCQ has excellent reliability, indicating that all the items in the MSCQ indeed measured various aspects of the same construct. The high alpha coefficients in the four subscales confirm the internal consistency of these scales.

All the mean ratings were less than 4, suggesting a minimal level of multicultural supervision competence, because 3 is the mid-point, indicating Undecided. Some of the supervisors had ratings lower than 2 on most of the items, indicating a lack of multicultural competence.

Implications of Low MSCQ Scores for Minority Students

Interviews with three supervisees revealed that their supervisors abused their supervisory power and had harmed them both psychologically and professionally. For example, one Asian supervisee was severely criticized and terminated from her clinical training for no other reason than being "too directive and structured." No explanation was given why a directive approach constituted a severe impairment that warranted termination. Worse still, this Asian student was not given any opportunity to make adjustments in her counseling style. According to Berry et al.'s (1992) analysis, the action taken by her supervisor represents the absolutist position, which imposes the values and criteria of the dominant culture on other cultures. Pedersen (1997) points out that this kind of cultural bias "leads to encapsulation and exclusionism, the consequences of which are hurtful and profoundly dangerous" (p. 228).

In another case, an Asian student was negatively evaluated for being weak in empathy skills, because she did not adequately reflect on her client's feelings. The main difficulty for this foreign student was that she did not have enough English vocabulary to express emotions; furthermore, she was not used to talking about feelings.

Sue and Sundberg (1996) observed that "Openness and the revealing of inner emotions thought to be indicative of good counselor qualities reflect a Western framework. Other cultures may not value these characteristics as highly, and successful multicultural counseling may require a different set of skills" (p.326). Ironically, by criticizing the Asian student's alleged weakness in empathy, the supervisor revealed her own deficiencies in cross-cultural empathy, which requires a genuine respect for the values and communication styles of different cultures.

The above examples illustrate how a lack of multicultural competencies can lead to ineffective and unethical supervision of minority students. Leong and Chou (1996) pointed out the danger of the training biases of Western models: "The mindless application of these models without taking into account cultural variables for international students will be doomed to failure with, and perhaps cause harm to, international student clients" (p.229). Their observation is equally applicable to cross-cultural supervision of minority trainees.

Implications of Low MSCQ Scores for Majority Students

The low average MSCQ scores of the present sample also raised the question of multicultural counseling training for majority students. If supervisors are incompetent in cross-cultural counseling, how can they teach others? Most students tend to treat clients according to the models to which they have been exposed. Given the strong Western biases in all aspects of counselor education, where do students acquire cross-cultural competencies? Some counselors may acquire multicultural counseling competencies through attending workshops and/or experiential learning. But if counselors acquire cross-cultural counseling competencies primarily through a process of trial and error, some minority clients may become casualties of culturally biased therapy.

The only way to ensure that all counselors possess an acceptable level of cross-cultural competencies is to make multicultural counseling an integral part of counselor education, especially in the area of practicum and internship training. To implement such a program would require supervisors who are competent in cross-cultural counseling and supervision.

The present findings may be indicative of a larger problem that many supervisors do not have adequate multicultural competence. This seems to be a widespread problem because most experienced supervisors received their graduate training before multicultural counseling was widely recognized. Faculty resistance to multiculturalism in counselor education and counseling compounds this problem (Sue & Sue, 1990).

Fong and Lease (1996) have identified four challenges in multicultural supervision: 1) unintentional racism, 2) power dynamics, 3) communication issues, and 4) trust and the supervisory alliance. The MSCQ can help assess how well supervisors have met these challenges.

Usefulness of the MSCQ in Cross-Cultural Counseling Training and Research

To our knowledge, there are no published scales on multicultural supervision competencies. The present findings suggest that the MSCQ is a promising instrument for improving multicultural counseling training. At the very least, the four-dimensional model of the MSCQ makes supervisors aware of the cross-cultural issues in supervision. Ideally, the MSCQ may be used by individual supervisors, institutions and accrediting agencies to systematically assess multicultural supervision competencies as perceived by counseling trainees. Such assessment will not only provide an indication of progress in multicultural competence, but also identify areas that require special attention.

In their recent review of assessment in cross-cultural counseling, Lonner and Ibrahim (1996) have made a compelling case that clients' cultural characteristics must be taken into consideration as an integral part of counseling. The same logic needs to be extended to supervision in order to produce cross-culturally competent counselors.

We also want to emphasize that the MSCQ can be used as a research instrument to discover the role of culture in supervision. For example, research is underway to investigate the relationship between the MSCQ and supervision functions as well as supervision effectiveness. There is also the need to study the linkage between the MSCQ scores of supervisors and the multicultural counseling competencies of supervisees.

Given the increasing diversity of our student population and society at large, the need for multiculturally competent supervisors will continue to increase. This is one of the urgent challenges facing counselor education — cross-cultural competence must begin with supervisors. Judging from the program of the 106th Annual Convention of the American Psychological Association in San Francisco, August 1998, multicultural supervision has emerged as one of the focal points of research and clinical education. It seems perfectly logical that the next major step of development in cross-cultural counseling psychology is multicultural supervision competence. We have presented the case that the MSCQ can contribute to both research and education in this important new development.

References

Atkinson, D. R., Morten, G., & Sue, D. W. (1993). *Counseling American Minorities* (4th ed.). Dubuque, IA: Brown & Benchmark.

Bernard, J. M. (1994). Multicultural supervision: A reaction to Leong and Wagner, Cook, Priest, and Fukuyama. *Counselor Education and Supervision, 34*, 159-171.

Bernard, J. M., & Goodyear, R. K. (1998). *Fundamentals of clinical supervision* (2nd ed.). Needham Heights, MA: Allyn and Bacon.

Berry, J. W., Poortinga, Y. H., Segall, M. H., & Dasen, P. J. (1992). *Cross-cultural psychology: Research and applications*. Cambridge, England: Cambridge University Press.

Bradley, L. J. (1989). *Counselor supervision: Principles, process, practice*. Muncie, IN: Accelerated Press.

Cook, D. A., & Helms, J. E. (1988). Visible racial/ethnic group supervisees' satisfaction with cross-cultural supervision as predicted by relationship characteristics. *Journal of Counseling Psychology, 35*, 268-274.

Corey, G., Corey, M. S., & Callanan, P. (1998). *Issues and ethics in the helping professions*. Pacific Grove, CA: Brooks/Cole.

Fong, M. L., & Lease, S. H. (1996). *Cross-cultural supervision: Issues for the white supervisor*. Newbury Park, CA: Sage.

Fukuyama, M. A. (1994). Critical incidents in multi-cultural counseling supervision: A phenomenological approach to supervision. *Counselor Education and Supervision, 34*, 142-151.

Heppner, P. P., & Roehlke, H. J. (1984). Differences among supervisees at different levels of training: Implications for a developmental model of supervision. *Journal of Counseling Psychology, 31*, 76-90.

Ho, M. K. (1992). *Family therapy with ethnic minorities* (2nd ed.). Newbury Park, CA: Sage.

Holloway, E. L. (1995). *Clinical supervision: A systems approach*. Thousand Oaks, CA: Sage.

Kaiser, T. L. (1997). *Supervisory relationships: Exploring the human element*. Pacific Grove, CA: Brooks/Cole.

Leong, F. T., & Chou, E. L. (1996). Counseling international students. In P. B. Pedersen, J. G. Draguns, W. J. Lonner, & J. E. Trimble (Eds.) (1996). *Counseling across cultures*. (4th ed.) (pp. 210-242).Thousand Oaks, CA: Sage.

Leong, F. T. L., & Wagner, N. S. (1994). Cross-cultural counseling supervision: What do we know? What do we need to know? *Counselor Education and Supervision, 34*, 117-131.

Lonner, W. J. (1997). Three paths leading to culturally competent psychological practitioners. *International Journal of Intercultural Relations, 21*(2), 195-212.

Lonner, W. J., & Ibrahim, F. A. (1996). Appraisal and assessment in cross-cultural counseling. In P. B. Pedersen, J. G. Draguns, W. J. Lonner, & J. E. Trimble (Eds.) (1996). *Counseling across cultures*. (4th ed.) (pp. 293-322). Thousand Oaks, CA: Sage.

McNeill, B. W., Hom, K. L., & Perez, J. A. (1995). The training and supervisory needs for racial and ethnic minority students. *Journal of Multicultural Counseling and Development, 23*, 246-258.

Pedersen, P. B. (1997). *Culture-centered counseling interventions: Striving for accuracy*. Thousand Oaks, CA: Sage.

Pedersen, P. B., Draguns, J. G., Lonner, W. J., & Trimble, J. E. (Eds.) (1996). *Counseling across cultures* (4th ed.). Thousand Oaks, CA: Sage.

Pope-Davis, D. B., & Dings, J. G. (1995). The assessment of multicultural counseling competences. In J. G. Ponterotto, J. M. Casas, L. A. Suzuki, & C. M. Alexander (Eds.). *Handbook of multicultural counseling* (pp. 323-352). Thousand Oaks, CA: Sage.

Priest, R. (1994). Minority supervisor and majority supervisee: Another perspective of reality. *Counselor Education and Supervision, 34*, 152-158.

Ronnestad, M. H., & Skovholt, T. M. (1993). Supervision of beginning and advanced graduate students of counseling and psychotherapy. *Journal of Counseling and Development, 71*, 396-405.

Rubin, J. Z., Kim, S. H., Peretz, N. M. (1990). Expectancy effects and negotiation. *Journal of Social Issues, 46*, 125-139.

Sodowsky, G. R., Taffe, R. C., Gutkin, T. B., & Wise, S. L. (1994). Development of a multicultural counseling inventory: A self-report measure of multicultural competencies. *Journal of Counseling Psychology, 41*, 137-148.

Sue, D. Multicultural training. *International Journal of Intercultural Relations, 21*(2), 175-193.

Sue, D., & Sundberg, N. D. (1996). Research and research hypotheses about effectiveness in intercultural counseling. In P. B. Pedersen, J. G. Draguns, W. J. Lonner, & J. E. Trimble (Eds.) (1996). *Counseling across cultures*. (4th ed.). Thousand Oaks, CA: Sage, pp.323-352.

Sue, D. W., Arredondo, P., & McDavis, R. J. (1992). Multicultural competencies/standards: A pressing need. *Journal of Counseling and Development, 70(4)*, 477-486.

Sue, D. W., Ivey, A. E., & Pedersen, P. B. (1996). *A theory of multicultural counseling and therapy*. Pacific Grove, CA: Brooks/Cole.

Sue, D. W., & Sue, D. (1990). *Counseling the culturally different: Theory and practice*. New York, NY: Wiley.

Worthington, E. L., Jr. (1987). Changes in supervision as counselors and supervisors gain experience. A review. *Professional Psychology: Research and Practice, 15*, 457-461.

Comparison of Managing Cultural Diversity in German-Chinese Research and Business Cooperation

Alexander Thomas
University of Regensburg
Institute of Psychology

ABSTRACT

In more than two hundred interviews with German and Chinese managers, language teachers and students, many so called "critical incidents" were collected and analysed by German and Chinese researchers. As one part of the research project, the paper will present prototypical examples for two fields of cooperation in research and business. The analysis will show that there are similarities between the effectiveness of German and Chinese cultural standards (e.g., fact orientation vs. social harmony orientation or individual vs. social conformity orientation) and the styler of managing cultural diversity. Consequences of intercultural trainings especially in regard to use of culture assimilator, negotiation, and conflict resolution will be discussed. Interview methods and questionnaires used to analyze critical incidents" will also be presented as a way to examine how data collection and research methodology can be culturally adapted.

Many professional business firms are becoming international in their range of operations. More people are required to have experience and competence in international management at a steadily increasing level of quality. These requirements can only be met if effective intercultural sensitization training (e.g., cultural general assimilator, Brislin, 1996) and culture-specific competence training (e.g., China business and Culture Assimilator, Thomas & Schenk, 1999) are available. In order to develop such training and practice material, empirical studies are needed that will measure the effectiveness of training sessions. These represent a field of intercultural experience in themselves, therefore posing corresponding challenges regarding cooperative scientific research (Thomas, 1993, 1996).

Research Program "Culture-Standards"

Critical incidents (see figure 1) occurring in interactions between German and Chinese business persons were presented in semi-structured interviews. These were conducted by German interviewers questioning German managers, language teachers, and students in China. Likewise, for Chinese managers, language teachers, and students in Germany, the interview was conducted by a Chinese interviewer (see figure 1).

An analysis of the extracted critical incidents (see figure 2) resulted in the following German cultural-standards as seen by Chinese managers (see figure 3) and Chinese cultural-standards as seen by German managers.

Figure 1. Sample and number of critical incidents

Interviews with		managers	language teachers	students	total sum
Germans interviewed in: China	N =	40	32	25	**97**
	CI =	*92*	*181*	*186*	***459***
Taiwan	N =	26	19	25	**70**
	CI =	*183*	*132*	*201*	***516***
Hongkong	N =	18	10	**In Hongkong no German students were available.**	**28**
	CI =	*65*	*50*		***115***
total sum	N =	**84**	**61**	**50**	**195**
	CI =	***340***	***363***	***387***	***1090***
Chinese interviewed in: Germany	N =	22	10	32	**64**
	CI=	*60*	180		***240***

N = Number of interviewed persons
CI = Number of Critical Incidents reported by interviewed persons

Figure 2. Steps in generating culture standards

1. Semi-structured interviews with German managers in China on critical incidents experienced during encounters with Chinese business partners
2. Analysis of the content of the interviews
   - Identification of "critical" interactions and journalistic wording
   - Answering the question: "Why did the Chinese act in such an unusual manner?"
   - Identification of coping-strategies used during critical exchanges
   - Identification of situations which went smoothly
   - Information about the person interviewed, their field of work etc.
3. Experts' assessment of critical incidents
   - Chinese experts (2)
   - German experts (2)
   - Psychologist (1)
   - Interviewed person (1)
4. Analysis of the content of the experts' assessment
5. Temporary naming/assignment of culture standards which fit the critical situation
6. Critical incidents are categorized with respect to the culture standards extracted
7. Final naming of culture standards
8. Definition of the net of correspondences between culture standards
9. Founding the culture standards on respective social and cultural history; aided by expert opinion and literature on cultural history

Figure 3. German and Chinese Culture Standards

German culture standards (as seen by Chinese managers)	Chinese culture standards (as seen by German managers)
Rule orientation	Social harmony
Individualism	Face saving
Directness/ Sincerity	Hierarchy
Separation of work- and private life	Guanxi (network of social relationships)
Close following of contracts	Cunning, tactics
Systematic solving of tasks	Danwei (unity of life and work)
Planning appointments and available time	Etiquette
Bureaucratic organization structures	Bureaucracy
Way of treating bodily and physical matters	
Distanced attitude towards foreigners	

Cultural-standards are value orientations which are used to judge and regulate one‘s actions as well as those of others. They strongly influence perception, way of thinking, judgement, and action of the great majority of the members of a certain culture. Cultural standards can be seen as the specific building blocks of a respective cultures' distinct world view. They consist of general norms and include an area of tolerance for accepted deviation from the norm. In intercultural situations, cultural-standards become evident in critical incidents. Conflict ridden interactions may be frequent when people have strongly divergent cultural-standards (e.g., Chinese "social harmony" versus German "rule orientation").

Research Program "Intercultural Orientation Training"

The development of orientation training to prepare German managers for cooperation in Chinese context as well as Chinese for cooperation in German contexts was based upon the information gained through interviews, the results of analysis by experts, and judgements on selected critical incidents made by individuals with no personal experience with Chinese or Germans respectively. Interviews with managers experienced with Chinese who were trained for their intercultural work as well as interviews with untrained interviewees also provided important information (see figure 4).

The central element of training consisted of a Chinese business and culture assimilator which corresponded with the standard versions developed by Fiedler, Mitchell and Triandis (1971), Albert (1983), Albert and Adamopoulos (1980), Triandis (1984), and Heuvel and Meertens (1989). However, not only one culturally adequate explanation was required of the participants. They were asked to put the responses into an order of preference and work on all information and commentaries provided on every explanation, be they correct or incorrect. The following culture assimilators have been developed: Thomas and Schenk, 1999;

Schenk, Bauer, Schnabel and Thomas, 1999; Thomas and Schenk, 1999; Thomas and Schenk, 1996; Lindner, Schenk and Thomas, 1999.

Seven trainings were offered for German managers (total of 182 persons) preparing to work in China and five trainings for Chinese managers (total of 87 persons) preparing to

Figure 4. Intercultural orientation training for German managers working in the Peoples Republic of China

1. Construction of a specific culture assimilator, e.g. "China business and culture assimilator"
2. Videographing of critical incidents between German and Chinese managers ending with the question: "What is happening here?"
3. Role play: "Negotiations on the introduction of a new software system in a German-Chinese joint venture"
4. Lectures including demonstrations and discussions on:
   - German and Chinese management methods: leadership, negotiation, solving conflicts, quality preservation
   - Chinese history and culture
   - The meaning of values, gestures and rituals in German-Chinese encounters
   - Bureaucracy and the legal system in China

work in Germany. The trainer team consisted of five people: psychologists, a linguist, a jurist, and a master in China studies of either German or Chinese origin. The sessions were evaluated both quantitatively (questionnaire on acceptance) as well as qualitatively (interviews and explanations chosen for critical incidents after half a year in China or, likewise, half a year of working with German partners in China (see figure 5).

Further Results of the Evaluation:

While most interviewees showed obvious signs towards culturally adequate behavior (e.g. saving face), other interviewees came to the conclusion that, in order to be successful in business, many situations do not call for behavior that is in any way different from what would be called for in Germany. Managers who display a manner of superiority in interaction with their Chinese partners, who can build up and preserve asymmetric relationships can force their Chinese partners to adapt their behavior. Thus, under favorable circumstances, some German manager they can be successful in spite of their negotiation and management style while others fail.

Behavioral practices such as exchange of calling cards which were introduced during the training could be directly applied. The German interviewees also stated that the training helped them anticipate situations and led them towards more positive interactions with Chinese colleagues. Some interviewees stated that certain situations in China reminded them of the training, yet they nonetheless experienced them as different from

Figure 5. Acceptance of elements of the training

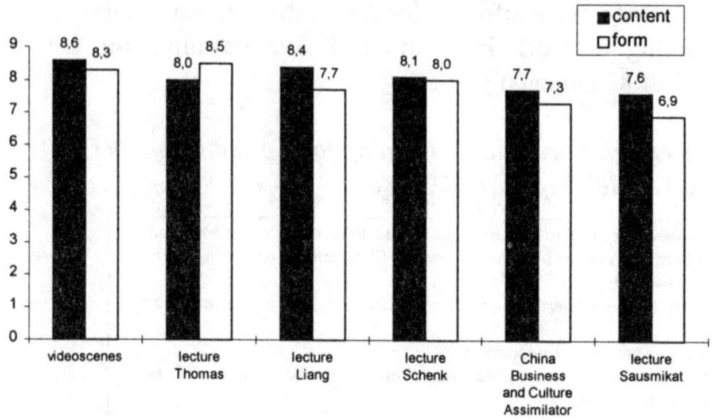

the training situations. Other managers explained that they acted according to the culture standard "face saving" which had been introduced during the training as well as exchanging calling cards.

Elements of training the participants found helpful were: "The jungle of responsibility" (role play); "Chinese words, guests, rituals" (exercise and audio-based training); sensibility training "communication and style of leadership"; work in small groups,; lectures on "negotiation-between law and culture", "traditional and modern China: a history of ideas and culture"; and "intercultural competence training". Of the cultural standards, "face saving", "guanxi" and "danwei" were recalled. The video sequences, the "China business and culture assimilator" and the role plays were extremely useful. The training helped overcome a certain fear of China. It was especially effective for participants without prior experience with Chinese persons. Interviewees who already had experience in China stated that while their behavior had not greatly changed after the training, they could better understand reactions shown by Chinese associates.

It can therefore be concluded that working with video sequences offers a successful way to present flexible, highly generalized information on behavioral norms. It also has proven useful to evaluate training with qualitative as well as quantitative measures. Furthermore, it is of great importance to conduct the interviews used for evaluation in Germany and in China, while trainees are living in the foreign country. The experiences which were seen as related to the training can only be reported in a precise and differentiated way in the actual setting in which they occur.

The interviewed managers interpreted the interviews as a sort of information, memory, and learning test in which they felt pressured to do as well as possible. This resulted in tension and uneasiness during the interviews and inevitable negative effects on the quality of the interviews. Socially approved answers, a strong tendency towards impression management (I don't have any problems! I've got everything under control! I can deal with the Chinese easily!) as well as attempts to eloquently get through interviews while evading the questions could be observed. All these factors influenced the quality of the interviews in a way almost impossible to control. These tendencies remained even when interviewers actively tried to create a relaxed atmosphere. (Thomas & Schenk, 1996).

Cultural Aspects in Research Cooperation

During the collection of data as well as the trainings, close cooperation with Chinese scientists was necessary. The conditions for successful scientific cooperation seemed ideal for the following reasons.

1.)The Chinese partner was a psychology professor (social and organization psychology), had done research in Germany, was sufficiently fluent in German, and already had experience in intercultural research.

2.)The German partner had traveled through China, spent years working on intercultural topics, was interested in cooperation, had experience in the development of culture assimilator, and in management training.

3.)Both partners had identical scientific fields of interest and previous training. They jointly conceptualized the research project and the application for a research grant, agreed on the scientific foundations (theory, methods, consequences) and on research methods (who conducts which interviews; who analyses which parts?).

4.)Mutual openness could be observed in relation to the use of research funds (who receives how much for what work). However, in the course of the two-year cooperation, the following problems surfaced.

The Interview Manual

The Chinese partner was convinced that the interview manual which had been developed to cover critical incidents experienced by German managers and language teachers could be used to interview Chinese participants with no alterations. Discussions on the eventual necessity of adapting the interview manual, thus rendering it more culturally adequate, were not productive. If it were made clear to the Chinese interviewees that the interview was for scientific purposes and specific goal, that the questioning should remain on a scientific level and remain anonymous, no modification of the interview manual or interview procedure was necessary.

The results clearly showed that the interviews conducted by the Chinese partner disregarded standard guidelines and directions for correctly conducting semi-structured interviews. The main problem was that the Chinese interviewees answered the questions very hesitantly, if at all. This led the Chinese interviewer to describe his own experiences with Germans and thus demonstrate how critical incidents develop and how one should react. The interviewees gratefully accepted this support, underlined what had been said and added to the incident. In comparison with the German interviews, the Chinese interviews were characterized by dominance of the interviewer and evasive behavior of the interviewees.

Extrinsically Motivated Cooperation in Research

The mutual understanding and harmony which characterized the preparation of the project, from the first ideas through to the application for financial aid changed abrupt when the financial means allotted became clear. At the outset, the research partners both seemed intrinsically motivated, and interested in furthering scientific knowledge on the problems Germans and Chinese experience when doing business, and finding ways to ameliorate the situation. During the course of the work on the interviews and their analysis, the Chinese partner displayed steadily increasing extrinsic motivation. For example, funding was requested for the interviews conducted, and for Chinese post-graduates who were using the project for their dissertations. Computer equipment financed by the project and payments to the Chinese university in return for cooperation was requested. These requests had not been incorporated into the joint research proposal, and could not be fulfilled. After a couple of months, the Chinese partner permanently withdrew from the project.

Working with the Data Obtained

Agreements made at the beginning of the project had envisioned that data would be collected and analyzed in a manner parallel to previous studies. Everything which was obtained from interviews with German managers, language teachers, and students and incorporated into tested models of the cultural assimilator based trainings, should have been processed in an identical manner for Chinese managers, language teachers and students. All data, stemming from interviews with both German and Chinese interviewees, should have been given to the partner in a version translated into the respective language for use in in future trainings.

The dramatic changes in the Republic of China between 1992 and 1995 rendered the data for intercultural trainings unrealistic. The Chinese managers showed decreased interests in intercultural trainings. The widespread belief seemed to be that a Chinese manager need not prepare for cross-cultural interactions prior to cooperating with German managers. The interviews conducted in Chinese were not translated by the Chinese partner as had been planned. An external translator was commissioned to do the work. The proposed trainings in China to prepare Chinese managers for cooperation with Germans was turned down. A new partner had to be found.

The Language Barrier

The fact that the Chinese partner had knowledge of the German language was an invaluable asset, especially as the German research partner spoke no Chinese. It could not, however, solve all language-based problems in the research project. It became clear that the Chinese partner's German was limited. He could read and understand German texts but had great difficulty with precise and clear articulation and had limited ability to translate Chinese texts into German. In addition to the basic translation difficulties, the team had problems concerning the transcription of the German and Chinese interviews. The quality of the translation of the interviews and the texts developed for the trainings was not controlled. As a result, the German Business and Culture Assimilator which had been developed in Chinese and counterchecked several times, was rated as having been written in poor language and was hard to understand. The exact problem could not be explained. It was not clear if its content was unacceptable and this was indirectly articulated by criticizing the wording of the text.

Problems with Questioning on "Critical Incidents"

The analysis of interviews completed by the Chinese interviewer showed that the quality of the statements regarding "critical incidents" was meagre in comparison to the interviews analyzed by the German researchers. This result indicates that it is problematic for Chinese researchers to speak about "critical" incidents with other people. As a consequence, it was decided, that German interviewers resorted to questioning Chinese managers in China about critical incidents experienced with their German partners. The fact that the interviews were conducted in German posed no great difficulties as the Chinese participants had excellent knowledge of the German language, some even having lived, studied, and worked in Germany for over 10 years. These participants, interviewed in Shanghai, were asked to describe critical incidents either they or their Chinese colleagues had observed with Germans, why these incidents had been problematic, and how resulting difficulties in communication and interaction might be solved. At the beginning of these interviews, those questioned remained on the safe side, offering only very general statements. They indicated that while there may well be certain difficulties during encounters with Germans, these were in no way extraordinary. Problems also occurred when interacting with person from other nations.

When the interviewers insisted on descriptions of concrete situations in which critical incidents had occurred, the Chinese participants conveyed the situations in such a way that it seemed that it was not the Chinese who had difficulties in encounters with Germans, but rather Germans had problems when interacting with a Chinese partner. Thus, although the approximately 45-minute interview started with a question aimed at revealing situations with critical interactions, the line of questioning was lost. Rather, the conversation focused on analyzing the difficulties Germans experience in China when working with Chinese partners. The interviewers described the interviews as "strange", "somehow unclear" and "not leading towards a goal", with themselves "never really knowing, what the interviewee had actually meant".

Only after analyzing both the line of the interview and the different sequences of the conversation was it revealed that the Chinese interviewee had changed strategies. Starting with a strategy of evasion, avoiding direct answers, and playing down the importance of the topic, they had shifted to a strategy of reversed causality. Several explanations for this behavior may be considered. The Chinese participants may have experienced the following:

- a need for harmony, and to give and save face;
- insufficient competence or limited experience in talking about human behhavior on an abstract level;
- unwillingness to express negativity about others in interviews;
- pride in China and its culture, rendering it unseemly to speak openly about difficulties with foreigners;
- difficulty admitting to problems when dealing with German associates.

Critical Incidents in Culture Assimilator Training

The intercultural orientation trainings offered in China to prepare Chinese managers for cooperation with Germans invariably showed two extremes in reaction:

1. The Chinese managers responded to the trainer team in a compliant, passive manner. The style of learning was predominantly receptive rather than active engagement.
2. Written and oral training materials were resisted. The critical incidents described in the German Business and Culture Assimilator were

considered unrealistic and inventions of the German researchers. The diction used in the culture assimilator was also criticized . Explanations regarding elements of the critical incidents were viewed as purely academic and unrealistic. Concrete situations taken out of everyday business life (negotiations, solving conflicts, leadership behavior) were criticized as being rare, cases without importance for professional life in China. This opposing behavior was demonstrated not only by managers who were sent to the training by their firms, and by volunteer participants.

Several explanations may be considered.

- The Chinese participants preferred to develop the orientation training independent of the Germans
- An orientation training developed by Germans in order to prepare Chinese for cooperation with Germans basically can never be of any good, even if it was jointly developed with Chinese. If Chinese are to participate in training measures, these must be developed by Chinese.
- An intercultural orientation training based on situations containing critical interaction between Germans and Chinese that had not run smoothly and harmonically was not acceptable to the Chinese participants. The situations appeared to provoke embarrassment and fear.

Summary of Consequences

The following conclusions are drawn from the experiences cited.

1. For research in cultural comparisons and in the intercultural field, it is necessary for scientists from the respective cultures to work together as a team.
2. Difficulties arising in the research team may stem from exactly the same kind of conflicts the team is trying to examine.
3. Productive scientific cooperation in a multi-cultural research team is only possible if all team members take the time and effort to discuss and, if possible, reach a consensus on their culture-specific ideas regarding scientific standards and methods, the sharing of resources, and utilization of results. Differences should be acknowledged and mutually accepted. The project made use of the semi-structured interview which allows freedom to express ones experiences, opinions, thoughts and emotions. This frequently used method was not as "harmless" as it was thought to be. It was limited by concrete culture-specific influences and restrictions. A culture which views no speaking is an accepted and understandable way of "answering" embarrassing questions can only regard an interview on critical interactions as

intrusive and provocative. The interview was a difficult and aversive encounter between two people who both summoned their culture-specific repertoire of problem solving strategies to cope with the situation. The results of such experiences must be interpreted more as artifacts than as solid scientific data.

References

Albert, R.D. (1983). The intercultural sensitizer or culture assimilator: A cognitive approach. In D.Landis & R. W. Brislin (Eds.), *Handbook of intercultural training,* Vol. II (pp. 186-217). New York: Pergamon.

Albert, R.D. & Amadopoulos, J. (1980). An attributational approach to culture learning. In M. Hamnet & R. W. Brislin (Eds.), *Resarch in culture learning: Language and conceptional studies.* Honolulu: University Press.

Brislin, R.W. & Cushner, K. (19962). *Intercultural interactions: a practical guide.* Thousand Oaks: Sage.

Fiedler, F.E., Mitchell, T. & Triandis, H.C. (1971). The culture assimilator. An approach to cross-cultural training. *Journal of Applied Psychology, 55,* 95 - 102.

Heuvel, H. van den & Meertens, R.W. (1989). The culture assimilator: Is it possible to improve interethnic relations by emphasizing ethnic differences? In J.P. van Oudenhoven & T.M. Willemsen (Eds.), *Ethnic minorities: Social psychological perspectives.* Amsterdam: Swets & Zeitlinger.

Lindner, W., Schenk, E. & Thomas, A. (1999). *German Teaching and Culture Assimilator - Übungsmaterial zur Vorbereitung deutscher Dozenten und Ausbildungsleiter auf den Chinaaufenthalt.* Lengerich: Pabst (in Druck).

Schenk, E., Bauer, S., Schnabel R. & Thomas, A. (1999). *German Study and Culture Assimilator - Übungsmaterial zur Vorbereitung deutscher Studenten und Praktikanten auf den Chinaaufenthalt.* Lengerich: Pabst Verlag (in Druck).

Thomas, A. (1993). Entwicklungslinien und Erkenntniswert kulturvergleichender Psychologie. In A. Thomas (Hrsg.), *Kulturvergleichende Psychologie - Eine Einführung* (S. 27-51). Göttingen: Hogrefe.

Thomas, A. (1996). Analyse der Handlungswirksamkeit von Kulturstandards. In A. Thomas (Hrsg.), Psychologie interkulturellen Handelns (S. 107-135). Göttingen: Hogrefe.

Thomas, A. & Schenk, E. (1996). *Abschlußbericht zum Forschungsprojekt: Handlungswirksamkeit zentraler Kulturstandards in der Interaktion zwischen Deutschen und Chinesen.* Regensburg: unveröffentl. Manuskript.

Thomas, A. & Schenk, E. (1999). *China Business and Culture Assimilator - Übungsmaterial zur Vorbereitung deutscher Manager auf den Chinaaufenthalt.* Lengerich: Pabst Verlag (in Druck).

Thomas, A., Schenk, E. & Lindner, W. (1999). *German Business and Culture Assimilator - Übungsmaterial zur Vorbereitung chinesischer Manager auf den Deutschlandaufenthalt.* Lengerich: Pabst Verlag (in Druck).

Triandis, H.C. (1984). A theoretical framework for the more effective construction of culture assimilators. *International Journal of Intercultural Relations, 8*, 301-310.